NATIONAL ACADEMIES

*Sciences
Engineering
Medicine*

NATIONAL
ACADEMIES
PRESS
Washington, DC

Preventing and Treating Dementia

Research Priorities to Accelerate Progress

Tia Powell, Autumn Downey,
and Olivia C. Yost, *Editors*

Committee on Research Priorities for
Preventing and Treating Alzheimer's
Disease and Related Dementias

Board on Health Sciences Policy

Health and Medicine Division

Board on Behavioral, Cognitive,
and Sensory Sciences

Division of Behavioral and
Social Sciences and Education

Consensus Study Report

NATIONAL ACADEMIES PRESS 500 Fifth Street, NW, Washington, DC 20001

This activity was supported by a contract between the National Academy of Sciences and the National Institutes of Health, Department of Health and Human Services, and has been funded in whole or in part with federal funds under Contract No. HHSN263201800029I/75N98023F00003. Any opinions, findings, conclusions, or recommendations expressed in this publication do not necessarily reflect the views of any organization or agency that provided support for the project.

International Standard Book Number-13: 978-0-309-73151-5
International Standard Book Number-10: 0-309-73151-8
Digital Object Identifier: https://doi.org/10.17226/28588
Library of Congress Control Number: 2025931436

Suggested citation: National Academies of Sciences, Engineering, and Medicine. 2025. *Preventing and treating dementia: Research priorities to accelerate progress*. Washington, DC: The National Academies Press. https://doi.org/10.17226/28588.

The **National Academy of Sciences** was established in 1863 by an Act of Congress, signed by President Lincoln, as a private, nongovernmental institution to advise the nation on issues related to science and technology. Members are elected by their peers for outstanding contributions to research. Dr. Marcia McNutt is president.

The **National Academy of Engineering** was established in 1964 under the charter of the National Academy of Sciences to bring the practices of engineering to advising the nation. Members are elected by their peers for extraordinary contributions to engineering. Dr. John L. Anderson is president.

The **National Academy of Medicine** (formerly the Institute of Medicine) was established in 1970 under the charter of the National Academy of Sciences to advise the nation on medical and health issues. Members are elected by their peers for distinguished contributions to medicine and health. Dr. Victor J. Dzau is president.

The three Academies work together as the **National Academies of Sciences, Engineering, and Medicine** to provide independent, objective analysis and advice to the nation and conduct other activities to solve complex problems and inform public policy decisions. The National Academies also encourage education and research, recognize outstanding contributions to knowledge, and increase public understanding in matters of science, engineering, and medicine.

Learn more about the National Academies of Sciences, Engineering, and Medicine at **www.nationalacademies.org**.

COMMITTEE ON RESEARCH PRIORITIES FOR PREVENTING AND TREATING ALZHEIMER'S DISEASE AND RELATED DEMENTIAS[1]

TIA POWELL (*Chair*), Professor of Epidemiology and Psychiatry, Division of Bioethics, Albert Einstein College of Medicine, Montefiore Medical Center

RHODA AU, Professor of Anatomy and Neurobiology, Boston University Chobanian & Avedisian School of Medicine

RITA BALICE-GORDON, CEO, Muna Therapeutics

DANIEL BARRON, Director, Pain Intervention & Digital Research, Brigham & Women's Hospital and Spaulding Rehabilitation Hospital, Mass General Brigham

CHRISTIAN BEHL, Professor of Pathobiochemistry, Chair and Institute Director, University Medical Center of the Johannes Gutenberg University Mainz, Germany

JEFFREY L. DAGE, Senior Research Professor of Neurology, Indiana University School of Medicine

NILÜFER ERTEKIN-TANER, Chair, Department of Neuroscience and Professor of Neurology and Neuroscience, Mayo Clinic

MARIA GLYMOUR, Chair and Professor, Boston University School of Public Health

HECTOR M. GONZÁLEZ, Professor, University of California San Diego School of Medicine

SUSANNE M. JAEGGI, Professor of Psychology, Applied Psychology, and Music, Northeastern University

KENNETH LANGA, Cyrus Sturgis Professor of Medicine, University of Michigan

PAMELA LEIN, Professor of Neurotoxicology and Chair, University of California Davis School of Veterinary Medicine

DOREEN MONKS, Program Director (retired), Stroke Program, Saint Barnabas Medical Center

KRISSAN LUTZ MOSS, Clinical Education Manager (retired), Genentech; Advocate for National Council of Dementia Minds, Lewy Body Dementia Association, and Dementia Action Alliance

KENNETH S. RAMOS, Alkek Professor of Medical Genetics, Executive Director, Institute of Biosciences and Technology and Assistant Vice Chancellor, Texas A&M University System

REISA A. SPERLING, Professor of Neurology, Harvard Medical School

---

[1] See Appendix C, Disclosure of Unavoidable Conflicts of Interest.

CHI UDEH-MOMOH, Assistant Professor of Epidemiology and Prevention, Division of Public Health Sciences, Wake Forest University School of Medicine

LI-SAN WANG, Peter C. Nowell, M.D. Professor, University of Pennsylvania Perelman School of Medicine

JULIE ZISSIMOPOULOS, Professor, University of Southern California

Study Staff

OLIVIA C. YOST, Study Director
AUTUMN DOWNEY, Senior Program Officer
MOLLY CHECKSFIELD DORRIES, Senior Program Officer
LYDIA TEFERRA, Research Associate
ASHLEY BOLOGNA, Research Assistant
CLARE STROUD, Senior Director, Board on Health Sciences Policy
DANIEL WEISS, Director, Board on Behavioral, Cognitive, and Sensory Sciences

National Academy of Medicine International Health Policy Fellow

HEI MAN CHOW, Assistant Professor, School of Life Sciences, The Chinese University of Hong Kong

Consultants

PICO PORTAL, INC.
MICHELLE MIELKE, Wake Forest University

Reviewers

This Consensus Study Report was reviewed in draft form by individuals chosen for their diverse perspectives and technical expertise. The purpose of this independent review is to provide candid and critical comments that will assist the National Academies of Sciences, Engineering, and Medicine in making each published report as sound as possible and to ensure that it meets the institutional standards for quality, objectivity, evidence, and responsiveness to the study charge. The review comments and draft manuscript remain confidential to protect the integrity of the deliberative process. We thank the following individuals for their review of this report:

ADAM L. BOXER, University of California, San Francisco
ROBERTA DIAZ BRINTON, University of Arizona
FIONA E. DUCOTTERD, University College London
HOWARD FILLIT, Alzheimer's Drug Discovery Foundation
CARL V. HILL, Alzheimer's Association
TIMOTHY J. HOHMAN, Vanderbilt University Medical Center
THOMAS K. KARIKARI, University of Pittsburgh
AMY J. H. KIND, University of Wisconsin
STORY LANDIS, National Institute of Neurological Disorders and Stroke (NINDS), retired
JESSICA LANGBAUM, Banner Alzheimer's Institute
ALLAN L. LEVEY, Emory University
KAREN MARDER, Columbia University Irving Medical Center
IOANNIS PASCHALIDIS, Boston University

LON S. SCHNEIDER, University of Southern California
RAJ C. SHAH, Rush University Medical Center
KRISTINE YAFFE, University of California, San Francisco

Although the reviewers listed above provided many constructive comments and suggestions, they were not asked to endorse the conclusions or recommendations of this report nor did they see the final draft before its release. The review of this report was overseen by **EILEEN M. CRIMMINS,** University of Southern California and **ALAN M. JETTE,** Boston University. They were responsible for making certain that an independent examination of this report was carried out in accordance with the standards of the National Academies and that all review comments were carefully considered. Responsibility for the final content rests entirely with the authoring committee and the National Academies.

Acknowledgments

The committee would like to acknowledge and thank the study sponsor—the National Institutes of Health, and particularly the National Institute on Aging and the National Institute of Neurological Disorders and Stroke—for their leadership in the development of this project. The committee also wishes to thank the many other individuals who gave presentations and participated in discussions with the committee.

Additionally, the committee would like to express its gratitude to the National Academies staff who worked on the study: Olivia Yost, Autumn Downey, Molly Dorries, Lydia Teferra, and Ashley Bologna, as well as National Academy of Medicine International Fellow, Hei Man Chow. The committee is also grateful for the contributions of Mark Goodin, editor; the team at PICO Portal, Inc. for their support with the scoping review; and Rebecca Morgan of the National Academies Research Center for her assistance with literature search strategy.

Contents

xi

Boxes, Figures, and Tables

BOXES

FIGURES

TABLES

Preface

Our understanding of dementia has changed in important ways and so should our research. We have learned so much in the last decade. We have learned that the majority of those who suffer from clinical dementia show a mix of different pathologies, rather than a single type. Though many living with clinical dementia show the amyloid plaques and tau tangles of Alzheimer's disease (AD), the majority of those people also show the hallmark pathologies of vascular, Lewy body, or other types of dementia. Interestingly, many older people without cognitive impairment also show plaques and tangles. So far, we do not know how these different pathologies interact to cause symptoms. We do not know the chain of causation for those different pathologies, and we do not know the best points in that chain for interventions that will prevent, delay, or even cure dementia. We have the start of therapeutics for Alzheimer's dementia, yet those with the *APOE4* gene variant, a large group with increased risk for AD, are at heightened risk for the side effects of current medications. Worse yet, we have no FDA-approved drugs for related dementias that are not Alzheimer's type beyond those for managing symptoms.

We have learned that the percentage of older people living with clinical dementia is decreasing in the United States, which is tremendous news. This improvement may result from changes in factors such as fitness, education, smoking cessation, and blood pressure control. We have not learned, however, how to ensure that those benefits reach populations who are disproportionately affected by dementia. For despite all we've learned, the risk of clinical dementia remains far greater among vulnerable populations. We need to continue working to address these health inequalities. We know that social isolation and loss of hearing and vision increase the risk of dementia, but we have yet to provide sufficient access to effective, widely available interventions to protect against these losses. We have learned that the process of diagnosing specific types of dementia can be time-consuming and too often inaccurate. We have not yet developed and validated sufficiently accurate, scalable, and affordable methods for use in clinical settings for assessing cognitive health and identifying how and when it starts to deteriorate. Without that knowledge, it will be difficult to develop and offer treatments tailored to individual needs.

This report's mandate is to assess the current state of research on Alzheimer's disease and related dementias (AD/ADRD), for both pharmacological and nonpharmacological interventions; to identify barriers to preventing and treating AD/ADRD; and to review the most promising areas of research—all with the goal of identifying appropriate research priorities for National Institutes of Health (NIH) funding. NIH and the many researchers it funds have produced an enormous increase, especially in the last decade, in the available knowledge regarding AD/ADRD. This report is the result of more than a year's effort by many people, ranging from dedicated National Academies of Sciences, Engineering, and Medicine staff, engaged and thoughtful committee members, experts presenting at our public meetings, and the author of a commissioned paper. We hope this report will build upon the good work already accomplished and guide NIH research priorities toward further explorations that will help prevent and treat AD/ADRD. For though the percentage of older people living with clinical dementia is decreasing, the overall numbers of those living with dementia in our aging population continue to increase. We are in dire need, today and in the future, for greater knowledge and more effective prevention and treatment for AD/ADRD.

Tia Powell, *Chair*
Committee on Research Priorities for Preventing and
Treating Alzheimer's Disease and Related Dementias

Prologue[1]

People are at the center of this report; they are the motivating factor behind each chapter. Doreen Monks and Krissan Lutz Moss are members of this committee who agreed to share their unique experiences living with cognitive impairment caused by neurodegenerative disease. Their stories are not intended to be representative of the experiences of all persons living with Alzheimer's disease and related dementias (AD/ADRD); rather, we use them to underscore key messages from this report and the importance of a person-centered approach to research on preventing and treating AD/ADRD. These are the people for whom the committee writes and hopes to benefit with the report.

Doreen Monks received her R.N. degree from Clara Maass Nursing School in Belleville, New Jersey, and later, her master's degree from Seton Hall University. She worked in various clinical and administrative positions, including a position at Cooperman Barnabas Medical Center where she collaborated with leading neurologists to develop a stroke program and taught nurses and doctors.

In late 2014, Doreen began noticing subtle cognitive changes and experiencing difficulties with performing tasks that had once been routine. These early signs of cognitive decline were initially easy to dismiss, but gradually, they worsened. It was not until October 2015, prompted by a conversation with a friend who had observed these changes, that Doreen sought medical

---

[1] Information provided by Doreen Monks and Krissan Moss, members of the Committee on Research Priorities for Preventing and Treating Alzheimer's Disease and Related Dementias, and stated here with their permission.

evaluation. This step marked the beginning of her journey on the complicated path of clinical diagnosis and management of cognitive impairment.

Over the next year, Doreen underwent a series of diagnostic tests, including magnetic resonance imaging and neuropsychological assessments. These evaluations revealed mild cognitive impairment, and she was diagnosed with early onset Alzheimer's disease in 2016. She was told that she would likely not survive beyond 8 or 9 years. Doreen initiated major life changes that had significant personal effects to prepare for this new future. She retired from the career she loved, leaving her with less for retirement than she had anticipated. She sold her home and entered an assisted living facility in preparation for rapidly worsening symptoms. After 11 months, she realized that she was too functional to live in an assisted living facility and eventually moved into a community for adults over 65 years of age. These were not simple logistical changes but deeply emotional ones, affecting her sense of self and autonomy. Desiring to help others facing similar circumstances and to make use of her past experiences as a nurse and educator, Doreen refocused her life around AD/ADRD advocacy and education to reduce the fear and stigma associated with these diseases and raise awareness regarding the importance of early diagnosis. She also sought to help advance research through participation in clinical trials.

In 2024, following preenrollment testing for a clinical trial for a new Alzheimer's disease drug, Doreen learned that although she had lived with a diagnosis of Alzheimer's disease for years, she was not qualified to participate in the trial owing to a lack of abnormal amyloid on her positron emission tomography scan—a prerequisite for many Alzheimer's disease drug trials. Further testing showed that her serum and cerebrospinal fluid (CSF) amyloid levels were also normal, but her serum and CSF levels of phospho-tau were elevated. Eight years after her initial diagnosis, Doreen was told that she does not have Alzheimer's disease but likely some form of mixed etiology featuring a tauopathy and possible Lewy bodies. As of this writing, she is still waiting on a new diagnosis.

Krissan Lutz Moss received her R.N. degree from Lutheran Hospital School of Nursing in Moline, Illinois, and her B.S.N. from the University of Illinois Chicago. Her career started in hospital oncology and intensive care units before exploring other clinical fields and positions, including leadership roles, clinical sales, and educational positions. The last 2 decades of her career were spent as a clinical education manager and thought leader liaison at Genentech. In each of her roles, patient advocacy was her focus.

In 2014, Krissan began noticing fluctuations in her cognitive abilities, such as difficulty learning new material, remembering words, and following conversations. As these cognitive difficulties progressed, she found herself withdrawing from core aspects of her job. Once able to teach complicated immunology, Krissan struggled to retain and relay scientific information.

She shifted to a new role with fewer demands, thinking that the stress of work travel and recent family illness was the driving factor in the cognitive fluctuations. Other symptoms, however, such as tremor, gait changes, severe constipation, and a loss of smell, became problematic. Krissan developed an inability to find words and noticed a change in personality, including a loss of filter and an uncharacteristic depression. Sleep disturbances and constant fatigue impaired her work performance and decision-making abilities. Eventually, multitasking and simple math were no longer possible.

In 2019, Krissan began to seek answers for her worsening symptoms. The path to her diagnosis included visits to multiple different specialists, ranging from gastroenterologists and speech therapists to sleep specialists and neurologists. In the fall of 2019, she was diagnosed with mild cognitive impairment, possible Lewy body dementia, Parkinsonism, and rapid eye movement (REM) sleep behavior disorder. While having an explanation for her symptoms provided relief, she had to begin the process of managing her disease, which included leaving a career she loved. Following her diagnosis, Krissan sought to help advance the state of the science on neurodegeneration through participation in observational studies such as the North American Prodromal Synucleinopathy study, which examines REM sleep behavior disorder and identifies potential biomarkers, genotypes, and phenotypes to improve diagnosis, early detection, and potential causes of Lewy body disease. She is currently diagnosed with prodromal Lewy body dementia, in addition to Parkinsonism, dystonia, and REM sleep behavior disorder. Krissan chooses to find joy in her moments and to live well with Lewy body disease, while participating in AD/ADRD research and working to change the stigma associated with neurodegenerative diseases. Being involved in advocacy and educational organizations allows Krissan to learn and teach strategies and adaptations to others so they too may live better with cognitive and physical changes.

Abstract

Accelerating the development of effective strategies for preventing and treating Alzheimer's disease and related dementias (AD/ADRD) is crucial to address the profound and growing public health crisis posed by dementia and to provide hope to millions of people at risk and those afflicted worldwide. In the last decade, spurred by the National Alzheimer's Project Act, the National Institutes of Health (NIH) has invested billions of dollars to support research on detecting, understanding, and developing interventions to prevent or treat AD/ADRD. These investments have led to many scientific advances, including the first treatments to slow the progression of Alzheimer's disease in some individuals, creating a foundation of knowledge to guide future research and interventions. However, the pace of progress has not matched the growing urgency for interventions that can prevent or cure AD/ADRD and reduce the emotional and financial toll on individuals, families, and communities.

The Committee on Research Priorities for Preventing and Treating Alzheimer's Disease and Related Dementias, convened by the National Academies of Sciences, Engineering, and Medicine, reviewed the research landscape and identified 11 scientific priorities with the potential to catalyze breakthroughs in the near and midterm that should be a focus of NIH-funded AD/ADRD research for the next 3 to 10 years (Recommendation 1). These research priorities, which are applicable across all causes of dementia and advance the committee's broader goal of optimizing brain health across the life course, fall into the following three broad areas:

5

1. Quantify brain health across the life course and accurately predict risk of, screen for, diagnose, and monitor AD/ADRD.
2. Build a more comprehensive and integrated understanding of the disease biology and mechanistic pathways that contribute to AD/ADRD development and resilience over the life course.
3. Catalyze advances in interventions for the prevention and treatment of AD/ADRD spanning from precision medicine to public health strategies.

The committee also developed recommendations to NIH and others in the AD/ADRD research ecosystem aimed at overcoming barriers to progress on the research priorities. The recommendations highlight investments and actions needed to maximize the knowledge generated from longitudinal research and accelerate clinical research (Recommendations 2 and 3). Other recommendations focus on breaking down silos to enable multidisciplinary, multisector, and collaborative research efforts (Recommendation 4) and fostering inclusive research practices that increase the accessibility and generalizability of AD/ADRD research (Recommendations 5 and 6). The recommendations also address the need to enhance the accessibility and usability of biological samples, data, and knowledge (Recommendations 7, 8, and 9). Finally, the committee suggests opportunities for NIH to promote innovation in AD/ADRD research to achieve transformational change (Recommendation 10).

Addressing the research priorities and recommendations will require sustained and dedicated resources and needs to be guided at all stages by those with lived experience to ensure synergy between scientific priorities and the priorities of those directly affected by dementia. Through the collaborative efforts of NIH, academic researchers, private industry, health care professionals, funders, policy makers, advocates, and people living with AD/ADRD, it is possible to envision a future where dementia is a preventable and treatable condition.

Summary[1]

Dementia exacts a weighty emotional and financial toll on individuals, families, and communities. Every person will have a unique experience of dementia influenced by their individual context, and many find ways to adapt to cognitive changes and enjoy meaningful lives for many years. Over the long run, however, the effects of dementia can be devastating, with advanced stages often robbing individuals of their sense of self, their memories and independence, their emotional and financial well-being, and ultimately, their lives. Moreover, the societal impacts, including the effects on families and communities and the enormous health and long-term care costs, are likely to grow with an aging population in the United States and globally. Accelerating the development of effective strategies for preventing and treating Alzheimer's disease and related dementias (AD/ADRD)—a collection of neurodegenerative conditions that can cause cognitive impairment and ultimately lead to clinical dementia—is therefore crucial to address the growing public health crisis posed by dementia and to provide hope to millions of people at risk and those afflicted worldwide.[2] Offering a chance to

---

[1] This summary does not include references. Citations for the discussion presented in this summary appear in the subsequent report chapters.

[2] The committee uses the terms *AD/ADRD* and *related dementias* throughout the report for consistency with its Statement of Task. The term *AD/ADRD* refers to all causes of neurodegeneration that are included in the study scope and *related dementias* refer to all causes of neurodegeneration that are included in the study scope with the exception of Alzheimer's disease. Additionally, for the purposes of this report and for consistency with commonly used terminology in the field, the term *dementia* refers to this group of neurogenerative diseases. The term *clinical dementia* will be used where referring to impairment that meets the clinical criteria for diagnosis of dementia. See Box S-1 and Chapter 1 for a discussion of terminology.

preserve cognitive function, reduce morbidity, and improve quality of life for individuals and their families is vital.

In the last decade, spurred by the National Alzheimer's Project Act, the National Institutes of Health (NIH) has invested billions to support research on detecting, understanding, and developing interventions for AD/ADRD. These investments have led to many scientific advances, including the first pharmacological treatments to slow the progression of AD in some individuals, creating a foundation of knowledge from which much more can be learned. However, the pace of progress has not matched the growing urgency for interventions that can prevent or cure AD/ADRD and reduce the societal costs of these diseases.

At the direction of the U.S. Congress, the National Institute on Aging (NIA) and the National Institute of Neurological Disorders and Stroke (NINDS) asked the National Academies of Sciences, Engineering, and Medicine to convene an expert committee to examine and assess the current state of biomedical research and recommend research priorities to advance the prevention and treatment of AD/ADRD. The committee was charged with identifying specific near- and medium-term scientific questions that can be addressed through NIH funding in the next 3 to 10 years, as well as opportunities to overcome major barriers to progress on these scientific questions. Box S-1 describes the collection of neurodegenerative disorders encompassed by the term *AD/ADRD* for the purposes of this report.

Of note, the committee was not asked to comprehensively catalog and assess NIH's programmatic activities related to AD/ADRD or to evaluate and make recommendations on the current strategic planning process used by NIH to set priorities. Rather this report is intended to

---

BOX S-1
Descriptions of Alzheimer's Disease and Related Dementias

Alzheimer's disease and related dementias (AD/ADRD): The committee's task is broadly focused on a group of progressive cognitive disorders, which develop over the life course and are characterized by an acquired loss of cognitive function that influences memory, thinking, and behavior and eventually is severe enough to interfere with independence and daily tasks. For the purposes of this report and for consistency with the Statement of Task, the term AD/ADRD includes Alzheimer's disease and the following related dementias: Lewy body dementia, frontotemporal dementia, limbic-predominant age-related TDP-43 encephalopathy, vascular dementia, and multiple etiology dementia. As understanding of

**BOX S-1
Continued**

the biological basis for this group of diseases continues to evolve, the inclusion and distinction of different disorders that fall under AD/ADRD may change. Brief descriptions of each, including distinguishing features related to brain pathologies and cognitive and behavioral characteristics, are included below.

Alzheimer's disease (AD) dementia: AD is defined by the specific presence and location of amyloid plaque and tau neurofibrillary tangle pathologies. The condition primarily affects individuals 65 and over. Individuals diagnosed prior to turning 65 are described as having early-onset AD and some of these will have genetic causes and be referred to as familial AD. Due to an extra copy of chromosome 21, which includes the *APP* gene, there is another form of early-onset AD called Down syndrome-related AD. Common symptoms of AD include memory loss; difficulty completing familiar tasks; impaired judgment; misplacing objects; changes in mood, personality, or behavior; and, eventually, difficulty walking, talking, and swallowing.

Lewy body dementia (LBD): LBD is associated with abnormal deposits of a protein called alpha-synuclein in certain regions of the brain (e.g., substantia nigra). These deposits, called Lewy bodies, may also be found in other types of dementia, including Alzheimer's dementia and Parkinson's disease dementia. Clinical symptoms of LBD typically begin to show at age 50 or older and can include visual or auditory hallucinations; changes in concentration, attention, alertness, and wakefulness; severe loss of other cognitive abilities that interfere with daily activities; REM sleep behavior disorder, impaired autonomic function, and impaired mobility with parkinsonian features (e.g., shuffling walk, stooped posture, balance problems and repeated falls, muscle rigidity, stiffness, tremors).

Frontotemporal dementia (FTD): FTD consists of a group of disorders caused by progressive nerve cell loss in the brain's frontal or temporal lobes, leading to loss of function in these brain regions and deterioration in behavior, personality, and/or difficulty with producing or comprehending language. Some patients with FTD may also have motor neuron disease (also known as amyotrophic lateral sclerosis or Lou Gehrig's disease) and vice versa. The two most prominent causes of FTD involve the proteins tau and TDP-43, although there are other types of FTD caused by specific genetic mutations and different protein inclusions. Unlike AD, FTD is more commonly diagnosed in midlife, among people between 40 and 60 years of age. The three major types of FTD include

continued

BOX S-1
Continued

behavioral variant frontotemporal dementia, which involves changes in personality, behavior, and judgment; primary progressive aphasia, which involves changes in the ability to use language to speak, read, write, name objects, and understand what others are saying; and movement disorders, which produce changes in muscle (motor neuron disease) or motor functions (parkinsonism). The latter can include symptoms associated with such atypical parkinsonian disorders as corticobasal syndrome and progressive supranuclear palsy. Mixed clinical presentations involving a combination of these symptoms are common in FTD.

Vascular dementia: Vascular dementia is caused by disruptions to vital blood and oxygen supply that also disrupt brain neurotoxin clearance, resulting in neuronal and glial injury and cell death culminating in cognitive decline and impairment. Vascular dementia is characterized by the presence of arteriolosclerosis and neuro-glio-vascular injuries to blood–brain barrier integrity. Cerebrovascular injuries include infarcts (micro or large vessel), hemorrhages (micro or lobar), myelin abnormalities due to small vessel disease, and cerebral amyloid angiopathy. Vascular dementia presents with similar symptoms to other types of dementia and can include confusion, challenges with organizing thoughts, difficulty with planning and communication, and physical symptoms such as reduced coordination and unsteady gait. Some but not all patients with vascular dementia may have an abrupt onset due to stroke or hemorrhage.

Limbic-predominant age-related TDP-43 encephalopathy (LATE): LATE was clinically recognized in 2019 as a type of dementia that is similar to AD in clinical presentation but involving a distinct pathology characterized by the accumulation of TDP-43 in the limbic system in the brain of older adults, typically among those over the age of 80 years. Symptoms of LATE can include memory loss and impaired cognition and decision making. Misdiagnosis as AD is believed to be widespread and co-occurrence with other types of dementia is also thought to be common; some patients diagnosed with AD may instead have LATE or a combination of both brain pathologies.

Multiple etiology dementia: Multiple etiology dementia occurs when two or more pathologies (mixed pathologies) co-occur in the brain of a person living with clinical dementia. The prevalence of such co-occurrence is widespread, and it is thought that most dementia cases among those over the age of 65 years are multiple etiology dementia. Symptoms reflect those associated with the distinct pathologies and may vary based on the type and extent of neuropathological changes present.

complement those efforts, highlighting opportunities to accelerate the translation of discoveries emerging from the vast and growing body of knowledge on AD/ADRD into effective strategies for prevention and treatment. The research priorities presented in this report represent the committee's consensus views on the areas of scientific inquiry with the greatest promise to catalyze significant advances and maximize return on investment in the form of improved population health. These research priorities are summarized in Recommendation 1 and detailed in Table S-1. The committee's Recommendations 2–10 are aimed at overcoming key, cross-cutting barriers to progress on those research priorities (see Figure S-1). Although the report is focused on opportunities to advance the science, the ultimate objective is to ensure that research investments translate to societal benefit by improving the lives of those already living with cognitive and other forms of impairment from AD/ADRD and preventing many more from developing these conditions. Addressing both the research priorities and the recommendations will require sustained and dedicated resources and need to be guided at all stages by those with lived experience to ensure synergy between scientific priorities and the priorities of those directly affected by dementia.

STATE OF THE SCIENCE ON PREVENTING AND TREATING AD/ADRD

At present there are no interventions that prevent or cure AD/ADRD, and there is an urgent need for treatments that substantially improve the lives of people living with dementia and those of their families, care partners, and caregivers—a difficult reality that shaped much of the committee's deliberations. However, the past few decades have brought significant advances in the understanding of AD/ADRD and in the development of tools and methods that can drive further progress. Noteworthy milestones include the ability to detect specific AD-related pathologies (amyloid and tau) years before symptoms emerge, the discovery of many new genes linked to AD/ADRD that shed light on pathogenic mechanisms, and the recognition that pathologies previously thought to distinguish different forms of dementia often co-occur. In addition, the recent approval of monoclonal anti-amyloid antibodies for early symptomatic stages of AD has given rise to optimism that AD and related neurodegenerative disorders can be treated to slow or halt disease progression and perhaps even prevented. Many researchers in the AD/ADRD field are encouraged by this momentum, hopeful that decades of inquiry and increased investment in research will soon lead to further breakthroughs in preventing and more effectively treating AD/ADRD, ultimately improving the lives of those affected by these disorders.

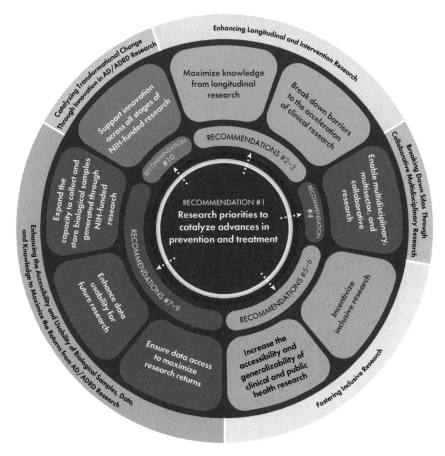

FIGURE S-1 Committee recommendations for advancing the prevention and treatment of AD/ADRD.
NOTE: AD/ADRD = Alzheimer's disease and related dementias.

Yet, the contrast between this potential future and the current state is stark, and progress has not been even across the different types of dementia. Cutting-edge tools and technologies such as fluid and digital biomarkers, multiomics methods, and artificial intelligence are poised to radically change the research and clinical practice landscape. However, some current tools for cognitive and other clinical assessments are not able to detect early, more subtle changes in cognition and are, in some cases, biased. Furthermore, while digital assessments show promise, most still lack validation as reliable biomarkers. Advances enabling early detection and subtyping of AD have yet to be realized for related dementias. Although the approval of anti-amyloid therapies for early symptomatic AD patients has generated optimism regarding the ability to slow cognitive decline, the clinical benefit of these therapies remains modest and has raised questions for many within the research community regarding their scope of application, long-term consequences, and the effect of their use in people living with mixed dementia. Further, people living with forms of dementia other than AD continue to have no treatments available that are approved by the U.S. Food and Drug Administration (FDA) beyond those for managing symptoms, crushing news for someone newly diagnosed with one of these forms today. Numerous studies on nonpharmacological strategies for preventing and mitigating AD/ADRD have also failed to provide definitive guidance on which approaches work and for whom, creating uncertainty for the public about how to protect cognitive health as they age. Despite considerable media coverage of health behaviors such as diet and exercise, definitive recommendations remain elusive. Consequently, the substantial scientific advances in AD/ADRD research have not translated into a widespread perception of progress among the public and policy makers.

The sense of stalled progress arises, in part, from a failure to effectively communicate the iterative and nonlinear nature of scientific advancement. Important achievements, such as declines in dementia prevalence and incidence rates, are not effectively communicated to audiences outside of the scientific community. The perception of stalled progress also underscores an urgent need—driven by compassion for those affected by these devastating disorders—for more rapid development of interventions to prevent or cure AD/ADRD, as well as treatments that substantially enhance the lives of those affected. Even if the accomplishments achieved to date were better recognized, the reality remains that there is a lack interventions to prevent or cure AD/ADRD and an urgent need for treatments that significantly improve the lives of individuals living with dementia and those close to them. The impact of dementia remains profound, despite the strides that have been made.

Based on its review of the research landscape, the committee identified the following scientific gaps that represent key bottlenecks that significantly impede progress toward preventing and treating AD/ADRD:

- There is a lack of rigorous evidence to support the identification of effective public health strategies for preventing AD/ADRD. Epidemiological research has yielded a large set of dementia risk factors (e.g., health behaviors, social isolation, socioeconomic disadvantage) based on statistical correlations. However, gaps in longitudinal data, data infrastructure, and study designs have resulted in limited understanding of causal relationships and the identification of exposures and system-level factors that, if mitigated, would have the greatest effect on the incidence of dementia. This impedes the development of effective public health approaches that could be implemented at a population scale to promote brain health across the life course and prevent AD/ADRD in diverse and especially disproportionately affected populations.

- There is an incomplete understanding of the biological basis and multiple etiologies underlying cognitive decline and dementia, as well as the mechanisms of resilience. There is still much that is not understood about AD/ADRD, conditions that may be characterized by decades of life-course health insults to brain and peripheral systems contributing to the development and detectable progression of neuropathology in the absence of clinical symptoms. Key knowledge gaps include how life-course exposures and other risk factors relate to pathobiology in diverse populations and the connections between molecular pathways that contribute to AD/ADRD and resilience (the maintenance of cognitive function despite the presence of brain pathology). This lack of understanding impedes drug discovery and the development of effective preventive and therapeutic intervention strategies. It also makes it difficult to predict the effect of risk factor reduction and drugs focused on single pathology targets on dementia incidence.

- There is a lack of effective, validated, and accessible tools and methods (e.g., novel biomarker tests, digital assessment technologies) for detecting early changes in brain health and accurately diagnosing, subtyping, and monitoring AD/ADRD in diverse populations. This foundational capability is essential to trace how the natural history of AD/ADRD differs from "healthy" brain aging. Progress made in the development of tools for AD needs to be expanded beyond amyloid and tau and extended to the multiple etiologies leading to dementia. The current capability gap impedes efforts to measure disease incidence and prevalence, to intervene early when chances of preventing and mitigating disease are greatest, to detect when treatments modify the trajectory of AD/ADRD, and to target specific interventions to the right populations (precision medicine).

Within each of these major scientific gaps of knowledge, there is also promising research that suggests opportunities to break current bottlenecks as new discoveries emerge. The discovery of imaging and fluid biomarkers for AD has catalyzed a shift in phenotyping procedures used in research and needs to be tested now in clinical practice. With the identification of risk genes/loci and the discovery of additional biomarkers, particularly for related dementias, current barriers to early detection, diagnosis, prognosis (e.g., the likelihood of progression to clinical dementia), and longitudinal monitoring may be overcome, and it will be possible to quantify and better understand multiple etiology dementia. The combination of digital tools and computational methods such as artificial intelligence/machine learning that may be able to identify changes in traits (e.g., speech, gait, sleep behavior) that may precede current measures of cognitive decline similarly shows promise for enabling early detection of changes in brain health, early diagnosis, and prognosis. Digital tools have also opened new opportunities for passive and remote data collection and are changing the way investigators engage with study participants, particularly those from underresourced and underrepresented populations, and the public.

Investments in basic science and longitudinal cohort studies have led to a significant expansion of the therapeutic pipeline with novel promising interventions that are not specific to any single dementia type by uncovering shared molecular pathways contributing to AD/ADRD (e.g., autophagic and lysosomal, immune, metabolic, myelination), as well as resilience factors. Multiomics methods are creating new opportunities to (1) evaluate disease mechanisms in diverse populations and (2) to identify molecular disease subtypes and endophenotypes, thereby creating the foundation for precision medicine approaches to prevention and treatment in the future.[3] Increased understanding of the links between AD/ADRD and chronic diseases such as hypertension and diabetes, along with encouraging evidence for multicomponent interventions focused on health behaviors, has highlighted the potential for public health strategies to reduce dementia risk.

SCIENTIFIC PRIORITIES FOR ADVANCING THE PREVENTION AND TREATMENT OF AD/ADRD

Building on the aforementioned examples of momentum and lines of promising research, the committee identified 11 research priorities and associated near- and medium-term scientific questions that it believes should be a focus of NIH-funded AD/ADRD biomedical research for the next 3 to 10 years. These research priorities, which are summarized in Recommendation 1 and detailed in Table S-1, fall into three broad areas:

1. Quantify brain health across the life course and accurately predict risk of, screen for, diagnose, and monitor AD/ADRD.
2. Build a more comprehensive and integrated understanding of the disease biology and mechanistic pathways that contribute to AD/ADRD development and resilience over the life course.

---

[3] Multiomics methods involve the integrative analysis of multiple "-omics" datasets, such as those generated from genomic, proteomic, transcriptomic, epigenomic, and metabolomic methods.

TABLE S-1 Committee-Identified Research Priorities to Advance the Prevention and Treatment of Alzheimer's Disease and Related Dementias (AD/ADRD)

Research Priority	Key Scientific Questions	Near-Term Research Opportunities to Address Key Scientific Questions
Research priorities to quantify brain health across the life course and accurately predict risk of, screen for, diagnose, and monitor AD/ADRD		
2-1: Develop better tools, including novel biomarker tests and digital assessment technologies, to monitor brain health across the life course and screen, predict, and diagnose AD/ADRD at scale.	• How can brain health be precisely measured at scale across a diverse population (universally scalable)? • Can diagnostic biomarkers help identify potential causes for changes in personalized brain health? • Which data are essential to collect across the life course? • What alternative measures can assess changes in cognition and other related behaviors (e.g., ability to learn)? • How can existing cohorts be used to understand key transition points in brain health across the life course?	• Establish criteria to evaluate the diagnostic and clinical utility of newly developed tools (e.g., cognitive, clinical, fluid or digital biomarkers, imaging). • Discover and validate novel measures that capture early changes in brain health from a person's baseline. • Discover and validate new diagnostic, prognostic, predictive, and treatment response biomarkers (molecular and digital). • Carry out analyses within and across existing cohorts, including those cohorts developed to characterize brain health and those created for examining other health outcomes. • Perform large-scale, multiomics cohort studies of peripheral and brain signatures in diverse populations. • Perform large-scale cohort studies of digital signatures in diverse subpopulations.
2-2: Implement advances in clinical research methods and tools to generate data from real-world clinical practice settings that can inform future research.	• What are the facilitators of and barriers to the adoption of clinical research tools and methods? • How does the performance of novel tools (e.g., biomarker-based diagnostics, digital health technologies) differ across real-world settings and research settings? • What are the harms and benefits of identifying those with a specific pathology but who may never develop any symptoms?	• Rapidly implement novel tools (e.g., biomarker tests, digital technologies) in current, cross-institute studies. • Educate about the use and utility of emerging tools and technologies. • Evaluate potential harms of false positive or incorrect diagnoses and stigma related to early diagnoses before meaningful cognitive or other clinical symptoms manifest.

continued

- How are the risks and benefits of biomarker testing and preclinical diagnosis balanced?
- How can the negative social and legal consequences of early detection or diagnosis of AD/ADRD be mitigated?

Research priorities to build a more comprehensive and integrated understanding of the disease biology and mechanistic pathways that contribute to AD/ADRD development and resilience over the life course

3-1: Identify factors driving AD/ADRD risk in diverse populations, particularly understudied and disproportionately affected groups, to better understand disease heterogeneity—including molecular subtypes and disparities in environmental exposures—and to identify prevention opportunities and advance health research equity.	• What are the determinants of AD/ADRD risk in diverse population groups (e.g., racial/ethnic, sex/gender, socioeconomic, geographic)? • Why are differences in pathology observed in diverse populations, and how does that influence risk of clinical disease? • What are the relative roles of modifiable social, economic, environmental, clinical, and behavioral mechanisms that might contribute to population differences in AD/ADRD? • How does the ability to modify risk factors vary across populations and their socioeconomic contexts? • What can be learned from the observed heterogeneity in severity (e.g., level of cognitive decline) and patterns of cognitive and other clinical symptoms among people who have similar levels of AD/ADRD-related pathology? • What genetic and other multiomics factors determine individuals' responses to interventions, modifiers, and exposures (e.g., exercise, diet, air pollution)? • What is required to increase interest in brain donation in diverse populations?	• Carry out a comprehensive survey of genetic and multiomics architecture in diverse well-characterized populations, using existing cohorts and infrastructure, to identify genomic determinants of risk. • Generate data to inform polygenic risk scores in people of non-European ancestry. • Use artificial intelligence and other computational tools to integrate multiple data types (e.g., multiomics, social, environmental) and identify commonalities across disease types and diverse populations and translate risk factors into biological mechanisms. • Across diverse populations, evaluate variations in the associations of life-course social, behavioral, and environmental exposure with longitudinal cognitive and biomarker data. • Identify opportunities to use natural experiments to evaluate exposure effects across the life course on clinical and biomarker outcomes in diverse populations.

TABLE S-1 Continued

Research Priority	Key Scientific Questions	Near-Term Research Opportunities to Address Key Scientific Questions
3-2: Characterize the exposome and gene–environment interactions across the life course to gain insights into biological mechanisms and identify opportunities to reduce AD/ADRD risk and increase resilience.	• Are there sensitive or critical periods across the life course when social, behavioral, or environmental exposures have a greater effect on different etiologic processes driving AD/ADRD risk? • What is the role of early- and midlife exposures in resilience and disease progression and do these vary for specific pathologies? • Do early- and midlife exposures result in brain circuitry changes that affect later life, and are these modifiable? • Which exposures have the largest effects on AD/ADRD risk and resilience (e.g., affect the largest proportion of the population) and should be prioritized for future investigations? • Are the gene–environment interactions that influence AD/ADRD risk and resilience different among diverse populations?	• Identify profiles (e.g., biochemical, multiomics) that reflect and capture individuals' exposures and link them to AD/ADRD outcomes to better understand exposure risk factors. • Investigate gene–exposure interactions using exposure data that are already available. • Link complex combinations of life-course social, behavioral, and environmental exposure measures to evaluate how these exposures synergistically influence longitudinal cognitive and biomarker data across diverse populations. • Evaluate how features of the social and environmental exposome or gene–environment interactions influence specific pathologies contributing to AD/ADRD using a life-course framework.
3-3: Elucidate the genetic and other biological mechanisms underlying resilience and resistance to identify novel targets and effective strategies for AD/ADRD prevention and treatment.	• What are the key factors that contribute to the resilience observed in positive or negative outliers (e.g., exceptional cases, including supercentenarians)? • What can be learned from individuals who do not develop pathologies (resistance) and those who develop pathologies but do not develop clinical symptoms within their lifetimes (resilience)? • What changes occur over time (i.e., with aging) in the way the brain deals with pathology (brain plasticity and adaptability), and is that process modifiable? • How do interactions between organ systems, including brain–body axes, contribute to resilience?	• Apply human tissue models from diverse groups of patients, including those with related dementias, and animal models to elucidate genes, multiomics factors, and molecular processes contributing to AD/ADRD resilience. • Investigate the role of brain–body axes (e.g., brain–gut and brain–renal axes) in resilience. • Establish a collection of resilient brains (organ collection) as a basis for the systematic comparative analysis of the causes of selective vulnerability and selective resilience and resistance to identify key factors and determinants of vulnerability and resilience, including a focus on disease-decisive factors.

3-4: Develop integrated molecular and cellular causal models to guide the identification of common mechanisms underlying AD/ADRD and their validation as novel targets for prevention and treatment.	• What are the primary interactions and sequential cascading effects that translate molecular and cellular dysregulation into disease? • How do distinct pathologic processes combine to culminate in clinical manifestations of AD/ADRD? • When do the different molecular factors and processes begin to disturb cellular, organ, or system function that leads, eventually, to disease onset (age dependent)? Considering multiple etiologic processes contributing to AD/ADRD individually and jointly, is there a particular point of no return? • How do the different cell types in the brain (e.g., glial cells, endothelial cells, neurons) interact with each other on a timescale, ultimately leading to neurodegeneration? • How do genome-wide association studies (GWAS)-based risk genes set the stage for alterations in brain cell physiology, predisposing the brain to dysfunction and disease later in life? • What is the functional effect of defined identified risk genes or defined groups of risk genes on neuronal and glial physiology and function? • How do exposome factors affect physiology of cell types contributing to disease? • How do amyloid-independent interventions (e.g., lysosomal stabilizers, autophagy inducers, neuroprotective compounds) change cellular biology? • What are the molecular and cellular mechanisms mediating interactions between organ systems, including brain–body axes, that lead to brain pathologies?	• Identify the earliest biological changes related to pathologic processes. • Investigate the function of glial, endothelial, neuronal, and other relevant types of brain cells during aging employing aged cell types and aged cell cultures. • Study the interactions of the different types of cells and mediators and the consequences of such interactions in appropriate cell and tissue models to identify a potential point of no return. • Include *aging* as the central risk factor of many dementia types into all cellular and molecular studies (e.g., aged glial cells, induced neurons from older individuals) and employ multiomics technologies. • Generate a framework based on grouping certain GWAS risk loci; identify functionally causal genes in these loci, and study their cellular and molecular effect on functions. • Systematically study the functional consequences of AD/ADRD risk genes in cellular models (extending beyond *APOE4* studies to a wider array of risk genes derived from GWAS and other omics studies). • Study the effect of exposomal factors (individually and in combination) on the physiology of glial and endothelial cells, neurons, and other relevant brain cell types in cellular and animal models. • Analyze the effect of experimental approaches and compounds on molecular pathways beyond those involved in the amyloid cascade, and employ amyloid-independent cellular and in vivo models.

continued

TABLE S-1 Continued

Research Priority	Key Scientific Questions	Near-Term Research Opportunities to Address Key Scientific Questions
3-4: Continued	• How do molecular and cellular mechanisms that contribute to development of neuropsychiatric symptoms interact with those that underlie the development of neuropathology? • Are there important differences in pathologic, molecular, and multiomics features that are shared across AD and related dementias?	• Employ comparative studies using histology and multiomics to identify commonalities among AD and related dementias. • Evaluate mediating and modifying pathways linking genetic and genomic risk factors and biomarker measures of disease with clinical manifestations. • Investigate the role of the brain–body axes (e.g., brain–gut and brain–renal axes) in the development of AD/ADRD pathology.
Research priorities to catalyze advances in interventions for the prevention and treatment of AD/ADRD spanning from precision medicine to public health strategies		
4-1: Integrate innovative approaches and novel tools into the planning, design, and execution of studies to accelerate the identification of effective interventions.	• What outcomes and biomarkers can be used to assess the interactive effects of mixed pathologies (e.g., vascular, alpha-synuclein, TDP-43, and AD pathology)? • What biological markers can be used to show that the intended pathway is engaged and the therapy is having the expected effect? • How can trial design be improved to determine whether late-stage trial failures are the result of ineffective interventions versus limitations in trial designs or execution? • How can trials be designed to incorporate and test innovative methodologies in ways that do not pose risks to the primary objective of the trial and the timely execution of clinical research?	• Incorporate innovative substudies into ongoing clinical trials to pilot novel approaches (e.g., new biomarkers as secondary outcomes, digital tools for remote data collection). • Create mechanisms to share successes and failures from innovative operational trial design aspects. • Optimize proof-of-concept trials with informative biomarkers and outcomes. • Identify and evaluate causal evidence on the role of past and ongoing public health initiatives, clinical care changes, and policy changes on AD/ADRD prevention at a population level (e.g., trial emulations using real-world data). • Use existing data (e.g., electronic health data) to identify subpopulations.

	• What innovative approaches can be used to increase the value of observational studies to inform prevention, including short- and long-term effects? • Can risk profiles based on biomarker testing of asymptomatic individuals decrease required sample sizes and accelerate trials?	• Use platform randomized trials to evaluate multiple interventions in parallel. • Conduct long-term follow-up of early- and midlife prevention strategies using networked data infrastructure. • Develop and use social determinants of health metrics in clinical research.
4-2: Advance the development and evaluation of combination therapies (including pharmacological and nonpharmacological approaches) to better address the multifactorial nature of AD/ADRD.	• Which combinations of interventions (drug combinations and combinations of drugs and nonpharmacological interventions [NPIs]) will work synergistically to prevent AD/ADRD or slow its clinical progression? • What are the long-term effects of combination interventions? • How does the sequencing of interventions affect their combined effectiveness and safety? • How do different combinations of interventions interact, and how can their effects be maximized? • Can combination interventions targeting multiple mechanistic pathways improve the effectiveness of treatment for people with mixed pathologies? • For combination trials that include NPIs, how can the trial be designed with adequate blinding and appropriate control groups? What are the relevant endpoints?	• Explore and understand the independent and/or synergistic mechanisms of multidomain interventions and combination therapies.
4-3: Evaluate precision medicine approaches for the prevention and treatment of AD/ADRD to better identify interventions likely to benefit specific groups of individuals.	• Can an understanding of the exposome guide population stratification to facilitate precision approaches to AD/ADRD interventions? • What criteria and molecular or multiomics factors and biomarkers are appropriate for use in (1) identifying subtypes and endophenotypes and (2) stratifying populations at a population and an individual level?	• Integrate findings from multiomic approaches and other modalities to characterize AD/ADRD subtypes that can be used to identify commonalities and stratify across different subtypes. • Use innovative research designs (e.g., platform trials, personalized interventions) that support precision medicine approaches.

continued

TABLE S-1 Continued

Research Priority	Key Scientific Questions	Near-Term Research Opportunities to Address Key Scientific Questions
4-3: Continued	• Does giving people more agency in how they implement interventions (e.g., personalized approaches to NPIs) affect trial outcomes?	• Conduct intervention trials that include study populations living with multiple pathologies. • Invest in longer-term studies of postintervention outcomes in diverse populations, including in populations with different comorbidities and levels of adherence. • Conduct follow-up studies of individuals treated with anti-amyloid antibodies to better understand the effects of copathologies on patient symptoms and to identify key targets to include in combination interventions. • Collaborate with safety registries to evaluate safety outcomes from real-world evidence.
4-4: Advance the adoption of standardized outcomes for assessing interventions that are sensitive, person-centered, clinically meaningful, and reflect the priorities of those at risk for or living with AD/ADRD.	• What outcomes matter most for people living with AD/ADRD and their caregivers and care partners? • How do intermediate outcomes such as biomarkers and risk scores translate to outcomes that are clinically meaningful? • What metrics are most important for assessing quality of life, well-being, and functional outcomes in diverse populations? • What are the continued clinical and biological outcomes in those who received an intervention? • How can study designs incorporate research questions around maximizing adherence to interventions?	• Develop and validate intermediate outcomes, including biomarkers and risk scores, that are robustly linked to cognitive, functional, or quality-of-life outcomes. • Use metrics that can be personalized for desired individual outcomes. • Conduct ethnographic and other similar studies to identify person-centered outcomes for use in clinical research. • Engage clinicians (e.g., primary care providers, geriatricians) and people living with AD/ADRD in the identification of clinically meaningful outcomes for use in clinical research. • Evaluate factors that influence adherence to interventions and how it affects outcomes.

| 4-5: Evaluate the causal effects of public health approaches on overall dementia incidence and incidence in understudied and/or disproportionately affected populations. | • What is the potential effect of a population approach (e.g., modifying exposure to an adverse environmental or social factor or behavior) on dementia incidence and inequalities relative to a precision medicine or high-risk individual-level approach (i.e., targeting risk reduction in individuals with the highest level of an adverse risk factor)?
• Considering mediating mechanisms and spillover effects, what are the most effective strategies for population interventions to reduce dementia incidence?
• What interventions can be most easily scaled to reduce risk of dementia at a population level in the near and medium terms? | • Estimate population-attributable fractions associated with identified risk factors for all-cause dementia risk, dementia subtypes, and on social inequalities in dementia risk.
• Compare plausible population-attributable fractions for AD/ADRD cases prevented associated with high-risk/precision medicine versus population approaches.
• Evaluate the evidence for causality of known risk factors with high population prevalence, with specificity regarding dose, duration, timing (age), and other possible sources of heterogeneity in exposure effects.
• Evaluate whether there are important distinct determinants of dementia that are common in groups historically underrepresented in AD/ADRD research (e.g., Black, Latino, Asian, or Indigenous populations; rural populations; and individuals from low socioeconomic backgrounds) and may be targets for public health approaches.
• Evaluate how specific policies or interventions that can be scaled to large populations influence dementia risk overall and inequalities in dementia risk.
• Evaluate how changes in existing policies shaping social and environmental determinants of health (e.g., policies shaping food security, economic security, healthy housing access, educational experiences across the life course, safe working conditions, retirement policies, violence exposure, air pollution and other environmental toxins, and community climate resilience) influence biomarkers associated with AD/ADRD risk and clinical AD/ADRD. |

continued

TABLE S-1 Continued

Research Priority	Key Scientific Questions	Near-Term Research Opportunities to Address Key Scientific Questions
4-5: Continued		• Contrast the near- and medium-term impact of clinical care strategies (e.g., hypertension treatment, access to amyloid-targeting therapies, or management of comorbid conditions and infectious diseases) versus behavior change strategies (e.g., dietary or physical activity interventions) versus policy interventions (e.g., changes in retirement age or clean air and water standards). • Incorporate estimates of spillover effects of modifying risk factors and of prevented dementia cases on family and other social network members.

NOTE: The numbering of research priorities in this table reflects the numbering in the report chapters.

3. Catalyze advances in interventions for the prevention and treatment of AD/ADRD spanning from precision medicine to public health strategies.

Importantly, the committee recommended research priorities that are not focused on gaps specific to individual dementia types. In an effort to move away from siloed thinking and toward more integrative research, the committee sought to emphasize opportunities that would be applicable across the spectrum of AD/ADRD and respond to the high prevalence of mixed pathologies in older individuals, as well as advance the committee's broader goal of optimizing brain health and cognitive function across the life course. It remains essential, however, to continue to advance research focused on specific pathologies in parallel (e.g., discovery of biomarkers and development of outcome measures for specific pathologies) to improve the detection, diagnosis, and subtyping of AD/ADRD (see Chapter 2) and advance precision medicine approaches (see Chapter 4).

Intervention strategies to optimize brain health and cognitive function across the life course include population-scale public health approaches aimed at preventing dementia through risk factor reduction and increasing resilience. Although the mechanisms are not well understood, the decline in age-specific clinical dementia incidence in high-income countries such as the United States suggests such approaches have already yielded success. Improved understanding of the contributors to the observed decrease in clinical dementia incidence may open opportunities to accelerate prevention efforts and to better leverage public health investments not specifically targeted to AD/ADRD (e.g., initiatives aimed at improving cardiovascular health). Such efforts can be pursued now even in the absence of a complete understanding of the underlying biological mechanisms that mediate the effects of public health strategies.

Another approach to maximize the effect of research investments across multiple dementia types is to target interventions to common (shared) mechanisms for pathogenesis (e.g., neuroinflammation, lysosomal failure, vascular disease, dysmyelination, mitochondrial and metabolic dysfunction) and resilience. Such strategies will rely on an improved understanding of the multiple and likely intersecting molecular pathways that contribute to AD/ADRD. While NIH has been critiqued for an overemphasis in past decades on AD and amyloid-related research, the recognition in recent years of the multifactorial nature of AD/ADRD and the predominance of multiple pathologies has led to a greater appreciation of the need for efforts beyond amyloid and more focus on a diversity of pathways and their integration. By enabling the identification of initial molecular and environmental triggers, downstream pathophysiology, and biological mechanisms that promote resilience and healthy aging, an integrated understanding of disease can guide combination approaches to AD/ADRD prevention and treatment that target multiple underlying pathways. Such an approach has the potential to achieve greater effect sizes and more meaningful patient outcomes.

Recommendation 1: Research priorities to catalyze advances in prevention and treatment
The National Institutes of Health (NIH) should focus on the research priorities and associated near- and medium-term scientific questions detailed in Table S-1 to advance a person-centered, multidisciplinary, and integrative research approach that will catalyze advances in the prevention and treatment of Alzheimer's disease and related dementias (AD/ADRD). These research priorities cover the following areas:

- Develop better tools, including novel biomarker tests and digital assessment technologies, to monitor brain health across the life course and screen, predict, and diagnose AD/ADRD at scale (Research Priority 2-1)
- Implement advances in clinical research methods and tools to generate data from real-world clinical practice settings that can inform future research (Research Priority 2-2)
- Identify factors driving AD/ADRD risk in diverse populations, particularly understudied and disproportionately affected groups, to better understand disease heterogeneity—including molecular subtypes and disparities in environmental exposures—and to identify prevention opportunities and advance health research equity (Research Priority 3-1)
- Characterize the exposome and gene–environment interactions across the life course to gain insights into biological mechanisms and identify opportunities to reduce AD/ADRD risk and increase resilience (Research Priority 3-2)
- Elucidate the genetic and other biological mechanisms underlying resilience and resistance to identify novel targets and effective strategies for AD/ADRD prevention and treatment (Research Priority 3-3)
- Develop integrated molecular and cellular causal models to guide the identification of common mechanisms underlying AD/ADRD and their validation as novel targets for prevention and treatment (Research Priority 3-4)
- Integrate innovative approaches and novel tools into the planning, design, and execution of studies to accelerate the identification of effective interventions (Research Priority 4-1)
- Advance the development and evaluation of combination therapies (including pharmacological and nonpharmacological

approaches) to better address the multifactorial nature of AD/ADRD (Research Priority 4-2)

- Evaluate precision medicine approaches for the prevention and treatment of AD/ADRD to better identify interventions likely to benefit specific groups of individuals (Research Priority 4-3)
- Advance the adoption of standardized outcomes for assessing interventions that are sensitive, person-centered, clinically meaningful, and reflect the priorities of those at risk for or living with AD/ADRD (Research Priority 4-4)
- Evaluate the causal effects of public health approaches on overall dementia incidence and incidence in understudied and/or disproportionately affected populations. (Research Priority 4-5)

The committee acknowledges that NIH has already made investments in each of these priority research areas to varying degrees. Given the breadth of the NIH AD/ADRD research portfolio, it is unsurprising that the committee did not identify any research priorities for which there had been no prior NIH investment. In some cases, research priorities identified by the committee, such as the development of biomarkers for monitoring brain health and the identification of factors driving risk in diverse populations, are already the focus of major NIH-funded research programs and initiatives, many of which are described in this report. Other identified research priorities, such as the characterization of the exposome and gene–environment interactions, the development of integrated molecular and cellular causal models, and the development of digital tools represent scientific areas of more recent or limited NIH investment. Relatedly, efforts to achieve associated near-term research opportunities, which are detailed in the right-hand column of Table S-1, may indeed be underway but have not yet been fully realized. Significant investment in the totality of the priority research areas is needed to address the knowledge gaps laid out in this report. Critically, beyond financial investment, success in tackling each of these research priorities will require an emphasis on the intentional expansion of research efforts beyond AD and the inclusion of diverse and understudied and/or disproportionately affected populations.

Importantly, Table S-1 is not intended as a prescribed research agenda. Nor is the identification of these priority areas meant to imply that lines of scientific inquiry outside of these areas are not of value or that work in all other areas should be suspended. There is a great deal of uncertainty in the process for scientific investigation regarding which discoveries from current research will lead to transformational advances in the future, and no guarantees can be offered regarding the ultimate fruitfulness of any specific line of inquiry. The committee's intention, however, is that the priorities will be used as a guide in the rebalancing of NIH funding for AD/ADRD.

These are near- and medium-term priorities in the sense that investment and expansion in these priority areas should occur in the near and medium term. The timeline for realization of scientific advancements from these investments is inherently harder to predict. Closing the scientific knowledge gaps raised by these priorities can occur by working to answer the committee's proposed scientific questions and acting on opportunities to overcome barriers to progress, as detailed in the recommendations that follow.

ENHANCING LONGITUDINAL AND INTERVENTION RESEARCH

Studies that follow individuals longitudinally and test interventions across time are needed to address the research priorities and associated scientific questions identified in Table S-1. Longitudinal cohort studies represent an important mechanism for identifying data that provide a comprehensive view of brain health and AD/ADRD development over the life course (including risk and resilience factors). Knowledge gained from such studies can be translated into protocols and sensitive tools (e.g., digital health technologies, biomarker assays) that can be deployed in research and practice for ongoing clinical monitoring and AD/ADRD prediction, detection, prognostication, and diagnosis. NIH has made significant investments to expand and leverage longitudinal research related to aging, resilience, and AD/ADRD.

Many datasets relevant to brain health and AD/ADRD have already been generated through longitudinal research focused on other health conditions, such as the Bogalusa Heart Study, which focuses on cardiovascular disease. A concerted effort to integrate those data with AD/ADRD outcomes could yield important insights into prevention and treatment strategies now while newer cohort studies remain ongoing. Progress to this end has been made through supplemental funding provided by NIH and other NIH funding mechanisms to incorporate an AD/ADRD focus into some existing cohorts, but the expansion of such efforts to other cohorts could help to fill current data gaps (e.g., data for younger age ranges and populations underrepresented in AD/ADRD research) and expand the set of measures that can be linked to brain health trajectories. Additionally, there remain opportunities to improve cohort representativeness, better capture data across the life course, bank samples for future analysis, and enable multicohort analyses through data harmonization.

Recommendation 2: Maximize knowledge from longitudinal research
To maximize knowledge from longitudinal research and enable future discoveries, the National Institutes of Health should prioritize investments in longitudinal research to address existing knowledge gaps regarding factors that influence brain health over the life course. These efforts should include the following:

- Invest in data infrastructure (see Recommendation 7), data harmonization (see Recommendation 8), and the cultivation of specialized expertise to enable the collection of data and conduct of analyses within and across existing cohorts, including those cohorts developed to characterize brain health and those created for examining other health outcomes.
- Create new, multidimensionally diverse (e.g., multilanguage, ethnoracial, geographic, socioeconomic) cohorts.
- Strategically add data points important to assessing brain health into existing cohorts constituted for research on other health conditions.
- Routinely collect early- and midlife exposure data (e.g., residential and work history, environmental toxicants, nutrition, education) from cohort study participants.
- Ensure that the data generated from shared biological samples are stored, searchable, and sharable.

Many entities (government, private, philanthropic, and academic) contribute to research for advancing interventions for AD/ADRD with complementary resources and expertise. While private industry is active in the development and evaluation of pharmacological agents and is often responsible for bringing therapeutics to market, other kinds of interventions and certain trial designs may be less appealing to industry owing to financial risk or the lack of financial incentives. This may be the case, for example, with many nonpharmacological interventions, repurposed drugs, and combination interventions, which are difficult to monetize. NIH plays a critical role in this complex research ecosystem by funding research on such interventions, incentivizing industry participation in collaborative efforts designed to develop and bring new and combination interventions to scale (see Recommendation 10), and supporting essential basic and translational research (e.g., target identification and validation) that feeds into the private-sector drug development pipeline. Increased collaboration and seamless transition between academia and industry throughout the research continuum could reduce the time to develop effective interventions. Likewise, fostering and incentivizing rapid and transparent data sharing from industry to nonindustry researchers would accelerate solutions.

NIH infrastructure investments for clinical research, such as the Alzheimer's Clinical Trials Consortium, the Dominantly Inherited Alzheimer Network Trials Unit, and the Alzheimer's Prevention Initiative, have facilitated increased collaboration with industry, philanthropy, and other partners (e.g., by using public–private partnerships) and innovation in AD/ADRD clinical trials (e.g., decentralization of trials using hub-and-spoke models, piloting platform trials, virtual engagement of participants, and digital data collection). However, to accelerate the pace of discovery, these efforts to increase collaboration need to be expanded to a much greater scale as NIH continues to support clinical research to evaluate AD/ADRD interventions in the coming years.

As drug discovery and target validation efforts are scaled, phase 1b and phase 2 clinical trials in particular need to be expanded. Increasing the quantity and quality of small phase 1b and phase 2 proof-of-concept trials with a focus on mechanisms, informative biomarkers (e.g., target engagement, biomarkers for copathologies), and outcomes (e.g., pharmacokinetics and pharmacodynamics, surrogate outcomes) is needed to smooth the transition to and better guide decision making for larger, later-stage trials.

In anticipation of the increased demand for clinical trial investigators, attention is needed to address current gaps in the workforce (e.g., investigators with specialized expertise in pharmacology trials). Ensuring investigators new to conducting trials utilize existing training programs with best practices can help to improve the rigor of earlier-stage trials. NIH-funded clinical trial consortia, if adequately supported, could provide training for clinical trial sites to disseminate knowledge, standards, and best practices.

> **Recommendation 3: Break down barriers to the acceleration of clinical research**
>
> The National Institutes of Health (NIH) should continue to lead efforts across a multiplicity of relevant entities (e.g., pharmaceutical and biotechnology companies, academia, foundations) to accelerate the movement of promising interventions for Alzheimer's disease and related dementias (AD/ADRD) into clinical trials and to expand the use of innovative approaches to improve the efficiency of clinical trials. These efforts should include the following:
>
> - Organize NIH investments in basic and translational research related to potential molecular targets for intervention into a portfolio to create a pipeline of validated targets that can be transitioned into drug development.
> - Expand the use of innovative trial designs (e.g., master protocols, platform, combination, adaptive trials) and increase investment in both early-phase (phase 1b and 2) proof-of-concept trials and later-stage pragmatic trials.
> - Identify and promulgate best practices for decreasing the barriers to, and time for, the clinical trial startup phase (e.g., decentralized participant screening, creation and use of pre-screened cohorts and screen-enroll mechanisms, use of electronic consenting procedures, centralized contracting, and institutional review board processes).

- Continue investing in innovative funding models, such as public–private partnerships, shared funding for global trials, and combined-phase funding, that support the progression of candidate interventions across the early-stage clinical research pipeline.
- Maximize coordination between NIH-funded AD/ADRD clinical trial programs and NIH-funded AD/ADRD centers (e.g., Alzheimer's Disease Research Centers) and evaluate these centers for representative participant clinical trial enrollment.

STRATEGIES FOR ADDRESSING CROSSCUTTING BARRIERS THAT IMPEDE PROGRESS

The committee was asked to identify key barriers to advancing AD/ADRD prevention and treatment and to highlight opportunities to address these barriers to catalyze advances across the field. In its examination of the AD/ADRD research landscape, several impediments to progress were consistently identified across the continuum from basic to clinical research. These crosscutting barriers include

- siloing within the AD/ADRD field and across related domains of research (e.g., aging, neurodegenerative diseases more broadly, exposure science);
- insufficient population representativeness and generalizability of research;
- inadequate infrastructure and support for management and analysis of data, samples, and knowledge generated from AD/ADRD research; and
- inadequate support for innovative methods capable of realizing transformational progress.

The committee recognizes the significant NIH investment to address each of these key barriers. It should also be acknowledged that many barriers are not unique to dementia research, and other scientific fields are also working to overcome similar challenges. Accordingly, in considering the implementation of the recommendations below, NIH and other research funders should continuously monitor the broader research landscape for examples of how such challenges have been successfully tackled in other fields and consider opportunities to apply those strategies in AD/ADRD research.

Breaking Down Silos Through Collaborative, Multidisciplinary Research

The heterogeneity of AD/ADRD, the prevalence of mixed pathologies, and the multifactorial and intersecting nature of the diverse pathways that

lead to disease all suggest that the path to effective strategies for preventing and treating this group of neurodegenerative diseases lies in collaborative, multidisciplinary research. Yet, throughout its information-gathering
process the committee encountered numerous silos, commonly reinforced
by funding structures. Current funding strategies that target individual
diseases, which have historically favored AD, fail to address the reality of
overlapping and mixed pathologies that contribute to neurodegenerative
disease, and they have contributed to the current dearth of effective therapies for related dementias. Research on pharmacological and nonpharmacological interventions are not well integrated, and as a result there have
been few efforts to date to evaluate the effect of combination approaches
despite a high likelihood that risk reduction and drug therapies will both
be necessary elements of a strategy to reduce the incidence and effect of
dementia. Moreover, the efforts of federal agencies supporting related areas
of research are not adequately coordinated, resulting in missed opportunities to collaborate and effectively use existing investments in studies and
infrastructure.

Innovative funding strategies and other incentives that encourage collaboration will be needed to address the current siloing of research and
accelerate the development of interventions for preventing and treating
AD/ADRD. Examples that have shown promise in AD/ADRD that could
be expanded include

- multi-institute research consortia that facilitate harmonization,
  coordination, and data sharing;
- public–private partnerships that leverage the respective talents of
  investigators in academia and industry;
- challenge programs that encourage team science approaches and
  risk taking while bringing new talent into the field; and
- community-based participatory research approaches that include
  and engage research participants, people with lived experience, and
  the public.

Coordination and collaboration at the program and project levels are
facilitated and may be incentivized by analogous efforts at the federal level.
Recognizing the existing mechanisms already in place and the challenges
of establishing new interagency bodies (e.g., time for agency personnel),
the committee encourages NIA, NINDS, the National Institute of Mental
Health, and other NIH funders of AD/ADRD research to identify further
opportunities to maximally leverage the strengths, resources, and unique
capacities of other agencies to advance shared focus areas. Examples of
collaborations with other federal agencies might include collaborating with
the Census Bureau to expand access to federal statistical research data

centers (FSRDCs) and facilitate the linkage of multiple data types relevant to AD/ADRD within the FSRDCs; working with the Centers for Medicare & Medicaid Services or FDA to tie expedited review processes for industry to data sharing policies; and working with the Centers for Disease Control and Prevention to generate a more robust evidence base for public health-level interventions. Building on the AMP model, collaboration with the Foundation for NIH can facilitate academic–industry research partnerships without creating financial conflicts of interest for academic researchers.

Recommendation 4: Enable multidisciplinary, multisector, and collaborative research
The National Institutes of Health (NIH) should expand mechanisms and leverage existing resources to break down silos and encourage multidisciplinary and integrative Alzheimer's disease and related dementias (AD/ADRD) research efforts, including the following:

- Expand trans-NIH initiatives and cofunded projects focused on healthy aging and neurodegenerative diseases to reduce the siloing of research efforts by individual institutes and centers, better cross-link and use existing resources, and address inconsistencies in data sharing policies across NIH institutes and centers while prioritizing data access.
- Prioritize research funding for projects with multidisciplinary research teams (e.g., basic and clinical researchers, population scientists, data scientists and artificial intelligence specialists, and those with lived experience) that address community-informed research questions.
- Expand collaborations globally, including but not limited to low- and middle-income countries and other countries less often involved in such collaborations, for both longitudinal research and clinical trials to better understand the biology of AD/ADRD and enhance the generalizability of findings to diverse populations.
- The National Institute on Aging and the National Institute of Neurological Disorders and Stroke should collaborate with the National Center for Advancing Translational Sciences and others to speed up the translation of research advances to clinical and public health practice and, in turn, expand new research inquiries through the collection of real-world evidence.

Fostering Inclusive Research

A comprehensive understanding of disease heterogeneity and the role of population differences (e.g., in genetic/genomic risk and social factors such as poverty, stress, and education) is crucial to developing broadly effective preventive and therapeutic intervention strategies for AD/ADRD. However, the populations that are disproportionately affected by dementia (e.g., certain ethnic/racial groups, people with low socioeconomic status or educational attainment) are persistently underrepresented in AD/ADRD research, both in observational studies and clinical trials. The result is limited generalizability of clinical research findings—including intervention safety and efficacy data—to the broader target population, impaired trust in the research enterprise, reduced understanding of disease biology (e.g., risk factors and causal mechanisms), clinical trial failures at later stages, and the compounding of existing health disparities.

Increasing the participation of underrepresented populations in dementia research has been a focus of past recommendations to NIH, and it is clear that NIA, NINDS, and other funders of dementia research are committed to and actively working on closing this gap. These efforts have included identifying best practices for engaging with and retaining diverse and underrepresented populations and connecting researchers to resources that can support more inclusive research. While there is some evidence to suggest that the efforts of NIH and those of the broader scientific community are starting to move the needle with regards to representation in AD/ADRD research, progress has been slow. Some measures of diversity in AD/ADRD-related studies are improving as compared to past decades, but this may not be consistent across all types of research or populations. It is imperative that NIH and AD/ADRD researchers continue to prioritize and incentivize inclusive research and increase accessibility for populations that are historically underrepresented despite being disproportionately affected by dementia.

Effective engagement with communities requires understanding and sensitivity to the different perspectives and cultures represented therein and this cannot be achieved without diverse and multidisciplinary research teams. Acknowledging the work NIH is already doing to foster a diverse and well-trained research workforce, continued efforts are needed to overcome barriers to entry (e.g., inadequate compensation for trainee and postdoctoral researchers on NIH awards) and ongoing career advancement. Such efforts not only help to address challenges related to underrepresentation in research but ensures the development of a skilled research workforce that benefits from the nation's rich diversity of people and their broad range of perspectives and experiences.

Given the multiple, interrelated factors that are associated with chronic underrepresentation of certain populations, achieving greater inclusivity and accessibility in AD/ADRD research will require a multipronged approach. This should include (1) ensuring adequate resources are budgeted for community engagement, recruitment, and the development of culturally appropriate research tools; (2) consideration of ways to overcome or work around common factors that contribute to attrition at the screening stage (exclusion criteria), particularly for members of underrepresented groups; (3) regular analysis of recruitment, enrollment, and retainment outcomes; and (4) building a diverse research workforce at all levels. Accountability—for NIH and NIH-funded investigators—will be a key determinant of future success in these endeavors.

Recommendation 5: Incentivize inclusive research
The National Institutes of Health should incentivize and guide the use of inclusive research practices to increase the accessibility of clinical and public health research and ensure that study populations are representative of populations at risk for and living with Alzheimer's disease and related dementias (AD/ADRD). These efforts should include the following:

- Strengthen requirements for the recruitment of diverse populations as a condition for initiating data collection (e.g., use of sampling frames as a best practice for targeted and intentional outreach).
- Support research to further understand participant and institutional barriers to involvement in clinical research at all levels.
- Develop social determinants of health metrics to be used as measures of diversity.
- Incentivize the incorporation of standardized benchmark measurements that can be used to evaluate and correct selection bias into new and ongoing research studies.
- Work with the Centers for Medicare & Medicaid Services to explore Medicare and Medicaid enrollment as opportunities for data collection and for enrollees to receive information about participation in AD/ADRD research studies using an opt-in model.
- Support initiatives to identify and overcome barriers to entry and continued professional advancement for a diverse clinical research workforce.

Recommendation 6: Increase the accessibility and generalizability of clinical and public health research
Investigators supported by the National Institutes of Health (NIH) should adopt inclusive research practices to increase the accessibility of clinical and public health research and ensure that study populations are representative of populations at risk for and living with Alzheimer's disease and related dementias (AD/ADRD). To increase research accessibility and generalizability, NIH-supported investigators should do the following:

- Reduce barriers to research participation (e.g., directing ineligible research volunteers to other studies, offering fair compensation,

expanding opportunities for virtual participation and passive and/or remote data collection, using in-home testing kits).
- Eliminate unnecessarily restrictive exclusion criteria that screen out diversity in the study population.
- Invest in the development of long-term, mutually beneficial relationships between research institutions and communities, and embed trials sites in communities with underrepresented populations (decentralized trials).
- Meaningfully engage and incorporate the perspectives of research participants and their communities throughout the research design and execution process (e.g., through patient or community advisory councils, codesigning research, community-based participatory research methods, use of community members such as *promotoras* or health navigators to collect data).

Enhancing the Accessibility and Usability of Biological Samples, Data, and Knowledge to Maximize the Returns from AD/ADRD Research

The billions of dollars in funding from NIH and others that has supported scientific investigations in the dementia field and the development of a robust AD/ADRD research infrastructure represents a significant national investment. Careful stewardship of that investment requires ensuring that the products of research—including biological samples, raw data, and findings—are accessible to, and usable by, the broader scientific community for the purpose of knowledge generation. When data and samples are siloed and sequestered within individual research groups, the kind of collaborative and integrative research called for by the committee cannot be achieved. Importantly, an advantage of stored raw data collected through digital technologies (e.g., voice recordings, data from wearable devices and in-home sensors) over banked biosamples is that digital data are not a finite resource. If properly stored, these data can be used indefinitely and simultaneously by multiple users without losing value over time. Thus, the return on collection and storage can be exponential. Also critical is the compilation and synthesis of knowledge in such a manner that it can be easily accessed and used to draw insights to guide future research and inform clinical care.

AD/ADRD data infrastructure investments by NIH have included a number of different platforms and repositories to support storage and accessibility of diverse data types (e.g., fluid biomarker, neuroimaging, neuropathology, genomic and other omics data). A key challenge before NIH is to link its major data hubs (e.g., NIA Genetics of Alzheimer's Disease Data Storage Site, National Alzheimer's Coordinating Center,

AD Knowledge Portal) into an agile, integrated data ecosystem while preserving the autonomy of the individual platforms and their respective strengths and networks. This integrated system should enable researchers without deep data analytics expertise to locate, access, and query existing data from NIH-funded research and, when available, data submitted by other investigators. This is a formidable undertaking but critical to maximizing insights from AD/ADRD research and returns from NIH's various investments.

Given the diversity of data types, data sources, and constraints such as privacy protection needs, there is no single solution to data management and accessibility. It will be important for NIH to work with investigators to identify solutions to data access challenges. While many datasets can and should be made publicly available, for others, such as clinical datasets with protected health information generated by private health systems, data accessibility may need to be achieved through other means.

Accessibility is necessary but not sufficient to ensure that data from past AD/ADRD research are usable to the fullest extent possible. Also critical is the expansion of data standardization and harmonization efforts to address the lack of interoperability and comparability of data from different studies, which impede data integration and cross-study analyses. Furthermore, increasingly complex tools for data integration and analysis are required to accommodate the growing volume and diversity of data being generated through AD/ADRD research. Artificial intelligence/machine learning and other computational methods (e.g., network analysis) hold great promise for enabling the linkage and subsequent extraction of insights from large and complex datasets, but there is a need for national-level resources that can support the development of such tools and analytic methods. The continued evolution of technology, tools, and analytic methods will create new opportunities to analyze data in ways that are unknown at present. Such future analyses may lead to the discovery and development of novel therapeutics or biomarkers.

Recommendation 7: Ensure data access to maximize research returns
Using the National Institutes of Health (NIH) Data Management and Sharing Policy as a foundation, NIH should convene and support an NIH workgroup to work with NIH-funded investigators to identify and implement solutions to barriers that impede access to data from Alzheimer's disease and related dementias research. Specific issues that should be addressed by the NIH workgroup include but are not limited to the following:
- the need for a centralized and continuously updated NIH-managed system for locating and searching existing data sources across different (NIH and non-NIH) data platforms;

- provision of incentives and clear procedures for ensuring compliance with the Data Management and Sharing Policy;
- approaches to maximize access to data from initiatives funded by multiple NIH institutes and centers;
- incentivization of transparent reporting and the synthesis of findings from negative studies, including observational studies and clinical trials, ideally with accompanying data release;
- provision of project-specific supplemental funding, including additional administrative supplements, commensurate with the anticipated level of data and code sharing;
- formulation of guidance for subsets of data within any given dataset to be categorized into access levels based on the access controls needed to protect sensitive data (e.g., participant health information) such that the portion of data requiring no permission for use can be made publicly available;
- return of derived data and analysis code from data users, as well as the return of newly collected data from ancillary studies, to the parent study while respecting the need to protect intellectual property and innovation;
- approaches to facilitate access to data from international collaborations; and
- expansion of capacity for storing raw digital data (e.g., unstructured data such as images and high-velocity voice recordings and sensor data).

Recommendation 8: Enhance data usability for future research
To enable the usability of data generated by Alzheimer's disease and related dementias research funded by the National Institutes of Health (NIH), NIH should do the following:
- Invest in data harmonization and interoperability efforts (e.g., use of common data elements) across data platforms and through collaborations across institutions and organizations, ensuring that levels of harmonization are aligned with the needs of different analytic approaches.
- Set requirements for user-intuitive data dictionaries.
- Explore new approaches, such as natural language processing, to automate the integration of different data types (e.g., clinical phenotype, multiomics data, exposure data).
- Fund the development and dissemination of novel open-source tools and analytic methods (e.g., large language models and other artificial intelligence/machine learning methods, statistical transport methods, data fusion approaches, synthetic data) to

collect, link, explore, and query existing data and support efficient analyses when data privacy rules create barriers.
- Provide dedicated grants for investigators working in settings with proprietary data that are difficult to share (e.g., major clinical datasets) focused on data curation or supporting analyses by external researchers.

Consideration of the future value of biological samples collected from research participants or donated by other members of the public is also important when investing in infrastructure and plans for collection and storage. Furthermore, stored samples have little value if they are not accessible to the scientific community. Ensuring accessibility entails the development of transparent inventories of samples that are available to external investigators and clear processes for sample requests and decision making on sample sharing. NIH has made substantial investments in infrastructure for biobanking, but critical gaps remain. Initiatives and resources appear fragmented. Capacity to collect tissues through autopsy and to store biological samples—both cost-intensive undertakings—is limited. As a result, precious samples may be discarded at the completion of studies. Maximizing the use and value of participant samples will require a more structured and standardized system for collection, archiving, and access.

Recommendation 9: Expand the capacity to collect and store biological samples generated through National Institutes of Health (NIH)-funded research
The National Institute on Aging, along with the National Institute of Neurological Disorders and Stroke, should expand support for the collection and storage of valuable biological samples from NIH-funded Alzheimer's disease and related dementias research in a manner that maximizes opportunities for future use. This should include the following:
- Provide supplements to researchers that meet the actual cost of storing and sharing samples following study completion.
- Expand support for the collection and storage of highly characterized biological samples (e.g., antemortem and postmortem blood and cerebrospinal fluid, donated brains) from participants of any longitudinal research studies and clinical trials, and from the public.
- Use standardized sample collection, assessment, and storage practices with careful consideration of the implications of different storage approaches for future value.
- Facilitate access to biological samples from international collaborations.

- Support digitized neuropathology to enable quantitative analysis using artificial intelligence and other computational methods.

Catalyzing Transformational Change Through Innovation in AD/ADRD Research

Accelerating progress in AD/ADRD prevention and treatment will require transformational change that can only be achieved through greater support for innovation in NIH-supported research. This may look different at different stages in the research continuum, as highlighted by the following examples:

- Basic research: developing and applying novel models and tools, seeking potential points of connection and commonalities with related fields (e.g., aging, other neurodegenerative diseases).
- Translational research: increasing the viability of innovative research targets and approaches.
- Clinical research: adopting innovative trial designs and participant recruitment and engagement mechanisms.
- Population research: identifying and integrating novel data sources that can be used to evaluate population-level strategies (e.g., policies or exposures that vary across larger geographic units) and effects on inequalities.

The current system for peer review at NIH favors investigators and projects for which there are strong track records and evidence for likely success based on existing preliminary data. Although the current process has many advantages, it is not ideally suited to promoting innovation and truly novel methods. Incentives are needed to promote more disruptive research approaches that may lead to significant steps forward. Agencies such as the Defense Advanced Research Projects Agency and the Advanced Research Projects Agency for Health are specifically focused on high-risk, high-reward research. Similarly, relatively new philanthropic funders have developed creative methods to identify and fund pilot-scale approaches to challenging scientific and medical problems. These groups may provide insight into how NIH can further enhance innovation, while working within its constraints. While an in-depth evaluation of funding structures and processes is beyond the scope of this report, the committee offers the following recommendation with suggestions for increasing innovation in AD/ADRD research.

Recommendation 10: Support innovation across all stages of National Institutes of Health (NIH)-funded research

NIH should use existing funding structures and other incentive mechanisms to stimulate innovation across all stages of Alzheimer's disease and related dementias (AD/ADRD) research. This could include the following:

- Implement advances and tools generated by the Advanced Research Projects Agency for Health and others into NIH-funded AD/ADRD research, including advances that are specific to dementia and those that can be applied from other fields.
- Field a program-wide review of the opportunities and barriers to interdisciplinary and transformational research at NIH-funded AD/ADRD centers and infrastructure programs (e.g., the Alzheimer's Disease Research Centers) and their capacity to prioritize the inclusion of diverse populations and foster innovative research with high potential for population impact.
- Capitalize on the best-in-class practices and technologies of other fields that are applicable to, and may address, current AD/ADRD research needs (e.g., data infrastructure and knowledge management, social engagement for recruitment).
- Prioritize support for research inquiries that have clear potential for future scalability and uptake.
- Build partnerships with foundations and other research funders to coordinate seamless funding pathways for fast-tracked phase 1–2 high-risk research opportunities.
- Identify and provide short-term funding for specific, highly innovative components of otherwise unsuccessful new and competing award applications.
- Identify past funded projects in the NIH portfolio that have progressed to real-world clinical implementation and adapt the grant review process to include criteria that promote real-world clinical implementation.

CONCLUDING REMARKS

The last decade of research has seen encouraging progress in the capability to detect early signals of changes in brain health, to understand the pathophysiologic mechanisms underlying AD/ADRD, and to develop and evaluate preventive and therapeutic interventions. Accelerating progress in AD/ADRD prevention and treatment will require transformation and new direction. With continued strategic research investments as outlined by the committee, there is good reason to hope that the coming years will see significant progress in the capability to prevent and treat AD/ADRD. Through the continued and collaborative efforts of NIH, academic researchers, private industry, health care professionals, funders, policy makers, advocates, and people living with cognitive and other forms of impairment from AD/ADRD, it is possible to envision a future where dementia is not inevitable for millions of people across the globe but is preventable and treatable.

1

Introduction

Dementia exacts a weighty emotional and financial toll on individuals, families, and communities. As with any disease, the experiences of people living with dementia vary, and many find ways to adapt to cognitive changes and enjoy meaningful lives for many years. Over the long run, however, the effects of dementia can be devastating, with advanced stages often robbing people of their sense of self, their memories and independence, their emotional and financial well-being, and ultimately, their lives. Moreover, the societal impacts, including the effects on families and communities and the enormous health and long-term care costs, are likely to grow with an aging population in the United States and globally. The development of effective strategies for preventing and treating Alzheimer's disease and related dementias (AD/ADRD), a collection of neurodegenerative diseases that may ultimately lead to clinical dementia, is thus considered one of the most pressing biomedical research needs at present. There remains no cure, and recently approved therapies for slowing Alzheimer's disease (AD), including lecanemab and donanemab, offer only modest clinical benefit to select AD patients; no approved treatments are available for people living with other forms of dementia beyond those for managing symptoms. A multitude of studies on the numerous nonpharmacologic strategies under investigation for preventing AD/ADRD have failed to provide definitive evidence on which strategies are effective and for whom.

And yet, the last couple of decades have witnessed encouraging and sometimes transformational scientific advances that are providing reason for optimism. Research investments by the National Institutes of Health (NIH) and other funders have led to improved understanding of the molecular and cellular biology underlying AD/ADRD, including genetic contributions to risk and resilience, as well as the discovery of biomarkers that enable early identification of changes in brain health that may lead to AD/ADRD. In addition to creating opportunities for earlier intervention, biomarker discoveries have led to the identification of a new form of dementia (limbic-predominant age-related TDP-43 encephalopathy) and the awareness that the majority of dementia cases feature a mix of pathologies. With the increased understanding of AD/ADRD has come a substantial expansion of the therapeutic pipeline (Cummings et al., 2024).

These past successes have built momentum and a foundation for accelerating the pace of discovery and catalyzing breakthroughs needed to develop effective prevention and treatment strategies for AD/ADRD. This report identifies research priorities focused on addressing current knowledge gaps that represent key bottlenecks impeding progress toward that goal. While the report is focused on opportunities to advance the science, the ultimate objective is to ensure that research investments translate to societal benefit by improving the lives of those already living with cognitive and other forms of impairment from AD/ADRD and preventing many more from developing these conditions.

STUDY ORIGIN AND STATEMENT OF TASK

Since passing the National Alzheimer's Project Act in 2011,[1] the U.S. Congress has made unprecedented investments in AD/ADRD research through targeted annual appropriations. In its Consolidated Appropriations Act of 2023,[2] Congress directed the National Institute on Aging (NIA), in collaboration with the National Institute of Neurological Disorders and Stroke (NINDS), to commission an independent National Academies study to identify promising areas of research and generate recommendations on research priorities to advance the prevention and treatment of AD/ADRD. The committee's full Statement of Task is presented in Box 1-1.

STUDY SCOPE AND KEY TERMINOLOGY

The research and practice landscape related to brain health and dementia is exceptionally broad and multifaceted. While each element of the landscape is critically important, an examination and analysis of

---

[1] Public Law 111-375.

[2] The congressional language requesting this consensus study can be found in Division H of the Joint Explanatory Statement that accompanied H.R. 2617, the Consolidated Appropriations Act, 2023 (Public Law 117-328) on PDF page 496 here: https://www.congress.gov/117/cprt/HPRT50348/CPRT-117HPRT50348.pdf (accessed October 24, 2023).

BOX 1-1
Statement of Task

An ad hoc committee of the National Academies of Sciences, Engineering, and Medicine will conduct a study and recommend research priorities to advance the prevention and treatment of Alzheimer's Disease and Related Dementias (AD/ADRD). In conducting its study, the committee will:

- Examine and assess the current state of biomedical research aimed at preventing and effectively treating AD/ADRD, along the research and development pipeline from basic to translational to clinical research.
- Assess the evidence on nonpharmacological interventions (e.g., lifestyle, cognitive training) aimed at preventing and treating AD/ADRD.
- Identify key barriers to advancing AD/ADRD prevention and treatment (e.g., infrastructure challenges that impede large-scale precision medicine approaches, inadequate functional measures and biomarkers for assessing response to treatment, lack of diversity in biobanks and clinical trials), as well as opportunities to address these key barriers and catalyze advances across the field.
- Review and synthesize the most promising areas of research into preventing and treating AD/ADRD.

Building on its review of past AD/ADRD strategic planning and related activities, existing literature and analyses, and other expert and public input, the committee will develop a report with its findings, conclusions, and recommendations on research priorities for preventing and treating ADRD, including identifying specific near- and medium-term scientific questions (i.e., in a 3- to 10-year period) that may be addressed through National Institutes of Health (NIH) funding. The report will also include strategies for addressing major barriers to progress on these scientific questions.

The committee's study will include dementia caused by Alzheimer's disease as well as related conditions such as frontotemporal disorders, Lewy body dementia, vascular contributions to cognitive impairment and dementia, and multiple etiology dementias; dementias with a clear etiology (e.g., incident stroke, acquired immunodeficiency syndrome [AIDS], traumatic brain injury) are outside the scope of this study. Dementia care and caregiving research, including care coordination, is outside the scope of this study.

the entire field is not feasible given the time and resources available to the committee. The Statement of Task limits this study to the area of AD/ADRD research and specifically research focused on prevention and treatment. During its first meeting on October 2, 2023, the committee had the opportunity to clarify remaining questions regarding the scope of the study with representatives from NIH. Specific points of clarification, which are described below, included the types of dementia and the types of AD/ADRD research that were within the study scope.

The Statement of Task specifies that the study's scope includes Alzheimer's disease and a number of other specific conditions that can ultimately cause clinical dementia. While *Alzheimer's disease (AD)* is a major contributor to clinical dementia, other common causes that fall within the study scope include *frontotemporal dementia (FTD), Lewy body dementia (LBD),* and *vascular dementia.* Excluded from the scope are nonneurodegenerative causes of clinical dementia—such as acquired immunodeficiency syndrome (AIDS) and traumatic brain injury—for which prevention and treatment strategies would follow from the known causes. Also excluded from the scope is clinical dementia arising acutely following incident stroke. Of note, vascular dementia developing in the years subsequent to a stroke was not excluded. *Multiple etiology dementia,* which is characterized by the identification of mixed pathologies in the brain of an individual experiencing clinical dementia symptoms, is also within the study scope (see descriptions of these disorders in Box 1-2). It should be noted, however, that the high prevalence of multiple etiology dementia (see Figure 1-1)—increasingly believed to be the predominant form in older individuals—and limited understanding of the connections among, and joint consequences of, distinct neuropathologies and overlapping clinical presentations and symptomatology results in complexity in the use of these terms both in the clinical and research settings. Such complexity also has consequences for individuals struggling to receive accurate and timely diagnoses and care.

The committee chose to use the terms *AD/ADRD* and *related dementias* throughout the report for consistency with its Statement of Task. *AD/ADRD* refers to all causes of neurodegeneration that are included in the study scope. Consistent with common terminology in the field, the report will also use the term *dementia* to refer to this group of neurodegenerative diseases. In contrast, *related dementias* refer to all causes of neurodegeneration that are included in the study scope with the exception of AD. The committee acknowledges concerns that the term *related dementias* may be viewed as implying that these are secondary in importance to AD and therefore dismissive of the experiences of those living with these diseases. The committee underscores that all forms of neurodegeneration are equally important, and many aspects of the committee's report are designed to be broadly applicable across all types of dementia. Where discussion is specific

BOX 1-2
Descriptions of Alzheimer's Disease and Related Dementias

Alzheimer's disease and related dementias (AD/ADRD): The committee's task is broadly focused on a group of progressive cognitive disorders, which develop over the life course and are characterized by an acquired loss of cognitive function that influences memory, thinking, and behavior and eventually is severe enough to interfere with independence and daily tasks (Alzheimer's Association, 2024a,b; NASEM, 2021b). For the purposes of this report and for consistency with the Statement of Task, the term AD/ADRD includes Alzheimer's disease and the following related dementias: Lewy body dementia, frontotemporal dementia, limbic-predominant age-related TDP-43 encephalopathy, vascular dementia, and multiple etiology dementia. As understanding of the biological basis for this group of diseases continues to evolve, the inclusion and distinction of different disorders that fall under AD/ADRD may change. Brief descriptions of each, including distinguishing features related to brain pathologies and cognitive and behavioral characteristics, are included below.

Alzheimer's disease (AD) dementia: AD is defined by the specific presence and location of amyloid plaque and tau neurofibrillary tangle pathologies (Alzheimer's Association, 2024b). The condition primarily affects individuals 65 and over. Individuals diagnosed prior to turning 65 are described as having early-onset AD, and some of these will have genetic causes and be referred to as familial AD. Due to an extra copy of chromosome 21, which includes the *APP* gene, there is another form of early-onset AD called Down syndrome-related AD. Common symptoms of AD include memory loss; difficulty completing familiar tasks; impaired judgment; misplacing objects; changes in mood, personality, or behavior; and, eventually, difficulty walking, talking, and swallowing (CDC, 2020; Alzheimer's Association, 2024b).

Lewy body dementia (LBD): LBD is associated with abnormal deposits of a protein called alpha-synuclein in certain regions of the brain (e.g., substantia nigra). These deposits, called Lewy bodies, may also be found in other types of dementia, including Alzheimer's dementia and Parkinson's disease dementia (Alzheimer's Association, 2024c). Clinical symptoms of LBD typically begin to show at age 50 or older and can include visual or auditory hallucinations; changes in concentration, attention, alertness, and wakefulness; severe loss of other cognitive abilities that interfere with daily activities; REM sleep behavior disorder; impaired autonomic function; and impaired mobility with parkinsonian features (e.g., shuffling walk, stooped posture, balance problems and

continued

BOX 1-2 Continued

repeated falls, muscle rigidity, stiffness, tremors) (Lewy Body Dementia Association, 2022).

Frontotemporal dementia (FTD): FTD consists of a group of disorders caused by progressive nerve cell loss in the brain's frontal or temporal lobes, leading to loss of function in these brain regions and deterioration in behavior, personality, and/or difficulty with producing or comprehending language. Some patients with FTD may also have motor neuron disease (also known as amyotrophic lateral sclerosis or Lou Gehrig's disease) and vice versa. The two most prominent causes of FTD involve the proteins tau and TDP-43, although there are other types of FTD caused by specific genetic mutations and different protein inclusions. Unlike AD, FTD is more commonly diagnosed in midlife, among people between 40 and 60 years of age (Alzheimer's Association, 2024d). The three major types of FTD include behavioral variant frontotemporal dementia, which involves changes in personality, behavior, and judgment; primary progressive aphasia, which involves changes in the ability to use language to speak, read, write, name objects, and understand what others are saying; and movement disorders, which produce changes in muscle (motor neuron disease) or motor functions (parkinsonism). The latter can include symptoms associated with such atypical parkinsonian disorders as corticobasal syndrome and progressive supranuclear palsy (FTD Talk, 2024). Mixed clinical presentations involving a combination of these symptoms are common in FTD (Alzheimer's Association, 2021).

Vascular dementia: Vascular dementia is caused by disruptions to vital blood and oxygen supply that also disrupt brain neurotoxin clearance, resulting in neuronal and glial injury and cell death culminating in cogni-

to a particular disease or type of dementia, the specific conditions of relevance are noted.

It is important to acknowledge that *dementia* in the clinical sense represents the culmination of a progressive process that begins with pathologic changes in the brain that eventually result in cognitive impairment and may also include the development of behavioral, psychiatric, motor, and functional impairments. Over time these impairments may reach a level of severity such that the individual can no longer function independently. Symptoms may progress to the point where individuals may not be able to walk, maintain continence, or even swallow. Ultimately dementia is a fatal condition. For the purposes of this report, the term *clinical dementia* will

tive decline and impairment. Vascular dementia is characterized by the presence of arteriolosclerosis and neuro-glio-vascular injuries to blood–brain barrier integrity. Cerebrovascular injuries include infarcts (micro or large vessel), hemorrhages (micro or lobar), myelin abnormalities caused by small vessel disease, and cerebral amyloid angiopathy. Vascular dementia presents with similar symptoms to other types of dementia and can include confusion, challenges with organizing thoughts, difficulty with planning and communication, and physical symptoms such as reduced coordination and unsteady gait. Some but not all patients with vascular dementia may have an abrupt onset caused by stroke or hemorrhage (Linton et al., 2021).

Limbic-predominant age-related TDP-43 encephalopathy (LATE): LATE was clinically recognized in 2019 as a type of dementia that is similar to AD in clinical presentation but involving a distinct pathology characterized by the accumulation of TDP-43 in the limbic system in the brain of older adults, typically among those over the age of 80 years. Symptoms of LATE can include memory loss and impaired cognition and decision making. Misdiagnosis as AD is believed to be widespread, and co-occurrence with other types of dementia is also thought to be common; some patients diagnosed with AD may instead have LATE or a combination of both brain pathologies (Nag and Schneider, 2023).

Multiple etiology dementia: Multiple etiology dementia occurs when two or more pathologies (mixed pathologies) co-occur in the brain of a person living with clinical dementia. The prevalence of such co-occurrence is widespread, and it is thought that most dementia cases among those over the age of 65 years are multiple etiology dementia. Symptoms reflect those associated with the distinct pathologies and may vary based on the type and extent of neuropathological changes present (NINDS, 2024).

be used when referring to impairment that meets the clinical criteria for a diagnosis of dementia.[3]

Importantly, cognitive impairment exists on a continuum and different people may experience impairment in different cognitive domains (e.g., executive function, memory) (NASEM, 2021a,b). Several different categorizations are commonly applied to describe levels of progressive impairment

---

[3] Throughout the report the committee endeavored to specify where the research cited was referring to clinical dementia. In some cases, it was not clear from the cited reference whether the authors referred to clinical dementia or a specific cause of dementia. In those cases, the committee used the same terminology as the reference.

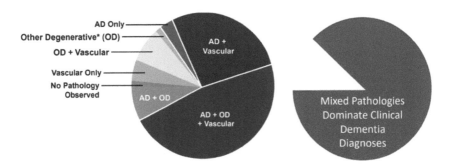

FIGURE 1-1 Proportions of different combinations of amyloid beta, tau, TDP-43, alpha-synuclein, and vascular pathologies in older adults with probable AD as confirmed by autopsy.
NOTE: These data are from 447 participants of the Religious Orders Study and the Memory and Aging Project. Other degenerative (OD) includes neurodegenerative disease pathologies: Lewy bodies, TDP-43, and hippocampus sclerosis. AD = Alzheimer's disease.
SOURCE: ASPE, 2023.

that do not meet the clinical criteria for dementia. *Mild cognitive impairment* (MCI) denotes a level of deterioration from normal cognitive function that is identifiable (e.g., by the individuals themselves, close contacts, or clinicians) but that does not significantly impair functions related to activities of daily living (McKhann et al., 2011; NASEM, 2017). MCI increases the risk of developing clinical dementia in the future (NIA, 2021). Other categorizations of cognitive decline include *age-related cognitive decline* (or cognitive aging), which is deterioration in cognitive performance that can be a normal part of aging (NASEM, 2017; Toepper, 2017), and *subjective cognitive decline*, which is a self-perceived decline in cognitive function in individuals without measurable cognitive decline (Jessen et al., 2020). The development of strategies for primary and secondary prevention of dementia need to consider MCI and the pathologic processes that precede it.[4] Thus, the populations of interest to the committee include those with clinical dementia, MCI, and neuropathologic changes in the absence of clinically measurable symptoms.

While probable diagnoses of different forms of dementia have historically been made based on clinical syndromes and confirmed definitively

---

[4] *Primary prevention* aims to prevent the onset of a condition and in the context of this report may include those interventions focused on making the brain more resilient and those aimed at preventing underlying processes that result in pathology. *Secondary prevention* aims to prevent the progression of an asymptomatic or early-stage condition.

postmortem by the observation of pathology at autopsy, the discovery of biomarkers that can be evaluated premortem is enabling the development of a biological definition for Alzheimer's (Jack et al., 2018) and, potentially, related neurodegenerative diseases (Simuni et al., 2024).[5] This allows for the potential diagnosis of disease in the absence of clinical symptomology, as discussed further in Chapter 2. *Biomarkers*—measurable indicators of biological processes in the body that may be measured through imaging, genetic testing, and testing of blood or cerebrospinal fluid (NIA, 2022)—are not only employed in the prediction and diagnosis of AD/ADRD but are also used in the stratification of populations into subgroups with shared characteristics (i.e., *biological subtypes*) and to assess response to prevention and treatment strategies.

The committee was charged with examining and assessing the current state of biomedical research aimed at preventing and effectively treating AD/ADRD, including research on pharmacological and nonpharmacological interventions. *Intervention* refers to any program or treatment applied at an individual or population level, including pharmacological and nonpharmacological approaches, that is designed to prevent or modify the condition under investigation (NASEM, 2017). The Statement of Task excludes from the study scope research on dementia care and caregiving interventions, including care models (e.g., care coordination). These topics have been the focus of other recent National Academies studies.[6] However, the distinction between dementia care and treatment of AD/ADRD was an early point of discussion for the committee, particularly in the context of treatments for *neuropsychiatric symptoms*—noncognitive core features of AD/ADRD that are included within diagnostic criteria and may include apathy, anxiety, and depression, among others (Cummings, 2021).

Treatments for neuropsychiatric symptoms are commonly classified as care interventions, distinct from *disease modifying therapies (DMTs)*, which are being defined in this report as pharmacological and nonpharmacological interventions that can produce a lasting change in the trajectory of AD/ADRD by targeting an underlying pathophysiologic mechanism of the disease that results in cell death (Cummings and Fox, 2017). Applications of DMTs may include both primary and secondary prevention, and DMTs need not be limited to pharmacological treatments; they may also include, for example, nonpharmacological neuroprotective strategies that

---

[5] A biological definition has been proposed for neuronal alpha-synuclein disease, which would include Parkinson's disease and dementia with Lewy bodies.

[6] Recent analyses of the research landscape related to dementia care and caregiving can be found in *Meeting the Challenge of Caring for Persons Living with Dementia and their Care Partners and Caregivers: A Way Forward* (NASEM, 2021a) and *Reducing the Impact of Dementia in America: A Decadal Survey of the Behavioral and Social Sciences* (NASEM, 2021b).

are implemented early in the life course (i.e., childhood, adolescence, and midlife) to prevent pathophysiologic processes. Given the current incomplete neurobiological understanding of AD/ADRD, the distinction between DMTs and treatments for neuropsychiatric symptoms may not be as clear as may be assumed.

An association between neuropsychiatric symptoms and acceleration in cognitive decline has been widely reported in the literature (Burhanullah et al., 2020; David et al., 2016; Defrancesco et al., 2020; Pink et al., 2023), although questions remain regarding the role of reverse causality (i.e., the contribution of cognitive decline to neuropsychiatric symptoms). Consequently, there is likely some overlap in interventions aimed at improving the well-being of persons living with AD/ADRD by seeking to alleviate such neuropsychiatric symptoms as depression and anxiety and interventions aimed at preventing, delaying, or slowing the progression of AD/ADRD. Given their potential to not only change the trajectory of disease but also to improve quality of life, reduce care costs, and enable persons living with AD/ADRD to remain in their homes or with family care partners and caregivers, the committee included in its evaluation of promising interventions those therapeutic approaches targeting neuropsychiatric symptoms that may also result in the preventing, delaying, or slowing of AD/ADRD.

In examining the state of the science and identifying research priorities to advance the prevention and treatment of AD/ADRD, the committee was asked to consider research spanning basic, translational, and clinical phases of the continuum. While the development of recommendations related to the implementation and scaling of tools and interventions in clinical practice and community settings was outside the study scope, the committee recognizes that the research and development pipeline is not linear and unidirectional. Lessons from real-world implementation feed back to inform future research and guide the development of new or modified tools, technologies, and intervention strategies for AD/ADRD prevention and treatment. With this in mind, the committee included in its examination of the research landscape opportunities to integrate implementation considerations early in the research and development process and to incorporate real-world evidence following implementation into the research pipeline. As the field advances and novel tools and interventions are developed and approach readiness for implementation, a deeper review of strategies and priorities for implementation in an impactful and equitable manner may be needed.

Consistent with the Statement of Task, this report focuses on the state of the science and research priorities for the prevention and treatment of AD/ADRD. However, the committee acknowledges that there are broader forces at play that impede access to effective prevention and treatment, including the need for a robust and diverse clinical workforce that has the training and capacity to deliver interventions and provide compassionate and high-quality care. While the committee was not asked to make recommendations related to the provision of care, it is within the scope of the committee's work to examine opportunities to develop tools and technologies that can enable the clinical workforce to detect, accurately diagnose, and continuously monitor AD/ADRD and select effective prevention and treatment strategies.

A final critical point regarding the study scope relates to the timescale indicated in the Statement of Task, which specifies that the committee should identify near- and medium-term scientific questions that may be addressed through NIH funding over the next 3 to 10 years. The committee interpreted this to mean that it should identify research areas that should be a high-priority focus over the next decade but not necessarily brought to completion within that time frame. Science evolves in a nonlinear, iterative manner, and there is still a great deal we still do not understand about the basic disease processes for AD/ADRD. Moreover, the building of necessary infrastructure and resources (e.g., research cohorts) is a time-intensive endeavor. While some goals may take more than a decade to realize, it is important to emphasize that this does not reflect a lower urgency than those that may be more reasonably achieved within the next 10 years.

STUDY CONTEXT

AD/ADRD Research at an Inflection Point

The AD/ADRD field stands at a crossroads—there is a palpable sense that decades of scientific inquiry and more recent increased investment in research are near to paying off with significant advances in diagnostic and intervention capabilities, generating excitement and momentum. Still, the juxtaposition of the near-term future potential and the current reality is striking. In the wake of recent approvals of new drugs for AD, there is growing hope regarding the ability to prevent and slow the progression of early disease through intervention, but even the modest benefits provided by these drugs apply only to a small proportion of the target population and little progress has been made toward effective treatments for those living with advanced disease and related dementias. Similarly, cutting-edge tools and technologies such as fluid and digital biomarkers, multiomic methods, and artificial intelligence are poised to radically change the research and clinical practice landscape, but some current tools for fundamental clinical cognitive assessments are not able to detect early, more subtle changes in cognition and are, in some cases, biased, posing barriers to linking emerging diagnostics to clinical outcomes.

An Urgent and Growing Need for Effective Prevention and Treatment Approaches

Few diseases have affected society on the scale at which AD/ADRD is exacting an emotional and financial toll for individuals, families, and communities. While the effects of dementia in terms of mortality, disability, and financial burden are staggering, no less devastating are its profound effects on the lives, livelihoods, and relationships of those affected by the disease. While every person will have a unique experience of dementia influenced by their individual context (NASEM, 2021a,b), for many, the suffering caused by dementia is further exacerbated by stigma, which stems in part from the fear and distress that often accompany diagnosis, particularly in the absence of effective treatments.

Currently, there are more than 6 million people living with clinical dementia caused by Alzheimer's disease in the United States (Manly et al., 2022) and more than 55 million people living with the dementia globally; the World Health Organization has recognized dementia as a global public health priority (WHO, 2023). Based on National Health Interview Survey data from 2022, 4 percent of adults in the United States self-reported having received a diagnosis of dementia, including AD, from a clinician. This proportion increased with age from 1.7 percent of respondents ages 65–74 years confirming a diagnosis of dementia to 13.1 percent among respondents age 85 years and older (Kramarow, 2024). Accurate data on the prevalence and incidence of the different types of dementia are lacking in part because these measures are reliant on the diagnostic definitions in use, which poorly account for related dementias and the presence of mixed pathologies. Measures such as cumulative lifetime incidence, which describe the probability that an individual will be affected by a clinical syndrome before their death, may provide a better understanding of the public health impact and inequities of AD/ADRD across the population. One prospective study in a diverse Northern Californian cohort reported a cumulative 25-year risk of clinical dementia (including AD, vascular dementia, and nonspecific dementia) at age 65 of 38 percent for African Americans, 35 percent for American Indians and Alaska Natives, 32 percent for Latinos, 25 percent for Pacific Islanders, 30 percent for Whites, and 28 percent for Asian Americans (Mayeda et al., 2016).

While deaths from some other major causes of mortality in the United States decreased or remained stable over the last 2 decades, deaths from AD more than doubled during this period (see Figure 1-2).[7] These phenomena are likely linked—increasing life expectancies resulting from progress

---

[7] Note that the accuracy of death certification for dementia has improved over time, but the reporting of dementia as a cause of death likely remains underreported based on the rate of clinical diagnosis (Adair et al., 2022).

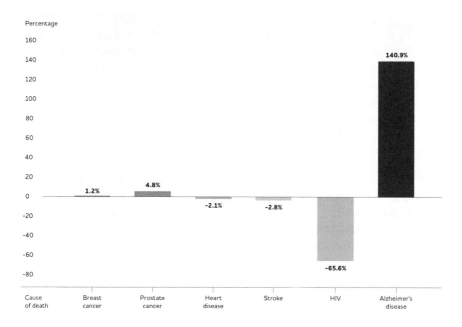

FIGURE 1-2 Percentage changes in selected causes of death (all ages) between 2000 and 2019.

NOTE: Data collected by the National Center for Health Statistics from death certificates listing Alzheimer's disease as an underlying cause of death. No information available on how cause of death determinations were made or whether other neuropathologies were present.

SOURCE: Alzheimer's Association, 2023.

reducing mortality from chronic conditions increases the lifetime risk of developing dementia (Zissimopoulos et al., 2018). Recent models predict that the number of older Americans (ages 65 and older) living with dementia will grow to nearly 12 million in 2040 in the absence of a change to the status quo (Zissimopoulos et al., 2018).

It is also well established that the impacts of dementia are not experienced uniformly across populations. In the United States, racial and ethnic disparities in dementia prevalence continue to persist; as compared to non-Hispanic White people, Black and Hispanic people are more likely to develop clinical dementia (Chen and Zissimopoulos, 2018). The lifetime risk of AD-type dementia for women has been estimated to be about twice that of men, but gender differences in risk may vary by dementia type; the incidence of vascular dementia, for example, is higher in men than in women in people 55–75 years of age (Mielke, 2024). Sex and gender differences in AD/ADRD are further discussed in Box 1-3. Social determinants of health significantly affect rates of dementia, as evidenced by increased AD/ADRD prevalence rates in lower-income and rural areas (Powell et al., 2020; Wing et al., 2020).

While these statistics are sobering, there is growing evidence of declining dementia prevalence and incidence in high-income countries (Farina et al., 2022; Wolters et al., 2020).[8] The prevalence of U.S. adults ages 70 years and older living with dementia declined between 2011 and 2019 from 13 percent to 9.8 percent (Freedman et al., 2021); however, it remains unclear to what degree different factors are driving that decline and to what degree the trends will continue. Additionally, as the baby boom generation continues to reach ages at which the risk of dementia significantly increases, the absolute number of people with dementia will continue to rise, along with the societal burden.

The estimated global societal cost of dementia in 2019, including the financial burden associated with unpaid caregiving, was more than $1 trillion (Wimo et al., 2023), although this is likely an underestimate. By 2030, total annual costs associated with dementia are estimated to rise to $624 billion in the United States alone (Zissimopoulos et al., 2014). Dementia cost estimates typically include medical costs and the cost of long-term services and support, as well as some indirect costs such as the value of unpaid caregivers' time for caring for persons living with dementia. Estimates of dementia costs, when based on a limited set of cost inputs, is likely a significant underestimate, particularly as it relates to costs associated with unpaid care provided by family and friends. Time spent caregiving may result in productivity losses and future income and wealth losses, and caregivers may experience challenges to their own health, quality of life, and finances associated with the challenges of caregiving. There may be other hidden costs, such as those associated with treatments, trial participation, or financial exploitation. Importantly, the costs of dementia are not static, and estimates require annual updates and consideration of health, treatment innovation, care, and cost dynamics to be useful for planning and prioritizing (Zissimopoulos et al., 2014).

Given the demographic shifts that are expected to occur in the coming decades, including the doubling of the population of older adults, the development of effective approaches for the prevention and treatment of AD/ADRD is of great importance to people at risk for dementia and those living with the disease, their family members, caregivers, and communities,

---

[8] Prevalence is the proportion of a population with the characteristic of interest at a specific point in time (NIMH, 2024). Incidence is the rate of new cases in a defined population occurring over a given period of time (Tenny and Boktor, 2023).

BOX 1-3
Sex and Gender Differences in Alzheimer's
Disease and Related Dementias (AD/ADRD)

Sex and gender differences have been observed for many aspects of AD/ADRD (e.g., epidemiology, risk factors, treatment effects). Sex (a biological construct related to genetics, anatomy, and physiology) and gender (a social construct) are often used interchangeably. However, many factors have both sex and gender components, and it is often challenging to tease apart the relative contributions of each (Mielke, 2024).

Differences between men and women in the risk of developing Alzheimer's disease or a related dementia have been reported across many studies (Andersen et al., 1999; Beam et al., 2018; Ruitenberg et al., 2001), although the literature is inconsistent (Kawas et al., 2000; Mielke et al., 2022; Wolters et al., 2020). The observation of gender differences in dementia risk varies across countries, and it remains unclear how much of this difference is due to the greater longevity of women as compared to men and the contributions of other sociodemographic factors (e.g., education and occupational opportunities) (Huque et al., 2023). Gender differences in dementia incidence also vary by dementia type (Akhter et al., 2021; Lucca et al., 2020).

In addition to risk, sex and gender differences in disease trajectory have also been reported. As a result of better baseline cognition in memory-related domains, women may be diagnosed with amnestic forms of dementia later and may therefore appear to progress to dementia more quickly as compared to men (Lin et al., 2015; Nebel et al., 2018). It has also been proposed that women's resilience to neuropathology may change over the course of disease progression, with diminished resilience at later stages resulting in steeper cognitive declines as compared to men (Arenaza-Urquijo et al., 2024).

Potential explanations for observed differences in AD/ADRD between men and women include a combination of biological (e.g., genetics, pregnancy, menopause) and sociocultural factors (e.g., caregiving roles, occupational opportunities) (Mielke, 2024). Such factors may contribute to sex and gender differences in certain AD/ADRD risk factors, such as cardiometabolic disorders (Gerdts and Regitz-Zagrosek, 2019; Ramirez and Sullivan, 2018), depression (Artero et al., 2008; Kessler et al., 1993; Kim et al., 2015), and physical inactivity (Barha et al., 2020; Luchsinger, 2008). Moreover, some well-established determinants of cognitive resilience, such as education, have historically had a large gender component (Gilsanz et al., 2021).

continued

BOX 1-3 Continued

Understanding of sex and gender differences in AD/ADRD and inter-sections with other factors such as race/ethnicity and cultural identity has been hampered by inadequate attention to the consideration of sex and gender in the design, execution, analysis, and reporting of re-search. While representation of women in clinical studies has improved and studies are increasingly adjusting for gender, relatively few studies analyze data for or report differences by sex and gender, despite the existence of an NIH policy requiring the consideration of sex as a bio-logical variable (Mielke, 2024). Taking a more sex- and gender-aware approach to AD/ADRD research will not only help elucidate sex- and gender-differences in risk, resilience, and clinical progression, but is also needed to understand differences in the efficacy of interventions and inform precision medicine approaches.

---

as well as policy makers, clinicians, and social services providers, and soci-ety as a whole.

Reasons for Optimism

In June 2021, the U.S. Food and Drug Administration (FDA) approved the monoclonal antibody-based drug aducanumab for the treatment of AD (Cavazzoni, 2021).[9] While the approval of the drug under the agency's accelerated approval pathway was controversial,[10] it was also notable as the first drug approved for treatment of AD in nearly 2 decades and the only approved drug (at that time) targeting an underlying patho-physiologic process—specifically, the accumulation of amyloid beta. While aducanumab's manufacturer announced that the drug would be discon-tinued in 2024 (Alzheimer's Association, 2024e), the approval of two additional amyloid-targeted antibody-based drugs followed shortly after

---

[9] In July 2024, the European Medicines Agency (EMA) recommended the refusal of the mar-keting authorization for lecanemab because the benefits did not outweigh the risk of serious adverse effects. EMA raised concerns that the risk of serious adverse effects may be heightened in people who are carriers of the *APOE4* gene variant (EMA, 2024).

[10] The accelerated approval pathway enables FDA to approve a drug for a serious or life-threatening illness based on the drug's effect on a surrogate endpoint that is likely to predict a meaningful clinical benefit to patients (beyond the benefits that may be achieved through existing treatments) even if there remains some uncertainty about the drug's therapeutic benefit (Cavazzoni, 2021).

aducanumab. In January 2023, lecanemab received accelerated approval by FDA for treatment of AD, which was converted to a traditional approval in July of that year based on the results of a confirmatory study verifying clinical benefit (FDA, 2023). In contrast to aducanumab, which was determined to have insufficient evidence that the drug was reasonable and necessary (AlzForum, 2022), the Centers for Medicare & Medicaid Services (CMS) decided to broadly cover lecanemab under Coverage with Evidence Development (CED) following FDA traditional approval (CMS, 2023).[11] Most recently, donanemab was approved in July 2024.

Amyloid-targeted antibody-based drugs are not a panacea. The clinical benefits, which were evaluated in research participants in the early stages of AD, have been modest, and there are significant risks to the treatment (Budd Haeberlein et al., 2022; Sims et al., 2023; van Dyck et al., 2023), as discussed further in Chapter 4. High costs and a health care system unprepared to deliver such intravenous infusion therapies are major barriers to translation into clinical practice on a scale commensurate with the burden of disease (Mattke et al., 2024). For example, annualized per-beneficiary medication costs for lecanemab were estimated at $25,851 for Medicare beneficiaries with an additional $7,330 in ancillary costs (e.g., infusions, imaging). Annual out-of-pocket costs for individual beneficiaries may be in the thousands of dollars (Arbanas et al., 2023). Importantly, anti-amyloid antibody-based therapeutics are not relevant to other forms of dementia that do not involve the accumulation of amyloid plaques, such as frontotemporal and Lewy body dementia, for which there remain no approved treatments beyond those for managing symptoms.

Despite their limitations, the availability of approved therapies for AD has given rise to optimism among patients and researchers that AD and related neurodegenerative disorders can be treated to slow or halt disease progression and perhaps even prevented. It is also driving renewed interest in investment in AD/ADRD drug development, interest that had waned in the face of a high clinical trial failure rate (98 percent over the last 2 decades) (Cummings, 2018; Kim et al., 2022; Mehta et al., 2017; WHO, 2021). The creation of NIH-funded research initiatives to diversify the drug development pipeline, such as the Accelerating Medicines Partnership® Program for Alzheimer's Disease (AMP-AD) consortium and the Target Enablement to Accelerate Therapy Development for Alzheimer's Disease (TREAT-AD) centers (discussed further in Chapter 3), have resulted in the nomination of over 900 potential targets for further therapeutic development for AD (Agora, 2024). Similar initiatives (e.g., the Accelerating

---

[11] Under Coverage with Evidence Development (CED), the treating clinical team must contribute to the collection of evidence on how the therapeutics work in the real world through participation in a CMS registry (CMS, 2023).

Medicines Partnership® Program for Parkinson's Disease and Related Disorders) are driving advances for other dementia types. Additionally, with ongoing private-sector investments in treatments for AD/ADRD and the expansion of public–private partnerships (Cummings et al., 2021), new waves of therapies could emerge in the next decade.

Over the last decade, significant advances have been made in the understanding of modifiable risk factors (e.g., physical inactivity, hypertension, diet, social isolation) common across multiple types of dementia. Based on these modifiable risk factors, it has been estimated that approximately 40 percent of dementia cases may be preventable (Livingston et al., 2020, 2024). Additionally, interventions that target modifiable risk factors (i.e., healthy behaviors) may extend the number of healthy years of life and, among those who do ultimately develop dementia, compress the number of years living with disease (Livingston et al., 2024). Findings such as these have opened new opportunities for the development and evaluation of multicomponent intervention approaches that are designed to simultaneously target multiple factors common across AD/ADRD and be implemented in combination with other therapeutics (discussed further in Chapter 4).

The use of innovative randomized controlled trials to assess the cognitive and quality-of-life effects of these lifestyle and health behavior interventions in diverse populations, such as the Finnish Geriatric Intervention Study to Prevent Cognitive Impairment and Disability and the Systematic Multi-domain Alzheimer's Risk Reduction Trial, have demonstrated the potential and feasibility of these study designs and interventions and are continuing to expand understanding of how these approaches can be optimized for maximum benefit based on individual and population preferences and characteristics (Ngandu et al., 2015; Yaffe et al., 2024). The continuation of this work may realize opportunities in the near and medium term to accelerate tailored AD/ADRD prevention and resilience-building efforts at individual and population levels.

Additionally, intensive research on the development of biomarkers, particularly for AD, have led to a number of exciting advances poised to radically change the research and clinical practice landscape. Advances in the development and validation of fluid, imaging, and digital biomarkers are allowing for better linking of interventions to target populations and measurement of intervention response. Developing tools such as blood-based biomarkers and digitally based assessments may provide for earlier detection of changes in brain health as compared to traditional cognitive assessments and reduce reliance on invasive and expensive tests. For the first time, a blood test is now commercially available for AD based on blood amyloid levels and a plasma phospho-tau biomarker has been demonstrated to be clinically equivalent to FDA-approved cerebrospinal fluid biomarker tests used to detect AD pathology (Barthelemy et al., 2024). While not yet available clinically, ongoing research is exploring biomarkers available for alpha-synuclein and TDP-43 pathologies. As additional biomarkers are discovered and validated, particularly for related dementias, current barriers to early detection, diagnosis, prognosis (e.g., the likelihood of progression to clinical dementia), and longitudinal monitoring may be overcome, and it will be possible to quantify and better understand multiple etiology dementia.

These past successes, among others, provide the foundation to accelerate future scientific and clinical progress. There is significant opportunity and need to expand the repertoire of interventions that can be used to effectively treat AD/ADRD and ultimately prevent disease development. Investments in basic mechanistic and epidemiological research have yielded returns in an expanded set of targets now being evaluated in clinical trials, as well as other breakthroughs, such as the development of blood-based biomarkers that hold promise for early diagnosis and precision medicine approaches (Sarkar et al., 2024). Such advances are poised to transform the landscape for AD/ADRD research.

The Role of NIH in Advancing AD/ADRD Research

Strategic Planning Guided by the National Plan to Address Alzheimer's Disease

The enactment of the National Alzheimer's Project Act in 2011 provided an unprecedented opportunity to undertake a national-level strategic planning initiative aimed at addressing the challenges of AD/ADRD. The Act required the Secretary of the U.S. Department of Health and Human Services (HHS) to work collaboratively with the newly established Advisory Council on Alzheimer's Research, Care, and Services to create and maintain a National Plan to Address Alzheimer's Disease (National Plan) (HHS, 2024). The first National Plan was released in 2012 and has since been updated annually, with these efforts led by the HHS Assistant Secretary for Planning and Evaluation (ASPE). Three overarching principles have guided each iteration of the National Plan:

- Optimize existing resources, and improve and coordinate ongoing activities.
- Support public–private partnerships.
- Transform the way we approach AD/ADRD (HHS, 2024).

The National Plan includes six foundational goals, the first of which—of particular relevance to this committee's report—is "Prevent and effectively treat Alzheimer's disease and related dementias by 2025" (HHS,

2024).[12] Interim milestones developed by HHS help to track progress toward achieving this goal (HHS, 2024). For each goal, the National Plan specifies individual strategies and associated action steps (see Box 1-4 for the strategies under Goal 1 and Goal 6, which are most closely linked to the committee's charge). The National Alzheimer's Project Act was reauthorized in October 2024, supporting the continuation of efforts to meet the six foundational goals of the National Plan until 2035.[13]

NIH has a lead role in research efforts supporting the goals of the National Plan, with a particular emphasis on Goal 1 (HHS, 2024; Kelley, 2023). While multiple institutes, centers, and offices within NIH are engaged in efforts to achieve the research goals of the National Plan, NIA and NINDS are leading many of the action steps, with NIA generally leading efforts related to Alzheimer's disease and with NINDS focused on related dementias.

To support the identification of research priorities, NIH convenes annual research summits, the focus of which rotates among Alzheimer's disease (led by NIA); related dementias (led by NINDS); and research on care, services, and supports for persons living with dementia and their care partners/caregivers (led by NIA) over a 3-year period. These summits serve as key opportunities to gather broad input for NIH's strategic planning efforts (depicted in Figure 1-3) and ensure that scientific input is gathered from diverse multisector partners and participants to inform the development of an integrated, comprehensive research agenda (Kelley, 2023). In addition to showcasing progress to date, the summits serve to identify research gaps, bottlenecks that impede progress, priorities, and opportunities to translate AD/ADRD research findings into practice. In addition to the summits, NIH gathers input from the external community through various other forums, including workshops, meetings, and other activities.

NIH research priorities are outlined as a series of research implementation milestones (NIA, 2024a), which identify activities to address the goals of the National Plan and together form a blueprint for an integrated research agenda. Success criteria and specific implementation steps are defined for each milestone, and progress is tracked through a publicly available AD/ADRD milestone database. The milestones are updated annually based on the input from the summits and other sources, including National Academies reports and NIH-hosted workshops, among others (Kelley, 2023). At present there are more than 200 milestones in the AD/ADRD research implementation milestone database that are divided among

---

[12] Goals 2–6 of the National Plan are: 2. Enhance Care Quality and Efficiency; 3. Expand Supports for People with Alzheimer's Disease and Related Dementias and Their Families; 4. Enhance Public Awareness and Engagement; 5. Improve Data to Track Progress; and 6. Accelerate Action to Promote Healthy Aging and Reduce Risk Factors for Alzheimer's Disease and Related Dementias (HHS, 2024).

[13] NAPA Reauthorization Act, Public Law 118-92, 118th Cong. (October 1, 2024).

BOX 1-4
Strategies for Goals 1 and 6 of the National
Plan to Address Alzheimer's Disease

Goal 1 of the National Plan is to "Prevent and Effectively Treat Alzheimer's Disease and Related Dementias by 2025" and includes five strategies, listed below, each accompanied by a series of action steps.

Strategy 1.A: Identify research priorities and milestones.

Strategy 1.B: Expand research aimed at preventing and treating Alzheimer's Disease and Related Dementias.

Strategy 1.C: Accelerate efforts to identify early and presymptomatic stages of Alzheimer's Disease and Related Dementias.

Strategy 1.D: Coordinate research with international public and private entities.

Strategy 1.E: Facilitate translation of findings into medical practice and public health programs.

Goal 6 of the National Plan is to "Accelerate Action to Promote Healthy Aging and Reduce Risk Factors for Alzheimer's Disease and Related Dementias" and includes six strategies, listed below, each accompanied by a series of action steps.

Strategy 6.A: Identify Research Priorities and Expand Research on Risk Factors for Alzheimer's Disease and Related Dementias.

Strategy 6.B: Facilitate Translation of Risk Reduction Research Findings into Clinical Practice.

Strategy 6.C: Accelerate Public Health Action to Address the Risk Factors for Alzheimer's Disease and Related Dementias.

Strategy 6.D: Expand Interventions to Reduce Risk Factors, Manage Chronic Conditions, and Improve Well-Being Through the Aging Network.

Strategy 6.E: Address Inequities in Risk Factors for Alzheimer's Disease and Related Dementias Among Marginalized Populations.

Strategy 6.F: Engage the Public About Ways to Reduce Risks for Alzheimer's Disease and Related Dementias.

SOURCE: HHS, 2024.

---

six research categories spanning basic, translational, clinical, and health services research:

1. Epidemiology/population studies
2. Disease mechanisms
3. Diagnosis, assessment, and disease monitoring
4. Translational research and clinical interventions

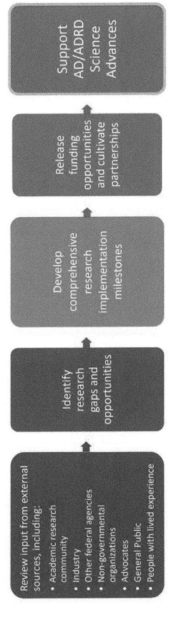

FIGURE 1-3 Overview of NIH AD/ADRD strategic planning process.
SOURCE: Kelley, 2023.

5. Dementia care and impact of disease
6. Research resources (NIA, 2024a)

The research blueprint formed by the milestones guides NIH funding opportunities but is also used for other purposes, such as informing priorities for cultivating partnerships and collaborations.

NIH Support for AD/ADRD Research

As noted earlier in this chapter, congressional appropriations related to AD/ADRD increased substantially following the enactment of the National Alzheimer's Project Act, resulting in a significant expansion of NIH investment in AD/ADRD research. While relative funding increases from fiscal year (FY) 2015 to FY2022 for specific related dementias were similar to and in some cases exceeded those for AD, absolute funding for AD represents the vast majority of support for AD/ADRD research (see Table 1-1). Some funding categorized as dedicated to AD research may also benefit and apply to related dementias, such as in the case of research on shared underlying mechanisms.

The vast majority of NIH funding support for AD/ADRD research comes from NIA (approximately $3.2 billion in FY2022), followed by NINDS (approximately $127.7 million in FY2022) (NIH RePORT, 2024).[14] Other institutes and offices that ranked within the top five for funding AD/ADRD research in FY2022 include the Office of the Director; the National Institute of General Medical Sciences, and the National Heart, Lung, and Blood Institute. While NIA provides the majority of the funding for AD research, NIA and NINDS both provide significant funding for research on related dementias (approximately $607.3 million and $84.6 million, respectively in FY2022) (NIH RePORT, 2024).

With increased appropriations from Congress, NIH has in the last decade significantly expanded its portfolio of supported projects across the full continuum of basic to clinical research, both in terms of numbers and diversity of projects, as exemplified by the graphs in Figure 1-4. Figure 1-5 shows the distribution of NIH funding for FY2022 across the eight Common Alzheimer's Disease Research Ontology Research Categories, which cover various aspects of basic, translational, and clinical research. These investments are complemented by support provided by

---

[14] FY2022 funding levels from individual NIH institutes, centers, and offices were obtained through the selection of relevant Research, Condition, and Disease Categorization (RCDC) categories—Alzheimer's Disease, Alzheimer's Disease Related Dementias (ADRD), and Alzheimer's Disease including Alzheimer's Disease Related Dementias (AD/ADRD)—in the RCDC system, which can be accessed at https://report.nih.gov/funding/categorical-spending#/.

TABLE 1-1 AD/ADRD Spending at NIH for Fiscal Years 2019 to 2022

Research/Disease Areas	FY2015	FY2016	FY2017	FY2018	FY2019	FY2020	FY2021	FY2022	Difference – FY2015 to FY2022
AD/ADRD[a]	$631	$986	$1,423	$1,911	$2,398	$2,869	$3,251	$3,514	5.6-fold increase
Alzheimer's disease (AD)	$589	$929	$1,361	$1,789	$2,240	$2,683	$3,059	$3,314	5.6-fold increase
Alzheimer's disease related dementias (ADRD)[b,c,d]	$120	$175	$249	$387	$515	$600	$725	$730	6.1-fold increase
Lewy body dementia	$15	$22	$31	$38	$66	$84	$113	$118	7.9-fold increase
Frontotemporal dementia	$36	$65	$91	$94	$158	$166	$164	$169	4.7-fold increase
Vascular cognitive impairment/ dementia	$72	$89	$130	$259	$299	$362	$455	$445	6.2-fold increase

NOTE: Funding levels are shown as U.S. dollars in millions
[a] The category Alzheimer's Disease including Alzheimer's Disease Related Dementias (AD/ADRD) reflects the sum of the two existing Research, Condition, and Disease Categorization (RCDC) categories—Alzheimer's Disease (AD) and Alzheimer's Disease Related Dementias (ADRD)—where duplicates are removed.
[b] The category ADRD reflects the sum of three existing RCDC categories—Frontotemporal Dementia, Lewy Body Dementia, and Vascular Cognitive Impairment/Dementia—where duplicates are removed.
[c] These categories were established pursuant to Section 230, Division G of the Consolidated and Further Continuing Appropriations Act of 2015 as related to reporting of NIH initiatives supporting the National Alzheimer's Project Act (NAPA), https://aspe.hhs.gov/national-alzheimers-project-act.
[d] NIH uses the term Alzheimer's disease-related dementia (ADRD) in some contexts.
SOURCE: Kelley, 2023.

A. NIH-supported projects related to molecular pathogenesis and physiology of AD/ADRD

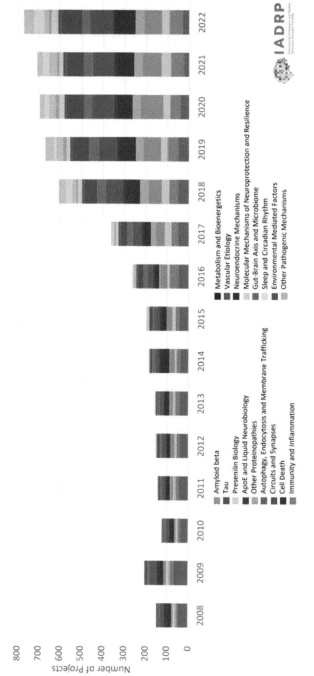

continued

B. NIH-supported projects related to early-stage clinical drug development

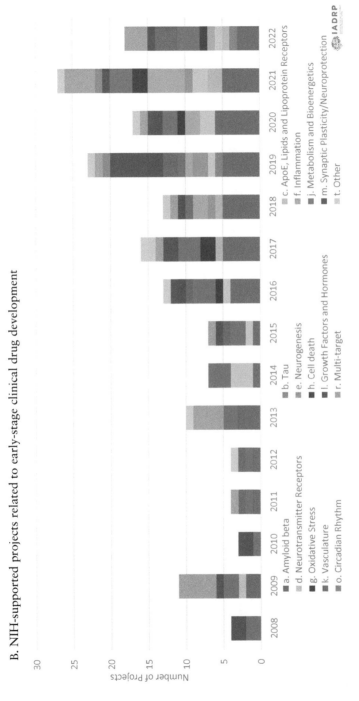

FIGURE 1-4 Trends in the number of new NIH-supported AD/ADRD projects related to (A) molecular pathogenesis and physiology, and (B) early-stage clinical drug development.
SOURCE: Kelley, 2023.

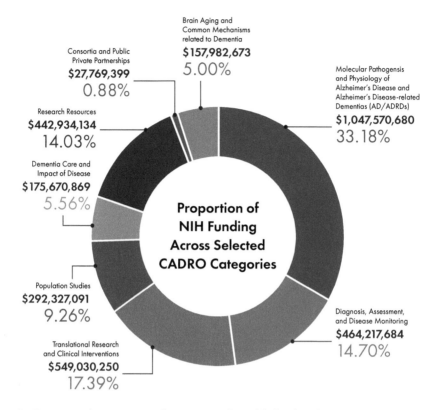

FIGURE 1-5 Relative National Institutes of Health funding for AD/ADRD across Common Alzheimer's Disease Research Ontology (CADRO) research categories, FY2022.
SOURCE: IADRP, 2024.

other funders within the research enterprise, including private industry and philanthropic groups.[15] As discussed later in this report, public–private partnerships, such as AMP-AD,[16] are increasingly bridging gaps at the interface of basic, translational, and clinical research, thereby helping to accelerate breakthroughs in the diagnosis, prevention, and treatment of

---

[15] AD/ADRD research supported by public and private organizations in the United States and abroad is captured in the International Alzheimer's and Related Dementias Research Portfolio (IADRP), a searchable database available at https://iadrp.nia.nih.gov/ (accessed January 11, 2024).

[16] AMP-AD is a public–private partnership between NIH, FDA, private industry, and nonprofit organizations focused on developing new diagnostics and treatments by working collaboratively to identify and validate promising biological targets (NIA, 2024b).

AD/ADRD. The expansion of funding support for AD/ADRD research to levels more commensurate with the scope of the problem has opened new opportunities and avenues for scientific breakthroughs that may not have been possible in a more resource-limited environment. Still, the importance of sustaining these research investments is apparent when considering the scope of dementia research relative to that of cardiovascular disease and cancer. For example, a search of clinicaltrials.gov yielded 272 active (nonrecruiting) dementia-focused clinical trials. In comparison, the number of trials for cardiovascular disease and cancer were near to 2,500 (nearly 10-fold higher) and 7,700 (nearly 30-fold higher), respectively (ClinicalTrials.gov, 2024a,b,c).[17]

The diversification of the NIH research portfolio, which has been guided by the strategic planning processes described above, reflects a paradigm shift that has emerged with the growing understanding of the scientific community regarding the complex, multifactorial nature of AD/ADRD. The committee was not asked to comprehensively catalog and assess NIH's programmatic activities related to AD/ADRD or to evaluate and make recommendations on the current strategic planning process used by NIH to set priorities. Rather this report is intended to complement those efforts, highlighting opportunities to accelerate the translation of discoveries emerging from the vast and growing body of knowledge on AD/ADRD into effective strategies for prevention and treatment. This report provides the committee's consensus views on the research areas with the greatest promise to catalyze significant advances and maximize return on investment in the form of improved population health.

STUDY APPROACH

To address the Statement of Task, the National Academies convened a 19-member committee of individuals with expertise spanning basic to clinical research and covering different aspects of AD/ADRD, including risk factors and epidemiology, biological mechanisms and intervention strategies, clinical trial design and implementation, precision medicine, health economics, and lived experience. Biographies of the committee members can be found in Appendix B.

---

[17] The search of clinicialtrials.gov for dementia, cardiovascular, and cancer trials did not restrict the results to trials of interventions for disease prevention and treatment. These cited numbers may therefore include trials on care interventions (e.g., care coordination) and other interventions not applicable to the scope of this report.

Guiding Themes

Early in the study process, the committee converged around a life-course approach to addressing the Statement of Task, consistent with another recent dementia-focused National Academies report (NASEM, 2021b), and applied this lens throughout the course of its work. The life-course approach is grounded in the understanding that aging is not something that just happens in the later decades of life—it happens across the entire lifespan. Brain functions change over time as a reflection of the biological development stage it is in. Moreover, the growing body of evidence related to risk and protective factors for AD/ADRD has increasingly been shifting focus to earlier life stages, even as early as the prenatal period (Boots et al., 2023).

In the context of a life-course approach, the committee sought to balance the conventional disease-focused medical model with a framing around optimization of brain health and functioning at every life stage (WHO, 2022). Outcomes of the disease-focused approaches that have dominated both research and clinical practice have included growing health care costs and lower-quality health. With this health-oriented reframing, prevention of disease can be viewed as an incidental benefit of focusing on brain health optimization rather than its primary objective.

Health equity is another theme that guided the committee's approach and intersects with the life-course framework. As depicted in Figure 1-6, health disparities—systemic, structural, contextual, and individual—have a cumulative effect on outcomes of AD/ADRD over the life course (NINDS, 2022). Applying a health equity lens helped the committee to more intentionally consider the effect of health disparities on outcomes related to optimizing brain health and preventing and treating AD/ADRD and to highlight intervention strategies with the greatest potential to address those disparities.

The application of a health equity lens to the development of this report included consideration of health research equity, and specifically, the underrepresentation of different population groups in AD/ADRD research. Diversity and inclusion in research are critical for high-quality science and important to ensure that the research serves all individuals. Diversity in research is inclusive of a broad array of factors that include but are not limited to race, ethnicity, sex, gender, sexual orientation, age, socioeconomic status, language, education, and profession. Historically many groups underrepresented in research have also been disproportionately affected by AD/ADRD and thus merit special prioritization in future research. For some groups, there is simply too little evidence currently available to know if they are disproportionately burdened by AD/ADRD, so these groups also merit prioritization in future research. Throughout this report, the committee thus

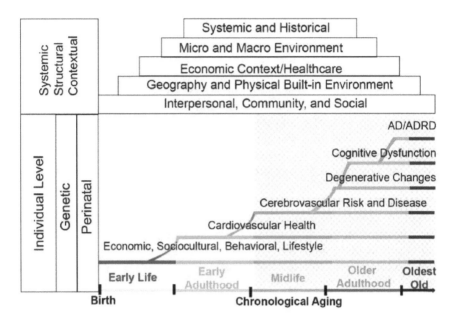

FIGURE 1-6 AD/ADRD life-course model showing the multiple components of health disparities that have a cumulative effect on AD/ADRD outcomes over the life course.
SOURCE: NINDS, 2022.

refers to "understudied and/or disproportionately affected populations" to emphasize the importance of expanding the evidence base for groups historically missing from AD/ADRD research and ensuring commitment to inclusion for groups with known disparities.

One additional aspect of health research equity that warrants attention is the imbalance in research among different types of dementias. As noted earlier in this chapter (see Table 1-1), the majority of funding support for AD/ADRD research has been focused on AD and, as a result, the literature base examined by the committee is similarly biased. This imbalance in research investment is to some degree reflected in the presentation of evidence in this report, although the committee endeavored to balance examples from AD research with examples for related dementias throughout. The continuation of increased focus on understudied related dementias will hopefully address such imbalances in the future, enabling a better understanding of these conditions as well as mixed etiology dementia.

The final theme that guided the committee in its deliberations is the imperative to innovate and to learn from successes and failures in biomedical research, both within and outside the AD/ADRD field. Innovation is inherently high risk, but failures hold equal potential as successes for expanding knowledge when embraced as an integral part of the scientific process and carefully deconstructed to extract insights. Ultimately, breakthroughs emerge when innovation enables us to break out of what is already being done. Other fields (e.g., cardiology, cancer) are well ahead of dementia in terms of prevention and precision medicine,[18] which is an evolving platform of health care delivery that "integrates investigation of mechanisms of disease with prevention, treatment, and cure, resolved at the level of the individual" (NAM, 2017). Such approaches will likely guide the next 10 years of medical research in AD/ADRD and other disease fields. The committee sought to understand the factors that led to paradigm shifts in those fields, to build from their successes, and to learn and apply effective strategies for translating failures into knowledge and progress.

Approach to Identifying Promising Areas of Research

The committee was charged with reviewing and synthesizing the most promising areas of research into preventing and treating AD/ADRD. To address this element of its task, the committee established criteria for different facets of what it could mean for research to be considered "promising." These were not intended as a checklist or a rigid rubric for evaluation but as a tool to shape the committee's thinking. As the committee explored and assessed the AD/ADRD research landscape, its efforts to identify promising research areas were guided by the following criteria:

- Multidisciplinary research that has the potential to open new lines of scientific inquiry and build on the successes of other fields;
- Research that maximizes inclusivity and minimizes exclusion as part of its methodology;
- Research that establishes baselines that would allow detection of differences across and within diverse populations and the identification of understudied and/or disproportionately affected populations;

---

[18] The goals of precision medicine are often interpreted through the lens of the disease- and treatment-focused medical model. Precision medicine in fact has a much broader scope that is inclusive of prevention and population-health approaches. The committee adopted this broader view that is aligned with the brain health optimization framing for this report. Throughout the report, there are times when the committee sought to emphasize the application of precision medicine approaches to maintenance of brain health (e.g., by continuously monitoring brain health and intervening prior to the development of disease) and in those contexts uses the term precision brain health. When referring to the application of precision medicine to specific preventive and therapeutic interventions, the committee uses the terms precision prevention and precision treatment, respectively.

- Research that has the potential to translate discoveries into a viable and diversified portfolio of interventions and biomarkers;
- Research that builds a foundation for precision medicine advances; and
- Research that maximizes the yields from existing research but also identifies opportunities to fill knowledge and data gaps.

Information Gathering

To complement its own expertise, the committee sought input from outside experts, advocates, and those with lived experience through a variety of mechanisms. The committee met and deliberated over a roughly 1-year period from October 2023 to November 2024. During this time, the committee held five public information-gathering sessions (October and November 2023, and January, April, and May 2024). During the October 2023 meeting, the committee received the charge from NIA and NINDS and clarified issues on the study's scope. During its November meeting the committee hosted a short public session on approaches for increasing innovation in biomedical research. A public workshop held in conjunction with the January 2024 meeting included sessions with nonfederal funders of, and advocacy groups involved in, AD/ADRD research, AD/ADRD academic and industry researchers based in the United States and abroad, researchers from outside the AD/ADRD field employing tools and approaches that could be applied to AD/ADRD research, and a keynote from an individual with lived experience.

A brief public session was held during the committee's fourth meeting to hear findings from and provide feedback to the author of a commissioned paper on sex and gender differences in AD/ADRD.[19] A fifth public meeting was held in May 2024 during which researchers and clinicians explored research discoveries, identified considerations for research priorities, and discussed barriers that impede the advancement of research for related dementias. Public session agendas can be found in Appendix D. The committee meetings in April and July 2024 were held in closed session. To inform its deliberations, the committee used several mechanisms to gather information, including (1) the review of information submitted to the committee from NIA and others; (2) examination of publicly available information; (3) a commissioned paper on sex and gender differences in

---

[19] The paper the committee commissioned on sex and gender differences in AD/ADRD addresses epidemiology, risk factors, clinical symptoms and diagnosis, clinical research, and treatment effects. While the committee's report does not include an in-depth review of sex and gender differences related to each of these areas, a brief synopsis of the paper is provided in Box 1-3 and key information from the commissioned paper was incorporated in relevant sections throughout the report. The full paper is available at https://nap.edu/28588.

AD/ADRD that included keys gaps in research; and (4) reviews of the published literature, including a scoping review of published systematic reviews on interventions for preventing and treating AD/ADRD. Multiple literature reviews were conducted throughout this study using PubMed and Scopus to support the committee's examination of the biomedical research landscape on AD/ADRD. These searches guided and provided references for content in this report. More information on the methods for the committee's scoping review of recent systematic reviews can be found in Appendix A.

Report Organization

The committee structured its report around the following three key elements necessary to catalyze advances in AD/ADRD prevention and treatment:

1. The ability to longitudinally track brain health and detect, diagnose, and monitor AD/ADRD development and progression (Chapter 2).
2. Advancing understanding of disease pathways to guide effective strategies for AD/ADRD prevention and treatment (Chapter 3).
3. The development and evaluation of interventions for prevention and treatment of AD/ADRD (Chapter 4).

The main report body concludes with a final chapter (Chapter 5) that summarizes the committee's research priorities, highlights crosscutting issues from the previous chapters that impede progress in AD/ADRD prevention and treatment, and provides recommendations for overcoming these barriers. The research priorities identified by the committee are presented in order of the chapters, but cumulatively address the report's goal of advancing the prevention and treatment of AD/ADRD. Of note, some key topics are inherently crosscutting and are therefore woven throughout the report chapters. These include equity, person centeredness, and opportunities to apply successful strategies for innovation from other fields.

REFERENCES

Adair, T., J. Temple, K. J. Anstey, and A. D. Lopez. 2022. Is the rise in reported dementia mortality real? Analysis of multiple-cause-of-death data for Australia and the United States. *American Journal of Epidemiology* 191(7):1270-1279.

Agora. 2024. *Nominated target list.* https://agora.adknowledgeportal.org/genes/nominated-targets (accessed August 22, 2024).

Akhter, F., A. Persaud, Y. Zaokari, Z. Zhao, and D. Zhu. 2021. Vascular dementia and underlying sex differences. *Frontiers in Aging Neuroscience* 13:720715.

AlzForum. 2022. *CMS plans to limit Aduhelm coverage to clinical trials.* https://www.alzforum.org/news/research-news/cms-plans-limit-aduhelm-coverage-clinical-trials (accessed August 13, 2024).

Alzheimer's Association. 2021. *What are frontotemporal disorders? Causes, symptoms, and treatment.* https://www.nia.nih.gov/health/frontotemporal-disorders/what-are-frontotemporal-disorders-causes-symptoms-and-treatment#typesandsymptoms (accessed August 13, 2024).

Alzheimer's Association. 2023. 2023 Alzheimer's disease facts and figures. *Alzheimer's and Dementia* 19:1598-1695.

Alzheimer's Association. 2024a. *2024 Alzheimer's disease facts and figures.* https://www.alz.org/alzheimers-dementia/facts-figures (accessed September 2, 2024).

Alzheimer's Association. 2024b. *What is Alzheimer's disease?* https://www.alz.org/alzheimers-dementia/what-is-alzheimers (accessed August 13, 2024).

Alzheimer's Association. 2024c. *Dementia with Lewy bodies.* https://www.alz.org/alzheimers-dementia/what-is-dementia/types-of-dementia/dementia-with-lewy-bodies (accessed August 13, 2024).

Alzheimer's Association. 2024d. *Frontotemporal dementia.* https://www.alz.org/alzheimers-dementia/what-is-dementia/types-of-dementia/frontotemporal-dementia (accessed August 13, 2024).

Alzheimer's Association. 2024e. *Aducanumab to be discontinued as an Alzheimer's treatment.* https://www.alz.org/alzheimers-dementia/treatments/aducanumab (accessed August 13, 2024).

Andersen, K., L. J. Launer, M. E. Dewey, L. Letenneur, A. Ott, J. R. Copeland, J. F. Dartigues, P. Kragh-Sorensen, M. Baldereschi, C. Brayne, A. Lobo, J. M. Martinez-Lage, T. Stijnen, and A. Hofman. 1999. Gender differences in the incidence of AD and vascular dementia: The EURODEM studies. EURODEM Incidence Research Group. *Neurology* 53(9):1992-1997.

Arbanas, J., C. Damberg, M. Leng, N. Harawa, C. Sarkisian, B. Landon, and J. Mafi. 2023. Estimated annual spending on lecanemab and its ancillary costs in the US Medicare program. *JAMA Internal Medicine* 183(8):883-885.

Arenaza-Urquijo, E. M., R. Boyle, K. Casaletto, K. J. Anstey, C. Vila-Castelar, A. Colverson, E. Palpatzis, J. M. Eissman, T. Kheng Siang Ng, S. Raghavan, M. Akinci, J. M. J. Vonk, L. S. Machado, P. P. Zanwar, H. L. Shrestha, M. Wagner, S. Tamburin, H. R. Sohrabi, S. Loi, D. Bartrés-Faz, D. B. Dubal, P. Vemuri, O. Okonkwo, T. J. Hohman, M. Ewers, R. F. Buckley, Reserve, Resilience and Protective Factors Professional Interest Area, Sex and Gender Professional Interest area and the ADDRESS! Special Interest Group. 2024. Sex and gender differences in cognitive resilience to aging and Alzheimer's disease. *Alzheimer's & Dementia* 20(8):5695-5719.

Artero, S., M. L. Ancelin, F. Portet, A. Dupuy, C. Berr, J. F. Dartigues, C. Tzourio, O. Rouaud, M. Poncet, F. Pasquier, S. Auriacombe, J. Touchon, and K. Ritchie. 2008. Risk profiles for mild cognitive impairment and progression to dementia are gender specific. *Journal of Neurology, Neurosurgery, and Psychiatry* 79(9):979-984.

ASPE (Assistant Secretary for Planning and Evaluation). Overview of the National Alzheimer's Project Act Implementation. 2023. Presentation at the NAPA Advisory Council Meeting on October 30. https://aspe.hhs.gov/collaborations-committees-advisory-groups/napa/napa-advisory-council/napa-advisory-council-meetings/napa-past-meetings/napa-2023-meeting-material.

Barha, C. K., J. R. Best, C. Rosano, K. Yaffe, J. M. Catov, and T. Liu-Ambrose. 2020. Sex-specific relationship between long-term maintenance of physical activity and cognition in the Health ABC study: Potential role of hippocampal and dorsolateral prefrontal cortex volume. *Journals of Gerontology: Series A, Biological Sciences and Medical Sciences* 75(4):764-770.

Barthelemy, N. R., G. Salvado, S. E. Schindler, Y. He, S. Janelidze, L. E. Collij, B. Saef, R. L. Henson, C. D. Chen, B. A. Gordon, Y. Li, R. La Joie, T. L. S. Benzinger, J. C. Morris, N. Mattsson-Carlgren, S. Palmqvist, R. Ossenkoppele, G. D. Rabinovici, E. Stomrud, R. J. Bateman, and O. Hansson. 2024. Highly accurate blood test for Alzheimer's disease is similar or superior to clinical cerebrospinal fluid tests. *Nature Medicine* 30(4):1085-1095.

Beam, C. R., C. Kaneshiro, J. Y. Jang, C. A. Reynolds, N. L. Pedersen, and M. Gatz. 2018. Differences between women and men in incidence rates of dementia and Alzheimer's disease. *Journal of Alzheimer's Disease* 64(4):1077-1083.

Boots, A., A. M. Wiegersma, Y. Vali, M. van den Hof, M. W. Langendam, J. Limpens, E. V. Backhouse, S. D. Shenkin, J. M. Wardlaw, T. J. Roseboom, and S. R. de Rooij. 2023. Shaping the risk for late-life neurodegenerative disease: A systematic review on prenatal risk factors for Alzheimer's disease-related volumetric brain biomarkers. *Neuroscience & Biobehavioral Reviews* 146:105019.

Budd Haeberlein, S., P. S. Aisen, F. Barkhof, S. Chalkias, T. Chen, S. Cohen, G. Dent, O. Hansson, K. Harrison, C. von Hehn, T. Iwatsubo, C. Mallinckrodt, C. J. Mummery, K. K. Muralidharan, I. Nestorov, L. Nisenbaum, R. Rajagovindan, L. Skordos, Y. Tian, C. H. van Dyck, B. Vellas, S. Wu, Y. Zhu, and A. Sandrock. 2022. Two randomized phase 3 studies of aducanumab in early Alzheimer's disease. *Journal of Prevention of Alzheimer's Disease* 9(2):197-210.

Burhanullah, M. H., J. T. Tschanz, M. E. Peters, J.-M. Leoutsakos, J. Matyi, C. G. Lyketsos, M. A. Nowrangi, and P. B. Rosenberg. 2020. Neuropsychiatric symptoms as risk factors for cognitive decline in clinically normal older adults: The Cache County study. *American Journal of Geriatric Psychiatry* 28(1):64-71.

Cavazzoni, P. 2021. *FDA's decision to approve new treatment for Alzheimer's disease.* https://www.fda.gov/drugs/our-perspective/fdas-decision-approve-new-treatment-alzheimers-disease (accessed September 2, 2024).

CDC (Centers for Disease Control and Prevention). 2020. *Alzheimer's disease and related dementias.* https://www.cdc.gov/aging/aginginfo/alzheimers.htm#:~:text=Alzheimer's%20disease%20is%20the%20most,thought%2C%20memory%2C%20and%20language (accessed August 13, 2024).

Chen, C., and J. M. Zissimopoulos. 2018. Racial and ethnic differences in trends in dementia prevalence and risk factors in the United States. *Alzheimer's & Dementia (NY)* 4:510-520.

ClinicalTrials.gov. 2024a. *Search results: Cancer.* https://clinicaltrials.gov/search?cond=cancer&aggFilters=status:act (accessed August 23, 2024).

ClinicalTrials.gov. 2024b. *Search results: Cardiovascular.* https://clinicaltrials.gov/search?cond=cardiovascular&aggFilters=status:act (accessed August 23, 2024).

ClinicalTrials.gov. 2024c. *Search results: Dementia.* https://clinicaltrials.gov/search?cond=dementia&aggFilters=status:act (accessed August 23, 2024).

CMS (Centers for Medicare & Medicaid Services). 2023. *Statement: Broader Medicare coverage of leqembi available following FDA traditional approval.* https://www.cms.gov/newsroom/press-releases/statement-broader-medicare-coverage-leqembi-available-following-fda-traditional-approval (accessed August 23, 2024).

Cummings, J. 2018. Lessons learned from Alzheimer disease: Clinical trials with negative outcomes. *Clinical and Translational Science* 11(2):147-152.

Cummings, J. 2021. The role of neuropsychiatric symptoms in research diagnostic criteria for neurodegenerative diseases. *American Journal of Geriatric Psychiatry* 29(4):375-383.

Cummings, J., and N. Fox. 2017. Defining disease modifying therapy for Alzheimer's disease. *Journal of Prevention of Alzheimer's Disease* 4(2):109-115.

Cummings, J., J. Bauzon, and G. Lee. 2021. Who funds Alzheimer's disease drug development? *Alzheimer's & Dementia: Translational Research & Clinical Interventions* 7(1):e12185.

Cummings, J., Y. Zhou, G. Lee, K. Zhong, J. Fonseca, and F. Cheng. 2024. Alzheimer's disease drug development pipeline: 2024. *Alzheimer's & Dementia: Translational Research & Clinical Interventions* 10(2):e12465.

David, N. D., L. Feng, A. P. Porsteinsson, and the Alzheimer's Disease Neuroimaging Initiative. 2016. Trajectories of neuropsychiatric symptoms and cognitive decline in mild cognitive impairment. *American Journal of Geriatric Psychiatry* 24(1):70-80.

Defrancesco, M., G. Kemmler, P. Dal-Bianco, G. Ransmayr, T. Benke, J. Marksteiner, J. Mosbacher, Y. Höller, and R. Schmidt. 2020. Specific neuropsychiatric symptoms are associated with faster progression in Alzheimer's disease: Results of the prospective dementia registry (PRODEM-Austria). *Journal of Alzheimer's Disease* 73(1):125-133.

EMA (European Medicines Agency). 2024. *Leqembi.* https://www.ema.europa.eu/en/medicines/human/EPAR/leqembi (accessed September 10, 2024).

Farina, M. P., Y. S. Zhang, J. K. Kim, M. D. Hayward, and E. M. Crimmins. 2022. Trends in dementia prevalence, incidence, and mortality in the United States (2000-2016). *Journal of Aging and Health* 34(1):100-108.

FDA (Food and Drug Administration). 2023. *FDA converts novel Alzheimer's disease treatment to traditional approval.* https://www.fda.gov/news-events/press-announcements/fda-converts-novel-alzheimers-disease-treatment-traditional-approval (accessed October 15 2024).

Freedman, V. A., J. C. Cornman, and J. D. Kasper. 2021. National Health and Aging Trends Study chart book: Key trends, measures and detailed tables. https://micda.isr.umich.edu/wp-content/uploads/2022/03/NHATS-Companion-Chartbook-to-Trends Dashboards-2020.pdf (accessed September 2, 2024).

FTD Talk. 2024. *Clinical syndromes.* https://www.ftdtalk.org/what-is-frontotemporal-dementia/clinical-syndromes/ (accessed October 15, 2024, 2024).

Gerdts, E., and V. Regitz-Zagrosek. 2019. Sex differences in cardiometabolic disorders. *Nature Medicine* 25(11):1657-1666.

Gilsanz, P., E. R. Mayeda, C. W. Eng, O. L. Meyer, M. M. Glymour, C. P. Quesenberry, and R. A. Whitmer. 2021. Participant education, spousal education and dementia risk in a diverse cohort of members of an integrated health care delivery system in northern California. *BMJ Open* 11(6):e040233.

HHS (U.S. Department of Health and Human Services). 2024. *National plan to address Alzheimer's disease: 2023 update.* https://aspe.hhs.gov/reports/national-plan-2023-update (accessed August 22, 2024).

Huque, H., R. Eramudugolla, B. Chidiac, N. Ee, L. Ehrenfeld, F. E. Matthews, R. Peters, and K. J. Anstey. 2023. Could country-level factors explain sex differences in dementia incidence and prevalence? A systematic review and meta-analysis. *Journal of Alzheimer's Disease* 91(4):1231-1241.

IADRP (International Alzheimer's and Related Dementias Research Portfolio). 2024. *Proportion of funding across selected CADRO by total.* https://iadrp.nia.nih.gov/visualization?t=&disease_op=or&disease%5B%5D=19045&disease%5B%5D=19046&disease%5B%5D=19047&disease%5B%5D=19048&disease%5B%5D=19049&class_op=or&class%5B%5D=73735&class%5B%5D=73736&class%5B%5D=73737&class%5B%5D=73738&class%5B%5D=73739&class%5B%5D=73740&class%5B%5D=73741&class%5B%5D=73742&p_title=&p_num=&p_type_op=or&f_mech_op=or&fun_year=2022&pi_ln=&pi_fn=&a_org_op=or&a_country_op=or&f_org_op=or&f_org%5B%5D=59956&f_country_op=or&field_program_official_op=or&spec_init_op=or&plot_by=funding&summarized=cadro_category_1&refine_by=total&cadro_category_1_children=&chart_type=pie (accessed August 23, 2024).

Jack, C. R., Jr., D. A. Bennett, K. Blennow, M. C. Carrillo, B. Dunn, S. B. Haeberlein, D. M. Holtzman, W. Jagust, F. Jessen, J. Karlawish, E. Liu, J. L. Molinuevo, T. Montine, C. Phelps, K. P. Rankin, C. C. Rowe, P. Scheltens, E. Siemers, H. M. Snyder, and R. Sperling. 2018. NIA-AA research framework: Toward a biological definition of Alzheimer's disease. *Alzheimer's & Dementia* 14(4):535-562.

Jessen, F., R. E. Amariglio, R. F. Buckley, W. M. van der Flier, Y. Han, J. L. Molinuevo, L. Rabin, D. M. Rentz, O. Rodriguez-Gomez, A. J. Saykin, S. A. M. Sikkes, C. M. Smart, S. Wolfsgruber, and M. Wagner. 2020. The characterisation of subjective cognitive decline. *Lancet Neurology* 19(3):271-278.

Kawas, C., S. Gray, R. Brookmeyer, J. Fozard, and A. Zonderman. 2000. Age-specific incidence rates of Alzheimer's disease: The Baltimore Longitudinal Study of Aging. *Neurology* 54(11):2072-2077.

Kelley, M. 2023. NIH strategic planning process overview. Presentation at Committee on Research Priorities for Preventing and Treating Alzheimer's Disease and Related Dementias. Meeting 1, Virtual. October 2, 2023.

Kim, C. K., Y. R. Lee, L. Ong, M. Gold, A. Kalali, and J. Sarkar. 2022. Alzheimer's disease: Key insights from two decades of clinical trial failures. *Journal of Alzheimer's Disease* 87(1):83-100.

Kim, S., M. J. Kim, S. Kim, H. S. Kang, S. W. Lim, W. Myung, Y. Lee, C. H. Hong, S. H. Choi, D. L. Na, S. W. Seo, B. D. Ku, S. Y. Kim, S. Y. Kim, J. H. Jeong, S. A. Park, B. J. Carroll, and D. K. Kim. 2015. Gender differences in risk factors for transition from mild cognitive impairment to Alzheimer's disease: A CREDOS study. *Comprehensive Psychiatry* 62:114-122.

Kramarow, E. A. 2024. *Diagnosed dementia in adults age 65 and older: United States, 2022. National Health Statistics Report* (203):1-9.

Kessler, R. C., K. A. McGonagle, M. Swartz, D. G. Blazer, and C. B. Nelson. 1993. Sex and depression in the national comorbidity survey. I: Lifetime prevalence, chronicity and recurrence. *Journal of Affective Disorders* 29(2-3):85-96.

Lewy Body Dementia Association. 2022. *Diagnosing and managing Lewy body dementia: A comprehensive guide for healthcare professionals.* Lilburn, GA: Lewy Body Dementia Association.

Lin, K. A., K. R. Choudhury, B. G. Rathakrishnan, D. M. Marks, J. R. Petrella, and P. M. Doraiswamy. 2015. Marked gender differences in progression of mild cognitive impairment over 8 years. *Alzheimer's & Dementia (N Y)* 1(2):103-110.

Linton, A. E., E. M. Weekman, and D. M. Wilcock. 2021. Pathologic sequelae of vascular cognitive impairment and dementia sheds light on potential targets for intervention. *Cerebral Circulation—Cognition and Behavior* 2:100030.

Livingston, G., J. Huntley, A. Sommerlad, D. Ames, C. Ballard, S. Banerjee, C. Brayne, A. Burns, J. Cohen-Mansfield, C. Cooper, S. G. Costafreda, A. Dias, N. Fox, L. N. Gitlin, R. Howard, H. C. Kales, M. Kivimäki, E. B. Larson, A. Ogunniyi, V. Orgeta, K. Ritchie, K. Rockwood, E. L. Sampson, Q. Samus, L. S. Schneider, G. Selbæk, L. Teri, and N. Mukadam. 2020. Dementia prevention, intervention, and care: 2020 report of the Lancet Commission. *Lancet* 396(10248):413-446.

Livingston, G., J. Huntley, K. Y. Liu, S. G. Costafreda, G. Selbæk, S. Alladi, D. Ames, S. Banerjee, A. Burns, C. Brayne, N. C. Fox, C. P. Ferri, L. N. Gitlin, R. Howard, H. C. Kales, M. Kivimäki, E. B. Larson, N. Nakasujja, K. Rockwood, Q. Samus, K. Shirai, A. Singh-Manoux, L. S. Schneider, S. Walsh, Y. Yao, A. Sommerlad, and N. Mukadam. 2024. Dementia prevention, intervention, and care: 2024 report of the Lancet Standing Commission. *Lancet* 404(10452):572-628.

Lucca, U., M. Tettamanti, P. Tiraboschi, G. Logroscino, C. Landi, L. Sacco, M. Garrì, S. Ammesso, A. Biotti, E. Gargantini, A. Piedicorcia, S. Mandelli, E. Riva, A. A. Galbussera, and A. Recchia. 2020. Incidence of dementia in the oldest-old and its relationship with age: The Monzino 80-Plus population-based study. *Alzheimer's & Dementia* 16(3):472-481.

Luchsinger, J. A. 2008. Adiposity, hyperinsulinemia, diabetes and Alzheimer's disease: An epidemiological perspective. *European Journal of Pharmacology* 585(1):119-129.

Manly, J. J., R. N. Jones, K. M. Langa, L. H. Ryan, D. A. Levine, R. McCammon, S. G. Heeringa, and D. Weir. 2022. Estimating the prevalence of dementia and mild cognitive impairment in the US: The 2016 Health and Retirement Study Harmonized Cognitive Assessment Protocol Project. *JAMA Neurology* 79(12):1242-1249.

Mattke, S., H. Jun, M. Hanson, S. Chu, J. H. Kordower, and E. M. Reiman. 2024. Health economic considerations in the deployment of an Alzheimer's prevention therapy. *Journal of Prevention of Alzheimer's Disease* 11(2):303-309.

Mayeda, E. R., M. M. Glymour, C. P. Quesenberry, and R. A. Whitmer. 2016. Inequalities in dementia incidence between six racial and ethnic groups over 14 years. *Alzheimer's & Dementia* 12(3):216-224.

McKhann, G. M., D. S. Knopman, H. Chertkow, B. T. Hyman, C. R. Jack, Jr., C. H. Kawas, W. E. Klunk, W. J. Koroshetz, J. J. Manly, R. Mayeux, R. C. Mohs, J. C. Morris, M. N. Rossor, P. Scheltens, M. C. Carrillo, B. Thies, S. Weintraub, and C. H. Phelps. 2011. The diagnosis of dementia due to Alzheimer's disease: Recommendations from the National Institute on Aging–Alzheimer's Association workgroups on diagnostic guidelines for Alzheimer's disease. *Alzheimer's & Dementia* 7(3):263-269.

Mehta, D., R. Jackson, G. Paul, J. Shi, and M. Sabbagh. 2017. Why do trials for Alzheimer's disease drugs keep failing? A discontinued drug perspective for 2010-2015. *Expert Opinion on Investigational Drugs* 26(6):735-739.

Mielke, M. 2024. Sex and gender differences in Alzheimer's disease and Alzheimer's disease related dementias. Commissioned Paper for the Committee on Research Priorities for Preventing and Treating Alzheimer's Disease and Related Dementias. https://doi.org/10.17226/28588.

Mielke, M. M., N. T. Aggarwal, C. Vila-Castelar, P. Agarwal, E. M. Arenaza-Urquijo, B. Brett, A. Brugulat-Serrat, L. E. DuBose, W. S. Eikelboom, J. Flatt, N. S. Foldi, S. Franzen, P. Gilsanz, W. Li, A. J. McManus, D. M. van Lent, S. A. Milani, C. E. Shaaban, S. D. Stites, E. Sundermann, V. Suryadevara, J. F. Trani, A. D. Turner, J. M. J. Vonk, Y. T. Quiroz, and G. M. Babulal. 2022. Consideration of sex and gender in Alzheimer's disease and related disorders from a global perspective. *Alzheimer's & Dementia* 18(12):2707-2724.

Nag, S., and J. A. Schneider. 2023. Limbic-predominant age-related TDP43 encephalopathy (LATE) neuropathological change in neurodegenerative diseases. *Nature Reviews: Neurology* 19(9):525-541.

NAM (National Academy of Medicine). 2017. *Vital directions for health & health care: An initiative of the National Academy of Medicine.* Washington, DC: The National Academies Press.

NASEM (National Academies of Sciences, Engineering, and Medicine). 2017. *Preventing cognitive decline and dementia: A way forward.* Edited by A. I. Leshner, S. Landis, C. Stroud, and A. Downey. Washington, DC: The National Academies Press.

NASEM. 2021a. *Meeting the challenge of caring for persons living with dementia and their care partners and caregivers: A way forward.* Edited by E. B. Larson and C. Stroud. Washington, DC: The National Academies Press.

NASEM. 2021b. *Reducing the impact of dementia in America: A decadal survey of the behavioral and social sciences.* Washington, DC: The National Academies Press.

Nebel, R. A., N. T. Aggarwal, L. L. Barnes, A. Gallagher, J. M. Goldstein, K. Kantarci, M. P. Mallampalli, E. C. Mormino, L. Scott, W. H. Yu, P. M. Maki, and M. M. Mielke. 2018. Understanding the impact of sex and gender in Alzheimer's disease: A call to action. *Alzheimer's & Dementia* 14(9):1171-1183.

Ngandu, T., J. Lehtisalo, A. Solomon, E. Levälahti, S. Ahtiluoto, R. Antikainen, L. Bäckman, T. Hänninen, A. Jula, T. Laatikainen, J. Lindström, F. Mangialasche, T. Paajanen, S. Pajala, M. Peltonen, R. Rauramaa, A. Stigsdotter-Neely, T. Strandberg, J. Tuomilehto, H. Soininen, and M. Kivipelto. 2015. A 2-year multidomain intervention of diet, exercise, cognitive training, and vascular risk monitoring versus control to prevent cognitive decline in at-risk elderly people (FINGER): A randomised controlled trial. *Lancet* 385(9984):2255-2263.

NIA (National Institute on Aging). 2021. *What is mild cognitive impairment?* https://www.nia.nih.gov/health/memory-loss-and-forgetfulness/what-mild-cognitive-impairment (accessed October 23, 2024).

NIA. 2022. *How biomarkers help diagnose dementia.* https://www.nia.nih.gov/health/alzheimers-symptoms-and-diagnosis/how-biomarkers-help-diagnose-dementia (accessed August 13, 2024).

NIA. 2024a. *AD and ADRD research implementation milestones.* https://www.nia.nih.gov/research/milestones (accessed August 22, 2024).

NIA. 2024b. *Accelerating Medicines Partnership Program for Alzheimer's disease (AMP AD).* https://www.nia.nih.gov/research/amp-ad (accessed August 22, 2024).

NIH RePORT. 2024. *Estimates of funding for various research, condition, and disease categories.* https://report.nih.gov/funding/categorical-spending#/ (accessed October 23, 2024).

NIMH (National Institute of Mental Health). 2024. *What is prevalence?* https://www.nimh.nih.gov/health/statistics/what-is-prevalence (accessed August 13, 2024).

NINDS (National Institute of Neurological Disorders and Stroke). 2022. *ADRD Summit 2022 report.* https://www.ninds.nih.gov/sites/default/files/documents/ADRD%20Summit%20 2022%20Report%20to%20NINDS%20Council%20FINAL.pdf (accessed October 31, 2024).

NINDS. 2024. *Focus on multiple-etiology dementias (MED) research.* https://www.ninds.nih.gov/current-research/focus-disorders/alzheimers-disease-and-related-dementias/focus-multiple-etiology-dementias-med-research#:~:text=Multiple%2Detiology%20 dementia%20symptoms%20may,mixed%20dementias%20(e.g.%2C%20Neurology (accessed August 13, 2024).

Pink, A., J. Krell-Roesch, J. A. Syrjanen, L. R. Christenson, V. J. Lowe, P. Vemuri, J. A. Fields, G. B. Stokin, W. K. Kremers, E. L. Scharf, C. R. Jack, D. S. Knopman, R. C. Petersen, M. Vassilaki, and Y. E. Geda. 2023. Interactions between neuropsychiatric symptoms and Alzheimer's disease neuroimaging biomarkers in predicting longitudinal cognitive decline. *Psychiatric Research and Clinical Practice* 5(1):4-15.

Powell, W. R., W. R. Buckingham, J. L. Larson, L. Vilen, M. Yu, M. S. Salamat, B. B. Bendlin, R. A. Rissman, and A. J. H. Kind. 2020. Association of neighborhood-level disadvantage with Alzheimer's disease neuropathology. *JAMA Network Open* 3(6):e207559.

Ramirez, L. A., and J. C. Sullivan. 2018. Sex differences in hypertension: Where we have been and where we are going. *American Journal of Hypertension* 31(12):1247-1254.

Ruitenberg, A., A. Ott, J. C. van Swieten, A. Hofman, and M. M. Breteler. 2001. Incidence of dementia: Does gender make a difference? *Neurobiology of Aging* 22(4):575-580.

Sarkar, S., N. Das, and K. Sambamurti. 2024. Development of early biomarkers of Alzheimer's disease: A precision medicine perspective. In *Comprehensive precision medicine*, 1st ed., Vol. 2, edited by K. S. Ramos. Elsevier, pp.511-525.

Sims, J. R., J. A. Zimmer, C. D. Evans, M. Lu, P. Ardayfio, J. Sparks, A. M. Wessels, S. Shcherbinin, H. Wang, E. S. Monkul Nery, E. C. Collins, P. Solomon, S. Salloway, L. G. Apostolova, O. Hansson, C. Ritchie, D. A. Brooks, M. Mintun, D. M. Skovronsky, and TRAILBLAZER-ALZ 2 Investigators. 2023. Donanemab in early symptomatic Alzheimer disease: The TRAILBLAZER-ALZ 2 randomized clinical trial. *JAMA* 330(6):512-527.

Simuni, T., L. M. Chahine, K. Poston, M. Brumm, T. Buracchio, M. Campbell, S. Chowdhury, C. Coffey, L. Concha-Marambio, T. Dam, P. DiBiaso, T. Foroud, M. Frasier, C. Gochanour, D. Jennings, K. Kieburtz, C. M. Kopil, K. Merchant, B. Mollenhauer, T. Montine, K. Nudelman, G. Pagano, J. Seibyl, T. Sherer, A. Singleton, D. Stephenson, M. Stern, C. Soto, C. M. Tanner, E. Tolosa, D. Weintraub, Y. Xiao, A. Siderowf, B. Dunn, and K. Marek. 2024. A biological definition of neuronal alpha-synuclein disease: Towards an integrated staging system for research. *Lancet Neurology* 23(2):178-190.

Tenny, S., and S. W. Boktor. 2023. Incidence. In *Statpearls*. Treasure Island, FL: StatPearls Publishing.

Toepper, M. 2017. Dissociating normal aging from Alzheimer's disease: A view from cognitive neuroscience. *Journal of Alzheimer's Disease* 57(2):331-352.

van Dyck, C. H., C. J. Swanson, P. Aisen, R. J. Bateman, C. Chen, M. Gee, M. Kanekiyo, D. Li, L. Reyderman, S. Cohen, L. Froelich, S. Katayama, M. Sabbagh, B. Vellas, D. Watson, S. Dhadda, M. Irizarry, L. D. Kramer, and T. Iwatsubo. 2023. Lecanemab in early Alzheimer's disease. *New England Journal of Medicine* 388(1):9-21.

WHO (World Health Organization). 2021. *World failing to address dementia challenge*. https://www.who.int/news/item/02-09-2021-world-failing-to-address-dementia-challenge (accessed August 13, 2024).

WHO. 2022. *Optimizing brain health across the life course: WHO position paper*. https://www.who.int/publications/i/item/9789240054561 (accessed August 13, 2024).

WHO. 2023. *Dementia*. https://www.who.int/news-room/fact-sheets/detail/dementia (accessed August 22, 2024).

Wimo, A., K. Seeher, R. Cataldi, E. Cyhlarova, J. L. Dielemann, O. Frisell, M. Guerchet, L. Jonsson, A. K. Malaha, E. Nichols, P. Pedroza, M. Prince, M. Knapp, and T. Dua. 2023. The worldwide costs of dementia in 2019. *Alzheimer's & Dementia* 19(7):2865-2873.

Wing, J., D. A. Levine, A. Ramamurthy, and C. Reider. 2020. Alzheimer's disease and related disorders prevalence differs by Appalachian residence in Ohio. *Journal of Alzheimer's Disease* 76(4):1309-1316.

Wolters, F. J., L. B. Chibnik, R. Waziry, R. Anderson, C. Berr, A. Beiser, J. C. Bis, D. Blacker, D. Bos, C. Brayne, J. F. Dartigues, S. K. L. Darweesh, K. L. Davis-Plourde, F. de Wolf, S. Debette, C. Dufouil, M. Fornage, J. Goudsmit, L. Grasset, V. Gudnason, C. Hadjichrysanthou, C. Helmer, M. A. Ikram, M. K. Ikram, E. Joas, S. Kern, L. H. Kuller, L. Launer, O. L. Lopez, F. E. Matthews, K. McRae-McKee, O. Meirelles, T. H. Mosley, Jr., M. P. Pase, B. M. Psaty, C. L. Satizabal, S. Seshadri, I. Skoog, B. C. M. Stephan, H. Wetterberg, M. M. Wong, A. Zettergren, and A. Hofman. 2020. Twenty-seven-year time trends in dementia incidence in Europe and the United States: The Alzheimer Cohorts Consortium. *Neurology* 95(5):e519-e531.

Yaffe, K., E. Vittinghoff, S. Dublin, C. B. Peltz, L. E. Fleckenstein, D. E. Rosenberg, D. E. Barnes, B. H. Balderson, and E. B. Larson. 2024. Effect of personalized risk-reduction strategies on cognition and dementia risk profile among older adults: The SMARRT randomized clinical trial. *JAMA Internal Medicine* 184(1):54-62.

Zissimopoulos, J., E. Crimmins, and P. St. Clair. 2014. The value of delaying Alzheimer's disease onset. *Forum of Health and Economic Policy* 18(1):25-39.

Zissimopoulos, J. M., B. C. Tysinger, P. A. St. Clair, and E. M. Crimmins. 2018. The impact of changes in population health and mortality on future prevalence of Alzheimer's disease and other dementias in the United States. *Journals of Gerontology: Series B, Psychological Sciences and Social Sciences* 73(Suppl 1):S38-S47.

2

Research Enabling the Longitudinal Evaluation of Brain Health and the Detection, Diagnosis, and Monitoring of AD/ADRD

The ability to precisely measure brain health over time and to accurately predict, detect, diagnose, and monitor changes in cognitive function is prerequisite to realizing significant advances in the prevention and treatment of Alzheimer's disease and related dementias (AD/ADRD). In most cases, changes in the brain that lead to clinical dementia occur slowly over a period of decades. Knowing when and how best to intervene to prevent early triggers and perturbations or to change disease trajectory through treatment relies on an understanding of the unfolding of this longitudinal process. While research in recent years has led to significant progress in the capability to detect early changes in brain health and to identify specific brain pathologies associated with different forms of dementia, which often co-occur, there is still much that is not understood about the processes that give rise to AD/ADRD over the life course and how to prevent, delay, and halt these diseases. Additionally, research advances have not been adequately translated into clinical practice.

The number of people living with AD/ADRD continues to grow rapidly as the U.S. population ages. People experiencing changes in brain health struggle to get an accurate and timely diagnosis—a challenge exacerbated by the contribution of multiple chronic conditions and mixed brain pathologies to mild cognitive impairment (MCI) and clinical dementia—and to know what steps to take to maintain their cognitive and functional abilities. Thus, despite the progress that has been made, there is a critical need to advance the capability to precisely monitor brain health and identify when changes are indicative of a neuropathological change, and to determine causes and track progression of AD/ADRD.

This chapter describes priority areas of research that can address current scientific gaps. It begins with an overview of the benefits and challenges related to the detection and diagnosis of AD/ADRD and the ongoing monitoring of brain health. It goes on to examine the opportunities for data collection across the life course to enable brain health monitoring and early detection and accurate diagnosis of AD/ADRD. The chapter ends with a discussion of opportunities and tools to integrate knowledge from research into clinical care to advance a precision brain health approach.

ADDRESSING THE CHALLENGES RELATED TO THE DETECTION, DIAGNOSIS, AND MONITORING OF AD/ADRD TO ADVANCE PRECISION BRAIN HEALTH

As exemplified by the experiences of two members of this committee described in the prologue of this report, the journey to a diagnosis is too often a long and painful process characterized by uncertainty, frustration, emotional distress, and a sense of urgency for the individuals living with AD/ADRD, as well as their loved ones (Grunberg et al., 2022). Many people who consult with a physician regarding subjective cognitive impairments will not receive a diagnosis (Roth et al., 2023).

Little has changed about the clinical diagnostic process for AD/ADRD in the last decade. Complicated diagnostic journeys such as those faced by the two members of this committee and countless others raise questions regarding how the diagnostic process could have been improved if better data had been available earlier and knowledge gained from research was better integrated into clinical care. Recent biomedical advances, including in the areas of biomarker discovery and digital health technologies (discussed later in this chapter), are providing opportunities to significantly change the way brain health is monitored over time and to move the detection and diagnosis of AD/ADRD much earlier in the disease course.

Importance of Brain Health Monitoring, Early Detection, and Accurate Diagnosis

In the context of a life-course brain health optimization model (discussed in Chapter 1), a key function of brain health monitoring is to allow early intervention to maintain brain health, such as through lifestyle or health behavior modification, to preserve and improve brain structure and function well before the age of risk when changes transition from within the range of normal to the point of disease development. The identification of early risk factors that can be used to predict later-life cognitive impairment or clinical dementia enables targeted preventive approaches that can be applied throughout the life course (e.g., mitigation of midlife risk factors) to optimize brain health in those most likely to benefit.

While maintaining brain health is the ideal goal, there are similarly benefits to early diagnosis, ideally before the onset of clinical symptoms (i.e., preclinical diagnosis; risks and benefits associated with preclinical diagnosis are discussed later in this chapter). The hope is that interventions (pharmacological and/or nonpharmacological) implemented at the preclinical disease stage,[1] either by the individual or under the guidance of a clinician, may delay or slow progression of AD/ADRD to prevent cognitive impairment and the eventual loss of function and independence. In the absence of disease modifying therapies, distinguishing AD from related dementias may have had little effect on clinical management of patients presenting with MCI or clinical dementia. However, with the approval of anti-amyloid treatments (aducanumab, lecanemab, and donanemab) and the likelihood that some future drugs will target pathologies that are specific to AD or a related dementia, accurate diagnosis is needed to inform decisions regarding the appropriate treatments.

Current evidence suggests that recently approved anti-amyloid therapies may work best for people in the early stages of Alzheimer's disease (AD) (see Chapter 4); the same may be true for future therapies for AD/ADRD. In the event that preclinical disease progresses to clinical symptoms, early diagnosis can enable the initiation of treatment early enough to maximize the chances of changing the disease trajectory. It can additionally provide people with the time and resources needed to plan for, and adapt to, eventual cognitive and behavioral changes associated with disease progression, including financial and decision-making implications (NASEM, 2021a).

Beyond the benefits to individuals, the ability to predict, detect, accurately diagnose, and phenotype AD/ADRD is critical to advancing research on preventive and therapeutic interventions and the development of precision medicine approaches. Accurate diagnosis and phenotyping allow for the identification of risk profiles and enable population stratification, which is a key factor in the success of precision medicine approaches, the aim of which is to ensure that the right people receive the right intervention(s) at the right time (discussed further in Chapter 4). Accurate diagnosis is also the basis for understanding trial results and designing future trials. The ability to longitudinally monitor disease allows the measurement of responses to interventions, which can help to identify effective interventions or inform changes to intervention strategies in the absence of evidence of benefit.

---

[1] In the context of AD/ADRD, preclinical disease is characterized by brain pathology in the absence of cognitive impairment.

Challenges Impeding Brain Health Monitoring and AD/ADRD Detection and Diagnosis

There are numerous challenges that impede ongoing brain health monitoring and early and accurate diagnosis of AD/ADRD. Key scientific gaps remain in the understanding of how best to define and measure brain health and AD/ADRD and in the availability of tools with the capability to ascertain brain health status throughout the life course, including the presence of pathophysiological features of AD/ADRD.

Clinical symptoms of AD and related dementias often overlap, making it difficult to accurately diagnose an individual based solely on cognitive, behavioral, or personality changes. Additionally, presentations of disease may be atypical, such as nonamnestic presentations of AD where memory impairment is not the primary cognitive deficit (McKhann et al., 2011), and may differ across subpopulations and individuals depending on the brain region affected, among other factors, all of which adds to the diagnostic complexity (Devi, 2023). Cognitive impairment is not dichotomous but occurs on a continuum. Early changes in cognition may be subtle and difficult to detect with many initial neuropsychological screening tools. Moreover, as cognitive assessments are rarely conducted during routine clinical visits (a notable gap in a brain health optimization paradigm), a lack of baseline for cognitive function can make it difficult to detect a decline. All of these factors may contribute to underdiagnosis.

Research in recent years has led to a paradigm shift in the understanding of the development of cognitive impairment and clinical dementia. It is now clear that the etiology is in most cases multifactorial, and mixed pathologies are predominant, with numerous potential combinations of amyloid plaques, tau tangles, cerebrovascular disease, and other pathologies (Dubois et al., 2021). The role of different pathologies in driving clinical symptoms remains unclear. This complexity makes it challenging to accurately diagnose patients, characterize disease phenotypes, and differentiate the individual diseases that contribute to clinical dementia—raising questions about the current systems for distinguishing these neurodegenerative disorders (Ritchie et al., 2015). The distinction of AD/ADRD from other neurodegenerative diseases such as amyotrophic lateral sclerosis or Parkinson's disease can also be difficult owing to disease co-occurrence and shared pathologic features, such as proteinopathies (Chu et al., 2023; Kawakami et al., 2019). Improved tools and methods are needed to better understand mixed pathologies, the connections between different pathologies, and clinical syndromes.

Given the diversity of potential pathologies that contribute to dementia, the challenges diagnosing AD/ADRD based on clinical symptoms, and the long period of silent pathophysiologic development prior to manifestation of clinical symptoms, significant research investments are focused on the development of biomarkers for AD/ADRD that can enable earlier and more accurate diagnosis, as discussed in more detail later in this chapter. Advances in the capability to detect specific neuropathologies has led to proposals to redefine AD and other neurodegenerative diseases based on biomarkers (see Box 2-1). The development of a biological definition is most advanced for AD but similar efforts are being pursued for neuronal alpha-synuclein disease, a group of diseases that includes Lewy body dementia (LBD). Ultimately, biomarker panels may enable the precise determination of specific co-occurring pathologies present. However, there is a notable gap between biomarker-based definitions of AD/ADRD being employed in research settings and current clinical diagnostic processes used in the United States, which, as described earlier, are in most cases based solely on symptoms and cognitive testing without confirmation by imaging or other biomarkers.

Of note, the use of cerebrospinal fluid (CSF) amyloid beta and tau (e.g., total tau, phosphorylated tau) biomarkers in dementia diagnosis is common in European countries (Hort et al., 2010). However, even with the availability of more precise diagnostic tools, a lack of effective treatments may also discourage physicians from pursuing a definitive diagnosis (Dubois et al., 2016), although this may change as more target-specific treatments approved by the U.S. Food and Drug Administration (FDA) become available on the market.

There are also social and systemic issues (e.g., socioeconomic and cultural barriers) that impede AD/ADRD detection and early diagnosis and may contribute to underdiagnosis. These include the following:

- Lack of public awareness regarding signs and symptoms that could indicate an early change in brain health and that may warrant discussion with a health professional;
- Access and equity issues such as lack of access to care because of costs and lack of insurance, transportation difficulties, and absence of specialists in certain geographic areas with the knowledge and resources to detect and diagnose AD/ADRD; and
- Resistance to seeking a diagnosis owing to the fear of being stigmatized (see Box 2-2) and fear of the resulting family burden and costs (Dubois et al., 2016; Stites et al., 2022).

Framing public education efforts as brain health rather than brain disease might have better penetration and help to overcome some (albeit not all) of these social and systemic barriers.

BOX 2-1
Biological Definitions for Alzheimer's Disease
and Related Dementias (AD/ADRD)

Symptoms of AD/ADRD are often overlapping, creating challenges to accurate diagnosis and, as more pathology-specific drugs become available, the appropriate targeting of treatments to people with mild cognitive impairment (MCI) and clinical dementia. In response to these challenges, there has been an effort in recent years to define AD and other neurodegenerative diseases using a biological definition. While these efforts are most advanced for AD (Dubois et al., 2021; Hampel et al., 2021; Jack et al., 2018, 2024), similar efforts are underway for neuronal alpha-synuclein disease, a group of diseases that includes Lewy body dementia (LBD) (Höglinger et al., 2024; Simuni et al., 2024).

The Definition of Alzheimer's Disease: The definition of AD and how it is diagnosed has evolved over the past century and has become a contentious topic. At the heart of the latest controversy is whether the definition of AD should be based on specific brain pathologies, in particular amyloid plaques and tau tangles, alone. Coupled with that are questions regarding the extent to which the clinical syndrome of cognitive decline and loss of functional independence should be considered. To illustrate this point, if a patient who had a clinical diagnosis of AD has an autopsy performed and is found to have TDP-43 pathology consistent with frontotemporal lobar dementia (FTLD-TDP) and a progranulin mutation, but no evidence of amyloid plaques or paired-helical filament tangles on neuropathological examination, did that patient really have AD?

In 2011 and 2018, the Alzheimer's Association and the National Institute on Aging convened workgroups to develop frameworks to guide diagnosis of AD, initially for use in clinical research and more recently to translate into clinical practice. In 2024, the Alzheimer's Association workgroup published an updated framework that endorsed a biological definition of AD and proposed guidelines for staging the disease with biomarkers and imaging (Jack et al., 2024). This framework differentiates the clinical syndrome of dementia from the currently proposed underlying etiologies and describes clinical staging for people with biological evidence of AD. The revised criteria in the 2024 framework define specific "Core 1" amyloid and tau biomarkers (e.g., amyloid-positron emissions tomography [PET], plasma phosphorylated (p)-tau217, and certain hybrid ratios such as CSF amyloid beta 42/40 and CSF p-tau 181/amyloid beta 42) that become abnormal early in the course of disease and can be used individually or in combination for the purposes of AD diagnosis (Jack et al., 2024). Other forms of tau reflecting deposits of aggregated tau in the brain that become abnormal later in the disease course (Core 2), along with AD-nonspecific biomarkers of neurodegeneration and inflammation, can be used in staging, prognosis, and as an indicator of biological treatment effect. Importantly, under the revised criteria, amyloid-PET alone is sufficient for AD diagnosis, a notable change from the 2018 criteria that required pathologic amyloid and tau (Jack et al., 2024).

Confirming whether a patient with MCI or mild clinical dementia has AD pathology has become particularly relevant in the setting of Food and Drug Administration (FDA)-approved anti-amyloid antibodies. Multiple studies have demonstrated that up to 37 percent of patients with an MCI diagnosis and up to 25 percent of patients with mild dementia diagnosed with clinical AD do not show evidence of AD pathology on biomarker testing or autopsy studies (Bangen et al., 2016; Cummings, 2019; Landau et al., 2016; Sevigny et al., 2016). Recent advances in blood-based biomarkers should enable a more accurate diagnosis of AD and avoid the need for PET imaging or lumbar puncture to obtain CSF measures in most cases.

Defining AD by the pathologic process in the brain, specifically amyloid and tau pathology, is viewed by some as too reductionist, and not in keeping with the lay public conception of AD as the clinical dementia syndrome. Perhaps the most controversial issue is that a biological definition of AD allows for the detection of AD in people who do not yet have symptoms (the preclinical stage of AD). The workgroup recommended against testing biomarkers in asymptomatic people outside of research studies until there is evidence from ongoing prevention trials that treating at this stage of disease is beneficial.

Although convergent evidence suggests that cognitively unimpaired individuals with high levels of amyloid, and especially combined with abnormal tau biomarkers, are at increased risk of decline over time (Cody et al., 2024; Ossenkoppele et al., 2022; Sperling et al., 2024), it is important to acknowledge that many individuals with detectable amyloid neuropathology (particularly if not accompanied by tau pathology) will not progress to dementia within their lifetime. This raises concern for significant "overdiagnosis" and costly and potentially harmful treatment in an estimated 47 million U.S. adults (Brookmeyer and Abdalla, 2018) with biomarker-defined preclinical AD. Additional work is needed to understand the mechanisms of cognitive resilience that allow people to remain cognitively intact in the setting of brain pathology, as well as resistance mechanisms that allow some individuals with high amyloid to avoid neocortical tau spreading that is more closely associated with imminent cognitive decline.

An additional issue arises from the findings from longitudinal observational cohorts that have included diagnostic biomarkers and autopsy

BOX 2-1 Continued

studies. These studies have made clear that multiple other neuro-degenerative processes contribute to cognitive decline, and that "pure" AD pathology—as defined by the presence of amyloid and tau—resulting in clinical dementia is relatively uncommon in older populations. Recent studies suggest that vascular pathology may exacerbate cognitive decline in the presence of amyloid pathology and potentially contributes to tau accumulation. This underscores the complexity of neurodegenerative disease, where multiple pathologies may coexist, leading to mixed pathology dementia. Currently, the lack of specific biomarkers for related dementias, such as vascular dementia, tauopathies such as frontotemporal dementia, and others makes it challenging to accurately diagnose these conditions. Consequently, individuals diagnosed with AD based solely on amyloid and tau positivity may actually have a different or mixed pathology dementia. In recognition that isolated AD is the exception in older populations with neuropathology, the revised criteria include biomarkers for copathologies that may commonly co-occur with AD, such as vascular brain injury as detected by magnetic resonance imaging and alpha-synuclein detected using seed amplification assays (Jack et al., 2024).

Beyond Alzheimer's Disease: Diagnosis and identification of other dementia syndromes are less controversial, but investment and advances in biomarkers have lagged behind AD. As biomarkers become available for related dementias, there has been interest in similar efforts to develop a biological definition of disease. In 2024, Simuni and colleagues (2024) proposed that Parkinson's disease and dementia with Lewy bodies be redefined as neuronal alpha-synuclein disease and suggested research criteria for a neuronal alpha-synuclein disease integrated staging system. Staging using the proposed system would be based on the presence of two biomarkers—neuronal alpha-synuclein and dopamine deficiency—the presence of pathogenic variants in the *SNCA* gene, and clinical signs and symptoms. Alternative research diagnostic criteria were proposed by Höglinger and colleagues (2024) that also included neuronal alpha-synuclein and genetic contributions (not limited to *SNCA*) but considered multiple forms of neurodegeneration beyond dopamine deficiency. As with the AD criteria, there remain many questions regarding the development of a biological definition for neurodegenerative diseases characterized by alpha-synuclein and the specific research criteria (Boeve et al., 2024). It is expected that criteria used in defining and staging AD/ADRD will continue to evolve as the development of biomarkers and disease modifying therapies advance.

BOX 2-2
Addressing the Stigma Associated with AD/ADRD

In surveys of middle-aged and older adults, dementia is commonly identified as one of the most feared health conditions of older age (Alzheimer Europe, 2011; Watson et al., 2023). Fear of dementia contributes to stigma associated with the disease, which can include patronization, stereotyping, social exclusion, and discrimination (ADI, 2012; Stites et al., 2022). Recent studies evaluating the social stigma associated with AD have illuminated its negative effects, which can include low self-esteem and isolation, along with poorer mental health outcomes and quality of life (Rosin et al., 2020; Stites et al., 2018). Stigma can also contribute to reduced health-seeking behaviors, resulting in later diagnosis, less use of health care services, and ultimately worse health outcomes (ADI, 2012; Rosin et al., 2020; Stites et al., 2018). For this reason, targeted efforts to reduce the stigma and harmful rhetoric surrounding this disease are of paramount importance to benefit those currently living with AD/ADRD along with individuals who may be at risk.

A LIFE-COURSE APPROACH TO BRAIN HEALTH AND DETECTION, DIAGNOSIS, AND MONITORING OF AD/ADRD: ADVANCING A NEW RESEARCH PARADIGM

AD/ADRD development, including its timeline and trajectory, need to be considered in the context of changes in brain health over time. Such knowledge may ultimately enable the linking of specific interventions for brain health optimization, disease prevention, and treatment to different stages across an individual's entire life course. However, understanding of brain health over the life course is currently limited. Improving our understanding of brain health and disease development will require the identification of specific types of data that should be collected across different spans of the life course (see Figure 2-1).

There are myriad types of data that can be collected and evaluated over time that, if integrated, can provide a more comprehensive view of brain health and disease development. Collection of data that can help address current data biases are particularly important. While some forms of data relevant to AD/ADRD, such as those from blood-based biomarker testing and other molecular data derived from biosamples, are just coming to the forefront, many other types, including cognitive and functional data that make up clinical phenotypes as well as more routine health data (e.g., longitudinal measures of cardiovascular health), are currently collected in

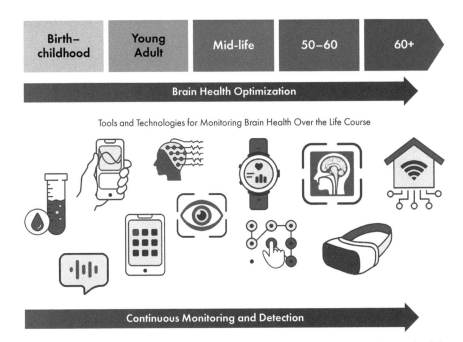

| Birth–childhood | Young Adult | Mid-life | 50–60 | 60+ |

Brain Health Optimization

Tools and Technologies for Monitoring Brain Health Over the Life Course

Continuous Monitoring and Detection

FIGURE 2-1 Data collection opportunities and approaches throughout the life course.
SOURCE: Adapted from a figure provided by Rhoda Au.

the clinical setting. However, siloing in the data collection and assessment process impedes efforts to develop a full clinical picture. For example, blood lipid levels and blood pressure may be routinely considered in assessing risk for cardiovascular disease (CVD) (Reitz, 2016) but not vascular dementia despite evidence connecting CVD and dementia risk.

Clinical assessments conducted by care providers may yield data on cognitive and psychological status, motor function, affect, sensory issues, patient history (e.g., social factors, exposures, clinical history), and patient experiences, such as sleep difficulties. Some of these data may be patient reported while for others standardized tools, such as screening assessments, provide an objective means for measuring change over time.

The accessibility of these types of data and their application to the ongoing monitoring of brain health and disease diagnosis continue to evolve as existing tests and tools are improved and as the development of new tools enables the detection and measurement of signs and symptoms that are currently missed. For example, although cognitive changes are often viewed as being toward the end of the disease trajectory (and generally later in the life course), with more sensitive measures, it may be found that these changes are not as downstream as once believed. By the time people notice symptoms of cognitive decline, often much has already changed in the brain. The ability to detect changes in an individual's capacity to learn, for example, could provide an early indicator of a change in brain health. This underscores the importance of a life-course approach whereby brain health is tracked and optimized over time and detection of a negative trajectory of decline is possible within a person's normal ranges of variability.

Digital tools are increasingly enabling some of these data (e.g., sleep disturbances, changes in motor function) to be collected outside of the clinic (e.g., via smartphone applications, wearables) and even in a passive manner (NIA, 2019), potentially providing a mechanism for alerting individuals and their clinicians when further assessment is warranted based on a change in status, and potentially facilitating earlier disease diagnosis. Sensitivity will need to be balanced with specificity and the implementation of such tools would need to consider the risk of alarm fatigue. This could be mitigated, for example, by alerting individuals based on trends involving multiple signals rather than single outlying data points, which would be a significant early detection advancement. By reducing reliance on subjective and self-reported measures, such tools may also help to address biases in clinical data.

While useful, these clinical and experiential data are not sufficient to elucidate the whole picture. It is also important to understand what is happening within the body, including biological signs of pathophysiology. At a gross level, this can be accomplished through imaging (e.g., positron emission topography [PET], magnetic resonance imaging [MRI]), which has been used to diagnose and monitor AD/ADRD. More recently, tests are being developed that can illuminate an individual's molecular and cellular landscape. Testing of blood, tissue, and CSF can provide information on peripheral and central biomarkers,[2] genetic risk, and epigenetic data that indicate how exposures have interacted with an individual's genetic makeup (Jia et al., 2024). Such data not only play a role in disease detection and diagnosis but can also contribute to an understanding of the mechanistic underpinnings for AD/ADRD (discussed further in Chapter 3). As understanding of what specific types of data need to be collected and when these data should be collected across the life course, and as tools and technologies are developed and validated, these can be integrated into personal and clinical care practices as part of a brain health approach (see Table 2-1).

---

[2] Peripheral biomarkers are measurable indicators of biological processes that may be measured less invasively from tissues outside the central nervous system, for example, using blood cells, skin fibroblasts, saliva, eyes (Htike et al., 2019). Central biomarkers, such as CSF samples and brain imaging (Hansson et al., 2018) are measurable indicators of biological processes occurring directly within the central nervous system.

TABLE 2-1 Example of Data Types and Collection Frequencies for the Purposes of Tracking Brain Health Across the Life Course

Example Data Types			Example Data Collection Frequency Across the Life Course
Biological measures	Blood	Genotype	Once
		Proteome	Set intervals throughout life
		Electrolytes	Set intervals throughout life
	Skin	Skin biopsy	Set intervals from mid to late life
	Brain	MRI	Set intervals throughout life
		PET	Set intervals from mid to late life
		CSF	Set intervals from mid to late life
Data on socioeconomic status		Parental income	Consistently throughout early life
		Developmental milestones	Consistently throughout early life
		Family stressors	Consistently throughout early life
		Personal income	Set intervals from mid to late life
		Education	Consistently throughout early life and young adult life
		Employment	Consistently throughout young adult to late life
		Relationships	Set intervals throughout life

Digital data	Wearable	Steps	Continuously from young adult to late life
		SpO$_2$ and VO$_2$ max	Continuously from young adult to late life
		Sleep	Continuously from young adult to late life
		6-min walk	Continuously from young adult to late life
	Smartphone	Video	Set intervals from mid to late life
		CLOX	Set intervals from mid to late life
		Audio	Set intervals from mid to late life
		EHR	Set intervals from mid to late life
Clinical data		Neuropsychiatric assessments	Consistently in later life
		Patient-reported outcome measures	Set intervals from mid to late life

NOTES: This table provides select examples of the potential types of data that could be integrated into personal and clinical care practices across the life course as part of a precision brain health approach. MRI = magnetic resonance imaging; PET = positron emission tomography; CSF = cerebrospinal fluid; SpO$_2$, VO$_2$ Max = oxygen saturation and maximum volume of oxygen; CLOX = clock drawing test; EHR = electronic health record.

Research is needed to identify and describe the essential data elements necessary to inform AD/ADRD prediction, detection, diagnosis, treatment (selection, dose adjustment, and cessation), and ongoing monitoring (e.g., risk and resilience factors, molecular biomarkers, clinical signs and symptoms) and to understand how those essential data elements relate to the health of a person over the life course.

Conclusion 2-1: The current, incomplete understanding of brain health throughout the life course impedes the development of accessible and sensitive clinical tools that can predict, diagnose, and monitor changes in cognitive function and inform strategies to maximize brain health and prevent and treat AD/ADRD.

Improving and Expanding Tools for Assessing Cognition, Function, and Other Measures

Recent biomedical advances are paving the way for a major paradigm shift in the detection, diagnosis, and management of AD/ADRD. Current processes that rely on identification of clinical symptoms are inherently late-stage focused, but in the near future, new and improved tools such as blood-based biomarkers and digitally based assessments may provide earlier signals of changes in brain health, as compared to traditional cognitive assessments, and reduce reliance on invasive and expensive tests such as PET imaging and CSF biomarker tests (see Figure 2-2). Earlier detection and diagnosis, better prediction of cognitive outcomes, and enhanced monitoring of AD/ADRD through biomarkers and digital technologies can guide decision-making algorithms for risk stratification and early intervention, thereby advancing a precision brain health approach (Hampel et al., 2022a).

This paradigm shift is already underway in the research setting but has yet to transition to the clinical environment where such issues as reimbursement and electronic health record integration influence the adoption of new tools (Cutler, 2024), as does uncertainty regarding their clinical usefulness (Hampel et al., 2022a). Investment in refining and developing tools for data collection should emphasize, though not solely focus on, universally scalable tools that can ultimately be incorporated into clinical practice. Universally scalable tools are appropriate for all populations and can be scaled for use at a population level, ideally without requiring specialized expertise. The case for investment rests on the ability to reduce cost of treatment at a population level (e.g., through prevention and thereby reducing the number of people requiring treatment or by reducing the amount of time for which treatment is needed). The real-world applicability and effects of a tool should therefore be a consideration in investment decisions.

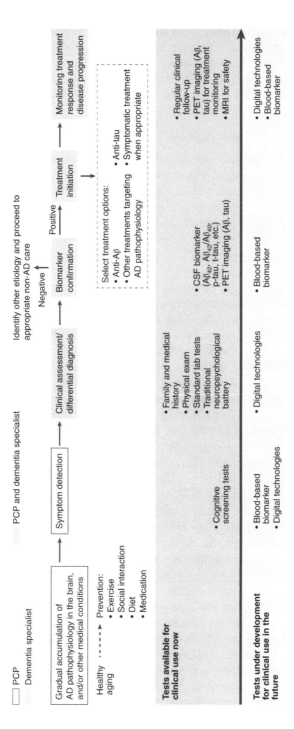

FIGURE 2-2 Incorporation of novel biomarkers and digital technologies into pathways for AD detection, diagnosis, and monitoring.
NOTE: AD = Alzheimer's disease; CSF = cerebrospinal fluid, PET = positron emission tomography, PCP = primary care provider.
SOURCE: Hampel et al., 2022a.

As discussed in the preceding section, variation in measures and methods is a major barrier to data aggregation. It will therefore be important to give early consideration to the harmonization and standardization of measures to accelerate advancements of new tests that are promising. Research consortia are well positioned to play a role in this harmonization process.

Traditional Clinical Assessment Tools

Several validated clinical assessment tools are commonly used in both research and clinical settings to objectively identify alterations in cognition, behavior, and function. These tools include patient-reported outcome measures (PROMs) and other clinician-administered tests for assessing cognitive function include the Mini-Mental State Examination, Montreal Cognitive Assessment, and Mini Cognitive Assessment Instrument. Functional and behavioral status may be assessed using an instrumental activities of daily living scale and the Neuropsychiatric Inventory Questionnaire, respectively. Such tools may be used by clinicians as part of routine screening or a diagnostic workup for patients presenting with subtle changes in cognition or behavior (Hampel et al., 2022a). They are also used in research studies to guide the selection of clinical trial participants and for evaluating outcomes following an intervention (Ng et al., 2018). In a research context, the diversity of available tests and measures impedes efforts to compare findings across studies and to pool data for analysis across multiple studies (NASEM, 2017; Ritchie et al., 2015), although these challenges are being addressed through efforts to develop composite scores (Crane et al., 2012) and harmonize data (Mukherjee et al., 2023).

Despite their widespread use, these clinical assessment tools suffer from a number of limitations. The most obvious limitation of PROMs is a reliance on a patient's ability to remember and report on their current state of function. Traditional modalities, such as clinician-administered pen-and-paper tests, are crude measures able to detect changes at later stages of cognitive impairment, but they are not able to detect early, more subtle changes in cognition. Such tests can also pose challenges for some individuals, including those with vision impairment, tremors, and similar physical impairments. Moreover, the data from such assessments may be biased; for example, such biases may be attributable to practice effects—although lack of a practice effect could be interpreted as an indicator of a cognitive issue (Öhman et al., 2021)—and the influences of cultural and language differences across populations that may skew test results and interpretations (Ng et al., 2018). The latter has been addressed through the development of visual-based cognitive screening tools that use culturally neutral pictures and figures and do not require language translation (Ng et al., 2018), but validation prior to clinical adoption is critical.

Furthermore, most clinical tests do not have gender-specific norms despite the fact that there are recognized gender differences in cognition throughout the lifespan. Women, for example, generally perform better on tests of verbal memory relative to men, which may reduce the likelihood of detecting amnestic MCI and result in the later diagnosis of women (Mielke, 2024). Recognizing these challenges, the National Institutes of Health (NIH) has invested in research infrastructure to develop and validate new tools that could be used in primary care and other similar care practice settings to detect cognitive impairment in diverse populations (see Box 2-3 for an example of such investments).

Digital Tools and Technologies

Digital tools and technologies have the potential to address some of the limitations of the traditional clinical assessment tools described above and are providing opportunities to answer questions that could not be addressed in the past. For example, a digital clock drawing test allows for real-time, highly sensitive assessment of neurocognitive behavior that would otherwise not be possible to obtain with the traditional pen-and-paper test currently used in clinical settings (Dion et al., 2020; Piers et al., 2017). Other examples include such technologies as tracking apps in smartphones and wearable fitness trackers, as well as home-based ambient sensing technologies (Cerino et al., 2021; NIA, 2019). The types of measures that can be collected using digital tools and technologies are broad and include sleep, gait, speech patterns, and typing behavior, changes in which may be indicators of early alterations in brain health or AD/ADRD development or progression. These technologies make it possible to collect data from environments in which people live (see Box 2-4), which allows that context to be captured and considered in analyses (Kaye, 2024). Moreover, by enabling frequent and even continuous data collection, data are less likely to be skewed by day-to-day variation in cognitive function (Cerino et al., 2021; Hampel et al., 2022a).

Digital tools and technologies enable passive data collection, which may reduce the cost and burden associated with data collection and help to reduce data bias. Passive data collection may also help overcome barriers to data collection arising from physical disabilities and sensory impairment, which may be common in some populations such as the oldest old (Corrada, 2024), as well as from those with advanced clinical dementia, for whom more active data collection may be challenging (Hampel et al., 2022a).

In the research setting, digital tools and technologies provide opportunities to increase inclusivity, allowing people interested in participating in research to collect and share data without the requirement (or with a

BOX 2-3
Consortium for Detecting Cognitive Impairment
Including Dementia

The National Institute of Neurological Disorders and Stroke (NINDS) and the National Institute on Aging (NIA)-funded Consortium for Detecting Cognitive Impairment, Including Dementia (DetectCID) is a collaborative research network established in 2017 and involves the collaboration of multidisciplinary research teams from the University of California San Francico, Albert Einstein College of Medicine, and Northwestern University (DetectCID, 2022). DetectCID is focused on improving the detection of cognitive impairment in primary care settings and in everyday clinical practice through the development, testing, and validation of novel paradigms, including new tools and protocols, to both increase the frequency and enhance the quality of patient evaluations. These efforts also prioritize addressing health disparities resulting from barriers to detection of cognitive impairment in diverse and underserved populations. The first phase of DetectCID focused on paradigm development and harmonization along with establishing interoperability among different evaluators and research sites.

The focus of the Consortium's second phase was on cohort and population testing along with optimizing and validating the novel paradigms, particularly primary-care and other everyday clinical contexts (DetectCID, 2022). Ultimately, each of the three research teams developed and piloted a paradigm for detecting incident cognitive impairment that included a user-friendly, short (less than 10 minutes) cognitive assessment and an implementation protocol for use in primary care. Features of the developed paradigms vary. For example, some tests can be performed on tablets and some are picture-based to meet the needs of low-literacy populations. One is available in multiple languages and another is designed to be self-administered (Bernstein Sideman et al., 2022). The MyCog Cognitive Screener developed by Northwestern University is being used in an NIH-funded pragmatic trial and is available through the NIH Toolbox (2024). TabCat-BHA developed by UCSF is available via an online platform (TabCAT, 2024).

reduced requirement) for traveling to study sites and submitting biosamples. This not only reduces the burden and barriers for people living with AD/ADRD who are interested in participating in research (Nicosia et al., 2023), but also moves the research enterprise closer to being able to use citizen science (Öhman et al., 2021).

NIH has made recent investments in resources to expand the accessibility of digital tools and technologies for use in research. The NIA-funded Mobile

---

BOX 2-4
In-Home Monitoring: Advances from the
Collaborative Aging Research Using Technology Initiative

The Collaborative Aging Research Using Technology (CART) Initiative is a multisite research initiative funded by National Institutes of Health (NIH) and the Department of Veterans Affairs (VA) that is using innovative new ways to study aging in place through the deployment of novel technologies and big data approaches to detect meaningful longitudinal changes in health across diverse populations of older adults. The four founding research sites for CART are Oregon Health and Science University (OHSU), Department of Veterans Affairs, Rush University, and University of Miami (OHSU, 2024a,b). The CART Initiative deploys a technology platform initially developed by OHSU's Oregon Center for Aging and Technology Life Lab (OHSU, 2024c). The system of in-home sensors, installed in participant homes at each site, continuously collects data in real time. Sensors are designed to be sensitive to the presence of people and to not interfere with the daily lives of participants. Data collected and analyzed by CART includes data on mobility (e.g., walking speed and movement between rooms), socialization (e.g., phone and e-mail use), medication adherence, sleeping behaviors, and physiologic functions (e.g., body mass index, pulse). The vast quantities of data produced through monitoring are then analyzed by researchers to understand subtle changes in activity and function over time (OHSU, 2024c). The CART Initiative has developed several collaborations to advance research on healthy aging using this platform and the data it collects. For example, the Ecologically Valid, Longitudinal, and Unbiased Assessment of Treatment Efficacy in Alzheimer Disease (EVALUATE-AD) Trial supported by NIH and Merck is using the CART platform to determine the feasibility of using in-home monitoring systems for detecting changes in meaningful outcomes in participants with mild cognitive impairment (MCI) or early-stage AD. CART is also collaborating with Emory University and Georgia Institute of Technology to assess the use of the CART platform as a modality for delivering interventions in the homes of participants enrolled in the MCI Empowerment Program (OHSU, 2024d).

Toolbox, for example, provides researchers with validated, digital cognitive and other health measures, such as digital measures derived from the Patient-Reported Outcomes Measurement Information System (PROMIS®), that can be integrated into remote cognitive assessments for research (Mobile Toolbox, 2024). The Mobile Toolbox also provides a platform to develop new smartphone applications, as well as to collect and manage digital data from participants (King and Wagster, 2024).

In the clinical context, digital tools and technologies may help reduce barriers to early detection and monitoring of changes in brain health, as well as early disease diagnosis (see Box 2-5). Health systems and clinical teams are already overwhelmed by the need for diagnosis and treatment of AD/ADRD given the time-sensitive nature of this group of diseases. As noted above, the routine clinical assessment (in its best case) with PROMs is time intensive on the part of both the patient and provider and relies on a patient's ability to remember and report on their current state of function.

BOX 2-5
Diagnostic Potential of Digital Data
Combined with Artificial Intelligence

Digital data combined with artificial intelligence (AI) approaches may provide novel, scalable, and cost-effective tools for screening and diagnosing Alzheimer's Disease and Related Dementias (AD/ADRD) in diverse populations regardless of language or sociocultural factors. Early efforts have included applying natural language processing methods to the assessment of digitized data from audio recordings of conventional neuropsychological exams. When the resulting data were combined with demographic data, models were able to classify participants into categories of normal cognition versus dementia, normal cognition or mild cognitive impairment (MCI) versus dementia, and normal cognition versus MCI (Amini et al., 2023; Paschalidis, 2024). Findings from this work suggest that this approach is effective in the identification of normal cognition from MCI and dementia and could be applicable as a remote tool that could be adapted to any language. This work did indicate less accuracy when differentiating normal cognition from MCI (Amini et al., 2023); however, other research demonstrated that a smartphone-based neuropsychological battery used to create a remote digital memory composite score could accurately and remotely distinguish cognitively healthy controls from participants living with MCI (Berron et al., 2024).

In addition to the described potential screening function, natural language processing techniques and machine learning methods are also being applied to digitized participant voice recordings from the Framingham Heart Study to predict progression from MCI to dementia—with an accuracy rate of 78.5 percent—within a 6-year span (Amini et al., 2024). This work demonstrates the potential use of digital data, such as digital voice data, in combination with AI methods to revolutionize the evaluation of brain health over time in ways that were not previously possible.

Digital tools that can offer continuous monitoring for alterations in brain health, such as changes identified in voice recordings or alterations in movement detected by smart watches and other wearables, may allow early intervention with nonpharmacological solutions when changes are still within the realm of normal, thereby potentially preventing disease development (Au et al., 2022; Öhman et al., 2021). Apps with digital versions of brief cognitive tests may help to identify early memory impairment associated with MCI (Berron et al., 2024; Cerino et al., 2021). By alerting individuals of a change in status that may indicate the need for a clinical assessment, such tools also offer opportunities to better support self-advocacy. They may also help to compensate for a lack of access to other diagnostic tools, such as some forms of imaging, that may not be available everywhere in the United States (e.g., rural areas), and they may improve the scalability and cost-effectiveness of regular screening for AD/ADRD (Öhman et al., 2021; Paschalidis, 2024). Despite the promising capabilities of digital tools and technologies, there remain several hurdles to their integration into clinical practice and mainstream use for ongoing brain health monitoring. With the notable exception of digital versions of existing clinical assessment tools, such as a digital Montreal Cognitive Assessment or Mini-Mental State Examination (Öhman et al., 2021), novel measures captured with these tools and technologies are not yet well accepted (Au et al., 2022). Validation efforts are needed to demonstrate the reliability of novel measures—that is, their accuracy relative to the outcome of interest. However, a challenge with the validation of digital tools and technologies is the lack of good reference data for benchmarking their performance (i.e., ground truthing). Given their own biases and other limitations, traditional clinical assessments may not be the best references against which to assess digital tools and technologies (Cook, 2024).

Another approach is to compare the digital data to fluid and/or imaging biomarker results (Öhman et al., 2021). In research contexts, digital tools and technologies are being used to collect data from people who often have not undergone biomarker or traditional clinical cognitive testing. Limiting data collection to those individuals who have undergone such testing would significantly limit the application and learning from digital tools and technologies. Another consideration is individuals' level of comfort with digital tools (Tsuang, 2024). Engaging people living with or at risk for AD/ADRD in the development of digital tools and technologies may increase acceptability and ensure the measures being captured are meaningful to those from whom the data will be collected.

Because we are unable to foresee which data will be useful for AD/ADRD detection, diagnosis, and monitoring, it is important to consider how raw data can best be stored and archived in digital repositories for future analysis. An advantage of stored digital data over banked biosamples is that digital data are not a finite resource. If properly stored, they can be used indefinitely and simultaneously by multiple data users without losing value over time. Thus, the return on collection and storage can be exponential.

There is also a need to consider and address data access, privacy, and confidentiality issues (Coravos et al., 2019) for different types of digital data. The use of commercial artificial intelligence (AI) and machine learning platforms for sharing and processing digital data, for example, may come with security and privacy concerns. De-identification, encryption, and the generation of synthetic data are potential approaches to data protection (Paschalidis, 2024). Developing the necessary data infrastructure that facilitates secure access to raw data in parallel to analytic methods is critical to realizing the full capabilities of these tools and technologies (Au et al., 2023).

Given the pace of technological advancements, investment in infrastructure and other resources may be needed to ensure academics can continue to push the cutting edge (Kaye, 2024; Paschalidis, 2024). For example, one needed resource to move digital tools forward is open-source digital data collection and processing tools for such functions as customizable applications, quality control, de-identification of data, and defining statistical summaries of the raw signal that capture some feature of clinical interest. Additional work is needed to rethink what data harmonization will need to look like given that (1) the technologies used to collect data will continue to evolve both for existing methods and still-to-emerge ones and (2) different analytic strategies have different definitions of what is analyzable (e.g., biostatistics versus automated AI analytics). Further, legacy methods of data sharing need to give way to new approaches that make data more easily and freely accessible and promote true democratization of data, without being hampered by outdated patriarchal governance and oversight policies or unnecessary data transfer fees.

Biomarkers

Biomarker discovery for AD/ADRD is a rapidly expanding area of research and holds considerable promise for accelerating the prevention, diagnosis, and treatment of AD/ADRD. Biomarkers have different uses across the clinical continuum, including the characterization of risk; detection, diagnosis, and staging of disease (focused on both prodromal and symptomatic phases); prognosis; and measurement of intervention effect (Figure 2-3). The clinical significance of biomarkers arises from their potential to aid in the early and accurate diagnosis of AD/ADRD and to guide treatment decisions based on subtyping, such that patients are matched with therapies that are likely to work best for them.

There are myriad types of diagnostic and prognostic biomarkers under investigation, including fluid biomarkers, novel imaging biomarkers, digital

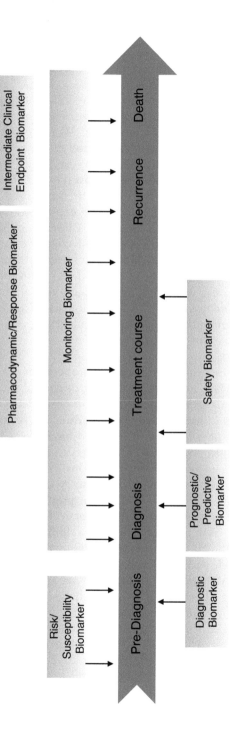

FIGURE 2-3 Biomarkers across the clinical continuum.
SOURCE: Cagney et al., 2018.

biomarkers, cognitive biomarkers, ocular biomarkers, and biomarkers of change in other areas (e.g., motor skills, sensory including vision and hearing). NIH has made significant investments in programs to support these biomarker discovery efforts (see Box 2-6).

It is important to keep in mind that many kinds of clinical data that may be collected are not biomarkers. Biomarkers need to be validated for their intended purpose (FDA-NIH Biomarker Working Group, 2020). A critical aspect of validation studies will be the evaluation of biomarker performance in diverse subpopulations (e.g., racial/ethnic, sex/gender, age) to understand any observed group-specific positivity differences. Variation in positivity across demographic groups has been observed for some biomarker types (e.g., PET imaging) but may be explained, for example, by inadequate stratification by disease status (MCI versus clinical dementia) or differences in the predominant etiology of cognitive impairment and dementia across groups, which may not be delineated by current diagnostic tools (Gao et al., 2023). The sections below describe promising advances and remaining gaps related to fluid, imaging, and digital biomarkers used to detect, diagnose, and monitor AD/ADRD. Biomarkers used in the context of clinical trials to demonstrate target engagement and evaluate responses to interventions are discussed in Chapter 4.

Fluid biomarkers   Tests to detect biomarkers of certain brain pathologies in AD using CSF or PET imaging are already in clinical use, but development of less invasive and more accessible and cost-effective blood-based biomarkers is an area of urgent need. Recent years have seen exciting progress in the discovery of peripheral, fluid-based biomarkers (Barthelemy et al., 2024; Gonzalez-Ortiz et al., 2023; Palmqvist et al., 2020; Zetterberg, 2022) that may help to address the limitations associated with imaging (e.g., cost, access in some regions of the country, coverage by insurance, need for highly trained analysts) and enable population-level screening. Although translation of these research advances to clinical practice has been slow, a blood test is now commercially available for AD based on blood amyloid levels, and the plasma phospho-tau biomarker p-tau217 has been demonstrated to be clinically equivalent to FDA-approved CSF biomarker tests used to detect AD pathology (Barthelemy et al., 2024). P-tau217 has been shown to detect AD neuropathological change in patients as many as 10 years before symptom onset and provides an opportunity to divide risks into AD versus non-AD risks. While more invasive than blood-based biomarkers, CSF biomarkers have also shown promise in detecting pathologic changes earlier than neuroimaging (Dubois et al., 2023)

At present, clinical recommendations indicate that blood-based biomarker tests and other AD diagnostics should not be used in clinical settings in asymptomatic patients; regardless, the potential to use simple finger stick

BOX 2-6
Examples of NIH Infrastructure Investments in Biomarker Discovery for Alzheimer's Disease and Related Dementias (AD/ADRD)

Centrally Linked Longitudinal Peripheral Biomarkers of Alzheimer's Disease in Multiethnic Populations (CLEAR-AD) Program: CLEAR-AD is an NIA-funded U19 program initiated in 2023 that focuses on discovering and validating centrally-linked peripheral molecular signatures (CLPMS) of Alzheimer's disease (AD) in multiethnic populations (CLEAR-AD, 2024a; NIH RePORTER, 2024a). The $41 million program is led by Mayo Clinic Florida and the Indiana University School of Medicine (CLEAR-AD, 2024b) and has the following aims:

1. "To discover CLPMS of the complex and heterogeneous AD pathophysiology and its copathologies.
2. To identify longitudinal CLPMS that detect and predict dynamic neuroimaging, fluid biomarker, and clinical changes across AD spectrum.
3. To characterize differences and similarities in CLPMS profiles across NHW [non-Hispanic White], African American (AA) and Latino American (LA) participants to uncover biomarker patterns in multi-ethnic groups.
4. To make these vast resources available to the scientific community to amplify and accelerate its impact" (CLEAR-AD, 2024a).

Through these efforts the program will advance the identification of novel AD biomarkers with mechanistic insights, support a precision medicine approach to the discovery and validation of multiomics biomarkers, discover new potential therapeutic targets, and create a harmonized resource of endophenotype and multiomics data in NIH-supported cohorts for sharing with the scientific community (CLEAR-AD, 2024a).

Alzheimer's Disease Neuroimaging Initiative (ADNI): ADNI was launched in 2004 as a longitudinal, multicenter study to validate biomarkers (e.g., imaging, genetic, biofluid) for AD (ADNI, 2024a). The ADNI study involves researchers across more than 60 sites in the United States and Canada who are collecting biomarker data to monitor the progression of AD in the brain across three disease stages: cognitively unimpaired, MCI, and clinical dementia (ADNI, 2024a). The primary goals of this initiative are to make this biomarker data, along with biospecimens, available to researchers and to improve how AD is diagnosed

continued

BOX 2-6 Continued

and treated. Moreover, investigators from related AD and collaborating studies, such as the ADNI depression study, the Department of Defense ADNI and Worldwide ADNI, have partnered with ADNI, leveraging its research network and study model while providing ADNI researchers access to data from a larger pool of cohort participants (ADNI, 2024a,b). ADNI has been operating under a series of phases since its initial launch. Its current phase, ADNI4, was initiated in 2022 and will receive over $147 million in NIA funding over 5 years with a primary goal of expanding the inclusion of historically underrepresented groups in AD research (ADNI, 2024a). Data generated through ADNI have been shared with over 45,000 researchers globally and have contributed to more than 5,500 scientific publications (ADNI, 2024a).

Biomarkers for Vascular Contributions to Cognitive Impairment and Dementia (MarkVCID): MarkVCID is a multisite NIH-funded consortium focused on the discovery and validation of "promising predictive, diagnostic, target engagement and progression biomarkers of the brain small-vessel diseases involved in the vascular contribution to cognitive impairment and dementia" (MarkVCID, 2017). The program is overseen by NINDS and in its second phase, MarkVCID2, consists of 9 performance sites located across 15 U.S. medical centers, along with a Coordinating Center and an External Advisory Committee. The Coordinating Center, led by Massachusetts General Hospital, facilitates collaboration among participating research sites, ensures the use of a standardized set of study procedures and data collection methods, and manages data and analyses at the consortium level (MarkVCID, 2017). Research sites are tasked with validating a selection of biomarkers identified in the first phase of this program. In the first 2 years of the program, each project site worked to enroll over 200 research participants from diverse backgrounds who were experiencing cognitive decline or exhibiting early symptoms of cognitive impairment that may be linked to cerebrovascular small vessel disease. Over the course of the program, these individuals would be followed through annual clinic visits to monitor their symptom progression while utilizing harmonized data acquisition procedures for biomarker validation (MarkVCID, 2017). The consortium ultimately aims to foster the identification and availability of biomarkers that successfully identify disease pathways that should be targeted to prevent cognitive impairment due to small vessel disease and signal whether particular treatments are effective.

tests in at-home kits appears to be on the horizon (Huber et al., 2023). To address concerns regarding such direct-to-consumer commercialization, education of clinicians and the public regarding the clinical significance of results (e.g., that a positive biomarker result does not mean the individual will necessarily progress to having clinical dementia) will be an urgent priority, as will the communication of available information about interventions that may target associated risk factors. In the near term, blood-based biomarkers will likely be useful for screening and to guide more comprehensive and resource-intensive diagnostic workups, but with further validation it is feasible that they could serve as confirmatory biomarkers comparable to CSF and PET and in the future could be used to predict disease risk, monitor disease progression, and evaluate intervention effects (Hampel et al., 2022b, 2023).

A challenge, however, is that currently available biomarkers reflect only a limited number of pathologies, such as amyloid beta, tau, and neurodegeneration. There are other pathologies for which blood-based biomarkers desperately need to be identified. Indeed, biomarker discovery for most of the related dementias (e.g., LBD and frontotemporal dementia [FTD]) are at roughly the same point where the AD field was 25 years ago. As described further in Box 2-7, ongoing research is expanding the types of biomarkers that can be evaluated from blood and CSF samples, including those for alpha-synuclein (a hallmark of LBD but also found in some AD cases) (Scott et al., 2021) and TDP-43 pathology, which is common in but not limited to FTD (Cordts et al., 2023; Gifford et al., 2023; Irwin et al., 2024a,b). Proteomic analyses of plasma proteins are aiding the identification of other potential fluid biomarkers for AD/ADRD (Guo et al., 2024; Katzeff et al., 2022; Teunissen, 2024). Importantly, studies conducted in brain tissue reveal perturbations in many biological pathways, including perturbations that do not involve protein pathology (e.g., neuroinflammation, demyelination, energetics/mitochondrial perturbations, innate immunity, adaptive immunity, blood–brain barrier dysfunction, synaptic change). Blood-based biomarkers that reflect these complex and heterogeneous brain molecular changes can help investigators better understand disease pathways (described further in Chapter 3). In some cases, such biomarkers may be used solely for research purposes, while others may play an essential role in guiding precision medicine approaches to AD/ADRD.

Blood-based biomarkers that capture the complexity and heterogeneity of AD/ADRD, including brain copathologies and molecular changes, are necessary for molecular subtyping (Teunissen, 2024), as well as following these changes longitudinally even before clinical symptoms become apparent, as has been done using CSF biomarkers (Jia et al., 2024). To identify such molecular biomarkers, large-scale studies that assess multiomic (e.g., transcriptome, epigenome, proteome) changes in longitudinal cohorts with

---

BOX 2-7
Progress in the Discovery of Fluid Biomarkers
for Related Dementias

Lewy Body Dementia (LBD)—At present, a definitive diagnosis of LBD—which includes dementia with Lewy bodies (DLB) and Parkinson's disease dementia—can only be made postmortem. Alpha-synuclein seed amplification assays, such as the Real-Time Quaking-Induced Conversion (RT-QuIC) assay for the ultrasensitive detection of self-propagating misfolded alpha-synuclein aggregates in cerebrospinal fluid (CSF) and peripheral tissues (e.g., skin), have demonstrated promise as an accessible and accurate biomarker for DLB and Parkinson's disease (Concha-Marambio et al., 2023; Gibson et al., 2023). A skin biopsy for the detection of phosphorylated alpha-synuclein deposition is also being evaluated for use in identifying synucleinopathies like DLB. As with the RT-QuIC assay, this approach for detecting the presence of alpha-synuclein shows promise in its sensitivity and specificity (Gibbons et al., 2024) as well as in its feasibility for use as a noninvasive test. The availability of a premortem diagnostic biomarker would advance opportunities in both research and in clinical care by providing a tool with which to understand LBD pathogenesis, support early and accurate diagnosis, and evaluate interventions (Bargar et al., 2021).

Frontotemporal Dementia (FTD)—Elevated levels of neurofilament light and phosphorylated neurofilament heavy in plasma and CSF are associated with the presence of neuronal injury and neurodegeneration for FTD and other neurodegenerative diseases such as amyotrophic lateral sclerosis and show promise as diagnostic and prognostic biomarkers (Gendron et al., 2022; Irwin et al., 2024b; Katzeff et al., 2022). While these potential markers are not specific to FTD, they could help to differentiate the disease from other types of dementia and neurodegenerative diseases, identify participants for clinical research, and provide earlier and more accurate diagnoses (Gendron et al., 2022; Katzeff et al., 2022).

---

validation in brain-based autopsy studies are necessary. Such studies will lay the foundation to detect peripheral molecular signatures that reflect brain molecular perturbations. Once validated in population-based and clinical studies, these signatures can become much-needed precision medicine biomarkers of AD/ADRD.

Although blood-based biomarkers are transforming early detection and diagnosis for AD/ADRD and are being assessed for use in AD risk screening (Palmqvist et al., 2019) and prognosis (Cullen et al., 2021; Palmqvist et al., 2021), there remain many areas for innovation and research. Specifically, there is an urgent need for fluid biomarkers associated with diagnosis of non-AD tauopathies as well as other related dementias. In most cases, related dementias are still diagnosed very late and such diagnoses are very error prone owing to the heterogeneity and overlapping nature of the pathologies and clinical symptoms. There also is a need for novel biomarkers related to the specific cell types and mechanisms affected across the clinical stages of AD/ADRD.

Imaging biomarkers Amyloid-PET is an imaging biomarker for AD that is used in both clinical and research settings for the detection of amyloid pathology and has played an important role in improving diagnostic accuracy (Hampel et al., 2022a). Tau PET tracers have also been approved by FDA (2020), and efforts are currently underway to evaluate their use for mapping the density and spatial distribution of tau pathology in the brain, which correlates with functional and cognitive outcomes in people living with AD (Fleisher et al., 2020; Hampel et al., 2022a). Tau imaging biomarkers may also be used to guide the selection of therapies and to monitor their effects. While Tau PET imaging is a valuable tool for diagnosing AD, it is costly and not widely accessible, and currently available tracers are insensitive to non-AD tauopathies. A study by Tsai et al. (2019) demonstrated that the Tau PET ^{18}F-flortaucipir tracer has limited sensitivity and specificity in patients with FTD-related tauopathy. PET imaging biomarkers for other AD-related pathologic features, including inflammation, synaptic dysfunction, and neuronal injury, are being developed but are not yet ready for integration into clinical care.

Imaging biomarkers for related dementias are not as advanced as those for AD but represent an area of active research and development given the lack of tools available for confirmation of related dementias. Computed tomography (CT) and structural MRI are both used to examine structural brain markers in patients with suspected FTD and LBD (e.g., to look for signs of atrophy), while PET, single-photon emissions computed tomography (SPECT), and functional MRI are used to evaluate functional parameters such as metabolic activity, dopamine transporter uptake, regional blood flow, or hemodynamic changes (Peet et al., 2021), all of which may be useful in a differential diagnosis process (Ishii, 2020; Mavroudis et al., 2019). PET with fluorodeoxyglucose F-18 (^{18}F-FDG-PET) has been used extensively in clinical and research settings to differentiate FTD from other pathologies through the examination spatial patterns of brain hypometabolism (Minoshima et al., 2022) and may also show promise in predicting near-term risk of developing clinical dementia (Heyer et al., 2024). Other functional neuroimaging tools such as electroencephalography (EEG) have been used alone or in combination with other approaches such as polysomnography to examine sleep activity and aid in the supporting diagnosis of dementia with Lewy bodies (Law et al., 2020) and may have prognostic value more broadly (Law et al., 2020; van der Zande et al., 2020). Interestingly, ^{123}I-meta-iodobenzylguanidine myocardial scintigraphy, which can be used to assess nerve damage in the peripheral nervous system, has shown promise for the diagnosis of LBD (Abdelmoaty et al., 2023; Blanc and Bousiges, 2022; Matsubara et al., 2022). Different imaging modalities may be more or less useful at prodromal versus clinical dementia stages of disease. Ongoing imaging biomarker discovery and validation is needed to address current challenges with a lack of specificity and sensitivity (Blanc and Bousiges, 2022).

The costs and capital requirements for the use of MRI reduce the accessibility of this neuroimaging modality. However, the advancement of emerging technologies such as low-field MRI may create more accessible options in certain use cases for extending neuroimaging in resource-limited settings because of the more portable nature and low power requirements of the equipment (Kimberly et al., 2023). In addition to the potential for clinical use, portable options such as low-field MRI could expand their feasibility in research settings and allow for use outside of traditional clinical settings, such as in a research participant's home or in a dedicated research vehicle, and enhance engagement with diverse populations often underrepresented in clinical research (Deoni et al., 2023).

Digital biomarkers   The slow and subtle development of AD/ADRD creates an urgent need for diagnostic and prognostic biomarkers that can be detected early enough in the pathophysiological process to guide early interventions with the capability of preventing or delaying disease onset (Öhman et al., 2021). As discussed earlier in this chapter, digital tools and technologies are enabling the collection of streams of myriad physiological and behavioral data that can provide insights into an individual's sensory, motor, and cognitive function. Importantly, digitally collected health-related data (e.g., gait, sleep, speech) does not necessarily translate to a digital biomarker, although this is a common mischaracterization (Au et al., 2022). The identification of digital biomarkers will require the same rigorous scientific investigation used to identify and validate fluid and imaging biomarkers.

At present, the regulatory framework for the validation and approval of biomarkers is not designed to accommodate the kinds of data being generated using digital tools and technologies, such as time-series data covering an extended period of time (Au et al., 2022). This regulatory misalignment may pose a barrier to the development and clinical translation of tools for evaluating digital biomarkers, such as by disincentivizing companies looking for assurance of a likely return on their investment. Even if it is possible to simplify multiple streams of data into a single measure to better fit the existing regulatory framework, such a step would likely represent a loss of important information. The value in using digital modalities is in the multidimensional nature of the data. Rather than seeking to condense these data, there needs to be an effort to adjust the regulatory framework to accommodate "digital biomarker trajectories" that comprise a mix of signals that show an evolving pattern predictive of cognitive impairment. Such an adjustment may require FDA to develop new pathways for validation and approval of digital biomarkers (Au et al., 2022). It is possible to imagine that an updated regulatory framework would include different processes for different categories of digital biomarkers—those that correlate with traditional clinical, imaging, or fluid biomarkers, which could be used as reference standards for validation, and novel digital biomarkers that lack a biological correlate.

Addressing the regulatory framework is necessary but not sufficient to advance the widespread acceptance and use of digital biomarkers for AD/ADRD. Strategies to promote adoption include increasing comfort levels with digital tools and technologies in clinical settings such as by promoting the use of FDA-approved and reimbursable technologies (Au et al., 2022) and demonstrating the usefulness of digital biomarkers through clinical trials (Coravos et al., 2019; Kaye et al., 2023).

Conclusion 2-2: The current FDA regulatory framework for the validation and approval of biomarkers and the current Centers for Medicare & Medicaid Services reimbursement model is not designed to accommodate the types of data that are produced by digital tools and technologies. New regulatory pathways, such as those that support distinct processes for different categories of digital biomarkers, are needed to realize the potential of these emerging tools and technologies.

Conclusion 2-3: The last 10 years has seen a transformational advancement in the detection of AD-related pathologies in living people. Some pathologies can be detected many years before symptoms are detectable and have enabled the development of novel therapies for AD. There remain major gaps in available biomarkers for related dementias and the ability to quantify and longitudinally monitor mixed pathologies. In addition, there remain pathways not associated with protein pathologies (e.g., neuroinflammation, demyelination, energetics/mitochondrial perturbations, innate immunity, adaptive immunity, blood–brain barrier dysfunction, and synaptic function) that lack accessible and efficient measures.

Leveraging Longitudinal Cohort Studies

There is still much that is not understood about AD/ADRD, which feature decades of clinical but not pathologic dormancy. The molecular inflection points and the extent to which modifiable risk factors influence risk and progression of disease or the life-course time points during which risk factors are important (e.g., early life, midlife) need to be better understood. Illuminating this will require looking longitudinally at the exposome and molecular changes and how they interact across the lifespan, as discussed further in Chapter 3.

Longitudinal cohort studies represent an important mechanism for identifying essential data types that, when integrated, can provide a comprehensive view of brain health and AD/ADRD development over the life course (including risk and resilience factors). It is reasonable to imagine that, when viewed longitudinally, individuals will have trajectories that are not captured by cross-sectional studies or detectable on a group level but are related to treatments that will be relevant to that individual at a specific time point on an individual's trajectory. Knowledge gained from such longitudinal studies can be translated into processes and tools, such as digital health technologies and biomarker assays, that can be used for ongoing monitoring and AD/ADRD prediction, detection, and diagnosis in clinical settings. Ultimately the goal of this research is to inform the development of more sensitive and accessible—across diverse social and cultural contexts—tools and methods that can be used in clinical settings to detect brain health changes at individual and population (aggregated data) levels. A notable example of such efforts is the ARTFL-LEFFTDS Longitudinal Frontotemporal Lobar Degeneration (ALLFTD). ALLFTD is a cohort of people with frontotemporal lobar degeneration from whom cognitive and behavioral data, imaging, and blood and CSF samples are being collected over time. This study aims to identify useful clinical measures and markers for predicting the onset of symptoms and use in future FTD treatment trials, in which cohort participants may be eligible to participate (ALLFTD, n.d.).

While some cohorts have been established specifically for the purpose of understanding brain health and the development of AD/ADRD, in other cases, measures of brain health and monitoring for AD/ADRD have been incorporated into cohorts designed for other purposes. For example, NIH provided funding for the addition of new cognitive and psychophysiological assessments and functional neuroimaging in the Midlife in the United States (MIDUS) study to improve understanding of the risk factors that lead to dementia and mechanisms to advance prevention (NIH RePORTER, 2024b). Box 2-8 provides descriptions of other examples of ongoing NIH-funded cohorts that were not established for the study of AD/ADRD but include a brain health component. Continuing to leverage these existing

---

BOX 2-8
Examples of NIH-Funded Cohort Studies Developed for Other Purposes that Provide Data on Brain Health and Alzheimer's Disease and Related Dementias (AD/ADRD)

The Women's Health Initiative (WHI): The WHI is a national health study that is funded by the National Heart, Lung, and Blood Institute (NHLBI) and was initiated in the 1990s (WHI, 2021a). Although the original study ended in 2005, WHI has since continued in the form of extension studies, which include annual health updates and outcomes for active participants. The WHI focuses on the prevention of major causes of death, disability, and frailty in older women, including cardiovascular disease, cancers, and osteoporotic fractures. With more than 161,000 women enrolled in the original study (WHI, 2021a), the WHI is one of the largest women's health projects in the United States. The WHI Memory Study (WHIMS) was initiated in 1995 and enrolled 7,427 women age 65 years and older to investigated the effects of hormone therapy on risk of cognitive impairment and probable dementia, as well as changes in global cognition over time (WHI, 2021b). Over the course of the WHI study, several WHIMS-related ancillary studies were conducted, including the Supplemental Case Ascertainment Protocol, which aims to identify probable dementia and mild cognitive impairment cases in participants who are deceased or proxy dependent, the Magnetic Resonance Imaging study, the WHI Study of Cognitive Aging, the WHI Memory Study of Younger Women, and a study on the Epidemiology of Cognitive Health Outcomes (WHI, 2021b).

All of Us Research Program: The framework for the All of Us Research Program was developed by the National Insitutes of Health's Precision Medicine Initiative Working Group of the Advisory Committee to the Director in 2015 (NIH, 2024b). The mission of the All of Us program is to "accelerate health research and medical breakthroughs, enabling individualized prevention, treatment, and care for all of us" (NIH, 2024a). The All of Us Research Program aimed to enroll at least one million U.S. participants as part of its efforts to build one of the largest and most diverse health databases of its kind (NIH, 2024c). The program collects different types of genetic and health data (e.g., data from surveys, electronic health records, and blood and urine tests). These data have been used to study various facets of brain health; for example, a recent study examined hypertension and type 2 diabetes as risk factors for dementia and underscored the value of this cohort for better understanding disease prevalence and risk factors (Nagar et al., 2022).

Framingham Heart Study (FHS): The FHS was launched in 1948 under the direction of what eventually became the National Heart, Lung,

continued

BOX 2-8 Continued

and Blood Institute (NHLBI, n.d.). The original goal of the FHS was to identify common factors that contribute to cardiovascular disease (CVD). The study's objectives are to understand the incidence and prevalence of and risk factors for CVD, to study trends in these rates and factors over time, and to examine familial patterns of CVD. The study initially recruited 5,209 men and women, ages 28–62 years, living in Framingham, MA from 1948 to 1952 (NHLBI, 2023) and has since become a multigenerational study that has gathered genetic information from more than 15,000 people across three generations (i.e., original participants, their children, and their grandchildren) (NHLBI, n.d.). The study continues to assess participants every 2 years under a contract to Boston University from the NHLBI, and receives grant support for specialized studies (NHLBI, 2023). The FHS Brain Aging Program (FHS-BAP) was established for the surveillance and evaluation of FHS participants for dementia using traditional and digital cognitive assessments and brain imaging (BU, n.d.a). The program has spurred the creation of three interrelated projects that are examining "vascular and inflammatory contributors to AD, identifying factors associated with AD risk and resilience, investigating the link between AD genetic vulnerabilities and chronic inflammation, and studying the impact of gene variants affecting immune function on AD-related changes" (BU, n.d.b). FHS-BAP is also establishing a robust platform to promote data sharing and collaboration for the purpose of accelerating AD research using FHS data. (BU, n.d.a). To accomplish this goal, the program offers tools that allow researchers to access and use FHS data; for example, a data dictionary is available to provide researchers with definitions and explanations for all variables and elements within datasets (BU, n.d.c).

Bogalusa Heart Study: The NHLBI-funded Bogalusa Heart Study is a longitudinal study focusing on cardiovascular risk factors among children and young adults living in a semirural parish of Bogalusa, Louisiana (NHLBI, 2018). The study collected data from approximately 14,000 people from birth to the age of 38 years in a population that is biracial (65 percent White and 35 percent Black) (American College of Cardiology, 2002). The study established that precursors of adult CVD begin as early as childhood. In 2019, researchers at Louisiana State University's Pennington Biomedical Research Center and Mary Bird Perkins Cancer Center received a $14.5 million grant from NIA to examine the impact of high blood sugar levels in early life on brain health (Yawn, 2023).

Strong Heart Study (SHS): The NHLBI-supported SHS is the largest epidemiological study of CVD in American Indians. The SHS was launched in the early 1980s and has included numerous phases, including a pilot study and later expansion of a family study focused on genetic contributions to CVD and its risk factors. The most recent phase includes follow-up examinations for approximately 3,500 SHS participants (SHS, 2017a). Several in-depth ancillary studies have been incorporated into this most recent follow-up examination phase that are relevant to aging and brain health. These include studies on resilience in brain aging; psychological risk factors, quality of life, community, and brain aging; social determinants of health and neurodegeneration; and targets for precision prevention of AD/ADRD in American Indians, among others (SHS, 2017b).

Multi-Ethnic Study of Atherosclerosis (MESA): MESA is an NHLBI-funded cohort study that was developed to examine characteristics of subclinical CVD and the risk factors that predict progression to clinical CVD in diverse populations. The study involves more than 6,000 men and women, ages 45–84 without known CVD, from six different communities in the United States (MESA, 2020). The field sites involved in MESA include Columbia University, Johns Hopkins University, Northwestern University, University of California Los Angeles, University of Minnesota, and Wake Forest University. MESA-MIND was created as an ancillary study that specifically focuses on understanding how subclinical vascular disease may increase dementia risk. Participants of the MESA-MIND study undergo detailed cognitive testing and brain imaging (i.e., MRI and amyloid-PET), in addition to other clinical assessments (MESA-MIND, 2024).

Health and Retirement Study (HRS): The HRS, led by the University of Michigan, is a longitudinal study supported by the National Institute on Aging and the Social Security Administration (HRS, 2021). The study began in 1992 and at present includes a representative, active study population of about 20,000 people (HRS, 2024). While not the sole focus of the HRS, a goal of the study is to understand changes in cognitive health with aging and the impact of AD/ADRD on people within the United States (HRS, 2021). The HRS aims to continue expanding the number of minority participants to continue to serve as a major resource for studying racial and ethnic disparities within AD/ADRD. The Aging, Demographics, and Memory Study (ADAMS) is an HRS supplemental study that involves additional data collection through in-person clinical assessments to obtain detailed information on the participants' cognitive status (HRS, 2024).

cohorts provides important opportunities for filling knowledge gaps, particularly regarding key transition points in the life course, and to prioritize the inclusion of data from underrepresented groups (e.g., data from the Black Women's Health Study), which help address biases in existing data.

Care must be taken to mitigate potential spotlight effects resulting from basing conclusions and models on the data and data sources currently available while failing to adequately explore other potential explanations and paradigms. For example, there is increasing interest in the vascular dimensions of AD/ADRD based in part on the availability of data from established sources such as the Framingham Heart Study, but other equally important contributors to AD/ADRD may yet to be discovered.

Conclusion 2-4: Longitudinal cohort studies, including those that have been specifically designed for the purpose of understanding brain health and those created for other purposes, are essential mechanisms for distinguishing what types of data can be integrated to advance a life-course understanding of brain health and disease across diverse populations. There are immediate opportunities to accelerate advances in research by leveraging existing cohorts to address knowledge gaps and biases in data.

Opportunities to Optimize Data Collection and Analysis from Longitudinal Cohorts

Improving cohort representativeness To ensure that data collection and evaluation strategies that emerge from cohort studies are not biased to certain subpopulations and have broad applicability, attention needs to be paid to ensuring cohort studies enroll diverse and representative populations. Some advances in cohort diversity have been achieved through NIH support for new cohorts (see Box 2-9) and increasing underrepresented populations in existing cohorts, such as the Health and Retirement Study (Nye et al., 2022), but these efforts need to be expanded. In doing so, representativeness should be considered across multiple dimensions including, but not limited to, race and ethnicity, occupation, geography (e.g., urban, rural), and socioeconomic status and social phenotypes.

While self-identified race and ethnicity data are often collected, use of genetic ancestry data can provide a more complete characterization of the diversity of cohorts and differences in risk across diverse groups (Reitz et al., 2023). Constructing cohorts solely of people from minoritized communities may better enable in-depth exploration of social factors that influence AD/ADRD risk and the understanding of heterogeneity in populations bearing increased risk of dementia (Weuve, 2024). For example, the Hispanic Community Health Study/Study of Latinos, the largest comprehensive study

---

BOX 2-9
The Health and Aging Brain Study: Health Disparities

The National Institute on Aging–funded Health and Aging Brain Study: Health Disparities (HABS-HD) was launched in 2022 and aims to understand the biological, social, and environmental factors that affect brain aging among diverse communities. This is the first large-scale, community-based project focusing on how biological, medical, environmental, and social factors, within a health disparities framework, contribute to AD risk within African Americans, Mexican Americans, and non-Hispanic Whites (NIH RePORTER, 2024c). One of the goals of the Health and Aging Brain Study is to identify racial/ethnic-specific risk profiles for cognitive loss among the diverse populations involved in the study (HCS Institute for Translational Research, 2022). The study will also collect life-course exposome and sociocultural data to examine how these factors affect biomarkers among diverse populations. Study data, including HABS-HD data, biofluid samples, and genomics data, will be available to the global scientific community (Toga et al., 2022).

---

of health and disease in people of Hispanic/Latino ancestry, assessed the risk and protective factors for chronic health conditions across more than 16,000 participants (NHLBI, 2024). Insights from this work have created opportunities for further research into health disparities and led to the dedicated investigation of aging and neurodegeneration within this population (González et al., 2019).

Another consideration for cohort diversity is the language spoken by participants. Cohorts have traditionally been restricted to a limited pool of spoken languages (e.g., English, Spanish, Chinese). As a result, tools developed and tested in existing cohorts may not translate well to a more diverse set of languages. Achieving more diverse cohorts will require investment in meaningful community engagement, which is discussed further in Chapter 5.

Capturing data from across the life course   While dementia is commonly thought of as a disease of old age based on the timing for the manifestation of the most severe symptoms, it is increasingly understood that dementia is often the culmination of a pathologic process that develops slowly over a period of decades and that AD/ADRD risk is a function of an individual's genetics, which are set at conception, along with the physical and social exposures that occur throughout the life course, including during gestational, childhood, adolescent, and adult life stages (Cadar, 2017; Whalley et al., 2006). To better understand the timing for key risk and protective factors related to AD/ADRD and to define data elements that should be included in a longitudinal data collection strategy, cohort studies need to enable the capture of data from across the entirety of the life course. While this may not be feasible for each individual cohort, multi-cohort analysis (discussed below) can allow a more complete picture to be developed from cohorts that include people of varying age ranges.

Early life is a critical period for the development of neuronal connections in the brain (WHO, 2022) and cognitive reserve (Livingston et al., 2020), which may lower the risk of dementia (Meng and D'Arcy, 2012). Although there has been some focus on the role of early-life education as a protective mechanism that functions through the development of cognitive reserve (Foverskov et al., 2020; McDowell et al., 2005; Meng and D'Arcy, 2012; Nguyen et al., 2016), less is known regarding the effect of other early-life exposures, both social (e.g., neglect and abuse) (Corney et al., 2022) and environmental (e.g., environmental neurotoxicants, such as lead) (Reuben, 2018). This stage of the life course has perhaps received the least attention, in part because of the large time lag between early life and AD/ADRD development. This gap may be addressed by ensuring routine data collection related to early-life exposures in cohort studies. Birth cohorts are of particular value for such endeavors. Such data would ideally be captured prospectively, as is being done in the NIH-funded National Longitudinal Study of Adolescent to Adult Health (Harris et al., 2019). However, it is also possible to fill data gaps retrospectively by collecting data from archival resources (Moceri et al., 2000).

The understanding of dementia as a disease that develops over many years has naturally shifted attention to the connection between events of midlife and late-life AD/ADRD development. Epidemiological studies of dementia risk have led to a particular focus on chronic diseases that manifest in midlife, such as hypertension and diabetes (Livingston et al., 2020; Whalley et al., 2006). Cohort studies focused on cardiovascular health are increasingly including outcomes related to brain health (see Box 2-8). However, there remain aspects of midlife, such as the effects of pregnancy and menopause on brain health and AD/ADRD in women, that are understudied (Barth and de Lange, 2020), and opportunities to better capture key data from this life period, including reproductive history, are being missed (Buckley, 2024).

Just as it is important to ensure cohort studies for AD/ADRD are inclusive of early life, much can be learned from prospective population-based studies of late life, when neuropathology, and particularly mixed pathologies, and cognitive impairment are far more prevalent (Corrada et al., 2012). Research focused on the oldest old, who are often excluded from studies owing to such issues as functional disabilities, frailty, and sensory impairment (Corrada, 2024), can yield insights into resilience factors for AD/ADRD (Andersen, 2020), and, for studies including a brain donation component, links may be found between cognitive function and the accumulation of neuropathologic changes over time for this population (Beker et al., 2021; Corrada et al., 2012).

Banking samples for future analyses   Biobanking provides a mechanism to maximize opportunities to learn from and effectively use the investments in existing cohorts to facilitate AD/ADRD research (Francis et al., 2018). As technology and analytic methods continue to evolve, there may be future opportunities to glean insights from banked samples that investigators cannot necessarily anticipate at the time of sample collection, potentially leading to the development of future tools or therapeutics. Banked samples from longitudinal cohorts have advantages over ad hoc donated biosamples resulting from the ability to link data derived from the analysis of the banked samples to clinical and other data (e.g., exposure history) collected premortem from the individuals in the cohort (Kind, 2024). A tradeoff should be noted, however, that data linked to biological samples may function to limit the accessibility of those samples due to privacy concerns. While individual cohort studies may be limited in size based on resource constraints, analyzing banked samples collected from diverse cohorts can not only increase the population size for a given analysis but also the diversity represented in the analyzed samples (Miller, 2024).

The collection of deeply phenotyped and well-characterized brain donor tissue samples can add significant value to cohort studies by enabling the validation of clinical diagnoses and imaging surrogates through neuropathologic examination and the association of neuropathology with premortem data from cohort participants (Cairns et al., 2010; Franklin et al., 2015). If banked brain samples can thus be used to identify prognostic markers, such information could guide early intervention strategies for those determined to be at high risk (Robinson et al., 2018). Increasing the availability of banked brain samples from diverse populations requires public education and outreach to convey the importance of brain donation to advancing AD/ADRD research and to clarify that brain donation for research involves a separate consent process from that used for organ donation intended to save lives. Also needed are resources to collect, analyze, and store the donated samples. Reaching potential donors can be facilitated by engaging advocacy groups and community members who are themselves or have family members living with AD/ADRD (Francis et al., 2018). NIH has developed resources for the public and the Alzheimer's Disease Research Centers (ADRCs) to support education efforts related to brain donation (NIA, n.d.a, 2022; NINDS, 2023), but inadequate resources have been a noted challenge to brain banking efforts, contributing to lost opportunities for future research (Franklin et al., 2015).

Similarly, banked blood samples linked to clinical and other data from cohort participants represent an invaluable resource as increasingly high-throughput assays are enabling multiomic and other analyses such as mass spectrometry for signatures of past exposures, at scales previously unachievable (Buckley, 2024; Miller, 2024). The Framingham Heart Study exemplifies the scientific value of banked blood samples collected before disease onset and their use years later in new forms of testing (e.g., genomics, proteomics, metabolomics) for potential disease-predictive biomarkers as technology evolved, resulting in opportunities to maximally leverage the cohort study. The emergence of blood-based biomarkers for AD/ADRD has been enabled in part through the analysis of banked blood samples, which set the stage for prospective studies focused on testing biomarkers for accuracy in predicting clinical disease onset years later (Au et al., 2023).

Ensuring that banked samples will continue to be a highly valuable resource for future AD/ADRD research will require consideration regarding, and funding for, harmonized sample collection processes and optimal storage, as well as systems for researcher access to these precious samples, including inventories of samples available for external use (discussed further in Chapter 5). Lack of transparency regarding sample availability has been a barrier to fully realizing the value of biobanking investments. An unfortunate result of the high cost of biobanking is that many donated samples will be discarded before they can be used. This not only represents a lost opportunity to gain valuable knowledge from the samples but also does a disservice to those who donated the specimens.

Some biorepositories may be able to step in as resources and opportunity allow to preserve valuable specimens from closed studies that cannot maintain their samples; however, this currently ad hoc process could be facilitated by the use of standardized consent forms and collection procedures. For example, the National Centralized Repository for Alzheimer's Disease and Related Dementias (NCRAD), an NIA-funded biorepository, was able to take in samples from the API Generation program, which was terminated prior to completing enrollment (NCRAD, 2024a), as well as samples that would have otherwise been lost from the Gingko Evaluation of Memory Study (NCRAD, 2024b). Further scaling of the capacity of this resource is needed to prevent further loss of precious biospecimens. See Box 2-10 for information on this and other NIH-funded biorepositories supporting AD/ADRD research.

BOX 2-10
Examples of National Institutes of Health (NIH)-
Supported Alzheimer's Disease and Related
Dementias (AD/ADRD) Biorepositories

NIH-funded biorepositories are critical research resources that support the collection, storage, and accessibility of essential biological specimens collected from NIH-funded studies and other biomedical research.

National Centralized Repository for Alzheimer's Disease and Related Dementias (NCRAD): NCRAD at the Indiana University School of Medicine is a National Institute on Aging (NIA)–funded biorepository established in 1990 for the purpose of supporting research on AD/ADRD etiology, detection, and development of therapeutics. NCRAD serves as a biorepository for a wide variety of biological sample types that have been generated by over 65 NIH-funded studies, such as the Alzheimer's Disease Neuroimaging Initiative, the 90+ Study, and the Alzheimer's Biomarker Consortium–Down Syndrome study, as well as clinic-based samples from Alzheimer's Disease Research Centers, accounting for 70,000 samples from over 118,000 participants and providing cutting-edge fluid biomarker analysis to investigators (NCRAD, 2024c,d,e).

Biospecimen Exchange for Neurological Disorders (BioSEND): BioSEND, based at the Indiana University School of Medicine, is a National Institute of Neurological Disorders and Stroke (NINDS)-funded biomarker repository established in 2015. The repository stores biospecimens from studies, including phase 2 and 3 trials, funded by or conducted in collaboration with NINDS. BioSEND collects a broad range of specimen types (e.g., DNA, RNA, plasma, serum, CSF, and whole blood) from studies on a wide variety of neurological and neuropsychiatric diseases, including Lewy body dementia and frontotemporal dementia. Samples from over 30 different studies are available for access by investigators (BioSEND, 2024).

NeuroBioBank: The NeuroBioBank was established in September 2013 and is supported by NIA, NINDS, the Eunice Kennedy Shriver National Institute of Child Health and Human Development, the National Institute of Mental Health, and the National Institute on Drug Abuse. The NeuroBioBank serves as a resource for researchers studying many different neurological, neuropsychiatric, and neurodevelopmental diseases and disorders. It provides centralized access to six biorepositories that are housed at academic and research centers throughout the United States and also partners with research centers (ADRCs) and not-for-profit organizations (e.g., the Brain Donor Project). In addition to supporting

continued

BOX 2-10 Continued

researchers' access to well-characterized, postmortem brain tissue and related biospecimens from across its network, the NeuroBioBank offers a centralized resource of best practices to guide the acquisition, preparation, and sharing of stored tissues (NeuroBioBank, 2024).

AgingResearchBiobank: Established by NIA in 2018, the AgingResearchBiobank is an inventory system designed to hold and distribute biospecimens and phenotypic and clinical data from relevant NIA-funded clinical trials and observational studies. The AgingResearchBiobank includes (1) a biorepository that is designed to receive, store, and distribute biospecimens from different study collections; and (2) a data repository that serves as a data coordinating center to receive, archive, maintain, and distribute images and databases from various study collections (NIA, n.d.b). While only relevant NIA-funded studies can submit biospecimens and data to the AgingResearchBiobank (at no cost to investigators), qualified investigators from around the world are eligible to apply for access to biospecimens and data from the AgingResearchBiobank, which facilitates the sharing of these resources with the broader research community (NIA, n.d.b, 2024a).

Aging Cell Repository: The NIA-funded Aging Cell Repository is located at the Coriell Institute for Medical Research, which holds a number of other repositories funded by the National Institute of General Medical Sciences, the National Human Genome Research Institute, and NINDS, among others (Coriell Institute, 2024). The Aging Cell Repository stores and shares cells and other biological samples derived from both older animals and humans to researchers. The cells and DNA samples, which are collected using strict diagnostic criteria, are stored in accordance with high-quality standards of cell culture and DNA purification. Researchers from over 40 countries have used the cell cultures from the Aging Cell Repository for both cellular and molecular research focusing on aging and neurodegeneration. Each year the Coriell Institute ships approximately 1,200 cell cultures and over 400 DNA samples from the cell bank to investigators at academic, nonprofit, or government institutions (Moro, 2018).

Conclusion 2-5: The potential value of, and uses for, biobanked samples, specifically those from longitudinal cohorts, may not be clear at the time of collection but may emerge as new analytic approaches and tools are developed. Therefore, careful consideration is needed to plan for how these samples can be collected and stored to avoid limiting future use opportunities and barriers to access and analysis.

Scaling data and sample collection: Balancing scientific opportunities and resource constraints Given the substantial costs of data and sample collection, storage, and analysis, data collection goals need to be balanced against resource restrictions and should consider the invasiveness of the testing procedure. Some data are easily collected with widely available tools and may form a minimal dataset for all cohorts while those of higher cost or burden to extract may need to be scaled down to smaller cohorts or subpopulations. As engineering and technological advances continue to increase the scale at which some data can be collected and analyzed cost-effectively, it may be possible to expand both cohort sizes and data collection. The shift to more virtual engagement with cohorts during the COVID-19 pandemic highlighted opportunities to reduce the burden and increase the scale of data collection (Buckley, 2024), providing a foundation for future cohort studies.

Enabling multicohort analysis through data access and harmonization Another way to maximally use the data collected from individual cohorts is to conduct multicohort analyses, which have the potential to increase the diversity of the population included in an analysis. For example, data from four cohorts featuring populations in different life stages were used to study the natural history of age-related cognitive decline over the life course and the effect of social disparities on trajectories (Yang et al., 2024). Barriers to multicohort analyses include data access issues and variation in measures and methods used across different cohorts. Of note, making data accessible differs in practice from active data sharing and distribution; the former may raise fewer concerns regarding data security. For example, on some platforms, data can be made accessible for analysis while restricting the downloading of raw datasets. This could help address such concerns as patient privacy and the potential for the commercialization of patient data. As discussed further in Chapter 5, tiering data access is another strategy that can be used to address privacy and data security concerns. Data with the lowest level of sensitivity, such as some fully de-identified data, can be made publicly available, while increasing levels of restrictions on access can be applied as the sensitivity of the data increases.

Data harmonization provides a means of pooling data from multiple studies despite heterogeneity in measures and test methods (Hampton et al., 2023; Mukherjee et al., 2023). As an example, the Phenotype Harmonization Consortium, a component of the Alzheimer's Disease Sequencing Project (ADSP) (see Chapter 3), was created to enable further genomic analyses through the intensive harmonization of rich endophenotypic data from 39 participating cohort studies on AD/ADRD and aging associated with the ADSP (ADSP, 2024; VMAC, 2024). However, given the complexity of post hoc harmonization and the need for specialized expertise and data infrastructure, coordination among study investigators during the planning stage could facilitate multicohort analyses by proactively addressing potential impediments related to data access and harmonization, thereby accelerating progress in AD/ADRD research. NIA funded the Harmonized Cognitive Assessment Protocol to realize the development and validation of harmonized measures for longitudinal cohorts to enable these cross-study comparisons and improve the understanding of dementia risk in diverse populations in high- and low-income countries (see Box 2-11).

Considerations Regarding Real-World Implementation of Emerging and Novel Tools to Guide Clinical Action

The overarching goal of all clinical research is to improve what happens when a patient meets with a clinician. To maximize the benefits to society from research, discoveries such as advancements in biomarkers, data collection methods, and interventions need to be translated to real-world settings.

Research investments have generated significant advances in the ability to more accurately diagnose AD/ADRD earlier in the life course and to monitor disease progression using biomarkers and other tools, but this capability has not yet been realized in most clinical settings. As a result, clinical decision making largely continues to rely on methods that leave considerable uncertainty regarding the best course of action. In addition to direct benefits to patients resulting from better-informed clinical decision making, the implementation of new tools for data collection in clinical practice also provides opportunities to further advance knowledge through the collection of real-world evidence. For example, more precise diagnostic capabilities would enhance knowledge regarding the prevalence and incidence of AD and related dementias, a current knowledge gap discussed in Chapter 1. In addition to considering the potential benefits to patients, the potential risks associated with the adoption of new tools needs to be considered.

Overcoming Barriers to Real-World Implementation

The implementation of new tools in real-world settings necessitates the consideration of barriers and facilitators to adoption and, for clinical settings, integration into existing workflows. Implementation science provides an approach for building the evidence base for such considerations. Investment in implementation testing, for example, in the form of pilot programs, can identify pain points and guide strategies to facilitate tool uptake in a broader rollout phase (NASEM, 2024).

Clinical uptake of new tools for AD/ADRD detection, diagnosis, and monitoring (e.g., biomarkers and digital technologies) has been slow, in

BOX 2-11
Harmonized Cognitive Assessment Protocol

The Harmonized Cognitive Assessment Protocol (HCAP) Network represents a major NIA investment in the harmonization of methods to measure cognitive function of older individuals from around the world (HCAP Network, 2023). The design of HCAP was led by the Health and Retirement Study (HRS) investigators in collaboration with a number of its sister studies worldwide. The HCAP is a harmonized cognitive battery that includes neuropsychological test items from previously validated cognitive test batteries along with an informant interview to help detect and diagnose mild cognitive impairment and dementia (Kobayashi et al., 2024). Ultimately, this effort yielded a flexible instrument for measuring late-life cognitive function that is being used to generate harmonized data for cross-national comparison analyses that are sensitive to cultural, linguistic, and educational differences across countries (Kobayashi et al., 2024). The work of the HCAP Network involves harmonization activities encompassing the entirety of the longitudinal research process including sample design, protocol development and administration, statistical harmonization of collected data, and diagnostic algorithms, among others (NIH RePORTER, 2024d). Importantly, the HCAP Network, a group of researchers who collaborate to support the harmonization of international studies using HCAP (HCAP Network, 2023), facilitates the use of pilot projects to continuously improve harmonization of studies.

A notable challenge is maintaining test and measure harmonization despite cross-country variations in life-course factors, such as poverty, diet, and educational attainment, that influence cognitive function and AD/ADRD risk (NIH RePORTER, 2024d). The HCAP network has begun to publish initial findings on cross-national differences (Kobayashi et al., 2024).

NIA also supported the creation of the HRS International Partner Study network to oversee continued harmonization using HCAP across large nationally representative samples throughout the world. As of 2024, the HCAP Network members include 13 longitudinal studies of aging and cognition, including the Longitudinal Aging Study in India, the Survey of Health, Aging, and Retirement in Europe, and the China Health and Retirement Longitudinal Study, among others (HCAP Network, 2024). Existing and planned HCAP studies capture an estimated 75 percent of the global population age 65 years or older (Kobayashi et al., 2024).

part because of uncertainty in the health care community. Other barriers to the widespread use of new tools in clinical settings include considerations related to insurance coverage, electronic health record integration, and out-of-pocket costs for patients. See Box 2-12 for examples of the integration of new tools into clinical diagnostic criteria for AD and LBD. A multipronged approach is needed to support implementation, including the education of primary care providers on the capabilities and limitations of tools, grants for workforce training, and the development of collaborations between community physicians and researchers. Parallel efforts should be focused on educating the public to help people understand the importance of research, to help them critically analyze research findings communicated in the media, and to better advocate for themselves when meeting with their clinicians. Such efforts should be informed by best practices from the science of outreach and engagement.

Awareness of the importance of implementation science has grown in recent decades, and dedicated resources to support improvements in research translation have been established by NIH. Most notably, NIH's National Center for Advancing Translational Sciences (NCATS) was established in 2011 and administers the Clinical and Translational Science Awards program, which is designed to provide funding support for research and workforce training to accelerate the translation of research discoveries into improved care (NCATS, 2024). To carry out its mission, NCATS collaborates with other NIH institutes and centers, including those involved in AD/ADRD research, as well as with other governmental agencies, private

---

BOX 2-12
Examples of the Integration of New Tools
into Clinical Diagnostic Criteria

Alzheimer's disease (AD): Initial criteria for the clinical diagnosis of AD were developed in 1984 (McKhann et al., 1984). A probable AD diagnosis could be made on the basis of clinical examination, including neuropsychological testing, and was supported by such factors as family history and the absence of other conditions that could explain the gradual and progressive deterioration of cognitive functions. The diagnostic criteria were updated in 2011 to reflect advances in tools and knowledge regarding AD (McKhann et al., 2011). The revised criteria retained but refined the categories of probable and possible AD dementia and allowed for an increased level of certainty when someone meeting the core clinical criteria were found to carry a causative AD genetic mutation (e.g.,

BOX 2-12 Continued

APP, PSEN1, PSEN2) or had imaging (PET) or fluid biomarker (CSF amyloid beta and tau) evidence of the AD pathophysiological process. The use of biomarker evidence in routine clinical diagnosis was not recommended given noted limitations in biomarker discovery and implementation at the time, but it was acknowledged as useful for clinical research and as an optional tool for clinicians (McKhann et al., 2011). Importantly, the 1984 and 2011 criteria are specific to clinical dementia caused by AD. Separate criteria address MCI caused by AD (Albert et al., 2011).

Dementia with Lewy bodies (DLB): The first consensus guidelines for the clinical and pathologic diagnosis for DLB were published in 1996 by the Consortium on Dementia with Lewy bodies and involved clinical assessment to confirm the presence of the central feature of progressive disabling cognitive impairment and the presence of at least one core clinical feature. The criteria included additional supportive and exclusion features that could make a possible or probable diagnosis more or less likely (McKeith et al., 1996). These consensus guidelines were updated in 2005 to reflect the addition of new knowledge of the clinical presentation of DLB and access to new biomarkers for clinical assessment (Yamada et al., 2020). The 2005 diagnostic criteria maintained a similar structure as the first edition with the central feature and three core clinical features to guide diagnosis, but added a category for suggestive features (e.g., REM sleep behavior; low dopamine transporter [DAT] uptake in basal ganglia, severe neuroleptic sensitivity). Importantly, for the first time, imaging biomarkers were included in categories for suggestive and supported features.

The most recent revised clinical criteria were released in 2017 and included specific criteria that distinguish diagnostic biomarkers from clinical features. The biomarkers were divided into two categories: indicative biomarkers (e.g., reduced DAT uptake in basal ganglia by SPECT/PET; abnormal MIBG myocardial scintigraphy and polysomnographic confirmation of REM sleep without atonia) and supportive biomarkers (e.g., preservation of the medial temporal lobe on CT/MRI, low uptake on SPECT/PET perfusion/metabolism scan with reduced occipital activity with or without cingulate island sign on FDG-PET, prominent posterior slow wave activity on EEG with periodic fluctuations in the pre-alpha/theta range). Looking forward, the development of novel imaging and skin biomarkers for alpha-synuclein and new fluid biomarkers (e.g., amplification assays for alpha-synuclein) may allow for the development of updated clinical criteria for the diagnosis of early stage/prodromal DLB (Yamada et al., 2020). Staging systems applying these new biomarkers are currently being explored for use in research (Simuni et al., 2024).

industry, academia, and patient-support organizations. Enhanced collabora-tion of NIA and NINDS with NCATS could yield opportunities to accel-erate the translation of cutting-edge research tools for the diagnosis and monitoring of AD/ADRD into clinical practice.

Research to Understand the Risks of Overtreatment in the Context of Preclinical Diagnosis

As described earlier in this chapter, numerous challenges—including scientific, technologic, social, and systemic barriers—impede the early and accurate detection and diagnosis of AD/ADRD. These factors may contribute to underdiagnosis. As biomedical advancements and changes in clinical prac-tice enable the detection and diagnosis of changes in brain health, it is also important to acknowledge the potential risks related to biomarker-based diagnosis of preclinical AD/ADRD (e.g., someone who has the hallmark neuropathologies of AD but no symptoms of cognitive decline; see Box 2-1). Beyond risks associated with any AD/ADRD diagnosis, such as psycho-logical distress and stigma, one important risk associated with diagnosis in asymptomatic individuals is overtreatment, which is of concern given the availability of FDA-approved anti-amyloid therapies for AD that have rare but substantial side effects and significant out-of-pocket costs. The relative benefits and risks of anti-amyloid treatment in asymptomatic individuals with AD pathologies are unclear as current treatments are only approved for use in people with MCI and early Alzheimer's dementia. In the case of AD, multiple studies have documented that not everyone with amyloid plaques in the brain will progress to MCI or clinical dementia within their lifetimes (Bennett et al., 2006; Knopman et al., 2003; Snowdon, 2003).

As discussed further in Chapter 3, the reasons for this are still under study but could include resilience factors or even death from another cause prior to clinical progression (Erickson et al., 2021; Langa and Burke, 2019; NASEM, 2021a,b). One modeling analysis estimated that the majority of the nearly 50 million Americans estimated to be living with elevated amyloid will not develop clinical dementia within their lifetimes (Brookmeyer and Abdalla, 2018). However, this analysis did not include the use of tau bio-markers, which more recent research indicates greatly improves prediction of cognitive decline. A recent large multicenter amyloid and tau PET study examined risk for future progression to MCI and clinical dementia in cog-nitively unimpaired cohort participants and found that participants with both amyloid and tau biomarkers had a much greater risk of progression to MCI and clinical dementia as compared to those who were negative for both biomarkers. Of those who were amyloid positive and positive for tau in the neocortical region, more than 50 percent progressed to MCI and 20 percent to clinical dementia within 6 years (Ossenkoppele et al., 2022). Several other recent studies have similarly found an increased risk of decline over time in cognitively unimpaired individuals with high levels of amyloid and abnormal tau biomarkers (Cody et al., 2024; Sperling et al., 2024).

Since there remains uncertainty in the true likelihood of transition from normal cognition to MCI and clinical dementia for those with different biomarker profiles, research in representative populations is urgently needed to better define these transition probabilities (e.g., presence of elevated amyloid to MCI to clinical dementia). This information, along with evidence on the efficacy of new treatments at preclinical disease stages, should inform education efforts for both the public and clinicians (Chin and Erickson, 2024; Largent et al., 2020). Such education will be essential to help clinicians and the public understand the evolving status of biomarker testing, particularly as diagnostic tools are commercialized and potentially marketed directly to consumers, and the risks and benefits of interventions for people with different combinations of biomarkers and cognitive symptoms. Ultimately, it is important to ensure that individuals have the information they require to make informed decisions, especially for those who meet the criteria for preclinical AD.

Real-World Data Integration to Guide Clinical Monitoring, Diagnosis, and Action

As novel research tools and methods are incorporated into clinical practice, it will be important to collect data to understand their performance in real-world settings and how implementation is addressing current knowledge gaps, guiding clinical management, and affecting the experiences of people living with AD/ADRD.

Data collection is not useful by itself; it must be used in decision models to guide clinical decision making (Barron et al., 2021). However, not all data are actionable. Actionable data are those that have a bearing on a specific clinical decision within a larger decision model. Some data that are not actionable at present may be actionable in the future, an issue that can be accounted for in a decision model. Certain data only become relevant at certain stages (e.g., after symptom development) or life experiences (see Table 2-1). This informs the timing for collection of specific types of data. Actionable data, therefore, must be gathered at the right time in the context of resolving a specific clinical question; that is, data have value in this context only if they resolve uncertainty and guide clinical decisions. So framed, data do not have equal utility in all clinical decisions and, especially in the context of finite resources, should be gathered only to resolve uncertainty within a specific clinical decision model. Additionally, the frequency of data collection may vary across the life course; during specific times, it may be desirable to take measurements more frequently or even continuously, which has been made feasible by technological advances. Within the context of a decision model, hypotheses regarding how different data interrelate may guide efforts to collect additional data as well as guiding decisions on how best to intervene across the life course.

Translating data into clinical action requires data integration and analysis, both longitudinal and cross-sectional. A notable gap is the absence of a framework or model for integrating disparate data sources (including structured and unstructured data) to generate knowledge regarding risk and to guide action. Given the diversity of potential data sources (e.g., clinical symptoms, molecular data, exposure data), addressing this gap will require data sharing and cross-disciplinary efforts.

In March 2023, NIH released a Request for Applications to fund an AD/ADRD Real-World Data Platform (HHS, 2023). The platform was intended to better capture and link data from multiple sources, thereby enhancing and accelerating the ability to answer scientific questions, particularly those not amenable to clinical trials, and increasing the engagement of and collection of data from diverse populations. However, in April 2024, NIH decided not to fund the platform, citing budgetary considerations and a desire to consider opportunities to leverage other federal large data initiatives (Wallin, 2024). The objectives of the original proposal remain important, but given the considerable investment and diversity of expertise that will be required to implement such a platform, consideration should be given to a precompetitive public–private partnership model. Existing public–private partnerships involving NIH, such as the Accelerating Medicines Partnership® Program for Alzheimer's Disease (AMP-AD program) (NIA, 2023a) and the NIH Science and Technology Research Infrastructure for Discovery, Experimentation, and Sustainability (STRIDES) Initiative,[3] which is providing NIH-supported investigators with affordable access to cloud services and environments, may serve as models.

> *Conclusion 2-6: To maximize the benefits to society from research, such discoveries as advancements in biomarkers, data collection methods, and interventions need to be translated to real-world settings. The implementation of such new tools into clinical practice in turn provides opportunities to further advance knowledge through the collection of real-world evidence.*

RESEARCH PRIORITIES

The ability to detect and track changes in brain health will be key to the development of rational strategies for the prevention and treatment of AD/

---

[3] https://datascience.nih.gov/strides (accessed June 12, 2024).

ADRD. Enabling the early and accurate identification of changes in brain health across diverse populations has been a major focus area for NIH. To this end, NIH has funded biomarker discovery and validation, as well as the development and implementation of digital tools and technologies to improve the capacity to diagnose and monitor AD/ADRD at its earliest stages and accurately distinguish the different forms of dementia (NIA, 2023b, 2024b). Infrastructure investments to support these efforts have included longitudinal cohort studies, as well as large, collaborative research programs (e.g., CLEAR-AD) and public–private partnerships. The committee identified two research priorities that align with and build upon this broad foundation of NIH investments. These research priorities are listed in Table 2-2 below and include key scientific questions and near-term research opportunities that would advance progress on the research priorities.

TABLE 2-2 Committee-Identified Research Priorities Related to Quantifying Brain Health Across the Life Course and Accurately Predicting Risk of, Screening for, Diagnosing, and Monitoring AD/ADRD

Research Priority	Key Scientific Questions	Near-Term Research Opportunities to Address Key Scientific Questions
2-1: Develop better tools, including novel biomarker tests and digital assessment technologies, to monitor brain health across the life course and screen, predict, and diagnose AD/ADRD at scale.	• How can brain health be precisely measured at scale across a diverse population (universally scalable)? • Can diagnostic biomarkers help identify potential causes for changes in personalized brain health? • Which data are essential to collect across the life course? • What alternative measures can assess changes in cognition and other related behaviors (e.g., ability to learn)? • How can existing cohorts be used to understand key transition points in brain health across the life course?	• Establish criteria to evaluate the diagnostic and clinical utility of newly developed tools (e.g., cognitive, clinical, fluid or digital biomarkers, imaging). • Discover and validate novel measures that capture early changes in brain health from a person's baseline. • Discover and validate new diagnostic, prognostic, predictive, and treatment response biomarkers (molecular and digital). • Carry out analyses within and across existing cohorts, including those cohorts developed to characterize brain health and those created for examining other health outcomes. • Perform large-scale, multiomics cohort studies of peripheral and brain signatures in diverse populations. • Perform large-scale cohort studies of digital signatures in diverse subpopulations.

continued

TABLE 2-2 continued

Research Priority	Key Scientific Questions	Near-Term Research Opportunities to Address Key Scientific Questions
2-2: Implement advances in clinical research methods and tools to generate data from real-world clinical practice settings that can inform future research.	• What are the facilitators of and barriers to the adoption of clinical research tools and methods? • How does the performance of novel tools (e.g., biomarker-based diagnostics, digital health technologies) differ across real-world settings and research settings? • What are the harms and benefits of identifying those with a specific pathology but who may never develop any symptoms? • How are the risks and benefits of biomarker testing and preclinical diagnosis balanced? • How can the negative social and legal consequences of early detection or diagnosis of AD/ADRD be mitigated?	• Rapidly implement novel tools (e.g., biomarker tests, digital technologies) in current, cross-institute studies. • Educate about the use and utility of emerging tools and technologies. • Evaluate potential harms of false positive or incorrect diagnoses and stigma related to early diagnoses before meaningful cognitive or other clinical symptoms manifest.

REFERENCES

Abdelmoaty, M. M., E. Lu, R. Kadry, E. G. Foster, S. Bhattarai, R. L. Mosley, and H. E. Gendelman. 2023. Clinical biomarkers for Lewy body diseases. *Cell & Bioscience* 13(1):209.

ADI (Alzheimer's Disease International). 2012. *World Alzheimer report 2012.* https://www.alzint.org/resource/world-alzheimer-report-2012/ (accessed August 20, 2024).

ADNI (Alzheimer's Disease Neuroimaging Initiative). 2024a. *About ADNI.* https://adni.loni.usc.edu/about/ (accessed August 14, 2024).

ADNI. 2024b. *Related and collaborative studies.* https://adni.loni.usc.edu/about/related-collaborative-studies/ (accessed August 14, 2024).

ADSP (Alzheimer's Disease Sequencing Project). 2024. *Alzheimer's Disease Sequencing Project Phenotype Harmonization Consortium (ADSP-PHC).* https://adsp.niagads.org/funded-programs/phenotype-harmonization/ (accessed August 22, 2022).

Albert, M. S., S. T. DeKosky, D. Dickson, B. Dubois, H. H. Feldman, N. C. Fox, A. Gamst, D. M. Holtzman, W. J. Jagust, R. C. Petersen, P. J. Snyder, M. C. Carrillo, B. Thies, and C. H. Phelps. 2011. The diagnosis of mild cognitive impairment due to Alzheimer's disease: Recommendations from the National Institute on Aging-Alzheimer's Association workgroups on diagnostic guidelines for Alzheimer's disease. *Alzheimer's & Dementia* 7(3):270-279.

ALLFTD (the ARTFL-LEFFTDS Longitudinal Frontotemporal Lobar Degeneration study). n.d. *Our Mission.* https://www.allftd.org/mission (accessed November 11, 2024).

Alzheimer Europe. 2011. *The value of knowing.* https://www.alzheimereurope.org/resources/publications/valueknowing?language_content_entity=en#:~:text=The%20survey%20on%20%22Value%20of,Public%20Health%20and%2Alzheimer%20Europe (accessed August 22, 2024).

American College of Cardiology. 2002. *Bogalusa Heart Study—Bogalusa.* https://www.acc.org/Latest-in-Cardiology/Clinical-Trials/2010/02/23/18/57/Bogalusa (accessed August 14, 2024).

Amini, S., B. Hao, L. Zhang, M. Song, A. Gupta, C. Karjadi, V. B. Kolachalama, R. Au, and I. C. Paschalidis. 2023. Automated detection of mild cognitive impairment and dementia from voice recordings: A natural language processing approach. *Alzheimer's & Dementia* 19(3):946-955.

Amini, S., B. Hao, J. Yang, C. Karjadi, V. B. Kolachalama, R. Au, and I. C. Paschalidis. 2024. Prediction of Alzheimer's disease progression within 6 years using speech: A novel approach leveraging language models. *Alzheimer's & Dementia* 20(8):5262-5270.

Andersen, S. L. 2020. Centenarians as models of resistance and resilience to Alzheimer's disease and related dementias. *Advances in Geriatric Medicine & Research* 2(3):e200018.

Au, R., V. B. Kolachalama, and I. C. Paschalidis. 2022. Redefining and validating digital biomarkers as fluid, dynamic multi-dimensional digital signal patterns. *Frontiers of Digital Health* 3:751629.

Au, R., Z. T. Popp, S. Low, P. H. Hwang, I. De Anda-Duran, S. Li, S. Rahman, H. Ding, A. Igwe, C. Karjadi, T. F. A. Ang, A. S. Devine, A. S. Gurnani, J. B. Mez, L. A. Farrer, P. Sunderaraman, H. Lin, and V. B. Kolachalama. 2023. Digital is the new blood: Enabling the present and the future. *Alzheimer's & Dementia* 19(S21):e078220.

Bangen, K. J., A. L. Clark, M. Werhane, E. C. Edmonds, D. A. Nation, N. Evangelista, D. J. Libon, M. W. Bondi, and L. Delano-Wood. 2016. Cortical amyloid burden differences across empirically-derived mild cognitive impairment subtypes and interaction with APOE ε4 genotype. *Journal of Alzheimer's Disease* 52(3):849-861.

Bargar, C., W. Wang, S. A. Gunzler, A. LeFevre, Z. Wang, A. J. Lerner, N. Singh, C. Tatsuoka, B. Appleby, X. Zhu, R. Xu, V. Haroutunian, W. Q. Zou, J. Ma, and S. G. Chen. 2021. Streamlined alpha-synuclein RT-QuIC assay for various biospecimens in Parkinson's disease and dementia with Lewy bodies. *Acta Neuropathologica Communications* 9(1):62.

Barron, D. S., J. T. Baker, K. S. Budde, D. Bzdok, S. B. Eickhoff, K. J. Friston, P. T. Fox, P. Geha, S. Heisig, A. Holmes, J. P. Onnela, A. Powers, D. Silbersweig, and J. H. Krystal. 2021. Decision models and technology can help psychiatry develop biomarkers. *Frontiers in Psychiatry* 12:706655.

Barth, C., and A. G. de Lange. 2020. Towards an understanding of women's brain aging: The immunology of pregnancy and menopause. *Frontiers in Neuroendocrinology* 58:100850.

Barthelemy, N. R., G. Salvado, S. E. Schindler, Y. He, S. Janelidze, L. E. Collij, B. Saef, R. L. Henson, C. D. Chen, B. A. Gordon, Y. Li, R. La Joie, T. L. S. Benzinger, J. C. Morris, N. Mattsson-Carlgren, S. Palmqvist, R. Ossenkoppele, G. D. Rabinovici, E. Stomrud, R. J. Bateman, and O. Hansson. 2024. Highly accurate blood test for Alzheimer's disease is similar or superior to clinical cerebrospinal fluid tests. *Nature Medicine* 30(4):1085-1095.

Beker, N., A. Ganz, M. Hulsman, T. Klausch, B. A. Schmand, P. Scheltens, S. A. M. Sikkes, and H. Holstege. 2021. Association of cognitive function trajectories in centenarians with postmortem neuropathology, physical health, and other risk factors for cognitive decline. *JAMA Network Open* 4(1):e2031654.

Bennett, D. A., J. A. Schneider, Z. Arvanitakis, J. F. Kelly, N. T. Aggarwal, R. C. Shah, and R. S. Wilson. 2006. Neuropathology of older persons without cognitive impairment from two community-based studies. *Neurology* 66(12):1837-1844.

Bernstein Sideman, A., R. Chalmer, E. Ayers, R. Gershon, J. Verghese, M. Wolf, A. Ansari, M. Arvanitis, N. Bui, P. Chen, A. Chodos, R. Corriveau, L. Curtis, A. R. Ehrlich, S. E. Tomaszewski Farias, C. Goode, L. Hill-Sakurai, C. J. Nowinski, M. Premkumar, K. P. Rankin, C. S. Ritchie, E. Tsoy, E. Weiss, and K. L. Possin. 2022. Lessons from detecting cognitive impairment including dementia (DetectCID) in primary care. *Journal of Alzheimer's Disease* 86(2):655-665.

Berron, D., W. Glanz, L. Clark, K. Basche, X. Grande, J. Gusten, O. V. Billette, I. Hempen, M. H. Naveed, N. Diersch, M. Butryn, A. Spottke, K. Buerger, R. Perneczky, A. Schneider, S. Teipel, J. Wiltfang, S. Johnson, M. Wagner, F. Jessen, and E. Duzel. 2024. A remote digital memory composite to detect cognitive impairment in memory clinic samples in unsupervised settings using mobile devices. *NPJ Digital Medicine* 7(1):79.

BioSEND. 2024. *About BioSEND*. https://biosend.org/about.html (accessed August 15, 2024).

Blanc, F., and O. Bousiges. 2022. Biomarkers and diagnosis of dementia with Lewy bodies including prodromal: Practical aspects. *Revue Neurologique* 178(5):472-483.

Boeve, B. F., A. A. Davis, Y. E. Ju, K. Kantarci, W. Singer, A. Videnovic, and NAPS coinvestigators. 2024. Concerns with the new biological research criteria for synucleinopathy. *Lancet Neurology* 23(7):659-660.

BU (Boston University). n.d.a. *Mission and objectives: Framingham Heart Study Brain Aging Program (FHS-BAP)*. https://www.bumc.bu.edu/fhs-bap/about-us/mission-fhs-bap/ (accessed August 14, 2024).

BU. n.d.b. *Evolution of the Framingham Heart Study and the birth of FHS-BAP*. https://www. bumc.bu.edu/fhs-bap/about-us/history/ (accessed October 25, 2024).

BU. n.d.c. *Access our data*. https://www.bumc.bu.edu/fhs-bap/for-researchers/access-our-data/ (accessed August 14, 2024).

Brookmeyer, R., and N. Abdalla. 2018. Estimation of lifetime risks of Alzheimer's disease dementia using biomarkers for preclinical disease. *Alzheimer's & Dementia* 14(8):981-988.

Buckley, R. 2024. *Panel discussion with committee*. Committee on Research Priorities for Preventing and Treating Alzheimer's Disease and Related Dementias Public Workshop, Hybrid. January 16-17, 2024.

Cadar, D. 2017. A life course approach to dementia prevention. *Journal of Aging and Geriatric Medicine* 1(2).

Cagney, D. N., J. Sul, R. Y. Huang, K. L. Ligon, P. Y. Wen, and B. M. Alexander. 2018. The FDA NIH Biomarkers, endpointS, and other Tools (BEST) resource in neuro-oncology. *Neuro-Oncology* 20(9):1162-1172.

Cairns, N. J., L. Taylor-Reinwald, J. C. Morris, and the Alzheimer's Disease Neuroimaging Inititative. 2010. Autopsy consent, brain collection, and standardized neuropathologic assessment of ADNI participants: The essential role of the neuropathology core. *Alzheimer's & Dementia* 6(3):274-279.

Cerino, E. S., M. J. Katz, C. Wang, J. Qin, Q. Gao, J. Hyun, J. G. Hakun, N. A. Roque, C. A. Derby, R. B. Lipton, and M. J. Sliwinski. 2021. Variability in cognitive performance on mobile devices is sensitive to mild cognitive impairment: Results from the Einstein Aging Study. *Frontiers in Digital Health* 3:78031.

Chin, N. A., and C. M. Erickson. 2024. Alzheimer's disease, biomarkers, and mAbs — What does primary care need? *New England Journal of Medicine* 390(24):2229-2231.

Chu, Y., W. Hirst, and J. Kordower. 2023. Mixed pathology as a rule, not exception: Time to reconsider disease nosology. *Handbook of Clinical Neurology* 192:57-71.

CLEAR-AD (Centrally-linked Longitudinal pEripheral biomARkers of AD). 2024a. *About.* https://clear-ad.org/index.php/about/ (accessed August 14, 2024).

CLEAR-AD. 2024b. *Home.* https://clear-ad.org/ (accessed August 14, 2024).

Cody, K. A., R. E. Langhough, M. D. Zammit, L. Clark, N. Chin, B. T. Christian, T. J. Betthauser, and S. C. Johnson. 2024. Characterizing brain tau and cognitive decline along the amyloid timeline in Alzheimer's disease. *Brain* 147(6):2144-2157.

Concha-Marambio, L., S. Pritzkow, M. Shahnawaz, C. M. Farris, and C. Soto. 2023. Seed amplification assay for the detection of pathologic alpha-synuclein aggregates in cerebrospinal fluid. *Nature Protocol* 18(4):1179-1196.

Cook, D. 2024. *Digital health.* Remarks at Committee on Research Priorities for Preventing and Treating Alzheimer's Disease and Related Dementias Public Workshop, Hybrid. January 16–17, 2024.

Coravos, A., S. Khozin, and K. D. Mandl. 2019. Developing and adopting safe and effective digital biomarkers to improve patient outcomes. *NPJ Digital Medicine* 2(1).

Cordts, I., A. Wachinger, C. Scialo, P. Lingor, M. Polymenidou, E. Buratti, and E. Feneberg. 2023. TDP-43 proteinopathy specific biomarker development. *Cells* 12(4).

Coriell Institute. 2024. *All biobanks.* https://www.coriell.org/1/Browse/Biobanks (accessed October 23, 2024).

Corney, K. B., E. C. West, S. E. Quirk, J. A. Pasco, A. L. Stuart, B. A. Manavi, B. E. Kavanagh, and L. J. Williams. 2022. The relationship between adverse childhood experiences and Alzheimer's disease: A systematic review. *Frontiers in Aging Neuroscience* 14:831378.

Corrada, M. 2024. *Envisioning the future of AD/ADRD research.* Presentation at Committee on Research Priorities for Preventing and Treating Alzheimer's Disease and Related Dementias Public Workshop, Hybrid. January 16–17, 2024.

Corrada, M., D. Berlau, and C. Kawas. 2012. A population-based clinicopathological study in the oldest-old: The 90+ study. *Current Alzheimer Research* 9(6):709-717.

Crane, P. K., A. Carle, L. E. Gibbons, P. Insel, R. S. Mackin, A. Gross, R. N. Jones, S. Mukherjee, S. M. Curtis, D. Harvey, M. Weiner, D. Mungas, and the Alzheimer's Disease Neuroimaging Initiative. 2012. Development and assessment of a composite score for memory in the Alzheimer's Disease Neuroimaging Initiative (ADNI). *Brain Imaging and Behavior* 6(4):502-516.

Cullen, N., A. Leuzy, S. Palmqvist, S. Janelidze, E. Stomrud, P. Pesini, J. A. Allue, N. K. Procter, H. Zetterberg, K. Blennow, J. Dage, N. Mattsson-Carlgren, and O. Hansson. 2021. Individualized prognosis of cognitive decline and dementia in mild cognitive impairment based on plasma biomarker combinations. *Nature Aging* 1(1):114-123.

Cummings, J. 2019. The role of biomarkers in Alzheimer's disease drug development. *Advances in Experimental Medicine and Biology* 1118:29-61.

Cutler, D. 2024. *Enhancing the use of tools for ADRD detection, diagnosis, and monitoring.* Presentation at Committee on Research Priorities for Preventing and Treating Alzheimer's Disease and Related Dementias Public Workshop, Hybrid. January 16–17, 2024.

Deoni, S. C. L., P. Burton, J. Beauchemin, R. Cano-Lorente, M. D. De Both, M. Johnson, L. Ryan, and M. J. Huentelman. 2023. Neuroimaging and verbal memory assessment in healthy aging adults using a portable low-field MRI scanner and a web-based platform: Results from a proof-of-concept population-based cross-section study. *Brain Structure and Function* 228(2):493-509.

DetectCID. 2022. *Advancing research towards the development of paradigms for detection of cognitive impairment and dementia that will benefit the public.* https://www.detectcid.org/overview#mission (accessed September 6, 2024).

Devi, G. 2023. A how-to guide for a precision medicine approach to the diagnosis and treatment of Alzheimer's disease. *Frontiers in Aging Neuroscience* 15:1213968.

Dion, C., F. Arias, S. Amini, R. Davis, D. Penney, D. J. Libon, and C. C. Price. 2020. Cognitive correlates of digital clock drawing metrics in older adults with and without mild cognitive impairment. *Journal of Alzheimer's Disease* 75(1):73-83.

Dubois, B., A. Padovani, P. Scheltens, A. Rossi, and G. Dell'Agnello. 2016. Timely diagnosis for Alzheimer's disease: A literature review on benefits and challenges. *Journal of Alzheimer's Disease* 49(3):617-631.

Dubois, B., N. Villain, G. B. Frisoni, G. D. Rabinovici, M. Sabbagh, S. Cappa, A. Bejanin, S. Bombois, M. Epelbaum, M. Teichmann, M. O. Habert, A. Nordberg, K. Blennow, D. Galasko, Y. Stern, C. C. Rowe, S. Salloway, L. S. Schneider, J. L. Cummings, and H. H. Feldman. 2021. Clinical diagnosis of Alzheimer's disease: Recommendations of the International Working Group. *Lancet Neurology* 20(6):484-496.

Dubois, B., C. A. F. von Arnim, N. Burnie, S. Bozeat, and J. Cummings. 2023. Biomarkers in Alzheimer's disease: Role in early and differential diagnosis and recognition of atypical variants. *Alzheimer's Research & Therapy* 15(1):175.

Erickson, C. M., N. A. Chin, S. C. Johnson, C. E. Gleason, and L. R. Clark. 2021. Disclosure of preclinical Alzheimer's disease biomarker results in research and clinical settings: Why, how, and what we still need to know. *Alzheimer's & Dementia* 13(1):e12150.

FDA (U.S. Food and Drug Administration). 2020. *FDA approves first drug to image tau pathology in patients being evaluated for Alzheimer's disease.* https://www.fda.gov/news-events/press-announcements/fda-approves-first-drug-image-tau-pathology-patients-being-evaluated-alzheimers-disease (accessed August 14, 2024).

FDA-NIH Biomarker Working Group. 2020. *BEST (Biomarkers, EndpointS, and other Tools) resource.* https://www.ncbi.nlm.nih.gov/books/NBK326791/ (accessed October 17, 2024).

Fleisher, A. S., M. J. Pontecorvo, M. D. Devous, Sr., M. Lu, A. K. Arora, S. P. Truocchio, P. Aldea, M. Flitter, T. Locascio, M. Devine, A. Siderowf, T. G. Beach, T. J. Montine, G. E. Serrano, C. Curtis, A. Perrin, S. Salloway, M. Daniel, C. Wellman, A. D. Joshi, D. J. Irwin, V. J. Lowe, W. W. Seeley, M. D. Ikonomovic, J. C. Masdeu, I. Kennedy, T. Harris, M. Navitsky, S. Southekal, M. A. Mintun, and A16 Study Investigators. 2020. Positron emission tomography imaging with [18F]Flortaucipir and postmortem assessment of Alzheimer disease neuropathologic changes. *JAMA Neurology* 77(7):829-839.

Foverskov, E., M. M. Glymour, E. L. Mortensen, M. Osler, G. T. Okholm, and R. Lund. 2020. Education and adolescent cognitive ability as predictors of dementia in a cohort of Danish men. *PLoS ONE* 15(8):e0235781.

Francis, P. T., H. Costello, and G. M. Hayes. 2018. Brains for dementia research: Evolution in a longitudinal brain donation cohort to maximize current and future value. *Journal of Alzheimer's Disease* 66(4):1635-1644.

Franklin, E. E., R. J. Perrin, B. Vincent, M. Baxter, J. C. Morris, N. J. Cairns, and the Alzheimer's Disease Neuroimaging Initiative. 2015. Brain collection, standardized neuropathologic assessment, and comorbidity in Alzheimer's Disease Neuroimaging Initiative 2 participants. *Alzheimer's & Dementias* 11(7):815-822.

Gao, Z., J. Li, L. Wang, and Y. Li. 2023. A systematic review of auricular therapy for poststroke cognitive impairment and dementia: A protocol for systematic review and meta-analysis. *Medicine (Baltimore)* 102(7):E32933.

Gendron, T. F., M. G. Heckman, L. J. White, A. M. Veire, O. Pedraza, A. R. Burch, A. C. Bozoki, B. C. Dickerson, K. Domoto-Reilly, T. Foroud, L. K. Forsberg, D. R. Galasko, N. Ghoshal, N. R. Graff-Radford, M. Grossman, H. W. Heuer, E. D. Huey, G. R. Hsiung, D. J. Irwin, D. I. Kaufer, G. C. Leger, I. Litvan, J. C. Masdeu, M. F. Mendez, C. U. Onyike, B. Pascual, A. Ritter, E. D. Roberson, J. C. Rojas, M. C. Tartaglia, Z. K. Wszolek, H. Rosen, B. F. Boeve, A. L. Boxer, ALLFTD Consortium, and L. Petrucelli. 2022. Comprehensive cross-sectional and longitudinal analyses of plasma neurofilament light across FTD spectrum disorders. *Cell Reports: Medicine* 3(4):100607.

Gibbons, C. H., T. Levine, C. Adler, B. Bellaire, N. Wang, J. Stohl, P. Agarwal, G. M. Aldridge, A. Barboi, V. G. H. Evidente, D. Galasko, M. D. Geschwind, A. Gonzalez-Duarte, R. Gil, M. Gudesblatt, S. H. Isaacson, H. Kaufmann, P. Khemani, R. Kumar, G. Lamotte, A. J. Liu, N. R. McFarland, M. Miglis, A. Reynolds, G. A. Sahagian, M. H. Saint-Hillaire, J. B. Schwartzbard, W. Singer, M. J. Soileau, S. Vernino, O. Yerstein, and R. Freeman. 2024. Skin biopsy detection of phosphorylated alpha-synuclein in patients with synucleinopathies. *JAMA* 331(15):1298-1306.

Gibson, L. L., C. Abdelnour, J. Chong, C. Ballard, and D. Aarsland. 2023. Clinical trials in dementia with Lewy bodies: The evolving concept of co-pathologies, patient selection and biomarkers. *Current Opinion in Neurology* 36(4):264-275.

Gifford, A., N. Praschan, A. Newhouse, and Z. Chemali. 2023. Biomarkers in frontotemporal dementia: Current landscape and future directions. *Biomarkers in Neuropsychiatry* 8(4):100065.

Gonzalez-Ortiz, F., M. Turton, P. R. Kac, D. Smirnov, E. Premi, R. Ghidoni, L. Benussi, V. Cantoni, C. Saraceno, J. Rivolta, N. J. Ashton, B. Borroni, D. Galasko, P. Harrison, H. Zetterberg, K. Blennow, and T. K. Karikari. 2023. Brain-derived tau: A novel blood-based biomarker for Alzheimer's disease-type neurodegeneration. *Brain* 146(3):1152-1165.

González, H. M., W. Tarraf, M. Fornage, K. A. González, A. Chai, M. Youngblood, M. L. A. Abreu, D. Zeng, S. Thomas, G. A. Talavera, L. C. Gallo, R. Kaplan, M. L. Daviglus, and N. Schneiderman. 2019. A research framework for cognitive aging and Alzheimer's disease among diverse US latinos: Design and implementation of the Hispanic Community Health Study/Study of Latinos-Investigation of Neurocognitive Aging (SOL-INCA). *Alzheimer's & Dementia* 15(12):1624-1632.

Grunberg, V. A., S. M. Bannon, P. Popok, M. Reichman, B. C. Dickerson, and A. M. Vranceanu. 2022. A race against time: Couples' lived diagnostic journeys to young-onset dementia. *Aging and Mental Health* 26(11):2223-2232.

Guo, Y., J. You, Y. Zhang, W. S. Liu, Y. Y. Huang, Y. R. Zhang, W. Zhang, Q. Dong, J. F. Feng, W. Cheng, and J. T. Yu. 2024. Plasma proteomic profiles predict future dementia in healthy adults. *Nature Aging* 4(2):247-260.

Hampel, H., J. Cummings, K. Blennow, P. Gao, C. R. Jack, Jr., and A. Vergallo. 2021. Developing the ATX(N) classification for use across the Alzheimer disease continuum. *Nature Reviews Neurology* 17(9):580-589.

Hampel, H., R. Au, S. Mattke, W. M. van der Flier, P. Aisen, L. Apostolova, C. Chen, M. Cho, S. De Santi, P. Gao, A. Iwata, R. Kurzman, A. J. Saykin, S. Teipel, B. Vellas, A. Vergallo, H. Wang, and J. Cummings. 2022a. Designing the next-generation clinical care pathway for Alzheimer's disease. *Nature Aging* 2(8):692-703.

Hampel, H., L. M. Shaw, P. Aisen, C. Chen, A. Lleó, T. Iwatsubo, A. Iwata, M. Yamada, T. Ikeuchi, J. Jia, H. Wang, C. E. Teunissen, E. Peskind, K. Blennow, J. Cummings, and A. Vergallo. 2022b. State-of-the-art of lumbar puncture and its place in the journey of patients with Alzheimer's disease. *Alzheimer's & Dementia* 18(1):159-177.

Hampel, H., Y. Hu, J. Cummings, S. Mattke, T. Iwatsubo, A. Nakamura, B. Vellas, S. O'Bryant, L. M. Shaw, M. Cho, R. Batrla, A. Vergallo, K. Blennow, J. Dage, and S. E. Schindler. 2023. Blood-based biomarkers for Alzheimer's disease: Current state and future use in a transformed global healthcare landscape. *Neuron* 111(18):2781-2799.

Hampton, O. L., S. Mukherjee, M. J. Properzi, A. P. Schultz, P. K. Crane, L. E. Gibbons, T. J. Hohman, P. Maruff, Y. Y. Lim, R. E. Amariglio, K. V. Papp, K. A. Johnson, D. M. Rentz, R. A. Sperling, and R. F. Buckley. 2023. Harmonizing the preclinical Alzheimer cognitive composite for multicohort studies. *Neuropsychology* 37(4):436-449.

Hansson, O., A. Mikulskis, A. M. Fagan, C. Teunissen, H. Zetterberg, H. Vanderstichele, J. L. Molinuevo, L. M. Shaw, M. Vandijck, M. M. Verbeek, M. Savage, N. Mattsson, P. Lewczuk, R. Batrla, S. Rutz, R. A. Dean, and K. Blennow. 2018. The impact of pre-analytical variables on measuring cerebrospinal fluid biomarkers for Alzheimer's disease diagnosis: A review. *Alzheimer's & Dementia* 14(10):1313-1333.

Harris, K. M., C. T. Halpern, E. A. Whitsel, J. M. Hussey, L. A. Killeya-Jones, J. Tabor, and S. C. Dean. 2019. Cohort profile: The National Longitudinal Study of Adolescent to Adult Health (ADD Health). *International Journal of Epidemiology* 48(5):1415-1415k.

HCAP Network. 2023. *About the HCAP network.* https://hcap.isr.umich.edu/ (accessed August 15, 2024).

HCAP Network. 2024. *HCAP network team.* https://hcap.isr.umich.edu/people/ (accessed October 17, 2024).

HCS Institute for Translational Research. 2022. *Health and Aging Brain Study—Health disparities.* https://apps.unthsc.edu/itr/research/habs (accessed August 22, 2024).

Heyer, S., M. Simon, M. Doyen, A. Mortada, V. Roch, E. Jeanbert, N. Thilly, C. Malaplate, A. Kearney-Schwartz, T. Jonveaux, A. Bannay, and A. Verger. 2024. (18)F-FDG PET can effectively rule out conversion to dementia and the presence of CSF biomarker of neuro-degeneration: A real-world data analysis. *Alzheimer's Research & Therapy* 16(1):182.

HHS (U.S. Department of Health and Human Services). 2023. *Alzheimer's disease (AD) and AD-related dementias (ADRD) real-world data platform.* https://grants.nih.gov/grants/guide/rfa-files/RFA-AG-24-009.html (accessed August 15, 2024).

Höglinger, G. U., C. H. Adler, D. Berg, C. Klein, T. F. Outeiro, W. Poewe, R. Postuma, A. J. Stoessl, and A. E. Lang. 2024. A biological classification of Parkinson's disease: The SynNeurGe research diagnostic criteria. *Lancet Neurology* 23(2):191-204.

Hort, J., A. Bartos, T. Pirttila, and P. Scheltens. 2010. Use of cerebrospinal fluid biomarkers in diagnosis of dementia across Europe. *European Journal of Neurology* 17(1):90-96.

HRS (Health and Retirement Study). 2021. *The health and retirement study: Telling the story of aging in America.* https://hrsonline.isr.umich.edu/sitedocs/databook-2021/HRS-Telling-the-Story-of-Aging-in-America.pdf (accessed October 28, 2024).

HRS. 2024. *Cognition data.* https://hrs.isr.umich.edu/data-products/cognition-data#adams (accessed October 23, 2024).

Htike, T. T., S. Mishra, S. Kumar, P. Padmanabhan, and B. Gulyas. 2019. Peripheral biomarkers for early detection of Alzheimer's and Parkinson's diseases. *Molecular Neurobiology* 56(3):2256-2277.

Huber, H., L. Montoliu-Gaya, K. Blennow, H. Zetterberg, M. B. Rovira, A. Jeromin, X. M. Arús, and N. J. Ashton. 2023. A finger prick collection method for detecting blood biomarkers of neurodegeneration—a pilot study (DROP-AD). *Alzheimer's & Dementia* 19(S14):e080275.

Irwin, K. E., P. Jasin, K. E. Braunstein, I. R. Sinha, M. A. Garret, K. D. Bowden, K. Chang, J. C. Troncoso, A. Moghekar, E. S. Oh, D. Raitcheva, D. Bartlett, T. Miller, J. D. Berry, B. J. Traynor, J. P. Ling, and P. C. Wong. 2024a. A fluid biomarker reveals loss of TDP-43 splicing repression in presymptomatic ALS-FTD. *Nature Medicine* 30(2):382-393.

Irwin, K. E., U. Sheth, P. C. Wong, and T. F. Gendron. 2024b. Fluid biomarkers for amyotrophic lateral sclerosis: A review. *Molecular Neurodegeneration* 19(1):9.

Ishii, K. 2020. Diagnostic imaging of dementia with Lewy bodies, frontotemporal lobar degeneration, and normal pressure hydrocephalus. *Japanese Journal of Radiology* 38(1):64-76.

Jack, C. R., Jr., D. A. Bennett, K. Blennow, M. C. Carrillo, B. Dunn, S. B. Haeberlein, D. M. Holtzman, W. Jagust, F. Jessen, J. Karlawish, E. Liu, J. L. Molinuevo, T. Montine, C. Phelps, K. P. Rankin, C. C. Rowe, P. Scheltens, E. Siemers, H. M. Snyder, and R. Sperling. 2018. NIA-AA research framework: Toward a biological definition of Alzheimer's disease. *Alzheimer's & Dementia* 14(4):535-562.

Jack, C. R., Jr., J. S. Andrews, T. G. Beach, T. Buracchio, B. Dunn, A. Graf, O. Hansson, C. Ho, W. Jagust, E. McDade, J. L. Molinuevo, O. C. Okonkwo, L. Pani, M. S. Rafii, P. Scheltens, E. Siemers, H. M. Snyder, R. Sperling, C. E. Teunissen, and M. C. Carrillo. 2024. Revised criteria for diagnosis and staging of Alzheimer's disease: Alzheimer's Association Workgroup. *Alzheimer's & Dementia* 20(8):5143-5169.

Jia, J., Y. Ning, M. Chen, S. Wang, H. Yang, F. Li, J. Ding, Y. Li, B. Zhao, J. Lyu, S. Yang, X. Yan, Y. Wang, W. Qin, Q. Wang, Y. Li, J. Zhang, F. Liang, Z. Liao, and S. Wang. 2024. Biomarker changes during 20 years preceding Alzheimer's disease. *New England Journal of Medicine* 390(8):712-722.

Katzeff, J. S., F. Bright, K. Phan, J. J. Kril, L. M. Ittner, M. Kassiou, J. R. Hodges, O. Piguet, M. C. Kiernan, G. M. Halliday, and W. S. Kim. 2022. Biomarker discovery and development for frontotemporal dementia and amyotrophic lateral sclerosis. *Brain* 145(5):1598-1609.

Kawakami, I., T. Arai, and M. Hasegawa. 2019. The basis of clinicopathological heterogeneity in TDP-43 proteinopathy. *Acta Neuropathologica* 138(5):751-770.

Kaye, J. 2024 *Development and use of digital tools to assess human health.* Presentation at Committee on Research Priorities for Preventing and Treating Alzheimer's Disease and Related Dementias Public Workshop, Hybrid. January 16–17, 2024.

Kaye, J. A., J. Marcoe, A. B. Mar, E. J. Hanna, A. Pierce, L. C. Silbert, Y. Shang, D. Schwartz, S. Gothard, N. Mattek, W. T. M. Au-Yeung, J. S. Steele, and Z. T. Beattie. 2023. DETECT-AD (Digital Evaluations and Technologies Enabling Clinical Translation for Alzheimer's Disease): A simulated anti-amyloid clinical trial using digital biomarkers as primary outcome measures. *Alzheimer's & Dementia* 19(S11):e082057.

Kimberly, W. T., A. J. Sorby-Adams, A. G. Webb, E. X. Wu, R. Beekman, R. Bowry, S. J. Schiff, A. de Havenon, F. X. Shen, G. Sze, P. Schaefer, J. E. Iglesias, M. S. Rosen, and K. N. Sheth. 2023. Brain imaging with portable low-field MRI. *Nature Reviews Bioengineering* 1(9):617-630.

Kind, A. 2024. *Discussant perspectives and committee discussion.* Presentation at Committee on Research Priorities for Preventing and Treating Alzheimer's Disease and Related Dementias Public Workshop, Hybrid. January 16–17, 2024.

King, J., and M. Wagster. 2024. *Mobile toolbox: Expand your cognitive assessment reach!* https://www.nia.nih.gov/research/blog/2024/06/mobile-toolbox-expand-your-cognitive-assessment-reach (accessed August 14, 2024).

Knopman, D. S., J. E. Parisi, A. Salviati, M. Floriach-Robert, B. F. Boeve, R. J. Ivnik, G. E. Smith, D. W. Dickson, K. A. Johnson, L. E. Petersen, W. C. McDonald, H. Braak, and R. C. Petersen. 2003. Neuropathology of cognitively normal elderly. *Journal of Neuropathology and Experimental Neurology* 62(11):1087-1095.

Kobayashi, L. C., R. N. Jones, E. M. Briceno, M. A. Renteria, Y. Zhang, E. Meijer, K. M. Langa, J. Lee, and A. L. Gross. 2024. Cross-national comparisons of later-life cognitive function using data from the Harmonized Cognitive Assessment Protocol (HCAP): Considerations and recommended best practices. *Alzheimer's & Dementia* 20(3):2273-2281.

Landau, S. M., A. Horng, A. Fero, and W. J. Jagust. 2016. Amyloid negativity in patients with clinically diagnosed Alzheimer disease and MCI. *Neurology* 86(15):1377-1385.

Langa, K. M., and J. F. Burke. 2019. Preclinical Alzheimer disease—early diagnosis or over-diagnosis? *JAMA Internal Medicine* 179(9):1161-1162.

Largent, E. A., K. Harkins, C. H. van Dyck, S. Hachey, P. Sankar, and J. Karlawish. 2020. Cognitively unimpaired adults' reactions to disclosure of amyloid PET scan results. *PLoS ONE* 15(2):e0229137.

Law, Z. K., C. Todd, R. Mehraram, J. Schumacher, M. R. Baker, F. E. N. LeBeau, A. Yarnall, M. Onofrj, L. Bonanni, A. Thomas, and J. P. Taylor. 2020. The role of EEG in the diagnosis, prognosis and clinical correlates of dementia with Lewy bodies—a systematic review. *Diagnostics (Basel)* 10(9):616.

Livingston, G., J. Huntley, A. Sommerlad, D. Ames, C. Ballard, S. Banerjee, C. Brayne, A. Burns, J. Cohen-Mansfield, C. Cooper, S. G. Costafreda, A. Dias, N. Fox, L. N. Gitlin, R. Howard, H. C. Kales, M. Kivimäki, E. B. Larson, A. Ogunniyi, V. Orgeta, K. Ritchie, K. Rockwood, E. L. Sampson, Q. Samus, L. S. Schneider, G. Selbæk, L. Teri, and N. Mukadam. 2020. Dementia prevention, intervention, and care: 2020 report of the Lancet Commission. *Lancet* 396(10248):413-446.

MarkVCID. 2017. *MarkVCID consortium overview.* https://markvcid.partners.org/about/m2-consortium-overview (accessed August 21, 2024).

Matsubara, T., M. Kameyama, N. Tanaka, R. Sengoku, M. Orita, K. Furuta, A. Iwata, T. Arai, H. Maruyama, Y. Saito, and S. Murayama. 2022. Autopsy validation of the diagnostic accuracy of ^{123}I-metaiodobenzylguanidine myocardial scintigraphy for Lewy body disease. *Neurology* 98(16):e1648-e1659.

Mavroudis, I., F. Petridis, and D. Kazis. 2019. Cerebrospinal fluid, imaging, and physiological biomarkers in dementia with Lewy bodies. *American Journal of Alzheimer's Disease & Other Dementias* 34(7-8):421-432.

McDowell, I., G. Xi, J. Lindsay, and M. Tierney. 2005. Mapping the connections between education and dementia. *Journal of Clinical and Experimental Neuropsychology* 29(2):127-141.

McKeith, I. G., D. Galasko, M. Kosaka, E. K. Perry, D. W. Dickson, L. A. Hansen, D. P. Salmon, J. Lowe, S. S. Mirra, E. J. Byrne, G. Lennox, N. P. Quinn, J. A. Edwardson, P. G. Ince, C. Bergeron, A. Burns, B. L. Miller, S. Lovestone, D. Collerton, E. N. H. Jansen, C. Ballard, R. A. I. de Vos, K. A. Jellinger, and R. H. Perry. 1996. Consensus guidelines for the clinical and pathologic diagnosis of dementia with Lewy bodies (DLB). *Neurology* 47(5):1113-1124.

McKhann, G., D. Drachman, M. Folstein, R. Katzman, D. Price, and E. M. Stadlan. 1984. Clinical diagnosis of Alzheimer's disease: Report of the NINCDS-ADRDA work group under the auspices of Department of Health and Human Services Task Force on Alzheimer's Disease. *Neurology* 34(7):939-939.

McKhann, G. M., D. S. Knopman, H. Chertkow, B. T. Hyman, C. R. Jack, Jr., C. H. Kawas, W. E. Klunk, W. J. Koroshetz, J. J. Manly, R. Mayeux, R. C. Mohs, J. C. Morris, M. N. Rossor, P. Scheltens, M. C. Carrillo, B. Thies, S. Weintraub, and C. H. Phelps. 2011. The diagnosis of dementia due to Alzheimer's disease: Recommendations from the National Institute on Aging—Alzheimer's Association workgroups on diagnostic guidelines for Alzheimer's disease. *Alzheimer's & Dementia* 7(3):263-269.

Meng, X., and C. D'Arcy. 2012. Education and dementia in the context of the cognitive reserve hypothesis: A systematic review with meta-analyses and qualitative analyses. *PLoS ONE* 7(6):e38268.

MESA (Multi-Ethnic Study of Atherosclerosis). *About.* https://internal.mesa-nhlbi.org/about (accessed November 11, 2024).

MESA MIND. *Study Overview.* https://www.mesa-nhlbi.org/MESAMind/StudyOverview (accessed November 11, 2024).

Mielke, M. 2024. Sex and gender differences in Alzheimer's disease and Alzheimer's disease related dementias. Commissioned Paper for the Committee on Research Priorities for Preventing and Treating Alzheimer's Disease and Related Dementias.

Miller, G. 2024. *Using exposomics to uncover the environmental contributors to AD/ADRD.* Presentation at Committee on Research Priorities for Preventing and Treating Alzheimer's Disease and Related Dementias Public Workshop, Hybrid. January 16–17, 2024.

Minoshima, S., D. Cross, T. Thientunyakit, N. L. Foster, and A. Drzezga. 2022. ^{18}F-FDG PET imaging in neurodegenerative dementing disorders: Insights into subtype classification, emerging disease categories, and mixed dementia with copathologies. *Journal of Nuclear Medicine* 63(Suppl 1):2S-12S.

Mobile Toolbox. 2024. *Measuring cognitive change where it matters.* https://mobiletoolbox. org/ (accessed October 15, 2024).

Moceri, V., W. Kukull, I. Emanual, G. van Belle, J. Starr, G. Schellenberg, W. McCormick, J. Bowen, L. Teri, and E. B. Larson. 2000. Using census data and birth certificates to reconstruct the early-life socioeconomic environment and the relation to the development of Alzheimer's disease. *Epidemiology* 12(4)383-389.

Moro, M. 2018. *The NIA aging cell repository: Facilitating research with aging cells.* https://www.nia.nih.gov/research/blog/2018/05/nia-aging-cell-repository-facilitating-research-aging-cells (accessed August 9, 2024).

Mukherjee, S., S. E. Choi, M. L. Lee, P. Scollard, E. H. Trittschuh, J. Mez, A. J. Saykin, L. E. Gibbons, R. E. Sanders, A. F. Zaman, M. A. Teylan, W. A. Kukull, L. L. Barnes, D. A. Bennett, A. Z. Lacroix, E. B. Larson, M. Cuccaro, S. Mercado, L. Dumitrescu, T. J. Hohman, and P. K. Crane. 2023. Cognitive domain harmonization and cocalibration in studies of older adults. *Neuropsychology* 37(4):409-423.

Nagar, S. D., P. Pemu, J. Qian, E. Boerwinkle, M. Cicek, C. R. Clark, E. Cohn, K. Gebo, R. Loperena, K. Mayo, S. Mockrin, L. Ohno-Machado, A. H. Ramirez, S. Schully, A. Able, A. Green, S. Zuchner, S. Consortium, I. K. Jordan, and R. Meller. 2022. Investigation of hypertension and type 2 diabetes as risk factors for dementia in the all of US cohort. *Scientific Reports* 12(1):19797.

NASEM (National Academies of Sciences, Engineering, and Medicine). 2017. *Preventing cognitive decline and dementia: A way forward.* Edited by A. I. Leshner, S. Landis, C. Stroud and A. Downey. Washington, DC: The National Academies Press.

NASEM. 2021a. *Reducing the impact of dementia in America: A decadal survey of the behavioral and social sciences.* Washington, DC: The National Academies Press.

NASEM. 2021b. *Meeting the challenge of caring for persons living with dementia and their care partners and caregivers: A way forward.* Edited by E. B. Larson and C. Stroud. Washington, DC: The National Academies Press.

NASEM. 2024. *Preventing and treating Alzheimer's disease and related dementias: Promising research and opportunities to accelerate progress: Proceedings of a workshop—in brief*, edited by A. Downey and O. Yost. Washington, DC: The National Academies Press.

NCATS (National Center for Advancing Translational Sciences). 2024. *About the CTSA program*. https://ncats.nih.gov/research/research-activities/ctsa (accessed October 17, 2024).

NCRAD (National Centralized Repository for Alzheimer's Disease and Related Dementias). 2024a. *API generation program*. https://ncrad.iu.edu/access-samples/available-samples/api (accessed August 15, 2024).

NCRAD. 2024b. *GEMS*. https://ncrad.iu.edu/access-samples/available-samples/gems (accessed August 15, 2024).

NCRAD. 2024c. *Who we are*. https://ncrad.iu.edu/about (accessed August 15, 2024).

NCRAD. 2024d. *Explore a multitude of research samples at NCRAD*. https://ncrad.iu.edu/access-samples/available-samples (accessed October 17, 2024).

NCRAD. 2024e. *Enhance your study with biomarker analysis at ncrad*. https://ncrad.iu.edu/biomarker-analysis (accessed October 17, 2024).

NeuroBioBank. 2024. *About the NIH NeuroBioBank*. https://neurobiobank.nih.gov/about/ (accessed August 15, 2024).

Ng, K. P., H. J. Chiew, L. Lim, P. Rosa-Neto, N. Kandiah, and S. Gauthier. 2018. The influence of language and culture on cognitive assessment tools in the diagnosis of early cognitive impairment and dementia. *Expert Review of Neurotherapy* 18(11):859-869.

Nguyen, T. T., E. J. Tchetgen Tchetgen, I. Kawachi, S. E. Gilman, S. Walter, S. Y. Liu, J. J. Manly, and M. M. Glymour. 2016. Instrumental variable approaches to identifying the causal effect of educational attainment on dementia risk. *Annals of Epidemiology* 26(1):71-76, e71-e73.

NHLBI (National Heart, Lung, and Blood Institute). n.d. *Framingham Heart Study (FHS)*. https://www.nhlbi.nih.gov/science/framingham-heart-study-fhs (accessed August 14, 2024).

NHLBI. 2018. *Bogalusa Heart Study (BHS)* https://biolincc.nhlbi.nih.gov/studies/bhs/ (accessed October 25, 2024).

NHLBI. 2023. *Framingham Heart Study—Cohort (FHS-Cohort)*. https://biolincc.nhlbi.nih.gov/studies/framcohort/ (accessed August 14, 2024).

NHLBI. 2024. *Hispanic Community Health Study/Study of Latinos (HCHS/SOL)*. https://www.nhlbi.nih.gov/science/hispanic-community-health-studystudy-latinos-hchssol (accessed August 22, 2024).

NIA (National Institute on Aging). n.d.a. *Brain donation*. https://www.nia.nih.gov/health/brain-donation (accessed August 15, 2024).

NIA. n.d.b. *AgingResearchBiobank*. https://agingresearchbiobank.nia.nih.gov/about/ (accessed August 22, 2024).

NIA. 2019. *National Institute on Aging Workshop on Applying Digital Technology for Early Diagnosis and Monitoring of Alzheimer's Disease and Related Dementias*.

NIA. 2022. *Brain donation resources for ADRCS*. https://www.nia.nih.gov/health/brain-donation/brain-donation-resources-adrcs (accessed October 17, 2024).

NIA. 2023a. *Accelerating Medicines Partnership program for Alzheimer's Disease (AMP AD)*. https://www.nia.nih.gov/research/amp-ad (accessed August 13, 2024).

NIA. 2023b. *Fiscal year 2024 budget*. https://www.nia.nih.gov/about/budget/fiscal-year-2024-budget (accessed August 22, 2024).

NIA. 2024a. *Data sharing resources for researchers*. https://www.nia.nih.gov/research/data-sharing-resources-researchers (accessed August 9, 2024).

NIA. 2024b. *Fiscal year 2025 budget*. https://www.nia.nih.gov/about/budget/fiscal-year-2025-budget (accessed August 22, 2024).

Nicosia, J., A. J. Aschenbrenner, D. A. Balota, M. J. Sliwinski, M. Tahan, S. Adams, S. S. Stout, H. Wilks, B. A. Gordon, T. L. S. Benzinger, A. M. Fagan, C. Xiong, R. J. Bateman, J. C. Morris, and J. Hassenstab. 2023. Unsupervised high-frequency smartphone-based cognitive assessments are reliable, valid, and feasible in older adults at risk for Alzheimer's disease. *Journal of the International Neuropsychological Society* 29(5):459-471.

NIH (National Institutes of Health). 2024a. *All of Us Research Program overview.* https://allofus.nih.gov/about/program-overview (accessed August 14, 2024).

NIH. 2024b. *All of Us—About.* https://allofus.nih.gov/about (accessed October 25, 2024).

NIH. 2024c. *FAQ.* https://allofus.nih.gov/about/faq (accessed October 25, 2024).

NIH RePORTER. 2024a. *Centrally-linked longitudinal peripheral biomarkers of AD in multi-ethnic populations.* https://reporter.nih.gov/search/aPaS7obQX0SvtsI_0JMY0A/project-details/10555723 (accessed October 23, 2024.

NIH RePORTER. 2024b. *Integrative pathways to cognitive, affective, and brain health.* https://reporter.nih.gov/search/atFWblv290KNG-3jZzxCPA/project-details/10558956 (accessed August 22, 2024).

NIH RePORTER. 2024c. *The Health and Aging Brain Study—Health Disparities.* https://reporter.nih.gov/search/SLCPkzy1o0umXa2JsO8B0Q/project-details/10493844 (accessed August 15, 2024).

NIH RePORTER. 2024d. *Research network for the harmonized cognitive assessment protocol.* https://reporter.nih.gov/search/15EEC00B468BC3D77598B8961CAA4A01A2FFCEB861BF/project-details/10663818 (accessed August 15, 2024).

NIH Toolbox. 2024. *MyCog: Overview of development.* https://nihtoolbox.org/mycog/ (accessed August 22, 2024).

NINDS (National Institute of Neurological Disorders and Stroke). 2023. *Consider donating your brain for neurological disease research.* https://www.ninds.nih.gov/health-information/patient-caregiver-education/consider-donating-your-brain-neurological-disease-research (accessed August 15, 2024).

Nye, E., H. Lamont, and L. Anderson. 2022. *Federal efforts to address racial and ethnic disparities in Alzheimer's disease and related dementias.* https://aspe.hhs.gov/sites/default/files/documents/5f3fc5aa6ae780f739265d40f20fc456/federal-racial-ethnic-disparities-adrd.pdf (accessed September 7, 2024).

Öhman, F., J. Hassenstab, D. Berron, M. Scholl, and K. V. Papp. 2021. Current advances in digital cognitive assessment for preclinical Alzheimer's disease. *Alzheimer's & Dementia* 13(1):e12217.

OHSU (Oregon Health and Science University). 2024a. *About us.* https://www.ohsu.edu/collaborative-aging-research-using-technology/about-us (accessed August 14, 2024).

OHSU. 2024b. *CART mission.* https://www.ohsu.edu/collaborative-aging-research-using-technology/cart-mission (accessed August 14, 2024).

OHSU. 2024c. *The CART home.* https://www.ohsu.edu/collaborative-aging-research-using-technology/cart-home (accessed October 15, 2024).

OHSU. 2024d. *For industry and community partners.* https://www.ohsu.edu/collaborative-aging-research-using-technology/industry-and-community-partners (accessed October 15, 2024).

Ossenkoppele, R., A. Pichet Binette, C. Groot, R. Smith, O. Strandberg, S. Palmqvist, E. Stomrud, P. Tideman, T. Ohlsson, J. Jogi, K. Johnson, R. Sperling, V. Dore, C. L. Masters, C. Rowe, D. Visser, B. N. M. van Berckel, W. M. van der Flier, S. Baker, W. J. Jagust, H. J. Wiste, R. C. Petersen, C. R. Jack, Jr., and O. Hansson. 2022. Amyloid and tau PET-positive cognitively unimpaired individuals are at high risk for future cognitive decline. *Nature Medicine* 28(11):2381-2387.

Palmqvist, S., S. Janelidze, E. Stomrud, H. Zetterberg, J. Karl, K. Zink, T. Bittner, N. Mattsson, U. Eichenlaub, K. Blennow, and O. Hansson. 2019. Performance of fully automated plasma assays as screening tests for Alzheimer disease-related beta-amyloid status. *JAMA Neurology* 76(9):1060-1069.

Palmqvist, S., S. Janelidze, Y. T. Quiroz, H. Zetterberg, F. Lopera, E. Stomrud, Y. Su, Y. Chen, G. E. Serrano, A. Leuzy, N. Mattsson-Carlgren, O. Strandberg, R. Smith, A. Villegas, D. Sepulveda-Falla, X. Chai, N. K. Proctor, T. G. Beach, K. Blennow, J. L. Dage, E. M. Reiman, and O. Hansson. 2020. Discriminative accuracy of plasma phospho-tau217 for Alzheimer disease vs other neurodegenerative disorders. *JAMA* 324(8):772-781.

Palmqvist, S., P. Tideman, N. Cullen, H. Zetterberg, K. Blennow, Alzheimer's Disease Neuroimaging Initiative, J. L. Dage, E. Stomrud, S. Janelidze, N. Mattsson-Carlgren, and O. Hansson. 2021. Prediction of future Alzheimer's disease dementia using plasma phospho-tau combined with other accessible measures. *Nature Medicine* 27(6):1034-1042.

Paschalidis, I. C. 2024. *Panelist Remarks*. Committee on Research Priorities for Preventing and Treating Alzheimer's Disease and Related Dementias Public Workshop, Hybrid. January 16–17, 2024.

Peet, B. T., S. Spina, N. Mundada, and R. La Joie. 2021. Neuroimaging in frontotemporal dementia: Heterogeneity and relationships with underlying neuropathology. *Neurotherapeutics* 18(2):728-752.

Piers, R. J., K. N. Devlin, B. Ning, Y. Liu, B. Wasserman, J. M. Massaro, M. Lamar, C. C. Price, R. Swenson, R. Davis, D. L. Penney, R. Au, and D. J. Libon. 2017. Age and graphomotor decision making assessed with the digital clock drawing test: The Framingham Heart Study. *Journal of Alzheimer's Disease* 60(4):1611-1620.

Reitz, C. 2016. Toward precision medicine in Alzheimer's disease. *Annals of Translational Medicine* 4(6):107.

Reitz, C., M. A. Pericak-Vance, T. Foroud, and R. Mayeux. 2023. A global view of the genetic basis of Alzheimer disease. *Nature Reviews Neurology* 19(5):261-277.

Reuben, A. 2018. Childhood lead exposure and adult neurodegenerative disease. *Journal of Alzheimer's Disease* 64:17-42.

Ritchie, C. W., G. M. Terrera, and T. J. Quinn. 2015. Dementia trials and dementia tribulations: Methodological and analytical challenges in dementia research. *Alzheimer's Research & Therapy* 7(1):31.

Robinson, A., R. McNamee, Y. S. Davidson, M. Horan, J. Snowden, L. McInnes, N. Pendleton, and D. Mann. 2018. Scores obtained from a simple cognitive test of visuospatial episodic memory performed decades before death are associated with the ultimate presence of Alzheimer disease pathology. *Dementia and Geriatric Cognitive Disorders* 45:79-90.

Rosin, E. R., D. Blasco, A. R. Pilozzi, L. H. Yang, and X. Huang. 2020. A narrative review of Alzheimer's disease stigma. *Journal of Alzheimer's Disease* 78(2):515-528.

Roth, S., N. Burnie, I. Suridjan, J. T. Yan, and M. Carboni. 2023. Current diagnostic pathways for Alzheimer's disease: A cross-sectional real-world study across six countries. *Journal of Alzheimer's Disease Reports* 7:659-674.

Scott, G. D., M. R. Arnold, T. G. Beach, C. H. Gibbons, A. G. Kanthasamy, R. M. Lebovitz, A. W. Lemstra, L. M. Shaw, C. E. Teunissen, H. Zetterberg, A. S. Taylor, T. C. Graham, B. F. Boeve, S. N. Gomperts, N. R. Graff-Radford, C. Moussa, K. L. Poston, L. S. Rosenthal, M. N. Sabbagh, R. R. Walsh, M. T. Weber, M. J. Armstrong, J. A. Bang, A. C. Bozoki, K. Domoto-Reilly, J. E. Duda, J. E. Fleisher, D. R. Galasko, J. E. Galvin, J. G. Goldman, S. K. Holden, L. S. Honig, D. E. Huddleston, J. B. Leverenz, I. Litvan, C. A. Manning, K. S. Marder, A. Y. Pantelyat, V. S. Pelak, D. W. Scharre, S. J. Sha, H. A. Shill, Z. Mari, J. F. Quinn, and D. J. Irwin. 2021. Fluid and tissue biomarkers of Lewy body dementia: Report of an LBDA symposium. *Frontiers in Neurology* 12:805135.

Sevigny, J., J. Suhy, P. Chiao, T. Chen, G. Klein, D. Purcell, J. Oh, A. Verma, M. Sampat, and J. Barakos. 2016. Amyloid PET screening for enrichment of early-stage Alzheimer disease clinical trials: Experience in a phase 1b clinical trial. *Alzheimer Disease and Associated Disorders* 30(1):1-7.

SHS (Strong Heart Study). 2017a. *About Strong Heart Study.* https://strongheartstudy.org/ About (accessed August 23, 2024).

SHS. 2017b. *Recently approved ancillary studies/collaborations by Strong Heart Study.* https:// strongheartstudy.org/Research/Ancillary-and-Sub-Studies/Approved-Ancillary-and-Sub-studies (accessed August 23, 2024).

Simuni, T., L. M. Chahine, K. Poston, M. Brumm, T. Buracchio, M. Campbell, S. Chowdhury, C. Coffey, L. Concha-Marambio, T. Dam, P. DiBiaso, T. Foroud, M. Frasier, C. Gochanour, D. Jennings, K. Kieburtz, C. M. Kopil, K. Merchant, B. Mollenhauer, T. Montine, K. Nudelman, G. Pagano, J. Seibyl, T. Sherer, A. Singleton, D. Stephenson, M. Stern, C. Soto, C. M. Tanner, E. Tolosa, D. Weintraub, Y. Xiao, A. Siderowf, B. Dunn, and K. Marek. 2024. A biological definition of neuronal alpha-synuclein disease: Towards an integrated staging system for research. *Lancet Neurology* 23(2):178-190.

Snowdon, D. A. 2003. Healthy aging and dementia: Findings from the Nun Study. *Annals of Internal Medicine* 139(5 Pt 2):450-454.

Sperling, R. A., M. C. Donohue, R. A. Rissman, K. A. Johnson, D. M. Rentz, J. D. Grill, J. L. Heidebrink, C. Jenkins, G. Jimenez-Maggiora, O. Langford, A. Liu, R. Raman, R. Yaari, K. C. Holdridge, J. R. Sims, and P. S. Aisen. 2024. Amyloid and tau prediction of cognitive and functional decline in unimpaired older individuals: Longitudinal data from the A4 and LEARN studies. *Journal of Prevention of Alzheimer's Disease* 11(4):802-813.

Stites, S. D., R. Milne, and J. Karlawish. 2018. Advances in Alzheimer's imaging are changing the experience of Alzheimer's disease. *Alzheimer's & Dementia* 10:285-300.

Stites, S. D., S. Midgett, D. Mechanic-Hamilton, M. Zuelsdorff, C. M. Glover, D. X. Marquez, J. E. Balls-Berry, M. L. Streitz, G. Babulal, J. F. Trani, J. N. Henderson, L. L. Barnes, J. Karlawish, and D. A. Wolk. 2022. Establishing a framework for gathering structural and social determinants of health in Alzheimer's disease research centers. *Gerontologist* 62(5):694-703.

TabCAT. 2024. *Detect cognitive changes earlier.* https://tabcathealth.com/ (accessed August 22, 2024).

Teunissen, C. 2024. *Biomarkers useful across the clinical continuum.* Committee on Research Priorities for Preventing and Treating Alzheimer's Disease and Related Dementias Public Workshop, Hybrid. January 16–17, 2024.

Toga, A., K. Yaffe, R. Rissman, L. Johnson, and S. O'Bryant. 2022. *The Health & Aging Brain Study—Health Disparities (HABS-HD).* https://experts.unthsc.edu/en/projects/the-health-aging-brain-study-health-disparities-habs-hd (accessed August 8, 2024).

Tsai, R. M., A. Bejanin, O. Lesman-Segev, R. LaJoie, A. Visani, V. Bourakova, J. P. O'Neil, M. Janabi, S. Baker, S. E. Lee, D. C. Perry, L. Bajorek, A. Karydas, S. Spina, L. T. Grinberg, W. W. Seeley, E. M. Ramos, G. Coppola, M. L. Gorno-Tempini, B. L. Miller, H. J. Rosen, W. Jagust, A. L. Boxer, and G. D. Rabinovici. 2019. ^{18}F-flortaucipir (AV-1451) tau PET in frontotemporal dementia syndromes. *Alzheimer's Research & Therapy* 11(1):13.

Tsuang, D. 2024. *Panelist remarks.* Committee on Research Priorities for Preventing and Treating Alzheimer's Disease and Related Dementias Public Workshop, Hybrid. January 16–17, 2024.

van der Zande, J. J., A. A. Gouw, I. van Steenoven, M. van de Beek, P. Scheltens, C. J. Stam, and A. W. Lemstra. 2020. Diagnostic and prognostic value of EEG in prodromal dementia with Lewy bodies. *Neurology* 95(6):e662-e670.

VMAC (Vanderbilt Memory and Alzheimer's Center). 2024. *Alzheimer's Disease Sequencing Project Phenotype Harmonization Consortium.* https://vmacdata.org/adsp-phc (accessed August 22, 2024).

Wallin, C. 2024. *Update from the NIA regarding Real-World Data Platform.* Document provided to the Committee on the Research Priorities for Preventing and Treating Alzheimer's Disease and Related Dementias on April 19, 2024. Available by request through the National Academies' Public Access Records Office.

Watson, R., R. Sanson-Fisher, J. Bryant, and E. Mansfield. 2023. Dementia is the second most feared condition among Australian health service consumers: Results of a cross-sectional survey. *BMC Public Health* 23(1):876.

Weuve, J. 2024. *Discussant perspectives and Committee Discussion.* Committee on Research Priorities for Preventing and Treating Alzheimer's Disease and Related Dementias Public Workshop, Hybrid. January 16–17, 2024.

Whalley, L. J., F. D. Dick, and G. McNeill. 2006. A life-course approach to the aetiology of late-onset dementias. *Lancet Neurology* 5(1):87-96.

WHO (World Health Organization). 2022. *Optimizing brain health across the life course: WHO position paper.* https://www.who.int/publications/i/item/9789240054561 (accessed August 13, 2024).

WHI (Women's Health Initiative). 2021a. *About WHI.* https://www.whi.org/about-whi (accessed October 25, 2024).

WHI. 2021b. *WHI Memory Study (WHIMS).* https://www.whi.org/md/39/whi-memory-study-whims (accessed August 14, 2024).

Yamada, M., J. Komatsu, K. Nakamura, K. Sakai, M. Samuraki-Yokohama, K. Nakajima, and M. Yoshita. 2020. Diagnostic criteria for dementia with Lewy bodies: Updates and future directions. *Journal of Movement Disorders* 13(1):1-10.

Yang, Y. C., C. E. Walsh, K. Shartle, R. C. Stebbins, A. E. Aiello, D. W. Belsky, K. M. Harris, M. Chanti-Ketterl, and B. L. Plassman. 2024. An early and unequal decline: Life course trajectories of cognitive aging in the United States. *Journal of Aging and Health* 36(3-4):230-245.

Yawn, A. 2023. *After 50 years of pioneering research in rural Louisiana, study pivots from heart to brain.* https://sph.tulane.edu/after-50-years-pioneering-research-rural-louisiana-study-pivots-heart-brain#:~:text=The%20Bogalusa%20Heart%20Study%20%E2%80%93%20in,lead%20to%20declines%20in%20brain (accessed August 14, 2024).

Zetterberg, H. 2022. Biofluid-based biomarkers for Alzheimer's disease-related pathologies: An update and synthesis of the literature. *Alzheimer's & Dementia* 18(9):1687-1693.

3

Understanding Disease Pathways to Guide Effective Strategies for Precision AD/ADRD Prevention and Treatment

Dementia etiology is multifactorial, involving complex interactions between genes, exposures, human physiology, and behaviors, all of which are influenced by the aging process. The brain is a dynamic and highly adaptive organ, and its capacity to meet the cognitive demands of daily life is influenced by the cumulative effects of growth, disease, and adaptation across the life course. Of course, the brain does not operate in isolation—all systems within the body interact with and are dependent on one another to keep an organism healthy (i.e., homeostasis) (Hampel et al., 2019). For example, the endothelial cells of the vascular system maintain the blood–brain barrier that regulates the brain–body exchange, the muscular system influences the beneficial effect of exercise on the brain, and the endocrine system links peripheral metabolic status to the functioning of the brain. More recently, the effect of the gut–brain axis on the body's—and brain's—physiology and pathophysiology has received increasing attention (Cocean and Vodnar, 2024; Zheng et al., 2023). Thus, a healthy body is essential to maintain a healthy brain and to support healthy aging.

Interventions to effectively prevent and treat Alzheimer's disease and related dementias (AD/ADRD) have seen limited success, in large part owing to immense gaps in our understanding of how chronic exposures (e.g., common chronic diseases such as hypertension, and social disadvantage), gene–environment interactions, and other biological pathways contribute to the different types of dementia. Moreover, while clinical symptoms of Alzheimer's disease (AD) and those of related dementias (e.g., Lewy body, frontotemporal, vascular) may present similarly (e.g., cognitive impairment), differences in the underlying causal biology and in the disease onsets and trajectories can be challenging to detect clinically. This poses an impediment to targeting and tailoring prevention and treatment approaches to the individual type of dementia.

Adding to this complexity is the predominance of mixed neuropathologies on autopsy, especially in older people, indicating that multiple pathological pathways are operating simultaneously and may require combinatorial interventions to achieve meaningful improvement. Consequently, different types of neurodegeneration as diagnosed clinically can show large overlaps in pathology at the brain tissue level (i.e., mixed pathology). Given the multiple and potentially intersecting pathways that contribute to AD/ADRD, diverse streams of research focused on individual pathogenetic processes and, most importantly, their integration, are needed to understand risk and resilience factors, as well as the biological processes leading to disease. The findings from such research will support the expansion of the current portfolio of prevention and treatment strategies (discussed in Chapter 4).

This chapter begins by framing the prevention and treatment of AD/ADRD in the context of healthy aging and the optimization of brain health across the life course. It goes on to explore key exposures and mechanistic pathways that may be intervened upon individually or in combination to optimize brain health over the life course and prevent and treat AD/ADRD. It focuses specifically on disease pathways that may be shared across AD/ADRD, as well as disease-agnostic (i.e., disease-nonspecific) resilience mechanisms. With this approach, the committee aims to identify opportunities to maximize the impact of AD/ADRD research investments and advocate for the transition away from the siloed study of individual causes of dementia that has dominated the research landscape and that fails to address the reality of mixed etiology dementia. The chapter ends by identifying research priorities directed at evidence gaps that, if addressed, could guide the development of population- and individual-level AD/ADRD intervention strategies.

HEALTHY AGING, RESILIENCE, AND BRAIN HEALTH ACROSS THE LIFE COURSE

Healthy aging can be defined as "a continuous process of optimizing opportunities to maintain and improve physical and mental health, independence, and quality of life throughout the life course" (PAHO/WHO, 2024). The later years of life present many new opportunities for older individuals, from pursuing new activities and long-neglected passions and even new career paths. Yet the chance to enjoy these opportunities depends to some degree on healthy aging.

As discussed further in this chapter, aging in the biological sense results from the deterioration of myriad molecular and cellular structures and processes over time. Importantly, however, these changes do not occur on a linear trajectory and do not strictly associate with a person's age in years (WHO, 2022). Chronological age represents the amount of time a person has been alive. Although there is no single definition for biological age, it is conceptualized in terms of various molecular and cellular changes that accumulate over time (Jazwinski and Kim, 2019). Building on the work of a 2014 trans-institute Geroscience Interest Group Summit sponsored by the National Institutes of Health,[1] López-Otín and colleagues (2023) recently proposed 12 hallmarks of aging, which spanned from the molecular to the meta-organism levels (see Figure 3-1). Manipulation of these hallmarks, which are interdependent, may accelerate or decelerate the biological aging process. Many of these hallmarks overlap with the biochemical and cellular pathologic pathways common to AD/ADRD (discussed later in this chapter), suggesting opportunities to use knowledge of biological aging processes in the development of interventions for AD/ADRD (Fillit et al., 2023).

Biological age is increasingly recognized as a better indicator of chronic health outcomes as compared to chronological age (Ho et al., 2023), with implications for lifespan and brain health span (the period of life during which an individual remains healthy) (Sierra, 2016). Biological age is not necessarily linked to chronological age, given that a person can be biologically younger or older than their chronological age suggests (Sierra et al., 2021; Zhang and Gladyshev, 2020). As a result, there is substantial diversity in the range of physical and cognitive ability seen in older age. While genetics plays a role, a large part of this variability arises from the physical and social environments in which people live and the effect of these environments on their opportunities and health behaviors (i.e., social determinants of health) (WHO, 2022), as supported by increasing evidence from animal and human studies (Durso et al., 2022; Horvath and Levine, 2015; Kalia et al., 2022; Liu et al., 2023a; Quach et al., 2017; Ward-Caviness et al., 2016). Complementary to biological hallmarks of aging, social hallmarks of aging, such as low socioeconomic status, minority status, adverse life events, adverse psychological states, and adverse behaviors, can accelerate aging, while reducing exposure to these social hallmarks can slow the onset of age-related poor health outcomes (Crimmins, 2020; Hooten et al., 2022).

The risk of sporadic forms of dementia increases as individuals age, typically accompanied by age-related biological changes in the brain and throughout the body that may not be observed in individuals with early-onset forms of the diseases (Scheltens et al., 2021). Some characteristics of neurodegenerative disease (e.g., neurodegeneration and cerebral atrophy,

---

[1] Geroscience is a transdisciplinary field focused on the relationship between biological aging and age-related diseases (Fillit et al., 2023; Hara et al., 2019).

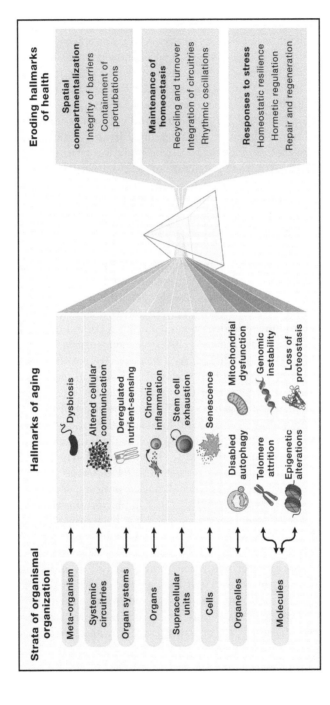

FIGURE 3-1 Twelve hallmarks of aging reflecting the erosion of hallmarks of health.
SOURCE: López-Otín et al., 2023. Reprinted with permission from Elsevier.

neuropathological protein accumulation, cognitive decline), gradually manifest over the life course even among individuals who do not develop clinical dementia (Zhang et al., 2023e). Thus, biological pathways underlying both aging and AD/ADRD exist on a continuum and are likely to overlap (Gonzales et al., 2022). Consequently, interventions targeting the underlying biological pathways associated with aging may be useful for delaying or even preventing the onset of AD/ADRD (Cummings et al., 2023a; Fillit et al., 2023; Hara et al., 2019; Sierra, 2016; Sierra et al., 2021).

It should be emphasized that the accumulation of neuropathologic changes with aging does not necessarily lead to cognitive decline. Studies to correlate neuropathologic changes with premortem cognitive function have demonstrated that cognitive health can be maintained despite the accumulation of high levels of neuropathology (Zhang et al., 2023e). This phenomenon has been defined as cognitive resilience, which refers to "the capacity of the brain to maintain cognition and function [despite the presence of] aging and disease" (Stern et al., 2023, p. 3).[2] The growing understanding of cognitive resilience and the implication for potential intervention strategies is important given that people generally care more about maintaining their cognitive and functional ability than about the neurobiological changes that may occur with aging. Building cognitive reserve or enhancing the brain's ability to compensate or adapt to neuropathology—which does not necessarily imply a return to a previous state of function but rather the ability to continue to function despite the presence of pathology—are strategies for increasing an individual's resilience (Stern et al., 2019), and may contribute to preventing, delaying, and/or slowing clinical disease progression.

Cognitive resilience is not dichotomous but rather exists on a continuum that includes better- and worse-than-expected performance for a given level of pathology (Zammit et al., 2023). Thus, mechanisms can either maintain or degrade resilience. For example, psychosocial risk factors such as depression, loneliness, and chronic distress increase risk of clinical dementia independent of effects on typical pathologic features such as amyloid plaques, tau tangles, Lewy bodies, or infarcts (Wilson et al., 2003, 2006, 2007a,b), indicating the existence of yet-to-be discovered mechanisms that degrade resilience. Other factors such as education, cognitive stimulation, socialization, sense of purpose, and physical activity may function in a protective manner to increase or maintain resilience, enabling the brain to

---

[2] Multiple definitions and frameworks have been proposed to clarify terminology and operationalize the concepts of resilience and resistance (Neuner et al., 2022; Stern et al., 2019, 2023; Zammit et al., 2023). For the purposes of this report, resistance to neuropathology is considered to be distinct from resilience and refers to the absence of neuropathology or lower levels than would be expected based on age and other risk factors (e.g., genetic risk) (de Vries et al., 2024; Zammit et al., 2023). This definition for resistance is similar to the definition for brain maintenance provided in one recently published consensus framework (Stern et al., 2023).

compensate for brain pathologies and maintain cognitive function (Zammit et al., 2023). As discussed later in this chapter, the discovery of protective genetic variants has shown that resilience can also be genetically mediated. Thus, there are both modifiable and nonmodifiable factors that contribute to resilience and may in fact interact. The neural mechanisms that underlie resilience are an active area of study (de Vries et al., 2024; Neuner et al., 2022). Understanding how protective variants and other mediators promote resilience may guide new strategies for interventions.

Strategies focused on avoiding *gerogens*—age-accelerating factors, such as pollution and stress (NASEM, 2020a,b)—and adopting resilience-promoting lifestyle factors, such as healthy diet, exercise, regular sleep patterns, and social activities, are applicable to both antiaging and AD/ ADRD prevention efforts and may support the extension of the health span and the optimization of brain health across the life course. Assessment of individuals' aging clocks using genetic, epigenetic, metabolomic, and other tools could in the future guide more personalized intervention strategies.

THE EXPOSOME AND BRAIN HEALTH ACROSS THE LIFE COURSE

Defining and Measuring the Exposome

The concept of the exposome emerged 2 decades ago and was originally described as encompassing "life-course environmental exposures (including lifestyle factors), from the prenatal period onwards" (Wild, 2005, p. 1848). In recognition of the public health importance of gene–environment interactions, the term was coined in an effort to draw attention to the need to characterize environmental exposures with the same scientific rigor and precision that was at the time being applied to the analysis of the human genome. Understanding the interplay between the genome and the environment depends on the ability to accurately assess environmental exposures (Siroux et al., 2016). Exposomics as a scientific discipline has continued to mature over the last 20 years and was recently defined as "a field that studies the comprehensive and cumulative effects of physical, chemical, biological, and psychosocial mediators that impact biological systems by integrating data from a variety of interdisciplinary methodologies and streams" in order to "enable discovery-based analysis of environmental influences on health" (Banbury Center, 2024). As suggested by this definition, exposures are considered broadly, extending well beyond environmental pollutants (e.g., air pollution, environmental lead) that may commonly be a focus of exposure assessments. Such factors as social determinants of health and health behaviors are also encompassed within the exposome.

For diseases for which genetic variants explain only a limited fraction of the variability in risk and that are presumed to be largely driven by gene–environment and age-associated interactions (i.e., acquired susceptibility), exposomics may provide one potential approach for better understanding disease pathways. The field relies on advanced data analytics and causal inference methods to identify the relationship between exposome factors and phenotypes of interest (e.g., disease outcomes) (Banbury Center, 2024). Findings from such efforts can guide and complement effective prevention strategies.

A notable challenge, however, relates to how the exposome is defined and comprehensively measured over the entire life course given its vastness of scale and inherent variability over time, as well as how it is linked to health (Siroux et al., 2016). Exposome measurement and evaluation methods use multiple technologies and multilayered data sources, including demographic surveys, administrative data (e.g., Social Security records, health care claims), historical information (e.g., geocoded residential histories), sensors and monitors, satellite data, and analysis of endogenous and exogenous compounds in the body that are biological indicators of exposures (Banbury Center, 2024; Miller, 2024). High-resolution mass spectrometry and other increasingly high-throughput multiomics approaches (e.g., epigenomics, transcriptomics, proteomics, metabolomics) are enhancing the identification of such biological exposure indicators, as well as early molecular changes that precede disease onset (Vineis et al., 2020).

Although a data-layering approach enables the exploration of interactions among different environmental exposures over the life course and consideration of high-risk exposure windows, such large-scale data collection, management, and analysis are costly and integration of these diverse data types requires sophisticated analytic tools (Siroux et al., 2016; Vermeulen et al., 2020). Moreover, the simultaneous analysis of multiple exposures and their effects on health raises concerns regarding risk of misattribution of the effect of one exposure to another (i.e., exposure misclassification) and can make it challenging to identify causal associations because of correlations between exposures in the exposome (Siroux et al., 2016). Data security and privacy considerations must also be considered given that exposome research may involve the linking of some forms of protected health information, such as residential history and genetic information (Safarlou et al., 2023).

Linking the Exposome to Brain Health and AD/ADRD

Findings from twin studies suggest that while genetics is a major contributor to AD/ADRD risk (Gatz et al., 2006), environmental and age-related factors also have a substantial influence (Maloney and Lahiri, 2016; Migliore and Coppedè, 2022; Paulson and Igo, 2011). Yet the role of environmental factors in AD/ADRD etiologies, either directly through effects on the brain or indirectly via altered brain–body interactions, remain poorly understood (Finch and Kulminski, 2019).

In the context of brain health, the exposome paradigm can be conceptualized in the form of the neural exposome, which encompasses a diverse array of non-genetic factors that influence neurodegenerative diseases (including AD/ADRD) and other neurological conditions (Tamiz et al., 2022). The neural exposome includes exogenous (e.g., originating from outside the organism such as environmental contaminants), behavioral (e.g., lifestyle), and endogenous factors (e.g., microbiome), as depicted in Figure 3-2. The brain's dynamic and adaptive nature, characterized by continual change as a function of experience and exposures across the life course, makes the study of the neural exposome complex. Additionally, just as genetic variants function together to influence genetic disease risk,

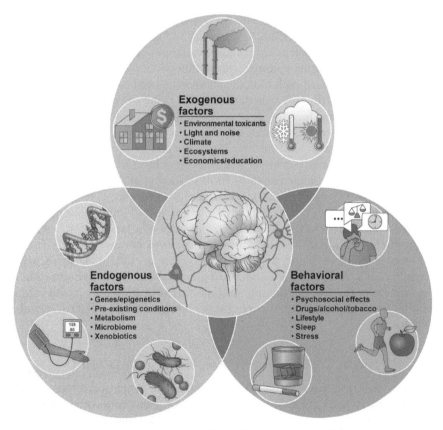

FIGURE 3-2 Facets of the exposome that influence brain health.
SOURCE: Tamiz et al., 2022. Reprinted with permission from Elsevier.

combined exposures from across the life course similarly are likely to have interactive effects on brain health (Tamiz et al., 2022). This complicates intervention efforts as strategies targeting a single factor may be expected to have limited effectiveness when different factors contribute additively or synergistically to the risk of AD/ADRD. Further complexity stems from the fact that exposures may be happening in early life (in so-called critical windows of development) but not manifesting until later in life. This is the basis for the developmental origins of health and disease hypothesis (Klocke and Lein, 2019; Migliore and Coppedè, 2022).

The human brain continues to develop through adolescence. Consequently, exposures (environmental and social) from gestation through teenage years can disrupt brain development in ways that will not be immediately apparent if the affected regions are not functional until later life or if compensatory mechanisms mask the effects until additional insults accumulate to a level that can no longer be compensated for. Though not related to neurodegeneration, an illustrative example is provided by the effects of monosodium glutamate, which, in high concentrations, can cause neuronal death in the hypothalamus of a developing brain. Deficits from the loss of those neurons does not become apparent until adolescence when the function of those cells is normally activated (Klocke and Lein, 2019). Whether and to what degree AD/ADRD have a developmental basis remains unclear but may be uncovered by further study of the exposome.

There has been growing investment in research on the exposome and, of particular interest to this report, its role in brain aging and disease, with the National Institute of Environmental Health Sciences (NIEHS), the National Institute on Aging (NIA), and the National Institute of Neurological Disorders and Stroke (NINDS) providing support for such research (Cavaliere and Gülöksüz, 2022; NIA, 2020; Tamiz et al., 2022). The growth of research on the exposome and AD/ADRD has created opportunities for greater interagency collaboration to advance critical research across multiple conditions. For example, in 2022, NINDS launched its Office of Neural Exposome and Toxicology, which is focused on interdisciplinary research on the neural exposome and the creation of partnerships within NINDS and across other National Institutes of Health (NIH) institutes, centers, and offices (ICOs), federal agencies (Centers for Disease Control and Prevention, Environmental Protection Agency), advocacy groups, and scientific societies (Tamiz et al., 2022). Additionally, several NIH ICOs (NIA, NINDS, NIEHS, the National Institute of Arthritis and Musculoskeletal and Skin Diseases, and the National Cancer Institute, among others) are cofunding a new coordinating center for exposome research to accelerate precision environmental health (Columbia University, 2024; NIH, 2023).

The contribution of exogenous environmental exposures to AD/ADRD is a topic of active investigation. For example, a growing body of evidence from epidemiological and experimental studies has linked air pollution (e.g., fine particulate matter, nitrogen dioxide, nitrous oxides) and other environmental pollutants (neurotoxic metals, pesticides) to increased risk of neurologic disorders, including dementia (Bakulski et al., 2012; Liu et al., 2023a; Migliore and Coppedè, 2022; NASEM, 2020a,b; Peters et al., 2019; Shi et al., 2021; Shih et al., 2007; Wilker et al., 2023; Zhang et al., 2023a), although data are lacking for the vast majority of chemicals to which humans are exposed. There is an opportunity to leverage existing databases, emerging technologies for high-throughput screening (Lefevre-Arbogast et al., 2024), and increased understanding of the pathogenesis of AD/ADRD to identify specific environmental chemicals that interact with biological pathways involved in neurodegeneration to promote disease, and conversely, resilience.

Research is also elucidating the influence of social, cultural, and behavioral factors on brain health. Behavioral factors such as physical inactivity, smoking, alcohol consumption, and diet are well-established risk factors for dementia (Livingston et al., 2024; Patten and Lein, 2019). However, recent studies focused on social and economic factors such as educational attainment, wealth, access to health care (Chen and Zissimopoulos, 2018), loneliness and social isolation (Huang et al., 2023), macro-level social systems, and structural influences have identified associations with cognitive impairment and dementia (Lamar et al., 2023; Powell et al., 2020; Reuben et al., 2024; Walsemann et al., 2023). Such research is critical to understanding how social disadvantage and disparities in exposures to environmental hazards (e.g., neighborhood proximity to landfills and major highways that generate traffic-associated air pollution) contribute to differences in AD/ADRD risk across diverse populations. There is also increasing evidence to suggest that gender roles (e.g., household, childrearing, and caregiving roles) and disparities (e.g., access to education, occupational opportunities, autonomy) contribute to gender differences in AD/ADRD incidence (Mielke, 2024). Continuing to uncover these kinds of associations and their interactions will require longitudinal cohort studies with in-depth exposome measurements and analysis.

To understand the exposome and how it interacts with molecular and cellular mechanisms to influence AD/ADRD risk, it is critical to capture the context in which exposures occurred over an individual's life course (e.g., socioeconomic status, locations in which individuals lived throughout their lives) (Melcher et al., 2024). Such contextual factors can significantly influence the exogenous, endogenous, and behavioral facets of the exposome, and are drivers of disparities in AD/ADRD outcomes (NASEM, 2024).

The linking of social phenotypes (e.g., social vulnerability) to biological phenotypes (e.g., neuropathology markers) can be done prospectively or retrospectively (Kind, 2024; Powell et al., 2020). As an example of the latter, public data tracing methods can be used to collect life-course residential histories for individuals whose brains were donated to Alzheimer's Disease Research Center brain banks, thereby linking historic population-level exposure data to existing biobank samples (Melcher et al., 2024). Retrospective approaches, however, are resource intensive and subject to the availability of accurate data. Collection of social phenotype data in parallel to biological data may be less costly and less labor-intensive. The Health and Retirement Study has been collecting social, economic, and demographic data on a nationally representative sample of middle-age and older Americans since 1992, as well as biomarker data on the study respondents (Biomarker Network, 2024). A structural and social determinants of health module has been developed and is being implemented in Alzheimer's Disease Research Centers to enable the linking of prospectively collected social determinants of health data to neuropathology findings, which will help improve understanding of how social determinants of health modify cognition and AD/ADRD risk (Stites et al., 2022). As noted earlier in this chapter, however, privacy laws and regulations and data security concerns related to protected health information can impede efforts to conduct such linking of studies. Research infrastructure addressing both administrative and legal challenges is needed to facilitate the intake and linkage processes for protected health information (Kind, 2023).

The findings from exposome studies suggest opportunities for individual-level, public health, and policy interventions aimed at primary prevention, such as reducing exposure to environmental contaminants, modifying lifestyle, and eliminating structural factors that contribute to social disadvantage. It is possible to imagine precision prevention approaches that stratify the population based on environmental exposures. However, important knowledge gaps regarding the timing for exposures and resultant changes in brain health remain, impeding efforts to develop life-course approaches to maximize AD/ADRD prevention. Acknowledging the NIH-supported research efforts already underway (NIA, 2023a; NINDS, 2024a), further investment is needed to identify and understand brain-critical exposures across the life course (from the prenatal period to late life); vulnerable age windows (Liu et al., 2023a), such as periods of neuro-development and major hormonal changes (e.g., adolescence, pregnancy, menopause); the dose-over-time dependency of effects; and how exposures correlate and interact (Tamiz et al., 2022). Cohort studies (discussed in Chapter 2) and natural experiments (e.g., city-level removal of lead pipes, policies aimed at air pollution reduction) provide opportunities to address these scientific priorities, but this requires multidisciplinary research (breaking down discipline-specific silos as discussed in Chapter 5) and attention to addressing current data gaps (e.g., early-life exposures, reproductive history, social determinants of health).

Conclusion 3-1: Understanding differences in pathways that contribute to AD/ADRD across diverse populations requires the expansion of multidimensional diverse cohorts, including cohorts focused on under-studied and/or disproportionately affected populations, paired with an investment in tools to generate and link the relevant life-course and exposome information. Also required are the data infrastructure and specialized expertise necessary to carry out complex data integration and analyses.

UNDERSTANDING THE BIOLOGICAL BASIS OF AD/ADRD

Risk and protective factors for AD/ADRD, from individual genes to macro-scale socioeconomic contexts, ultimately affect individuals through their effects on molecules, cells, and physiologic systems (e.g., neural circuits, multiorgan interactions). Molecular targets for pathogenesis (or resilience) include DNA (through mutation or other changes that affect gene expression), RNA, proteins (e.g., misfolding and aggregation, loss of enzymatic function), lipids, and metabolites. Molecular-level changes can affect cells in myriad ways, for example, inducing cell cycle arrest (senescence), cell death, or transition to an altered phenotype. At the organ level, neuronal cell loss and other cellular changes disrupt synaptic function and brain circuitry, as well as the systems that connect the brain with other organs of the body (e.g., vascular, neuromuscular), giving rise to the symptoms experienced by people living with AD/ADRD, including impaired cognitive and motor function and changes in personality and behavior. Despite considerable investment in basic research and resulting scientific advances, there is still much that is not understood regarding these multiscale effects. Continued investment in mechanistic research is needed to understand the biological basis for the effects of risk and protective factors on brain health and to determine whether associations are causal in nature (Tamiz et al., 2022). This needs to include elucidating the biological causes of the different forms of dementia, considering age-associated alterations and the interplay with an individual's risk factor profile.

The Genetic Architecture of AD/ADRD

While sporadic forms of AD/ADRD are predominant, some forms of dementia are inherited in an autosomal dominant fashion, as is the case for forms of early-onset AD that are mediated by mutations in the *APP*, *PSEN1*, and *PSEN2* genes (Cacace et al., 2016). As indicated in Table 3-1, there are also autosomal dominant forms of Lewy body dementia (LBD) and frontotemporal dementia (FTD) (Guerreiro et al., 2020). While the occurrence of autosomal dominant mutations is rare, such mutations have large effect sizes and can therefore be identified and investigated through family studies. Rare population cohorts (e.g., ARTFL-LEFFTDS Longitudinal Frontotemporal Lobar Degeneration [ALLFTD][3], the Dominantly Inherited Alzheimer's Network) have been established for the study of these dominantly inherited forms of dementia and have yielded invaluable insights on disease mechanisms, biomarkers, and potential treatment targets (Asken et al., 2023; Bateman et al., 2011; Zhang et al., 2023b).

Genetically determined forms of dementia are not limited to those that are inherited in an autosomal dominant manner. Down syndrome-related AD is another form of genetically determined early onset AD that results from a gene dose effect stemming from an extra copy of the *APP* gene, which is located on chromosome 21. Neuropathological hallmarks of AD (amyloid plaques and tau neurofibrillary tangles) are nearly universal in people with Down syndrome by the age of 40, and the lifetime risk of dementia in this population is estimated at greater than 90 percent (Fortea et al., 2021). As with autosomal dominant forms of AD/ADRD, the natural history of Down syndrome-related AD follows a predictable course (clinical and biomarker changes). Consortia such as the Alzheimer Biomarkers Consortium—Down Syndrome (NIA, 2024a) and the Alzheimer's Clinical Trials Consortium—Down Syndrome (ACTC-DS, 2024) are working to advance the development of AD biomarkers and therapies for people with Down syndrome.

A recently published analysis proposes that *APOE4* homozygotes may constitute a third form of genetically determined AD (Fortea et al., 2024). The E4 allele of the apolipoprotein E gene (*APOE*) has long been recognized as a major genetic risk factor for AD with a large effect size (Cacace et al., 2016; Lambert et al., 2023). APOE protein is known to be involved in lipid transport (Raulin et al., 2022), but the mechanisms by which *APOE4* increase dementia risk have yet to be fully elucidated and represent an area of intense research.[4] The proposal of *APOE4* homozygotes as a genetic form of AD is based on the near full penetrance of AD neuropathology, as well as the predictability of symptom onset and clinical and biomarker changes over time, characteristics that are also seen with autosomal dominant AD and Down syndrome-related AD. Furthermore, *APOE3* and *APOE4* heterozygotes exhibit intermediate phenotypes, suggesting the possibility of autosomal semidominant inheritance (Fortea et al., 2024; Genin et al., 2011).

---

[3] ALLFTD recruits people with autosomal dominant FTD syndromes, as well as people with sporadic FTD.

[4] NIA organized a workshop on *APOE* genetics as a major determinant of AD pathobiology in September 2024. More information is available at https://www.nia.nih.gov/research/dab-dgcg-dn/workshops/apoe-genetics-major-determinant-alzheimers-disease-pathobiology (accessed October 11, 2024).

TABLE 3-1 Loci/Genes Associated with Lifetime Risk for Alzheimer's Disease, Lewy Body Dementia, and Frontotemporal Dementia Across Multiple Populations

Dementia Type	Loci/Genes Associated with Lifetime Risk					
		Sporadic Form/ by Genetic Ancestry Groups (GWAS Reaching Gnome-Wide Significance)				
	Familial Form	European	African	Hispanic	Asian	
AD	APP, PSEN1, PSEN2 (Cacace et al., 2016)	SORT1, CR1, ADAM17, PRKD3, NCK2, BIN1, WDR12, INPP5D, MME, IDUA, CLNK, RHOH, ANKH, COX7C, TNIP1, RASGEF1C, HLA-DQA1, UNC5CL, TREM2, TREML2, CD2AP, HS3ST5, UMAD1, ICA1, TMEM106B, JAZF1, EPDR1, SEC61G, SPDYE3, EPHA1, CTSB, PTK2B, CLU, SHARPIN, ABCA1, USP6NL, ANK3, TSPAN14, BLNK, PLEKHA1, SPI1, MS4A4A, EED, SORL1, TPCN1, FERMT2, SLC24A4, SPPL2A, MINDY2, APH1B, SNX1, CTSH, DOC2A, BCKDK, IL34, MAF, PLCG2, FOXF1, PRDM7, WDR81, SCIMP, MYO15A, GRN, WNT3, ABI3, TSPOAP1, ACE, ABCA7, KLF16, APOE, SIGLEC11, LILRB2, RBCK1, CASS4, SLC2A4RG, APP, ADAMTS1 (Bellenguez et al., 2022)	ARRDC4/IGF1R, APOE, ABCA7, HMHA1, COBL, SLC10A2 (Mez et al., 2017; Reitz et al., 2013, 2023)	APOE (Reitz et al., 2023)	APOE (East Asians) FAM47E (Japanese), OR2B2 (Japanese+European) RHOBTB3/GLRX, CTC-278L1.1, CTD-2506J14.1, NECTIN2, CHODL, (Chinese) CACNA1A, LRIG1 (Korean) SORL1 (Japanese+Korean+ European) (Jia et al., 2021; Miyashita et al., 2013, 2023; Shigemizu et al., 2021)	

LBD[a]	SNCA, GBA, APOE (Guerreiro et al., 2020)	GBA, BIN1, TMEM175, SNCA-AS1, APOE (Chia et al., 2021)	None	None	None
FTD	GRN, MAPT, C9ORF72, TBK1, TARDBP, SQSTM1, CHMP2B, VCP, CHCHD10 (Guerreiro et al., 2020)	MAPT, MOBP, APOE (Manzoni et al., 2024) HLA-DRA/HLA-DRB5, BTNL2 (Ferrari et al., 2014) TMEM106B (FTD with TDP-43 inclusions) (Van Deerlin et al., 2010)	None	None	None

NOTES: This table provides a portrait of the genetic architecture of Alzheimer's disease (AD), frontotemporal dementia (FTD), and Lewy body dementia (LBD)—which includes dementia with Lewy bodies (DLB) and Parkinson's disease dementia (PDD)—across multiple populations. The table was generated by selecting recent reviews or representative genome-wide association study (GWAS) papers with very large sample size (excluding preprints). For familial forms of AD, LBD, and FTD, the table lists established loci with observed genetic mutations that were found to be significant in family or sequencing studies. For sporadic forms of AD, LBD, and FTD, only loci reaching genome-wide significance ($P \leq 5 \times 10^{-8}$) either using samples from one ancestry or after adding samples from multiple ancestries are listed. This is not a comprehensive or systematic review of the literature on risk loci, although it captures the current state of the field and the relative strengths in cohort size and statistical power across populations and diseases.

[a] Given that DLB and PDD have similar clinical features, Chia and colleagues (2021) examined both disorders together to increase sample size. The two disorders may have different molecular pathways and require different therapeutic strategies, and a better differential diagnostic strategy is needed (Jellinger et al., 2018).

SOURCES: Cacace et al., 2016; Bellenguez et al., 2022; Chia et al., 2021; Ferrari et al., 2014; Guerreiro et al., 2020; Jia et al., 2021; Manzoni et al., 2024; Mez, et al., 2017; Miyashita et al., 2013, 2023; Reitz et al., 2013, 2023; Shigemizu et al., 2021; Van Deerlin et al., 2010.

While requiring further evaluation, the confirmation of *APOE4* homozygotes as a form of genetically determined AD would have important implications for approaches to developing and evaluating therapies (e.g., trial participant screening and genetic counseling, population stratification and precision medicine approaches, analytic approaches used in clinical trials) (Fortea et al., 2024). It also underscores the need for continued research to deepen understanding of APOE biology and effects on neurodegeneration (e.g., the contribution of APOE to disease heterogeneity), as well as differences in effects by sex and ancestry. Such research needs to include longitudinal studies of individuals with different *APOE* genotypes, including not just *APOE4* homozygotes and heterozygotes, but also those with alleles (e.g., *APOE2*) and mutations (e.g., Christchurch mutation in *APOE3*)[5] observed to be protective against clinical dementia (Arboleda-Velasquez et al., 2019; Raulin et al., 2022). Importantly, the study of *APOE4* carriers who demonstrate resilience to clinical progression can be a means of identifying protective variants in genes other than *APOE* (Bhattarai et al., 2024; Huq et al., 2019). Understanding how these rare variants promote dementia resilience opens new avenues for developing treatments. Ensuring adequate inclusion of underrepresented groups in such studies will be important to address pressing scientific questions related to why effect sizes (particularly for *APOE4*) have been observed to vary across populations with different genetic ancestry. As *APOE4* is known to increase risk for related dementias (e.g., LBD) in addition to AD, continued efforts are needed to elucidate the role of APOE in amyloid-dependent and amyloid-independent disease pathways and implications for multiple etiology dementias (Raulin et al., 2022).

Even among those without autosomal dominant mutations or *APOE4* alleles, genetic predisposition is thought to be a predominant contributing factor for sporadic (typically late onset) forms of AD/ADRD (Patten and Lein, 2019; Reitz et al., 2023). Genome-wide association studies (GWAS) have identified more than 70 genes or loci associated with sporadic AD (Lambert et al., 2023; Reitz et al., 2023). In many cases, variants identified by GWAS may only have small individual effects on risk but cumulatively—and depending on aging—can contribute to changes in the functions of genes organized in specific molecular and cellular pathways, leading to pathogenic effects (Gan et al., 2018). The large number and diversity of risk genes and loci provide support for the role of multiple mechanistic pathways that may function independently and/or interact with each other or environmental risk factors to contribute to dementia, as discussed later in this chapter.

---

[5] The observation of a protective effect for the Christchurch mutation in *APOE3* for an individual with an autosomal dominant *PSEN1* mutation highlights the importance of *APOE* as a fundamental driver of AD neuropathology.

Given the large number of publications reporting risk genes and loci, efforts are underway to review published studies and evaluate the quality of the evidence for each reported locus or gene (ADSP, 2023). The gene verification committee of the Alzheimer's Disease Sequencing Project (see Box 3-1) is organizing loci and genes into tiers based on the quality of the evidence of an association. Though results are not yet published in the peer-reviewed literature, this effort will provide the scientific community with lists of loci supported by high-quality evidence that can be used to guide follow-on functional genomics efforts and increase confidence in the pursuit of potential therapeutic targets. The framework developed by the gene verification committee may also serve as a useful model for disease research outside of AD/ADRD.

Identified genetic variants have been used to generate polygenic risk scores that can be used to predict the individual risk of AD (Harrison et al., 2020) and may be helpful tools in the development of precision medicine approaches to prevention and treatment by informing stratification and intervention strategies (discussed further in Chapter 4). However, the majority of known variants were identified in non-Hispanic White individuals from North America and Europe (see Table 3-1), suggesting that additional genetic risk factors for other populations remain to be discovered and limiting the applicability of current polygenic risk scores to individuals of other ethnicities (Clark et al., 2022; Reitz et al., 2023). Additionally, there may be sex differences in genetic risk factors that would need to be accounted for (Mielke, 2024).

Far fewer risk loci have been identified for sporadic forms of LBD, FTD,[6] and vascular dementia—in part because of smaller sample sizes for GWAS as compared to AD. In contrast to risk loci with small effect sizes, strong risk loci, such as those associated with autosomal dominant forms, can be identified without the need for large sample sizes. As indicated in Table 3-1, there is some evidence of overlap in risk genes for these different forms of dementia (Chia et al., 2021; Ciani et al., 2019; Guo et al., 2022; Ikram et al., 2017; Rongve et al., 2019), but more studies are needed to firm up these relationships. Additionally, genes associated with common diseases, such as cardiovascular disease and stroke, are shared with AD/ADRD. Thus, there is a critical need to conduct further GWAS of adequate sample size and statistical power to detect additional genetic associations for sporadic forms of AD/ADRD (Bellenguez et al., 2022). It will be important in such efforts to use large study populations (to detect rare variants) representing

---

[6] Sporadic forms make up 70 percent of FTD, a smaller fraction as compared to AD and LBD (Greaves and Rohrer, 2019). A larger number of strong risk loci (i.e., those associated with autosomal dominant forms of disease) have been identified for FTD as compared to AD (see Table 3-1).

BOX 3-1
Alzheimer's Disease Sequencing Project

The NIA-funded Alzheimer's Disease Sequencing Project (ADSP) was established in 2012 following the enactment of the National Alzheimer's Project Act and has grown into a global collaboration focused on better understanding the genetic architecture of AD/ADRD (ADSP, 2024). The ADSP works to identify and explore new genes and genetic variations that are linked to increased risk of or protection against AD/ADRD with the goal of advancing findings into therapeutic targets for further development. The ADSP network of funded collaborations and programs includes infrastructure and expertise to genotype and sequence samples from existing studies from around the world; perform functional and computational analyses; and process, store, and share these high-quality data with researchers (ADSP, 2024). Since its initiation in 2012, ADSP has evolved over a series of phases. The first two phases included a majority of samples from participants of non-Hispanic White ancestry. ADSP received additional funding from NIA to diversify the existing ADSP dataset (NIA, 2024b). This most recent phase, ADSP Follow-Up Study 2.0: The Diverse Population Initiative, involves the whole-genome sequencing of 18,500 AD/ADRD cases and 18,500 controls each from Hispanics, African Americans and Africans, and Asians using samples from the U.S. and international collaborations in Africa, Central and South America, and Asia (NIA, 2024b). This expansion in diversity will enable the identification of genetically driven targets and improvements in the design of clinical trials (ADSP, 2024; NIA, 2024b). The ADSP Follow-Up Study 2.0 "follows on three other recent initiatives to enhance the ADSP's capability to identify new risk and protective genes:

- The Phenotype Harmonization Consortium is aggregating and harmonizing clinical, cognitive, imaging, and biomarker phenotype data from all participating ADSP cohorts.
- The Functional Genomics Consortium is generating "omics" experimental data to further characterize ADSP genetic findings and to help better define subtypes of Alzheimer's and related dementias.
- The Artificial Intelligence/Machine-Learning Consortium employs sophisticated computational methods to further integrate and analyze ADSP data and optimize subject selection for clinical trials based on participants' characteristics" (NIA, 2024b).

diverse ancestral backgrounds, as genetic analysis has shown that continental genetic ancestry plays an important role in AD risk and protection, as evidenced by the variation in risk effect for the *APOE4* allele across populations with diverse ancestral backgrounds (Reitz et al., 2023). Observing more population-specific variants increases statistical power in AD/ADRD gene discovery. The Alzheimer's Disease Sequencing Project has been a major NIA investment in improving understanding of the genetic architecture of AD/ADRD, and recent phases of the initiative have included a focus on expanding the genetic diversity of study populations (see Box 3-1).

Continued investment in understanding how different variants affect the functional role of each gene associated with disease risk can help to elucidate the biological mechanisms of AD/ADRD (discussed later in this chapter) and thereby guide the development of more targeted intervention strategies. For example, genetic studies have implicated lysosomal dysfunction and autophagy pathways in AD/ADRD (Bellenguez et al., 2022; Deng et al., 2017). However, caution is required when attempting pathway analysis using GWAS findings as it is not always clear which gene is linked to an identified locus and pathway annotation suffers from a number of limitations (Silberstein et al., 2021). Further development of tools and processes is needed to improve the translation of genetic signals to target pathways. In the meantime, triangulation using a combination of genetic findings and data from experimental studies (in vitro and in vivo) can increase confidence in the identification of affected pathways.

Understanding Gene–Environment Interactions

As noted earlier, there are various molecular and cellular targets through which exposome factors (e.g., lifestyle, social determinants of health, pollutant exposures) may exert pathogenic effects. For example, exposome factors can interact directly with proteins (e.g., bind to and/or alter the function of receptors, enzymes, and structural proteins), but may also alter protein levels or function through interactions with an individual's epigenome and/or genome. In framing brain health as a trajectory over the life course, an individual's genetics can be envisioned as defining the major bounds for that trajectory, while the exact course will be determined by the interactions between genes and exposome factors. Perhaps the best studied gene–environment interactions are those involving the *APOE* gene, but generally these interactions remain poorly understood (Dunn et al., 2019; Migliore and Coppedè, 2022). In fact, environmental and social factors (e.g., socioeconomic status) likely influence observed associations between genetic variants and AD (Reitz et al., 2023), making it challenging to disentangle risks from different sources, which is important for understanding the variation in AD/ADRD risk across diverse populations.

Although population-specific gene variations may have different levels of impact in disturbing disease pathways, another possibility is that population-specific exposures and gene–environment interactions contribute to observed population-specific differences. Deciphering the individual causes and trajectories of AD/ADRD is dependent on understanding an individual's specific profile of risk genes and their exposures (e.g., family resources, education, chemical exposures, inflammation, trauma), including comorbid conditions (e.g., metabolic disorders), across the life course.

The field of functional genomics is advancing understanding of the mechanisms by which the exposome interacts with an individual's genetic background (Reitz et al., 2023). Such knowledge will be critical to uncovering how gene–environment interactions contribute to the development of AD/ADRD. Quantification of messenger RNA (mRNA) and protein levels through transcriptomic and proteomic approaches, respectively, can provide information on gene expression levels that can be linked to specific exposures. Epigenetics methods can be used to directly examine allele-specific DNA methylation and histone acetylation, which modulate gene expression (Reitz et al., 2023). A growing body of evidence suggests gene–environment interactions commonly manifest through epigenetic mechanisms (a description of how epigenetic mechanisms influence gene expression and pathogenesis can be found in Box 3-2) (Cavalli and Heard, 2019; Maloney and Lahiri, 2016; Marsit, 2015; Migliore and Coppedè, 2022; Schrott et al., 2022). Air pollution exposure, for example, has been linked to the DNA methylation of genes involved in inflammation pathways, contributing to the risk of cerebrocardiovascular disease (Migliore and Coppedè, 2022; Vineis et al., 2020).

Early-life lead exposure has also been associated in animal models with decreased methylation at the promoter of *APP* and histone modifications that influence the expression of genes related to the AD pathway (*APP* and *BACE1*) (Mei et al., 2023). These kinds of epigenetic effects are not limited to exposures involving environmental contaminants. Lower folate and vitamin B12 levels, for example, have been linked to reduced methylation of genes involved in the production of amyloid (*PSEN1* and *BACE1*) in AD patients as compared to age-matched controls (Migliore and Coppedè, 2022). Proteomics can enable the identification of aberrant posttranslational modifications (e.g., phosphorylation, glycosylation, acetylation, and ubiquitination)—mechanisms that regulate the trafficking, function, and degradation of proteins in normal cellular processes—which may result from exposures and influence pathological pathways leading to AD/ADRD (Guan and Wang, 2023; Ramesh et al., 2019). Thus, the layering of multiomics data has great potential to elucidate gene–environment interactions in AD/ADRD. However, limited access to datasets that include both genetic and exposome data is a current barrier to these kinds of

BOX 3-2
Epigenetic Influences and Gene–Environment Interactions

The epigenome encompasses all of the chemical modifications that are added to the genome and the changes to histone proteins that influence chromatin structure. Epigenetic processes enable cells to incorporate external stimuli into their genetic material, thereby influencing gene expression without modifying the DNA sequence itself (Maloney and Lahiri, 2016; Rozek et al., 2014). These dynamic modifications are reversible in nature and encompass DNA methylation, chromatin remodeling, histone modification, and noncoding RNA, such as microRNAs. Changes to chromatin structure influence the accessibility of DNA by the cell's transcription machinery, thereby modulating gene expression. Similarly, DNA methylation—the reversible addition of a methyl group to the cytosine base of a cytosine-guanine pair, which are common in regulatory regions of genes (Rozek et al., 2014)—influences the binding of transcription factors that mediate the initiation of the transcription process. Transcription (and gene expression) may be up- or down-regulated depending on whether transcription factor binding affinity is increased or decreased by the methylated cytosine, but more commonly DNA methylation reduces gene expression (Maloney and Lahiri, 2016; Rozek et al., 2014).

Noncoding microRNAs can regulate gene expression through binding to mRNA but also play a role in epigenetic regulation processes through posttranscriptional regulation of important chromatin- and DNA-modifying enzymes responsible for the epigenetic modification of DNA. These miRNAs are themselves regulated through epigenetic mechanisms (methylation) (Favier et al., 2021; Migliore and Coppedè, 2022). Through these mechanisms, cells can respond and adapt to diverse environmental cues, which play a vital role in gene regulation and cellular function (Bufill et al., 2020). However, epigenetic mechanisms can contribute to pathogenesis by altering gene expression and the levels of the encoded protein.

It is possible that epigenetic changes induced in early life (e.g., from stress or environmental exposures) can generate susceptibility to other insults that accumulate over the life course, eventually leading to disease, consistent with the developmental origins of health and disease theory discussed earlier in this chapter (Migliore and Coppedè, 2022). Postmortem studies have identified altered epigenetic profiles in brain tissue from individuals diagnosed with AD and other forms of dementia premortem, and there is experimental evidence implicating epigenetic changes in the pathogenesis of AD and related dementias (Gao et al., 2022; Martinez-Feduchi et al., 2024; Nikolac Perkovic et al., 2021).

continued

BOX 3-2 Continued

The dynamic nature of the epigenome over the human lifespan and the tissue-specificity of epigenetic changes raises unique challenges related to standardization of epigenetic measurement methods and data analysis (Carter et al., 2017). Artificial intelligence and machine learning methods that are enabling integrated analysis of epigenetic and other omics data have the potential to overcome some data analytic challenges and advance precision medicine approaches (Hamamoto et al., 2020).

---

analyses (Pericak-Vance, 2024). Moreover, collaboration among biomedical science experts and experts in bioinformatics and information science will be needed to tackle the data analytic challenges related to managing and integrating these vast and complex datasets and developing tools to extract insights (Hamamoto et al., 2020).

In addition to research focused on understanding how interactions between exposures and genetics lead to disease, other studies are exploring the degree to which genetic risk can be offset by protective aspects of the exposome and the mechanisms behind those protective effects. For example, a recent observational study of associations by Lourida and colleagues (2019) found that a healthy lifestyle (e.g., regular exercise, healthy diet, no current smoking, and alcohol consumption in moderation) could lower but not eliminate dementia risk in individuals with a high genetic risk.

Understanding Molecular and Cellular Mechanisms Associated with Aging and AD/ADRD

Neurodegenerative diseases such as AD/ADRD exhibit a wide range of clinical manifestations, which arise from the loss of specific neurons and synapses in different areas of the brain. While different disorders display some tissue specificity (e.g., degeneration of cholinergic neurons for AD, degeneration of dopaminergic neurons for Parkinson's disease [PD], degeneration of motor neurons for amyotrophic lateral sclerosis [ALS]), they also feature some anatomical overlaps of affected brain regions and possess shared characteristics and mechanisms, particularly the regional aggregation and spreading of cytosolic or nuclear inclusion proteins. Thus, even when different diseases are associated with distinct genetic variants, common biological themes can be observed (Behl, 2023; Gan et al., 2018).

As discussed in Chapter 1, mixed pathologies are now believed to be predominant; based on the current biological definition of AD as plaques-and-tangles disease, "pure Alzheimer's is rare" (Robinson et al., 2021). There is a strong pathological overlap of AD with, for instance LBD, vascular dementia, or hippocampal sclerosis (Jellinger, 2022; Rabinovici et al., 2017). Similarly, Lewy bodies comprising alpha-synuclein protein are features of LBD and Parkinson's disease dementia (Mensikova et al., 2022). Given the prevalence of mixed pathologies in AD/ADRD and the potential for variation in aberrant protein aggregates found in different diseases, it may be possible to achieve broader effect through interventions targeting underlying biological pathways not specific to a single pathology. Such an approach may benefit from moving away from historical clinical classifications and definitions toward descriptions that reflect diseases at a molecular and cellular resolution (Balusu et al., 2023).

Genetic mutations and epigenetic alterations can lead to defects in a multiplicity of molecular and cellular pathways, depicted in Figure 3-3, that are common across neurodegenerative diseases and occur in an age-dependent manner (Behl, 2023; Gan et al., 2018; Schumacher et al., 2021). These shared molecular and cellular pathways include:

- chronic inflammation and immune dysfunction,
- vascular dysfunction and diminished blood–brain barrier integrity,
- aberrant proteostasis and deficiency in the endosomal–lysosomal (autophagy) pathway,
- mitochondrial and metabolic dysfunction,
- disturbed lipostasis and altered lipid metabolism,
- cellular senescence, and
- epigenetic dysregulation (Hara et al., 2019).

There is increasing evidence that each of these potentially pathogenic factors and processes can play a role in the development of AD/ADRD and exert effects in varying combinations over the life course. Currently lacking, however, is an understanding of the interactions and sequential cascading effects that translate dysregulation at any one level into disease. A better understanding and an integrated model (discussed later in this chapter) will be needed to guide intervention strategies that reflect the multifactorial nature of disease. As new therapeutics targeting these earlier-stage molecular and cellular pathways are developed, it will be important to have biological markers that could be used in trials to show that the intended pathway is engaged and the therapy is having the expected effect (Lamb, 2024).

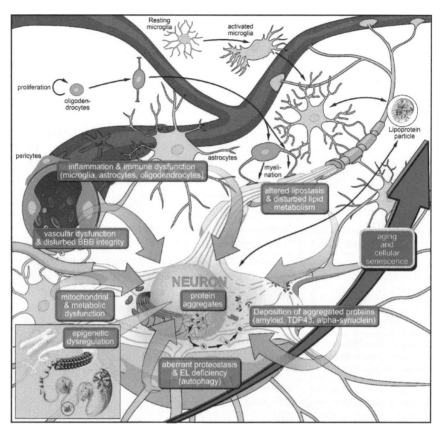

FIGURE 3-3 An integrative view of the complex array of molecular and cellular pathways that are altered in neurodegeneration.
NOTE: This is a network of interacting cells; a number of interacting factors and pathways affect neuronal function and, eventually, lead to dysfunction and degeneration. The pathogenic processes occur over time and can change during aging. BBB = blood–brain barrier; EL = endosome-lysosome; TDP43 = TAR DNA-binding protein 43.
SOURCE: Image reproduced with permission from Christian Behl.

Chronic Inflammation and Immune Dysfunction

Multiple studies have established links between the presence of pro-inflammatory mediators in the bloodstream and the advancement of neurodegenerative disorders, indicating that systemic inflammation may contribute to the emergence of persistent brain inflammation (Cao and Zheng, 2018; Italiani et al., 2018; Kim et al., 2018; Swardfager et al., 2010). Chronic inflammation, which plays a role in various age-related ailments, has been associated with decreased brain volume and impaired cognitive function in AD/ADRD (Franceschi and Campisi, 2014; Hara et al., 2019; Pilling et al., 2015).

As the resident immune cells in the brain, microglia play essential roles in maintaining homeostasis, including defense against infection or damage and phagocytosis of debris or dying cells (Salter and Stevens, 2017). Microglia also secrete tissue rebuilding factors (Vasic et al., 2019), a function that may be targeted by therapies aimed at stimulating brain tissue regeneration (discussed further in Chapter 4). During aging and in the context of some neurodegenerative diseases, microglia can acquire an activated proinflammatory phenotype characterized by morphological and functional changes, which include the release of proinflammatory cytokines and other neurotoxic mediators (Tejera et al., 2019; Wang et al., 2023). While pathways leading to microglial activation are not fully understood, there is some evidence that systemic inflammation can affect the inflammatory response of microglial cells in the brain and interfere with their clearance of aggregating proteins, such as amyloid beta in AD (Tejera et al., 2019). Environmental exposures such as brain chemical injuries or infection that trigger systemic inflammatory responses may thereby contribute to microglial activation (Ahmed et al., 2024; Greve et al., 2023; Jayaraj et al., 2017; Zhang et al., 2023c). Similarly, studies have found a link between proinflammatory microbial metabolites in the gastrointestinal tract and microglial activation and alpha-synuclein aggregation in the brain in PD (Sampson et al., 2016). Perivascular macrophages and astrocytes are also involved in the brain's innate immune response. Depending on the injury, astrocytes can demonstrate distinct activation states and transcriptional signatures that mediate neurotoxic or neurotrophic effects, which may be modulated by a microglia-astrocyte crosstalk mechanism (Gao et al., 2023; Liddelow et al., 2017).

While not as well studied as the role of the innate immune system in AD/ADRD, the adaptive immune system may also contribute to neurodegenerative disorders and may have both protective and pathogenic roles (Chen and Holtzman, 2022; Mayne et al., 2020). Studies of the adaptive immune system in dementia have primarily focused on the composition and roles of T-cell populations, which appear to infiltrate the brain from the periphery, potentially facilitated by changes to the blood–brain barrier (Chen and Holtzman, 2022). Activated T cells may perpetuate the inflammatory cascade and induce microglia into an activated phenotype by secreting proinflammatory and neurotoxic mediators. Further research is needed to understand the function of specific T-cell populations in different types of dementia. For example, proinflammatory CD4+ T_H17 cells have been implicated in neuronal degeneration in LBD (Gate et al., 2021). CD4+ T cells that exhibit an immune suppressive phenotype, known as Tregs, are thought to have a neuroprotective role in AD based on animal studies. However, alterations in Treg levels and immunomodulatory activity over the course of neurodegeneration are not well understood and some studies have suggested a detrimental effect of Tregs (Duffy et al., 2018; Gendelman and Appel, 2011; Mayne et al., 2020).

The role of B cells and humoral immune responses in neurodegeneration leading to dementia is less studied (Chen and Holtzman, 2022; Lutshumba et al., 2021), but research in mouse models suggests a role for B cells in AD progression (Kim et al., 2021). Similarly not well understood is the potential role of autoimmunity in neurodegenerative diseases that cause dementia. Some converging lines of evidence suggest that dementia may have an inflammatory autoimmune component (Lindbohm et al., 2022). Links between autoimmune disorders and subsequent dementia based on epidemiological studies, however, have not been as strong as the associations between infections and dementia (Janbek et al., 2023).

Genetic studies provide strong evidence for the link between immune dysfunction, inflammation, and AD/ADRD. Indeed, many genes associated with neurodegenerative diseases regulate responses of the innate immune system (Gan et al., 2018). For example, whole-genome sequencing studies helped identify rare variants in TREM2 (a transmembrane receptor highly expressed in immune system cells, including microglia and myeloid cells) that lead to a two- to threefold increase in AD risk (Gan et al., 2018; Guerreiro et al., 2013; Jonsson et al., 2013; Zhang et al., 2013). In familial FTD-TDP, genetic mutations that lead to insufficient production of the pro-granulin gene product, which is highly expressed in microglia, are associated with exacerbation of proinflammatory responses and the activation of microglial cells (Baker et al., 2006; Cruts et al., 2006; Yin et al., 2010). The immunomodulatory effects of these and other disease-associated gene mutations implicate aspects of the innate immune system in neurodegenerative diseases (Gan et al., 2018).

To further elucidate the role of inflammation and immune dysregulation in AD/ADRD, key knowledge gaps need to be addressed, including:

- pathways promoting various microglial states in neurodegeneration;
- connections between microglia, astrocytes, neurons, oligodendrocytes, and endothelial cells;
- the role of microglia in the clearance of protein aggregates; and
- the role of the adaptive immune system in neurodegeneration (Lamb, 2024).

Such research may suggest strategies for therapies targeting neuro-inflammation (Lin et al., 2023; Tejera et al., 2019). While broad-spectrum anti-inflammatory drugs have not been effective, specifically targeting some aspects of inflammation may be a more promising approach (Fillit et al., 2023).

Vascular Dysfunction

Vascular pathology is widely acknowledged as a contributing factor to the development of dementia (Gorelick et al., 2011; Hara et al., 2019). Epidemiological evidence supports an association between risk factors for cardiovascular disease, cerebrovascular dysfunction, and cognitive impairment (Corriveau et al., 2016; Pacholko and Iadecola, 2024). Vascular pathologies are thought to be widely prevalent. Findings from two longitudinal cohort studies showed that over 95 percent of individuals diagnosed with probable AD had mixed pathologies observed at autopsy. Approximately 90 percent of those with probable AD had vascular pathologies present (Kapasi et al., 2017).

Vascular contributions to cognitive impairment and dementia arise from age-related alterations in the neurovascular unit. The neurovascular unit consists of various components, including nonfenestrated endothelial cells,[7] pericytes, smooth-muscle cells, astrocytes, microglia, oligodendroglia, and neurons (see Figure 3-4). These components collectively contribute to the regulation of cerebral blood flow matched to neuronal metabolic demands (Claassen et al., 2021), maintenance of the blood–brain barrier, and communication between the vascular and neural compartments. Age-related changes within the neurovascular unit can disrupt these crucial functions, leading to cognitive impairment and the development of vascular dementia (Cai et al., 2017). During aging, and particularly in the context of neurodegenerative diseases, there is a notable decline in the population of pericytes, resulting in diminished cerebral blood flow delivery and subsequent downstream changes leading to neurodegeneration and dementia (Uemura et al., 2020).

One vascular pathology relevant to AD is vascular breakdown in the brain resulting from blood–brain barrier disruption (Fillit et al., 2023), which may be caused by pathological changes to the neurovascular unit. The integrity of the blood–brain barrier diminishes during normal aging, and this decline becomes even more pronounced in individuals with AD and related dementias, which often results in capillary leakage, brain leukocyte infiltration (Cai et al., 2017), ingress of toxic substances, and reactive response of astrocytes and microglia, which further aggravates neural dysfunction (Watanabe et al., 2020). Additionally, such breakdown also leads to the leakage of fibrinogen into the central nervous system (CNS),

---

[7] "Non-fenestrated endothelium is characterized by low permeability and a high abundance of tight junctions" (Gifre-Renom et al., 2022).

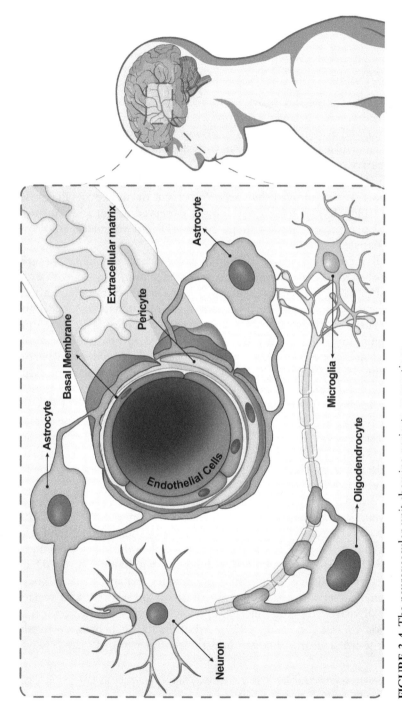

FIGURE 3-4 The neurovascular unit showing pericyte connections.
SOURCE: Wang and Chen, 2023. CC-BY-ND 4.0, https://creativecommons.org/licenses/by-nc-nd/4.0.

triggering neuroinflammation and causing insoluble fibrin clots to form (Bardehle et al., 2015; Fillit et al., 2023). Fibrinogen is not detectable in a healthy brain; in AD, however, it reaches detectable levels and interacts with amyloid, which then exacerbates clotting, fibrin deposition, and proinflammatory signaling (Fillit et al., 2023; Ryu and McLarnon, 2009; van Oijen et al., 2005; Viggars et al., 2011).

Decreased blood flow to the brain and the disruption of the blood–brain barrier can on their own contribute to neurodegeneration and the development of dementia, but may also be elements of what has recently been described as "multiple hits" models (which include vascular changes) contributing to dementia (Patrick et al., 2019; Steele et al., 2022). Multi-hit models (see Figure 3-5) describe the convergence of interconnected hits associated with age-related, genetic, vascular, and immune factors (e.g.,

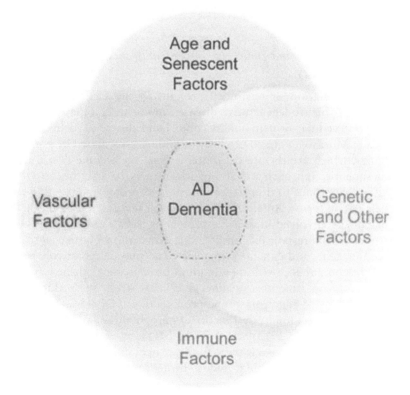

FIGURE 3-5 A multi-hit framework suggesting the convergence of vascular, immune, and other risk factors in AD.
SOURCE: Mehta and Mehta, 2023. CC BY 4.0.

neurovascular dysfunction, neuroinflammation, oxidative stress, endosomal trafficking dysfunction, changes in lipid metabolism, among others) to precipitate AD pathology, including extracellular amyloid plaques and intraneuronal neurofibrillary tangle formation, as well as other alterations that contribute to dementia (Steele et al., 2022).

One prominent NIH-supported effort in this area is the Molecular Mechanisms of the Vascular Etiology of Alzheimer's Disease (M²OVE-AD) initiative, which was established in 2016 and works to examine the link between vascular risk factors, cerebrovascular disease, and AD (NIA, 2016). This consortium brought together over 12 crossdisciplinary research teams from different institutes to use brain tissue and peripheral fluids collected from previous studies that have characterized neurodegeneration and vascular disease to generate various types of multiomics data. Integration of these data with cognitive, neuroimaging, and vascular physiology data is helping to better understand and predict the underlying molecular mechanisms behind vascular pathology and AD risk (AD Knowledge Portal, 2024a).

Aberrant Proteostasis and Deficiency in the Endosomal–Lysosomal (Autophagy) Pathway

The accumulation of misfolded proteins in the CNS is a common feature of many neurodegenerative diseases, implicating a major role for a breakdown in cellular protein quality control and clearance pathways (Gan et al., 2018; Morawe et al., 2012). Protein folding is mediated by molecular chaperones, which are themselves proteins that can become dysregulated. One therapeutic approach under investigation is to use the activity of molecular chaperones to disaggregate misfolded proteins and refold them into their native forms. An alternative approach involves targeting the cellular machinery involved in clearing protein aggregates. Autophagy is the cellular mechanism responsible for breaking down and recycling aggregated misfolded proteins and damaged organelles and plays a major role in proteostasis. In conjunction with the ubiquitin-proteasome and the lysosomal systems, autophagy functions to alleviate cellular stress by breaking down pathogenic forms of aggregate-prone proteins (i.e., TDP-43, amyloid, tau, and alpha-synuclein), lipids, dysfunctional mitochondria, and other organelles in cells (Hu et al., 2015; Scrivo et al., 2018).

This cellular mechanism is particularly critical in postmitotic cells such as neurons, as they are unable to reduce proteotoxic burden and eliminate cellular waste through cell division, rendering them more vulnerable to proteotoxic insults (Nixon, 2013). Thus, functional protein and organelle turnover as provided by a functional autophagy secures neuronal function, stability, and resistance. During the aging process, autophagy may become disrupted, resulting in intracellular buildup of various misfolded proteins. This age-associated effect can be magnified in the context of neurodegenerative disease (Bartlett et al., 2011; Gonzales et al., 2022).

Aberrant autophagy may contribute to the pathologic accumulation of amyloid plaques, tau tangles, and other protein aggregates found deposited in the brain (e.g., alpha-synuclein, TDP-43) in AD and other forms of neurodegenerative disorders (Fillit et al., 2023; Rubinsztein et al., 2011). Analysis of postmortem human brains affected by AD reveals abnormal autophagy (Lee et al., 2022; Loeffler, 2019). Propagation of misfolded proteins in animal models match observed progression patterns of neurodegeneration in the human brain (Yang et al., 2021). Endosomal–lysosomal dysfunction is one of the early pathophysiological changes that can be observed in neurodegeneration. The lysosome is the executor of autophagic clearance of proteins. Lysosomal dysfunction is acknowledged as a central catalyst of neurodegeneration (Nixon, 2020), and, consequently, lysosomal activity is a new pharmacological target.

Support for this pathway comes from observed mutations or perturbations in autophagy pathway genes in various neurodegenerative diseases. For example, genes implicated in Parkinson's disease (e.g., *PARK2, ATP13A2, PINK1, GBA*) encode lysosomal proteins or regulators of endolysosomal trafficking (Abeliovich and Gitler, 2016). In progressive supranuclear palsy, part of the FTD complex of neurodegenerative disorders, GWAS have implicated genes for components of the ubiquitin–proteasome system, including *TRIM11* (Jabbari et al., 2018), a gene that also has been shown to be downregulated in AD (Zhang et al., 2023d). While not fully understood, *APOE4* is thought to contribute to dysregulation in the endosome–lysosome and autophagy pathways, which may mediate increased AD risk in *APOE4* carriers (Asiamah et al., 2024).

Protein degradation and clearance mechanisms (e.g., stabilization of lysosomal function) are becoming prime pharmacologic therapeutic targets as they have the potential to affect multiple proteinopathies simultaneously (Knopman et al., 2021), which could be especially promising for those with multiple brain pathologies. This is in contrast to approaches such as a focused anti-amyloid or anti-tau immunotherapy that target only one type of protein aggregate.

Mitochondrial and Metabolic Dysfunction

Mitochondrial function is closely intertwined with cell viability, overall cellular function, and the various hallmarks associated with aging. Mitochondria not only play a critical role in cellular respiration—using oxygen to extract, transfer, and generate energy from such molecular substrates as glucose, fat, fatty acids, and amino acids—they are also involved in maintaining calcium and iron balance, regulating cell proliferation and cell death, facilitating cell signaling, and ensuring proteostasis (Gonzales et al., 2022; Lima et al., 2022). Neurons have a high metabolic demand, and dysfunctional mitochondria disturb the energy supply of neurons. For neurons and glial cells to function optimally, a plentiful and uninterrupted supply of adenosine triphosphate (ATP) is needed, which is best accomplished by oxidative phosphorylation of glucose. As compared to healthy aging, glucose consumption is reduced (i.e., hypometabolism) in AD/ADRD (Kato et al., 2016; Yan et al., 2020). Using fluorodeoxyglucose positron emission topography, disruption to cerebral glucose metabolism in specific brain regions has been detected (Bohnen et al., 2012; Kato et al., 2016; Yan et al., 2020). Reduced glucose utilization can occur prior to the presentation of clinical symptoms as demonstrated in a study involving participants with mild cognitive impairment due to AD (Drzezga et al., 2003; Yan et al., 2020). A longitudinal study assessing data from 128 participants found that glucose uptake in the precuneus, an area of the brain in which there is early amyloid deposition, is reduced in patients 10 years prior to the development of symptoms (Bateman et al., 2012; Yan et al., 2020).

Neurogenic glucose metabolism is perturbed by impaired insulin signaling, resulting in characteristics of AD that mirror the pathophysiology of non-CNS tissues in type 2 diabetes mellitus (Duelli and Kuschinsky, 2001). Moreover, reductions in glucose transporters GLUT1 and GLUT3 were observed in AD patient brains (An et al., 2018) and has been associated with a reduction in brain glucose consumption and cognitive impairment (Landau et al., 2010; Yan et al., 2020). Brain insulin resistance is acknowledged as an early and common feature of AD and can be closely linked to cognitive decline. In fact, there are many pathogenetic connections between brain disorders—including neurodegeneration—diabetes, and insulin resistance (de Galan, 2024).

Oxidation end products are pathological hallmarks of a variety of neurodegenerative pathologies. Mitochondria are a key source of oxidative stress resulting from respiratory chain activities and potential generation of superoxide radicals. Impairment of the activity of mitochondrial respiratory chain complexes are reported in AD, PD, and ALS (Golpich et al., 2017). Sublethal but progressive changes in mitochondrial function have been proposed to drive aging (i.e., the free radical theory of aging) (Harman, 1956) and AD (i.e., the "mitochondrial cascade" hypothesis of AD) (Swerdlow and Khan, 2004). Destabilized mitochondria create more free oxygen radicals than can be buffered sufficiently by the intrinsic antioxidant systems. A previous study reported that impaired mitochondrial function resulting from mitochondrial DNA (mtDNA) damage tends to increase with age, and levels of mtDNA damage were increased in individuals with AD as compared to age-matched controls (de la Monte et al., 2000). Single-cell analyses have revealed an increase in mtDNA deletions specifically within neurons affected by AD (Krishnan et al., 2012).

In experiments where mtDNA is transferred from donor cells to cells with identical nuclear DNA but lacking mtDNA, it has been demonstrated that mtDNA from individuals with AD is responsible for subtle variations in mitochondrial morphology, biogenesis, membrane potential, oxidative stress, and calcium buffering capacity (Swerdlow et al., 2017). Such distinct mitochondrial characteristics seen in peripheral tissues of individuals with AD, as opposed to control groups, implies that changes in mitochondrial status relevant to the brain can potentially be detected and monitored in peripheral samples. These findings suggest that mitochondrial dysfunction, which may be a cause rather than a result of AD neuropathology, could be an early event in the disease onset and progression (Theurey and Pizzo, 2018; Wilkins and Swerdlow, 2021).

Disturbed Lipostasis and Altered Lipid Metabolism

The brain has an abundance of lipid-rich myelin. Changes in the lipid composition of the brain are observed in both the natural process of aging and various neurodegenerative diseases (Gonzales et al., 2022). Genetic studies—including genetic linkage studies, GWAS, and exome sequencing studies—have repeatedly linked genes/loci related to lipid metabolism (including APOE) with AD (Andrews et al., 2020; Gonzales et al., 2022; Jones et al., 2010; Sims et al., 2020), suggesting a role for aberrations in lipid transport, lipid processing, and metabolism. The field of lipidomics, which involves the investigation of "pathways and networks of cellular lipids in biological systems" (Gonzales et al., 2022), has uncovered AD-associated lipid profiles (Han, 2010; Naudi et al., 2015). For instance, multiple research groups have consistently reported the early accumulation of ceramide levels in brains affected by AD (Cutler et al., 2004; Han et al., 2002). In contrast, sulfatides, a group of sulfoglycolipids highly enriched in myelin, have been shown to be significantly reduced at the earliest clinical stages of AD (Cheng et al., 2013; Gonzales et al., 2022; Han et al., 2003; Irizarry, 2003). Similarly, phospholipid plasmalogen was found to be reduced in the brains of individuals with AD and is associated with disease severity (Goodenowe et al., 2007).

Although the role of lipid metabolism in the pathogenesis of AD/ADRD is still under study, one interesting avenue of lipidomics research is the potential application of lipid mediators to resolve inflammation associated with proteinopathy. Free forms of proresolving lipid mediators made from the enzymatic oxygenation of polyunsaturated fatty acids have been found to be deficient in AD as a result of depletion in the pool of bound or esterified lipid mediators. Improving understanding of the regulation of lipid esterification and release could suggest effective therapeutic strategies for inflammation resolution (Shen et al., 2022; Taha, 2024).

Cellular Senescence

Cellular senescence can be defined as "a cell state triggered by stressful insults and certain physiological processes, characterized by a prolonged and generally irreversible cell-cycle arrest with secretory features, macromolecular damage, and altered metabolism" (Gorgoulis et al., 2019, p. 814). Senescent cells employ antiapoptotic pathways and halt the cell cycle as a means to evade cell death. Additionally, these cells release various substances such as proinflammatory cytokines, chemokines, growth factors, extracellular remodeling proteins, and other signaling molecules, collectively known as the senescence-associated secretory phenotype (SASP) (Gorgoulis et al., 2019). In the absence of efficient senescent cell clearance, SASP can lead to tissue damage, cell death, or even the conversion of other cells into a senescent state as a propagating phenotype (Yousefzadeh et al., 2020). As people age, senescent cells are found to accumulate throughout the body, including the brain (Yousefzadeh et al., 2020).

Nerve cells are aging over the lifetime and are only stable and functional if the nerve-cell intrinsic defense, repair, and recycling mechanisms are adequately working. Such repair mechanisms include local (axonal, synaptic, soma compartment) protein recycling pathways (see the section above on proteostasis and autophagy) but also DNA surveillance pathways. In postmortem human brain tissues of AD, various senescent cell types have been identified, including astrocytes (Bhat et al., 2012), neurons (Dehkordi et al., 2021; Musi et al., 2018), microglia (Streit and Xue, 2014), oligodendrocyte precursor cells (Zhang et al., 2019), and endothelial cells (Bryant et al., 2020). Unbiased single-cell transcriptomics analysis conducted on the dorsolateral prefrontal cortex of individuals with AD has shown that excitatory neurons are a predominant senescent cell type in the brain and are correlated with the coexistence of intracellular neurofibrillary tangles (Dehkordi et al., 2021). In healthy aging brains, however, analyses of transcriptomics data derived from bulk tissue revealed that the prevailing senescent cell types in the brain were endothelial cells and microglia (Xu et al., 2022). This finding underscores the potential disparities in senescent cell types observed in healthy versus diseased states, but it could also be attributable to the nature of the analyzed material and variations in the predetermined criteria used to define senescence.

While tracing the cause of brain senescent cell emergence in humans is not currently feasible, studies conducted on rodents revealed that such emergence could be triggered by the endogenous accumulation of tau (Bussian et al., 2018; Musi et al., 2018) or amyloid beta protein (Zhang et al., 2019), insulin resistance (Chow et al., 2019), and immune dysfunction (Yousefzadeh et al., 2021). Contributing exposomal factors may include a high-fat diet (Ogrodnik et al., 2019), chronic ethanol exposure from alcohol consumption (Sun et al., 2023), chronic unpredictable stress (Lin et al., 2021), and brain injury (Arun et al., 2020). Further elucidation of the role of cellular senescence may be achieved through comparative studies, including widescale multiomics studies, of brain regions that are normally spared in AD/ADRD (e.g., resistant) and vulnerable regions. Knowing that age is the prime risk factor for the most prominent neurodegenerative disorders in humans, the effect of age-related changes and the senescence status of different brain cell types need to be understood in more detail.

The Cellular Senescence Network (SenNet) is a collaborative research effort launched by the NIH Common Fund to comprehensively identify and characterize the heterogeneity of senescent cells in multiple human (and other model organism) tissues, in various states of health, and across the lifespan. Ultimately, the network aims to develop public atlases of these cells and create tools and technologies (e.g., biomarker panels, computer and experimental model systems, imaging tools) that build from other Common Fund programs to advance the development of therapeutics (NIH, 2024; SenNet Consortium, 2022).

Epigenetic Dysregulation

DNA methylation in the brain trends toward global decreases with aging, which has been associated with enhanced gene expression (De Jager et al., 2014; Pellegrini et al., 2021). The pattern and frequency of epigenetic changes—in particular, DNA methylation at cytosine-guanine pair sites—have been proposed as a mechanism for comparing chronological and biological age (i.e., an epigenetic clock) (Gonzales et al., 2022). Differential methylation patterns have been observed in genes associated with AD, such as *APP* and *MAPT*, among others, when comparing individuals with AD to control subjects (De Jager et al., 2014; Iwata et al., 2014; Yu et al., 2015). As age advances, increases in chromatin remodeling and chromatin heterogeneity are also observed. In addition to DNA methylation, histone acetylation typically decreases with aging, resulting in a chromatin structure that is more condensed and consequent changes in transcription (Gonzales et al., 2022; Peleg et al., 2016). By analyzing postmortem human brain tissue, a recent study uncovered an increase in the expression of two histone acetyltransferases, which were associated with both amyloid beta pathology and neurodegeneration (Nativio et al., 2018, 2020).

Alterations in levels of multiple mitochondrial RNAs have been found in AD cases, which may play a role in multiple aspects of pathology, such as modulating amyloid beta and tau production and function, synaptic plasticity, neuronal growth, apoptosis, and inflammatory response. Mitochondrial RNAs may therefore be useful as potential biomarkers and therapeutic targets (Zhang and Bian, 2021).

Understanding the relationships between the exposome, age, epigenetic and posttranslational changes, and such age-related diseases as AD/ADRD holds promise for disease prediction (Grodstein et al., 2020; Shireby et al., 2020) and intervention efforts. As potentially reversible contributors to AD/ADRD, epigenetic and posttranslational alterations are appealing targets for therapeutic interventions (Hara et al., 2019; Migliore and Coppedè, 2022). Realizing such potential will require the systematic analysis and comparison of epigenetic and posttranslational changes in aged and diseased (AD/ADRD) brain tissue and identification of areas of overlap.

Toward an Integrative Biological Framework for AD/ADRD

As illustrated in Figure 3-3 above and described throughout this section, the process of neurodegeneration is influenced by a number of cell types and pathogenic processes. Importantly, the factors and mechanisms affecting the onset and progression of disease act along the life course, meaning they occur to different extents as the brain ages, and may also interact with each other. These processes (e.g., inflammation, vascular dysfunction, altered proteostasis and autophagy, mitochondrial and metabolic changes) and cellular players (e.g., neurons, endothelial and glial cells) comprise a complicated biological framework for neurodegeneration. It is increasingly acknowledged that age-associated neurodegenerative diseases, such as AD/ADRD, are the result of complex and multifactorial events. However, all the pathways described are disease relevant and need to be taken into account when creating a more integrative understanding of events taking part in age-related neurodegeneration (Behl, 2023; Lehmann et al., 2023).

By enabling better discernment of the initial triggers, cascading pathophysiologic sequences, and biological systems working to counteract those perturbations to restore homeostasis, such a model could potentially guide combination approaches to AD/ADRD interventions that sequentially target key steps in the etiologic cascade and that integrate age-dependent changes. For example, nonpharmacological interventions implemented early in life for individuals at risk for dementia (e.g., based on genetic and exposome risks) could be followed later in life with an anti-inflammatory therapy, and potentially, a pathology-specific (e.g., amyloid) immunotherapy to avoid microglia activation. Such a combination approach may be necessary to achieve effect sizes greater than those observed to date for strategies targeting a single pathology and pathway.

Some progress has been made in the development of integrated models for molecular and cellular pathways contributing to neurodegeneration

(Balusu et al., 2023; De Strooper and Karran, 2016; Gan et al., 2018). In such models, a biochemical phase features perturbations in normal cellular processes that contribute to the protein aggregation commonly observed in neurodegenerative diseases; protein aggregation, on the other hand, is not part of the pathological process in dementia types based on vascular changes (vascular dementia). The biochemical phase is followed by a cellular phase during which cells in the brain react to the protein aggregates. A key element of the cascade proposed here is the generation of an innate inflammatory reaction mediated by microglia, which triggers reactions from other cells and ultimately leads to neuronal cell death. The resulting damage to the brain, some potentially irreversible, leads to the clinical phase (cognitive impairment and clinical dementia) (De Strooper and Karran, 2016; NASEM, 2024).

While described linearly for simplicity, within this cascade there are several feedback mechanisms, adding to the model complexity, as depicted in Figure 3-3 earlier in this chapter. On the other hand, this proposed sequence leaves behind the neuron-only modeling of neurodegeneration and considers also the effect of other nonneuronal cell types. As neuroinflammatory endophenotypes and biomarkers for different biochemical pathways are developed, it may be possible to further unravel the temporal relationship between inflammatory responses and other pathophysiological aspects of AD/ADRD (Arafah et al., 2023; Hampel et al., 2020).

While the aforementioned cascade provides a useful starting place for understanding the interdependent molecular and cellular processes contributing to AD/ADRD, a comprehensive model needs to account not only for pathologic factors occurring within the brain, but also the role of the exposome, brain–peripheral body interactions, and mechanisms of resilience.

The Role of the Exposome and Brain–Peripheral Body Interactions

Upstream of the intracellular biochemical events leading to the different pathogenic processes are the contributions of the exposome to pathogenesis, which need to be incorporated into an integrative model. While it is clear that genetic variants associated with AD/ADRD can increase susceptibility to and/or accelerate many of the hallmarks of aging, the contributions of exposome factors, mediated either through gene–environment interactions or through direct biochemical and/or cellular effects, have not been well characterized and are important for understanding differences in AD/ADRD across diverse populations. As discussed earlier in this chapter, efforts are needed to identify exposure-related pathways that modulate or converge with other AD/ADRD risk factors or pathways to mediate pathogenesis. For example, air pollution may alter the blood–brain barrier (Oppenheim et al., 2013) and has also been shown to reduce levels of esterified lipid mediators, which, as noted earlier, are involved in resolving inflammation and have been found to be deficient in AD (Shen et al., 2022; Taha, 2024), indicating the potential for synergistic deleterious effects.

A growing body of evidence suggests that infections, both CNS specific and systemic, can increase the risk of dementia and that these effects may be mediated in part by inflammation, although pathogen-specific pathways may also be involved (Itzhaki, 2021; Sipilä et al., 2021; Vestin et al., 2024), particularly for pathogens that can infect the brain, such as herpes simplex virus (Itzhaki, 2021) and SARS-CoV-2 (Liu et al., 2023b). Furthermore, behavioral factors such as diet and physical activity contribute to cardio-vascular risk factors, such as hypertension, diabetes, and obesity (Gonzalez et al., 2024; Marquez et al., 2024) and are increasingly understood to con-tribute to neurodegeneration through vascular pathways (NASEM, 2018), but behavioral factors may also affect AD/ADRD risk through epigenetic effects (Maloney and Lahiri, 2016; Migliore and Coppedè, 2022).

The potential for extra-CNS infections to increase dementia risk and the well-established cardiovascular risk factors for dementia underscore the need for brain–peripheral body interactions to be represented in a more holistic integrated model (Hampel et al., 2019). AD/ADRD are not dis-eases exclusive to neurons but involve the whole body since the brain and the (rest of the) body are tightly connected through metabolic, immune, and vascular systems (Hampel et al., 2019). As discussed earlier in this chapter, vascular dysfunction may be linked to such neurodegenerative mechanisms as neuroinflammation and impeded clearance of protein aggre-gates. Thus, targeting cardiovascular risk factors in the periphery (e.g., atherosclerosis, hypertension) has the potential to affect multiple potential AD/ADRD pathways in the brain in a disease-agnostic manner, in addi-tion to effects on cardiovascular diseases such as heart disease and stroke (preventive interventions targeting cardiovascular risk factors are discussed in Chapter 4).

Another notable example of such brain–peripheral body interactions is the gut microbiome and its potential contribution to AD/ADRD through the gut–brain axis. Microbial metabolites may exert effects on the brain through multiple pathways (e.g., immune, endocrine, enteric nervous sys-tem), and are thought to have a wide range of effects including altering neuronal transcription, compromising the blood–brain barrier integrity, and triggering neuroinflammation (Wang et al., 2021). Ongoing research is seeking to elucidate how gut microbiota interact with certain risk gene settings and exposome factors, such as air pollution (Dutta et al., 2022), to influence the onset and/or progression of AD/ADRD. In addition to the gut–brain axis, connections via the lung–brain and renal–CVD–brain axes have also been studied (Finch and Kulminski, 2019; Owaki et al., 2024).

The Role of Cognitive Resilience

Also critical for inclusion in an integrated model are pathways that provide an explanation for why many individuals with evidence of accumulated brain pathologies and neurodegenerative changes fail to develop cognitive impairment or clinical dementia (Aizenstein et al., 2008) and why others do not develop neuropathology, as can be observed in a cohort of centenarians (Zhang et al., 2023e). As an example, one-third of individuals in the Religious Orders Study and Rush Memory and Aging Project (ROSMAP) cohorts who met the diagnostic criteria for pathologic AD at the time of autopsy had no clinical signs of cognitive impairment at the time of death, suggesting the existence of resilience factors—endogenous (e.g., personality, life outlook, genetic factors) and/or exogenous (e.g., access to resources)—capable of offsetting the detrimental effects of brain pathologies (i.e., a cognitive reserve hypothesis) (Katzman et al., 1988; Zammit et al., 2023).

Genomics and other omics approaches are helping to identify resilience factors, elucidate their underlying biological mechanisms, and to relate them to neuropathology and changes in brain function (Box 3-3 describes the Resilience-AD program that is supporting some of this work) (de Vries et al., 2024). Proteomics studies using samples from ROSMAP cohorts have shown that synaptic function and mitochondrial activity are enriched by proteins associated with higher cognitive stability, while proteins associated with more rapid cognitive decline were enriched for inflammatory response, apoptosis, and endothelial function in glial cells (Zammit et al., 2023). Of interest, some proteins associated with cognitive resilience are pleiotropic, also conferring resilience to motor phenotypes of neurodegenerative diseases, underscoring the breadth of health benefits afforded by resilience factors. While specific mechanisms of action are still being uncovered, resilience factors may fall into three different mechanistic categories: (1) those affecting clinical phenotypes independent of brain pathologies, (2) those that interact with brain pathologies to attenuate or modify their effects, and (3) those directly affecting the magnitude of brain pathologies (i.e., conferring resistance to pathology) (Zammit et al., 2023).

The identification of modifiable resilience factors can guide the development of preventive and therapeutic approaches for AD/ADRD (Neuner et al., 2022). For instance, evidence regarding the contributions of physical activity and education to resilience provide support for individual-level and public health nonpharmacologic interventions focused on these factors (discussed further in Chapter 4). Moreover, advancing understanding of the biological mechanisms underlying cognitive resilience can inform drug discovery. For example, increased levels of Neuritin 1, a protein with an important role in plasticity and synaptic function, is associated with cognitive resilience

BOX 3-3
Resilience-AD

The Resilience-AD program was established with the goal of improving understanding of how gene–environment interactions contribute to cognitively resilient phenotypes in people at high risk for Alzheimer's disease (AD), with the ultimate objective of identifying novel therapeutic targets for pharmacological and nonpharmacological interventions aimed at prevention (AD Knowledge Portal, 2024b). Resilience-AD is intended to be complementary to and inform other efforts focused on the discovery of novel targets and biomarkers, including the Accelerating Medicines Partnership® Program for Alzheimer's Disease and M²OVE-AD Programs. The program will generate multiomic (e.g., genomic, proteomic, metabolomic) profiling data from samples collected from individuals who (1) are resistant to the development of AD/ADRD neuropathology despite high genetic risk (e.g., APOE4 homozygotes, people with Down Syndrome, autosomal dominant mutation carriers), (2) reach very old age (90 years of age or older) without developing dementia, or (3) remain cognitively normal despite the presence of neuropathologic disease biomarkers (AD Knowledge Portal, 2024b). Using network biology approaches, molecular, clinical, pathologic, and exposome (e.g., environmental, lifestyle, experiential) data collected from individuals exhibiting resilience to AD will be integrated and used to identify molecular networks that can predict cognitive resilience.

and has been identified as a therapeutic target for AD (Hurst et al., 2023; Zammit et al., 2023). Cellular studies aiming to define resistance and adaptive factors that provide protection against neurodegeneration-associated challenges and stress (e.g., oxidative and endoplasmic reticulum stress) may complement in vivo investigations (Chakraborty et al., 2019; Pham et al., 2023). To advance precision approaches to AD/ADRD interventions, resilience-focused research and an integrative biological framework for AD/ADRD need to consider the interplay of biological and sociocultural factors and the consequent potential for heterogeneity in resilience determinants and trajectories across different population groups. An important example is the observation of sex and gender differences in resilience, which may stem from myriad interrelated factors requiring further study, including neuroanatomy, genetic architecture, and influences of gender roles on modifiable risk factors (Arenaza-Urquijo et al., 2024).

Targeting resilience factors represents an appealing alternative to targeting individual AD/ADRD pathologies, especially given the prevalence of mixed pathologies. In the future, a cognitive resilience index based on the ability to measure known resilience factors could facilitate a precision medicine approach to interventions, which may include combinations of resilience behaviors, such as physical activity, and novel resilience therapies aimed at maintaining brain health and late-life cognitive function.

Conclusion 3-2: AD/ADRD has complex multifactorial origins. Fundamental gaps in the current understanding of the underlying biology of dementia and the siloed study of neurodegenerative diseases and mechanistic pathways impede efforts to develop effective prevention and treatment strategies. The investigation of pathways and mechanisms that are shared across neurodegenerative diseases will provide opportunities to identify targets for prevention and treatment that are not specific to a singular pathology.

Conclusion 3-3: The creation of a comprehensive biological framework that integrates knowledge of the shared molecular and cellular mechanistic pathways underlying neurodegenerative disease and their interplay with exposome, genetic, and resilience factors, among others, would provide a holistic model that could facilitate the translation of basic research into effective preventive and therapeutic interventions across multiple pathologies. Resilience and resistance factors that provide normal cognitive functions despite disease-like pathologies need to be uncovered.

Model Systems and Other Tools for Elucidating Molecular and Cellular Pathways Leading to AD/ADRD

Considering the various and interrelated molecular and cellular pathways discussed in the sections above, one central question remaining is how to model complex brain diseases that develop over decades and are affected by various sets of risk genes, as well as their interplay with peripheral organs (i.e., system health) and the environment (i.e., exposome). NIH has made substantial investments to support the creation of model systems to serve as an experimental basis for studying disease pathogenesis and facilitating drug discovery. As no single model is able to fully recapitulate the human condition, and each has its strengths and weaknesses, a variety of in vivo and in vitro models have been developed to answer different kinds of scientific questions. Thus, it is important to adequately define the key questions at the start of a scientific endeavor so they may drive the development and selection of an appropriate model. In the understandable absence of an ideal model, the use of multiple models in combination can enhance the robustness of the experimental findings.

As with other tools, all models need to be adequately validated to ensure reliability and reproducibility for a given context of use (i.e., how and when the model will be used). The stringency of the validation process depends on how the data will be used (NASEM, 2023). For example, different levels of stringency would be needed for validation of models used to understand mechanistic pathways through basic research versus those used to inform decisions regarding the safety of a novel therapeutic.

In Vivo Models

While AD/ADRD are explicitly human disorders and do not appear to occur naturally in conventional laboratory rodents, genetic engineering has enabled the development of mouse and rat models for use in elucidating pathogenic processes that lead to different types of neuronal dysfunction and evaluating potential therapeutic approaches (Sinclair et al., 2024). For AD alone, there are hundreds of mouse models available and each may have different trajectories and timelines related to the formation of plaques, tangles, neuronal dysfunction, gliosis, synaptic loss, and memory impairment (AlzForum, 2024). These mouse models are mostly based on amyloid and tau biology. Despite limitations stemming from differences in human and murine anatomy and physiology and potential artifacts from the genetic engineering process, mouse models have also played an important role in enhancing understanding of the role of various genes, such as *APOE4* (Padmanabhan and Gotz, 2023) or those encoding elements of the endosomal–lysosomal system (Lee et al., 2022; Terron et al., 2024) in AD/ADRD, as well as pathogenic processes such as the prion-like neuron-to-neuron spreading of amyloid and tau pathology (Padmanabhan and Gotz, 2023).

While many transgenic mouse models were generated using genetic alterations associated with dominantly inherited disease forms (e.g., familial AD and FTD), concerns regarding the applicability of such models to sporadic, late-onset disease forms and their failure to predict the clinical efficacy of therapies in clinical trials spurred efforts to create novel animal models for late-onset disease using genetic engineering methods such as CRISPR and other innovative approaches (Collins and Greenfield, 2024; Oblak et al., 2020; Padmanabhan and Gotz, 2023). One prominent NIA-funded effort is the Model Organism Development and Evaluation for Late-onset Alzheimer's Disease (MODEL-AD),[8] which is using computational analyses of human datasets made available from other NIH initiatives such as the Accelerating Medicines Partnership® Program for Alzheimer's Disease (AMP-AD), M²OVE-AD, ADSP, ADNI, and other sources to guide the development of novel models that recapitulate key hallmarks of late-onset

---

[8] Further information is available at https://www.model-ad.org/ (accessed June 5, 2024).

AD. Ultimately, the aim is to integrate these models into preclinical testing pipelines to identify and evaluate novel therapies (MODEL-AD, 2024; NIA, 2023b). MODEL-AD, like most animal model development to date, has primarily focused on AD, with a heavy bias toward amyloid pathways, although some models for LBD (Lim et al., 2011; Magen and Chesselet, 2011; Sander et al., 2023; Stylianou et al., 2020) and FTD (Ahmed et al., 2017; Kashyap et al., 2023; Roberson, 2012) have been created. To continue to expand the therapeutic pipeline to other nonamyloid targets and related dementias, there is a need for further investment in the creation and characterization of models that can inform those efforts, including mixed-pathology models. Animal models are also critical to understanding synaptic and cellular contributors to resilience (de Vries et al., 2024; Neuner et al., 2022).

In addition to mice, other animals with the potential to model AD/ADRD include fruit flies (Trotter et al., 2017); rats; dogs, which naturally develop amyloid plaques with age (Noche et al., 2024); and nonhuman primates (NHPs) (Padmanabhan and Gotz, 2023). Rats are commonly used in pharmacokinetic studies but also may be superior to mice in modeling inflammation (Du et al., 2017; Seok et al., 2013) and complex cognitive behaviors. NIA's intramural research program is conducting a longitudinal study of neurocognitive aging in rats—Successful Trajectories of Aging: Reserve and Resilience in RatS (STARRRS)—which will generate shareable resources of phenotypic and neuroimaging data, as well as biological samples (NIA, 2024c)

As compared to rodents, NHPs are more similar to humans with regards to neuroanatomy and neurophysiology (NASEM, 2023), which may make them useful models for neurodegenerative diseases such as AD/ADRD. Some NHPs (great apes, macaques) develop amyloid plaques with age but they do not appear to regularly spontaneously develop other features of human AD pathology that lead to dementia (e.g., neurofibrillary tangles) (Beckman et al., 2021). Consequently, there is interest in genetically engineering more human-relevant NHP models for AD/ADRD. NIH recently funded the Marmosets As Research Models of AD (MARMO-AD) program, which is exploring transgenic marmosets as models to study primate-specific cellular and molecular mechanisms that contribute to the pathogenesis and progression of AD (Sukoff Rizzo et al., 2023). Genetic engineering of new NHP models is still in its infancy, however, and may be slowed by the high cost and logistic hurdles of working with NHPs, as well as ethical considerations (Padmanabhan and Gotz, 2023).

Consistent with NIH policy requirements (NIH, 2015), NIH-funded AD/ADRD studies using animal models need to consider sex as a biological variable, beginning with the development of research questions and extending to analysis of results and reporting of findings (e.g., sex disaggregated).

In doing so, preclinical animal studies can help to improve understanding of sex-specific differences in AD/ADRD (Arenaza-Urquijo et al., 2024).

In Vitro Models

To complement AD/ADRD research using animal models, there has been increasing focus on the development of in vitro models derived from human cells in the hopes of generating more human-relevant findings. Cell-based systems for studying human diseases were revolutionized in the early 2000s by the discovery of human induced pluripotent stem cells (iPSCs) (Yamanaka, 2012), which can be used to generate most human tissue cell types. Patient-derived iPSCs have been used to develop human brain organoids and brain microphysiological systems (i.e., tissue chips), which are being explored as potential model systems to study AD/ADRD. The generation of iPSCs from participants involved in cohort studies provides opportunities to link data from the cell-based models to longitudinal clinical data (NIA, 2022a).

Additional and further advanced in vitro systems that can recapitulate patient-like pathophysiology are emerging and represent potential alternatives to conventional animal- and cell-based models (Amartumur et al., 2024). For example, brain or cerebral organoids are three-dimensional (3D) cellular aggregates that when generated from human iPSCs exhibit some similarities to the structural and functional features of specific regions of a human brain, including neural circuit formation and neuroimmune and neurovascular interactions. Such models have been used to compare amyloid clearance by microglia carrying the *APOE4* or the *APOE3* allele (Paşca, 2019) and to elucidate early pathogenic events resulting from mutations in the *MAPT* gene that gives rise to an inherited form (autosomal dominant) of FTD (Bowles et al., 2021). As their architecture and functionality more closely resemble an embryonic brain, brain organoids may generally be better suited to the study of neurodevelopment than age-related neurodegeneration (Paşca, 2019).

Microphysiological systems are similarly 3D cellular systems intended to recapitulate specific aspects of human physiology but differ from organoids in that they are formed on microfluidic chips, giving researchers more control over the development of the composition and architecture of the tissue and the ability to model such features as vascular perfusion (Hargrove-Grimes et al., 2021). Coculture systems that can enable the investigation of complex cellular interactions (e.g., among neurons, astrocytes, microglia, endothelial cells) (Cetin et al., 2022) have the potential to help answer pressing scientific questions regarding the perturbations in cellular activity that lead to the loss of homeostasis in the brain (De Strooper and Karran, 2016). For some scientific questions regarding AD/ADRD biology, such coculture systems may better model in vivo conditions and have greater translational relevance than cellular models involving only a single cell type (Cetin et al., 2022). Furthermore, the ability to connect chips with different tissues in a modular fashion can enable the study of interactions of peripheral body organs with the brain. A workshop hosted by NIH in 2022 focused on opportunities for microphysiologic systems to serve as alternatives to animal models for AD/ADRD and their potential role in drug discovery and development (NIA, 2022a). This workshop highlighted examples of efforts underway to develop 3D cell-based models for AD/ADRD including an organoid model for AD and tissue chip models for FTD and the blood–brain barrier.

An important limitation of iPSC-derived organoid and microphysiologic models is that the process of reprogramming patient-derived cells into iPSCs results in the loss of their somatic epigenetic patterns, including aging, exposure, and disease-related markers (Balusu et al., 2023). A promising complementary approach that may circumvent this limitation is induced neuron (iN) models, which are generated by converting already differentiated cells, commonly fibroblasts, into neurons (Balusu et al., 2023; Traxler et al., 2022). In contrast to iPSC models, iN models retain to some degree (albeit not well characterized) the epigenetic profile and metabolic state of the patients they are derived from and demonstrate enhanced expression of mature neuronal markers and improved functionality (Balusu et al., 2023). Employing iN models may lead to a better understanding of neuronal state and fate changes, which in turn could guide intervention approaches to manipulation of cell fate with the goal of promoting neuronal resilience, repair, and, potentially, rejuvenation (Traxler et al., 2023). Further comparative evaluations of iPSC and iN models are needed to better characterize the advantages and limitations of each and their use as complementary systems.

Of course, in vitro models are not suited to some aspects of AD/ADRD research, such as elucidating the underlying effects of such factors as exercise, hypertension, psychological stress, sociobehavioral factors, and sleep, which generally require the study model to be an integrated organism. Other considerations regarding findings from human-derived cell models include potential variability resulting from such factors as differences in cell sources, genetic backgrounds, and culture methods (including their ability to mimic physiologic conditions) (Slanzi et al., 2020), as well as how representative existing models are of the population and different dementia phenotypes.

Single-cell sequencing of samples from brains collected postmortem from individuals with AD/ADRD have the potential to generate data that are complementary to cell-based models, such as uncovering affected neuronal and nonneuronal cell types, vulnerable brain regions, and changes (e.g., somatic DNA mutations, altered gene expression) that precede neuronal dysfunction and death (Balusu et al., 2023; Miller et al., 2022). Advances in multiomics approaches are enabling the analysis of genomic, transcriptomic, metabolomic, lipidomic, and epigenomic information from single cells (Vandereyken et al., 2023), providing new opportunities to elucidate molecular pathways leading to dementia, especially when coupled with emerging spatial multiomics methods. In addition, multiomics approaches in combination with GWAS and genetic single-nucleotide polymorphism studies have the potential to define "a cluster of core alterations in AD" and can advance a more holistic approach in AD/ADRD research (Argyriou et al., 2024). As discussed later in this chapter, findings from studies using unbiased GWAS and multiomics approaches require significant investment in follow-on basic, mechanistic research (including studies using in vivo models) to understand their biology and how they might be targeted therapeutically.

One challenge with the high-dimensional analyses of single cells from postmortem brain samples is that the disease has generally already progressed to late or end stage and data can only be captured from the more resistant, surviving neurons. To address these limitations, data from single-cell analyses of human brain samples could be supplemented with single-cell multiomics data from animal models, which may provide insights into earlier-stage dysfunction (Balusu et al., 2023). Of note, the Brain Research Through Advancing Innovative Neurotechnologies® (BRAIN) initiative recently released a comprehensive single-cell spatial map of the mouse brain and identified thousands of cell types, underscoring the importance of leveraging large-scale resources developed by other institutions.

Conclusion 3-4: Animal and in vitro models have important roles to play in enhancing understanding of select molecular, biochemical, and physiological processes of AD/ADRD. While no model can recapitulate the full complexity of disease pathogenesis across the human life course, preclinical research can elucidate elements of this complexity and links between pathogenic factors and risk genes.

ACCELERATING THE TRANSLATION OF BASIC, EPIDEMIOLOGICAL, AND SOCIAL SCIENCES RESEARCH FOR THE DEVELOPMENT OF INTERVENTION STRATEGIES

As described in this chapter, diverse streams of epidemiological, social science, and mechanistic research have been pursued, funded by NIH and others (Stephan et al., 2024). An expansion beyond this breadth of inquiry is appropriate given the breadth of the exposome and the longitudinal and molecular complexity of pathways that lead to AD/ADRD. All of these factors contribute to the individuality of this group of neurodegenerative diseases, as increasingly supported by recent advances in biomarkers and subtyping studies (Tijms et al., 2024), as discussed further in Chapter 4.

Advances in the understanding of the risks associated with different types of dementia and the molecular and cellular pathways that mediate those risks need to be accompanied by efforts to translate this new knowledge into intervention strategies. These efforts can be guided by advancements in blood-based or other biomarkers to stratify risks into all-cause dementia, AD, or related dementia risks.

Translational Epidemiology Approaches: Moving from Risk Factors to Public Health Interventions and Back to Stratified Epidemiology

Research to guide interventions must evaluate causation, and yet for decades the statistical training typically offered to clinical researchers has emphasized "risk factor" epidemiology (i.e., the identification of correlates of disease without rigorous evaluation of causality). Revolutionary progress in conceptualization and methodology for causal inference started in the 1980s and created substantial debates in clinical research (Pearl, 2009). Technical tools to support causal inference in the absence of formal randomization continue to improve, alongside rigorous frameworks for recognizing the limitations of evidence from randomized and nonrandomized studies (Hernán, 2018). This progress is highly relevant to AD/ADRD research and yet very few researchers have adopted these tools. The slow adoption is attributable to a combination of statistical difficulty, the limited formal training available to many researchers (the field is deeply interdisciplinary), or training that occurred prior to the causality revolution and thus did not incorporate the tools. As a result, the quality of evidence available even for routine questions that have been tackled in countless studies, such as the effects of alcohol use on AD/ADRD, or common medications, remains thin.

Many observational studies are vulnerable to identical biases, so they offer little new evidence to complement one another. More formal frameworks to integrate evidence across study designs, populations, and data types are needed. This includes work on measurement harmonization and cross-walking, meta-analyses and meta-regression, and evidence triangulation (Lawlor et al., 2016; Thurmond, 2001). For example, randomized controlled trials are not always or even often feasible, especially for preventive interventions for a disease that develops over decades. As a result, conclusions about preventive strategies rest heavily on studies that were not intentionally designed randomized controlled trials.

There are two general strategies for evaluating causality in these settings: (1) control for confounders that might influence the exposure and also AD/ADRD or (2) identify a quasi-random source of variation in exposure and evaluate how that influences AD/ADRD risk (Matthay et al., 2020). Combining evidence from both approaches offers a far stronger basis for causal conclusions. Additional opportunities for evidence triangulation include identifying settings where the confounders are likely to be entirely different or finding negative control outcomes. These approaches align well with the policy emphasis in Chapter 4, highlighting the strategies of public and institutional policies to translate epidemiological findings into public health impact for prevention of AD/ADRD. Policies are often directly amenable to evaluation via quasi-experimental approaches, for example, leveraging approximately random variation in the timing of policy adoption and implementation. Major progress already achieved in declining age-specific incidence rates in many settings suggest rigorous evaluation of the changes that account for those declines may point the way to future breakthroughs.

In addition, as blood tests for AD/ADRD are implemented in real-world settings, the availability of biomarker data will enable epidemiological research to stratify the population and differentiate risk factors for AD from those for related dementias. This will enable the development of tailored interventions in both public health and therapeutics.

Conclusion 3-5: Despite substantial evidence, the translation of epidemiological research to public health interventions has been slow and has been hindered by insufficient evaluation of causation that can be addressed, in part, through intensive statistical work to triangulate evidence from different study designs, types of data, and populations.

Opportunities to Accelerate Discoveries into Interventions for AD/ADRD

At present there are more than 100 drugs being evaluated in clinical trials for effectiveness against AD (Cummings et al., 2023b), many targeting pathways not specific to any one AD/ADRD pathology, such as those described earlier in this chapter. More than 150 trials are evaluating nonpharmacological interventions (Kelley, 2023). Despite hope for each approach, the reality is that most phase 2 trials will fail. Thus, improving our ability to learn from failures, as well as improving the probability of success for the pharmacological interventions entering the clinic, needs to be a research priority as it has the greatest potential to improve the delivery of treatments for AD/ADRD. Negative clinical trials need to be analyzed to identify points of failure in translation and the potential causes, and this information needs to be fed back into earlier phases of the research and development pipeline, as discussed further in Chapter 4. However, this can only occur if trials are well designed and have specific and validated target engagement or pharmacodynamic biomarkers informing upon the hypothesized mechanism of action. Currently only 44 percent of clinical trials have fluid biomarkers fulfilling this role and the numbers drop in industry-sponsored trials (Marlies Oosthoek, 2024), and even fewer have imaging measures because of the associated costs.

This is a significant barrier to the translation of clinical research back to basic mechanisms.

Success of clinical drug discovery research can be seen two ways. First, success is achieving a positive primary outcome providing evidence of efficacy on an accepted endpoint. This type of success leads to phase 3 studies to demonstrate application across a larger and more diverse patient population. However, this does not occur often; instead, many drug discovery trials fail to meet their primary outcome. Outside of safety, the most important secondary outcome is that the intervention engages the mechanism and provides sufficient activity such that an efficacy response would have been observed if that mechanism was related to the disease. The majority of drug discovery trials do not invest sufficiently in this area and thus, despite the investment in clinical research, the field advances slowly and leaves many questions pertaining to why efficacy was not achieved.

Conclusion 3-6: Almost all early-phase clinical research (phase 1b and 2 trials) fails to achieve its primary efficacy outcomes. However, the return on the investment in clinical research can be dramatically improved through the focus on testing specific mechanistic hypotheses and employing specific and analytically validated measures in these early-phase trials. Where this is not yet possible, biobanking can facilitate future understanding if samples are easily accessible by academic researchers. Such an approach will improve the quality and value of the results obtained and ensure that the participants' involvement in drug trials achieves maximum benefit.

The probability of success for pharmacological interventions entering the clinic is low and requires improvements in target diversity, validation, and enablement. NIH has intensified infrastructure investments in these areas and has developed several interconnected translational research programs that support the identification, validation, and enablement of targets as part of a precision medicine approach to drug development for AD (see Figure 3-6) (NIA, 2023b). These strategic investments in the earliest phases of drug discovery and preclinical research have resulted in the generation of large and diverse (e.g., genetic, exposome, functional multiomics) datasets that can be used for the identification of novel targets.

The Accelerating Medicines Partnership® (see Box 3-4), a cross-sector partnership launched in 2014 and managed by the Foundation for the NIH has used several avenues to identify pathways and nodes specific to certain cell types that are affected in AD (NIA, 2024d). The Target Enablement to Accelerate Therapy Development for Alzheimer's Disease (TREAT-AD) centers function to bridge the efforts of AMP-AD and those to enable novel targets through early drug discovery using animal models developed

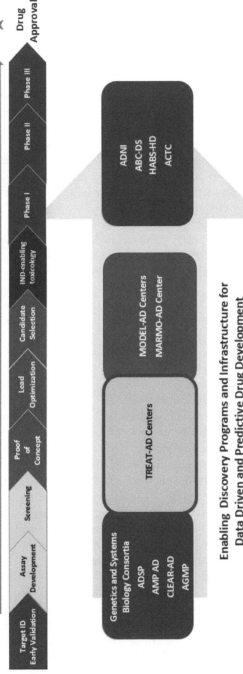

FIGURE 3-6 NIH-funded pipeline of translational research programs and infrastructure to diversify the therapeutic pipeline and enable a precision medicine approach to drug development.

NOTE: ABC-DS = Alzheimer Biomarkers Consortium–Down Syndrome; ACTC = Alzheimer's Clinical Trails Consortium; ADNI = Alzheimer's Disease Neuroimaging Imitative; ADSP = Alzheimer's Disease Sequencing Project; AMP-AD = Accelerating Medicines Partnership—Alzheimer's Disease Target Discovery and Preclinical Validation; CLEAR-AD = Centrally-linked Longitudinal pEripheral biomARkers of Alzheimer's Disease; IND = investigational new drug; TREAT-AD = Target Enablement to Accelerate Therapy Development for Alzheimer's Disease; HABS-HD = Health and Aging Brain Study—Health Disparities; MARMO = Marmosets as Research Models for Alzheimer's Disease; MODEL—AD = Model Organism Development and Evaluation for Late-onset Alzheimer's Disease. SOURCE: NIA, 2024e.

BOX 3-4
The Accelerating Medicines Partnership®

The Accelerating Medicines Partnership® (AMP) program is a public–private partnership that brings together federal agencies (NIH, FDA), industry (e.g., biopharmaceutical and life sciences companies), and non-profit organizations to reduce the time and costs associated with making new diagnostics and treatments available to patients by fostering joint efforts to identify and validate promising biological targets for therapeutics (NIA, 2024d). The cross-sector partnership was launched in 2014 and is managed through the Foundation for the NIH (FNIH). Several disease-specific AMP programs have been established, including but not limited to programs for AD (NIA, 2024d), PD (AMP-PD, n.d.), and ALS (NINDS, 2024b). Given the potential for commonalities and overlapping mechanisms among these neurodegenerative diseases, coordination will be important going forward to ensure siloing of efforts does not result in missed opportunities to leverage advances in knowledge, innovation, and infrastructure and to foster a more integrative approach.

Accelerating Medicines Partnership® Program for Alzheimer's Disease (AMP-AD)

Initiated in 2014, AMP-AD is part of a larger NIH effort to identify and validate novel biomarkers and therapeutic targets for AD (e.g., in conjunction with CLEAR-AD and TREAT-AD) (Kelley, 2023). All AMP-AD partners have agreed to making the data and analyses from this initiative publicly available for broad scientific use; these data can be accessed via a centralized data infrastructure and data-sharing platform, the AD Knowledge Portal, and through the open-source platform, Agora (NIA, 2024d). In its first iteration, AMP-AD was focused on identifying novel therapeutic targets and evaluating tau imaging as a biomarker for measuring disease progression and response to treatment. The second iteration, AMP-AD 2.0, was launched in 2021 to expand on the prior efforts to discover and validate new targets and biomarkers using a precision medicine approach (NIA, 2022b). Supported by a series of NIH foundational grants, specific strategic directions for AMP-AD 2.0 include the following:

- "Expand the molecular profiling in brain, CSF, and blood samples from diverse cohorts
- Generate longitudinal immunologic profiling data to enable dynamic modeling of the disease trajectory
- Expand the existing single-cell/single-nucleus molecular profiling efforts to build predictive models of the disease at single-cell resolution" (NIA, 2022b).

continued

BOX 3-4 Continued

Accelerating Medicines Partnership® Program for Parkinson's Disease and Related Disorders (AMP-PDRD)

The Accelerating Medicines Partnership® Program for Parkinson's Disease (AMP-PD) was established in 2018 as a partnership between NINDS, NIA, FDA, several industry partners, and the Michael J. Fox Foundation for Parkinson's Research (AMP-PD, n.d.). AMP-PD aims to identify and validate biomarkers (diagnostic, prognostic, and progression) biomarkers with the longer-term objective of improving clinical trial design and advancing the identification of new pathways for development of therapeutics. In pursuit of this goal, AMP-PD leverages samples and data from existing well-characterized cohorts including the NINDS Parkinson's Disease Biomarkers Program, the BioFIND study, and the International Lewy Body Dementia Genetics Consortium Genome Sequencing in Lewy body dementia case-control cohort, among others (AMP-PD, n.d.). Building on the work of AMP-PD, AMP-PDRD was initiated by FNIH in 2024 with the goal identifying and validating biomarkers that can be used to distinguish PD from related disorders with similar biological characteristics and symptoms (e.g., LBD, multiple system atrophy, progressive supranuclear palsy). Ultimately these efforts are intended to improve the success of clinical trials, expand therapies for these related conditions, and enable precision medicine approaches to treatment (FNIH, 2024).

---

through MODEL-AD (see Box 3-5). The Centrally Linked Longitudinal Peripheral Biomarkers of Alzheimer's Disease in Multiethnic Populations (CLEAR-AD) program is exploring through a diverse set of samples centrally linked and longitudinal peripheral biomarkers to enable personalized medicine approaches (see Box 2-6). Coupled with the investments in the Alzheimer's Disease Research Centers, these programs function to derisk novel targets and facilitate their translation toward clinical development (NIH, 2019) or the Small Business Innovative Research program. Considering the comparatively small number of clinical trials for dementia relative to other high-burden diseases such as cardiovascular disease and cancer (see Chapter 1), these programs are critical to enabling the expansion of early-phase trials of preventive and therapeutic interventions for AD/ADRD, as discussed further in Chapter 5.

However, the importance of considering both AD and related dementias cannot be overstated. As the field has expanded beyond amyloid-targeting mechanisms, investigators have found that the mechanistic hypotheses for

BOX 3-5
Target Enablement to Accelerate Therapy Development
for Alzheimer's Disease (TREAT-AD)

Two complementary TREAT-AD drug discovery centers—one led by researchers at the Indiana University School of Medicine and Purdue University, and the second by researchers at Emory University, Sage Bionetworks, and the Structural Genomics Consortium (NIA, 2023c)— were established with a mission to "improve, diversify and reinvigorate the Alzheimer's disease (AD) drug development pipeline by accelerating the characterization and experimental validation of next generation therapeutic targets and integrating the targets into drug discovery campaigns" (TREAT-AD, 2024). NIH support for the two centers is estimated at over $73 million over the course of 5 years (NIA, 2019). To achieve their mission, the TREAT-AD centers will "1) design, develop and disseminate tools that support target enabling packages (TEPs) for the experimental validation of novel, next generation therapeutic targets, including those emanating from the NIA-funded, target discovery programs such as Accelerating Medicines Partnership-Alzheimer's Disease (AMP-AD), and 2) initiate early stage drug discovery campaigns against the enabled targets" (TREAT-AD, 2024). In doing so, the program aims to de-risk potential therapies to incentivize industry to continue investment in their development. The data and experimental and analytic tools generated from the work of TREAT-AD are available to investigators from industry, academia, and other research organizations. For example, the TEPs, which include "validated commercial antibodies, protein structures, genetically modified cell lines, and assay protocols," and associated data can be accessed through the AD Knowledge Portal to aid researchers in validating novel and understudied targets (NIA, 2023c).

these conditions often overlap (as discussed earlier in this chapter). This overlap suggests a shared pathophysiology, which could potentially be targeted by similar therapeutic strategies. NIH-funded programs, such as AMP-AD, TREAT-AD, MODEL-AD, and CLEAR-AD, can be instrumental in this regard with the expansion of their mandate beyond AD and into related dementias. Where parallel programs for related dementias already exist (e.g., AMP-PDRD), opportunities for integration should be pursued to break down silos (discussed further in Chapter 5). This expansion and integration would not only enhance the understanding of shared disease mechanisms but also facilitate the development of novel therapeutic targets and personalized medicine approaches. By considering and prioritizing mechanisms that might have relevance across AD/ADRD and supporting research to develop mechanism-specific translational biomarkers, these programs can help to diversify and validate potential targets, thereby increasing the likelihood of successful clinical trials. This comprehensive approach is crucial for advancing the fight against these debilitating conditions.

Conclusion 3-7: The expansion of NIH-funded early-discovery and development programs to accelerate and diversify the therapeutic pipeline beyond AD to include related dementias will enhance understanding of healthy aging and neurodegeneration and support the development of novel therapeutic targets and personalized medicine approaches relevant to shared disease mechanisms.

Conclusion 3-8: The NIH-funded drug discovery programs and infrastructure for diversifying the therapeutic pipeline need to be strengthened with long-term support to develop and deliver critical drug discovery input and translational biomarkers that reflect changes in pathways under investigation.

A well-recognized barrier to advancing interventions for AD/ADRD and many other diseases is the so-called valley of death—the large gap that spans early-stage scientific research (generally in academic settings) that provides mechanistic insights and identifies promising therapeutic targets and the later-stage, lower-risk programs that are more attractive to pharmaceutical companies and investors (Parrish et al., 2019). As a result of the valley of death, many potentially effective therapeutic strategies are not pursued. Strategies to bridge the valley of death can include

- establishing challenge programs to spur innovation and the acceleration of translational research;
- strategically targeting public or philanthropic funding to de-risk novel intervention approaches to incentivize private-sector investment and advance research on strategies that the pharmaceutical industry may not have an interest in, such as repurposing generic drugs (Smith, 2024); and
- creating public–private partnerships, which can draw on the talents of academia in discovery and those of industry in bringing therapies to market (Atkinson et al., 2023; HHS, 2012).

Partnerships also have a role in accelerating translational research outside of the drug development space, as discussed further in Chapter 5. Partnerships between different public entities (e.g., NIH partnership with housing or education departments) can facilitate more cross-disciplinary approaches and better leverage existing investments that may affect brain health and AD/ADRD (Kremer, 2024).

RESEARCH PRIORITIES

The advancement of knowledge of risk and protective exposures for diverse populations, elucidation of the complex biological basis of AD/ADRD, and the rapid translation of basic and epidemiological research discoveries to clinical trials are essential to the development of effective strategies for the prevention and treatment of AD/ADRD. In recent years, NIH has made significant investments in basic research focused on elucidating diverse molecular and cellular processes of AD/ADRD vulnerability and resilience (NIA, 2023d, 2024f). Infrastructure investments to support these efforts have included the creation of large-scale, collaborative research programs to support the identification of disease mechanisms; application of emerging analytic approaches; development of novel therapeutic targets and open-science tools; and mechanisms to support early-stage clinical research. The committee identified four research priorities that build upon these existing efforts and investments. These research priorities are listed in Table 3-2 and include key scientific questions and near-term research opportunities that would advance progress on the research priorities.

TABLE 3-2 Committee-Identified Research Priorities Related to Building a More Comprehensive and Integrated Understanding of the Disease Biology and Mechanistic Pathways That Contribute to AD/ADRD Development and Resilience over the Life Course

Research Priority	Key Scientific Questions	Near-Term Research Opportunities to Address Key Scientific Questions
3-1: Identify factors driving AD/ADRD risk in diverse populations, particularly understudied and disproportionately affected groups, to better understand disease heterogeneity—including molecular subtypes and disparities in environmental exposures—and to identify prevention opportunities and advance health research equity.	• What are the determinants of AD/ADRD risk in diverse population groups (e.g., racial/ethnic, sex/gender, socioeconomic, geographic)? • Why are differences in pathology observed in diverse populations, and how does that influence risk of clinical disease? • What are the relative roles of modifiable social, economic, environmental, clinical, and behavioral mechanisms that might contribute to population differences in AD/ADRD? • How does the ability to modify risk factors vary across populations and their socioeconomic contexts? • What can be learned from the observed heterogeneity in severity (e.g., level of cognitive decline) and patterns of cognitive and other clinical symptoms among people who have similar levels of AD/ADRD-related pathology? • What genetic and other multiomics factors determine individuals' responses to interventions, modifiers, and exposures (e.g., exercise, diet, air pollution)? • What is required to increase interest in brain donation in diverse populations?	• Carry out a comprehensive survey of genetic and multiomics architecture in diverse well-characterized populations, using existing cohorts and infrastructure, to identify genomic determinants of risk. • Generate data to inform polygenic risk scores in people of non-European ancestry. • Use artificial intelligence and other computational tools to integrate multiple data types (e.g., multiomics, social, environmental) and identify commonalities across disease types and diverse populations and translate risk factors into biological mechanisms. • Across diverse populations, evaluate variations in the associations of life-course social, behavioral, and environmental exposure with longitudinal cognitive and biomarker data. • Identify opportunities to use natural experiments to evaluate exposure effects across the life course on clinical and biomarker outcomes in diverse populations.

TABLE 3-2 Continued

Research Priority	Key Scientific Questions	Near-Term Research Opportunities to Address Key Scientific Questions
3-2: Characterize the exposome and gene–environment interactions across the life course to gain insights into biological mechanisms and identify opportunities to reduce AD/ADRD risk and increase resilience.	• Are there sensitive or critical periods across the life course when social, behavioral, or environmental exposures have a greater effect on different etiologic processes driving AD/ADRD risk? • What is the role of early- and midlife exposures in resilience and disease progression and do these vary for specific pathologies? • Do early- and midlife exposures result in brain circuitry changes that affect later life, and are these modifiable? • Which exposures have the largest effects on AD/ADRD risk and resilience (e.g., affect the largest proportion of the population) and should be prioritized for future investigations? • Are the gene–environment interactions that influence AD/ADRD risk and resilience different among diverse populations?	• Identify profiles (e.g., biochemical, multiomics) that reflect and capture individuals' exposures and link them to AD/ADRD outcomes to better understand exposome risk factors. • Investigate gene–exposure interactions using exposure data that are already available. • Link complex combinations of life-course social, behavioral, and environmental exposure measures to evaluate how these exposures synergistically influence longitudinal cognitive and biomarker data across diverse populations. • Evaluate how features of the social and environmental exposome or gene–environment interactions influence specific pathologies contributing to AD/ADRD using a life-course framework.

continued

TABLE 3-2 Continued

Research Priority	Key Scientific Questions	Near-Term Research Opportunities to Address Key Scientific Questions
3-3: Elucidate the genetic and other biological mechanisms underlying resilience and resistance to identify novel targets and effective strategies for AD/ADRD prevention and treatment.	• What are the key factors that contribute to the resilience observed in positive or negative outliers (e.g., exceptional cases, including supercentenarians)? • What can be learned from individuals who do not develop pathologies (resistance) and those who develop pathologies but do not develop clinical symptoms within their lifetimes (resilience)? • What changes occur over time (i.e., with aging) in the way the brain deals with pathology (brain plasticity and adaptability), and is that process modifiable? • How do interactions between organ systems, including brain–body axes, contribute to resilience?	• Apply human tissue models from diverse groups of patients, including those with related dementias, and animal models to elucidate genes, multiomics factors, and molecular processes contributing to AD/ADRD resilience. • Investigate the role of brain–body axes (e.g., brain–gut and brain–renal axes) in resilience. • Establish a collection of resilient brains (organ collection) as a basis for the systematic comparative analysis of the causes of selective vulnerability and selective resilience and resistance to identify key factors and determinants of vulnerability and resilience, including a focus on disease-decisive factors.

continued

TABLE 3-2 Continued

Research Priority	Key Scientific Questions	Near-Term Research Opportunities to Address Key Scientific Questions
3-4: Develop integrated molecular and cellular causal models to guide the identification of common mechanisms underlying AD/ADRD and their validation as novel targets for prevention and treatment.	• What are the primary interactions and sequential cascading effects that translate molecular and cellular dysregulation into disease? • How do distinct pathologic processes combine to culminate in clinical manifestations of AD/ADRD? • When do the different molecular factors and processes begin to disturb cellular, organ, or system function that leads, eventually, to disease onset (age dependent)? Considering multiple etiologic processes contributing to AD/ADRD individually and jointly, is there a particular point of no return? • How do the different cell types in the brain (e.g., glial cells, endothelial cells, neurons) interact with each other on a timescale, ultimately leading to neurodegeneration? • How do genome-wide association studies (GWAS)-based risk genes set the stage for alterations in brain cell physiology, predisposing the brain to dysfunction and disease later in life? • What is the functional effect of defined identified risk genes or defined groups of risk genes on neuronal and glial physiology and function? • How do exposome factors affect physiology of cell types contributing to disease? • How do amyloid-independent interventions (e.g., lysosomal stabilizers, autophagy inducers, neuroprotective compounds) change cellular biology?	• Identify the earliest biological changes related to pathologic processes. • Investigate the function of glial, endothelial, neuronal, and other relevant types of brain cells during aging employing aged cell types and aged cell cultures. • Study the interactions of the different types of cells and mediators and the consequences of such interactions in appropriate cell and tissue models to identify a potential point of no return. • Include *aging* as the central risk factor of many dementia types into all cellular and molecular studies (e.g., aged glial cells, induced neurons from older individuals) and employ multiomics technologies. • Generate a framework based on grouping certain GWAS risk loci, identify functionally causal genes in these loci, and study their cellular and molecular effect on functions. • Systematically study the functional consequences of AD/ADRD risk genes in cellular models (extending beyond *APOE4* studies to a wider array of risk genes derived from GWAS and other omics studies). • Study the effect of exposomal factors (individually and in combination) on the physiology of glial and endothelial cells, neurons, and other relevant brain cell types in cellular and animal models.

continued

TABLE 3-2 Continued

Research Priority	Key Scientific Questions	Near-Term Research Opportunities to Address Key Scientific Questions
3-4: continued	• What are the molecular and cellular mediating interactions between organ systems, including brain–body axes, that lead to brain pathologies? • How do molecular and cellular mechanisms that contribute to development of neuropsychiatric symptoms interact with those that underly the development of neuropathology? • Are there important differences in pathologic, molecular, and multiomics features that are shared across AD and related dementias?	• Analyze the effect of experimental approaches and compounds on molecular pathways beyond those involved in the amyloid cascade, and employ amyloid-independent cellular and in vivo models. • Employ comparative studies using histology and multiomics to identify commonalities among AD and related dementias. • Evaluate mediating and modifying pathways linking genetic and genomic risk factors and biomarker measures of disease with clinical manifestations. • Investigate the role of the brain–body axes (e.g., brain-gut and brain–renal axes) in the development of AD/ADRD pathology.

REFERENCES

Abeliovich, A., and A. D. Gitler. 2016. Defects in trafficking bridge Parkinson's disease pathology and genetics. *Nature* 539(7628):207-216.

ACTC-DS. 2024. *Alzheimer's clinical trials consortium—Down syndrome.* https://www.actc-ds. org/ (accessed August 23, 2024).

AD Knowledge Portal. 2024a. *M²OVE-AD: Molecular mechanisms of the vascular etiology of Alzheimer's disease.* https://adknowledgeportal.synapse.org/Explore/Programs/ DetailsPage?Program=M2OVE-AD (accessed August 19, 2024).

AD Knowledge Portal. 2024b. *Resilience-AD: Cognitive resilience to Alzheimer's disease.* https:// adknowledgeportal.synapse.org/Explore/Programs/DetailsPage?Program=Resilience-AD (accessed October 22, 2024).

ADSP (Alzheimer's Disease Sequencing Project). 2023. *List of AD loci and genes with genetic evidence compiled by ADSP gene verification committee.* https://adsp.niagads.org/gvc-top-hits-list/ (accessed August 23, 2024).

ADSP. 2024. *ADSP overview.* https://adsp.niagads.org/about/adsp-overview/ (accessed August 16, 2024).

Ahmed, C., H. J. Greve, C. Garza-Lombo, J. A. Malley, J. A. Johnson, Jr., A. L. Oblak, and M. L. Block. 2024. Peripheral HMGB1 is linked to O_3 pathology of disease-associated astrocytes and amyloid. *Alzheimer's & Dementia* 20(5):3551-3566.

Ahmed, R. M., M. Irish, J. van Eersel, A. Ittner, Y. D. Ke, A. Volkerling, J. van der Hoven, K. Tanaka, T. Karl, M. Kassiou, J. J. Kril, O. Piguet, J. Gotz, M. C. Kiernan, G. M. Halliday, J. R. Hodges, and L. M. Ittner. 2017. Mouse models of frontotemporal dementia: A comparison of phenotypes with clinical symptomatology. *Neuroscience and Biobehavior Review* 74(Pt A):126-138.

Aizenstein, H. J., R. D. Nebes, J. A. Saxton, J. C. Price, C. A. Mathis, N. D. Tsopelas, S. K. Ziolko, J. A. James, B. E. Snitz, P. R. Houck, W. Bi, A. D. Cohen, B. J. Lopresti, S. T. DeKosky, E. M. Halligan, and W. E. Klunk. 2008. Frequent amyloid deposition without significant cognitive impairment among the elderly. *Archives of Neurology* 65(11):1509-1517.

AlzForum. 2024. *Research models.* https://www.alzforum.org/research-models/alzheimers-disease (accessed August 19, 2024).

Amartumur, S., H. Nguyen, T. Huynh, T. S. Kim, R. S. Woo, E. Oh, K. K. Kim, L. P. Lee, and C. Heo. 2024. Neuropathogenesis-on-chips for neurodegenerative diseases. *Nature Communications* 15(1):2219.

AMP-PD. n.d. *About AMP PD overview.* https://amp-pd.org/about (accessed October 23, 2024).

An, Y., V. R. Varma, S. Varma, R. Casanova, E. Dammer, O. Pletnikova, C. W. Chia, J. M. Egan, L. Ferrucci, J. Troncoso, A. I. Levey, J. Lah, N. T. Seyfried, C. Legido-Quigley, R. O'Brien, and M. Thambisetty. 2018. Evidence for brain glucose dysregulation in Alzheimer's disease. *Alzheimer's & Dementia* 14(3):318-329.

Andrews, S. J., B. Fulton-Howard, and A. Goate. 2020. Interpretation of risk loci from genome-wide association studies of Alzheimer's disease. *Lancet Neurology* 19(4):326-335.

Arafah, A., S. Khatoon, I. Rasool, A. Khan, M. A. Rather, K. A. Abujabal, Y. A. H. Faqih, H. Rashid, S. M. Rashid, S. Bilal Ahmad, A. Alexiou, and M. U. Rehman. 2023. The future of precision medicine in the cure of Alzheimer's disease. *Biomedicines* 11(2):335.

Arboleda-Velasquez, J. F., F. Lopera, M. O'Hare, S. Delgado-Tirado, C. Marino, N. Chmielewska, K. L. Saez-Torres, D. Amarnani, A. P. Schultz, R. A. Sperling, D. Leyton-Cifuentes, K. Chen, A. Baena, D. Aguillon, S. Rios-Romenets, M. Giraldo, E. Guzmán-Vélez, D. J. Norton, E. Pardilla-Delgado, A. Artola, J. S. Sanchez, J. Acosta-Uribe, M. Lalli, K. S. Kosik, M. J. Huentelman, H. Zetterberg, K. Blennow, R. A. Reiman, J. Luo, Y. Chen, P. Thiyyagura, Y. Su, G. R. Jun, M. Naymik, X. Gai, M. Bootwalla, J. Ji, L. Shen, J. B. Miller, L. A. Kim, P. N. Tariot, K. A. Johnson, E. M. Reiman, Y. T. Quiroz. 2019. Resistance to autosomal dominant Alzheimer's disease in an APOE3 Christchurch homozygote: A case report. *Nature Medicine* 25(11):1680-1683.

Arenaza-Urquijo, E. M., R. Boyle, K. Casaletto, K. J. Anstey, C. Vila-Castelar, A. Colverson, E. Palpatzis, J. M. Eissman, T. Kheng Siang Ng, S. Raghavan, M. Akinci, J. M. J. Vonk, L. S. Machado, P. P. Zanwar, H. L. Shrestha, M. Wagner, S. Tamburin, H. R. Sohrabi, S. Loi, D. Bartrés-Faz, D. B. Dubal, P. Vemuri, O. Okonkwo, T. J. Hohman, M. Ewers, R. F. Buckley, Reserve, Resilience and Protective Factors Professional Interest Area, Sex and Gender Professional Interest area and the ADDRESS! Special Interest Group. 2024. Sex and gender differences in cognitive resilience to aging and Alzheimer's disease. *Alzheimer's & Dementia* 20(8):5695-5719.

Argyriou, S., J. F. Fullard, J. M. Krivinko, D. Lee, T. S. Wingo, A. P. Wingo, R. A. Sweet, and P. Roussos. 2024. Beyond memory impairment: The complex phenotypic landscape of Alzheimer's disease. *Trends in Molecular Medicine* 30(8):713-722.

Arun, P., F. Rossetti, D. M. Wilder, S. Sajja, S. A. Van Albert, Y. Wang, I. D. Gist, and J. B. Long. 2020. Blast exposure leads to accelerated cellular senescence in the rat brain. *Frontiers in Neurology* 11:438.

Asiamah, E. A., B. Feng, R. Guo, X. Yaxing, X. Du, X. Liu, J. Zhang, H. Cui, and J. Ma. 2024. The contributions of the endolysosomal compartment and autophagy to APOEε4 allele-mediated increase in Alzheimer's disease risk. *Journal of Alzheimer's Disease* 97(3):1007-1031.

Asken, B. M., P. A. Ljubenkov, A. M. Staffaroni, K. B. Casaletto, L. Vandevrede, Y. Cobigo, J. C. Rojas-Rodriguez, K. P. Rankin, J. Kornak, H. Heuer, J. Shigenaga, B. S. Appleby, A. C. Bozoki, K. Domoto-Reilly, N. Ghoshal, E. Huey, I. Litvan, J. C. Masdeu, M. F. Mendez, B. Pascual, P. Pressman, M. C. Tartaglia, W. Kremers, L. K. Forsberg, B. F. Boeve, A. L. Boxer, H. J. Rosen, J. H. Kramer, and ALLFTD Consortium Investigators. 2023. Plasma inflammation for predicting phenotypic conversion and clinical progression of autosomal dominant frontotemporal lobar degeneration. *Journal of Neurology, Neurosurgery, and Psychiatry* 94(7):541-549.

Atkinson, P. J., M. Swami, N. Ridgway, M. Roberts, J. Kinghorn, T. T. Warner, J. M. Staddon, and A. K. Takle. 2023. Advancing novel therapies for neurodegeneration through an innovative model for industry–academia collaborations: A decade of theEisai-UCL experience. *Drug Discovery Today* 28(10):103732.

Baker, M., I. R. Mackenzie, S. M. Pickering-Brown, J. Gass, R. Rademakers, C. Lindholm, J. Snowden, J. Adamson, A. D. Sadovnick, S. Rollinson, A. Cannon, E. Dwosh, D. Neary, S. Melquist, A. Richardson, D. Dickson, Z. Berger, J. Eriksen, T. Robinson, C. Zehr, C. A. Dickey, R. Crook, E. McGowan, D. Mann, B. Boeve, H. Feldman, and M. Hutton. 2006. Mutations in progranulin cause tau-negative frontotemporal dementia linked to chromosome 17. *Nature* 442(7105):916-919.

Bakulski, K., L. Rozek, D. Dolinoy, H. Paulson, and H. Hu. 2012. Alzheimer's disease and environmental exposure to lead: The epidemiologic evidence and potential role of epigenetics. *Current Alzheimer Research* 9(5):563-573.

Balusu, S., R. Praschberger, E. Lauwers, B. De Strooper, and P. Verstreken. 2023. Neurodegeneration cell per cell. *Neuron* 111(6):767-786.

Banbury Center. 2024. Integrating exposomics into the biomedical enterprise. Summary Report of Conference, December 3-6, 2023. https://www.cshl.edu/wp-content/uploads/2024/03/Banbury_EXPOS_Output_Two-Pager-Final_20240205.pdf.

Bardehle, S., V. A. Rafalski, and K. Akassoglou. 2015. Breaking boundaries—coagulation and fibrinolysis at the neurovascular interface. *Frontiers in Cellular Neuroscience* 9:354.

Bartlett, B. J., P. Isakson, J. Lewerenz, H. Sanchez, R. W. Kotzebue, R. C. Cumming, G. L. Harris, I. P. Nezis, D. R. Schubert, A. Simonsen, and K. D. Finley. 2011. p62, Ref(2)P and ubiquitinated proteins are conserved markers of neuronal aging, aggregate formation and progressive autophagic defects. *Autophagy* 7(6):572-583.

Bateman, R. J., P. S. Aisen, B. De Strooper, N. C. Fox, C. A. Lemere, J. M. Ringman, S. Salloway, R. A. Sperling, M. Windisch, and C. Xiong. 2011. Autosomal-dominant Alzheimer's disease: A review and proposal for the prevention of Alzheimer's disease. *Alzheimer's Research & Therapy* 3(1):1.

Bateman, R. J., C. Xiong, T. L. Benzinger, A. M. Fagan, A. Goate, N. C. Fox, D. S. Marcus, N. J. Cairns, X. Xie, T. M. Blazey, D. M. Holtzman, A. Santacruz, V. Buckles, A. Oliver, K. Moulder, P. S. Aisen, B. Ghetti, W. E. Klunk, E. McDade, R. N. Martins, C. L. Masters, R. Mayeux, J. M. Ringman, M. N. Rossor, P. R. Schofield, R. A. Sperling, S. Salloway, and J. C. Morris; Dominantly Inherited Alzheimer Network. 2012. Clinical and biomarker changes in dominantly inherited Alzheimer's disease. *New England Journal of Medicine* 367(9):795-804.

Beckman, D., P. Chakrabarty, S. Ott, A. Dao, E. Zhou, W. G. Janssen, K. Donis-Cox, S. Muller, J. H. Kordower, and J. H. Morrison. 2021. A novel tau-based rhesus monkey model of Alzheimer's pathogenesis. *Alzheimer's & Dementia* 17(6):933-945.

Behl, C. 2023. *Alzheimer's disease research*. Springer Cham.

Bellenguez, C., F. Kucukali, I. E. Jansen, L. Kleineidam, S. Moreno-Grau, N. Amin, A. C. Naj, R. Campos-Martin, B. Grenier-Boley, V. Andrade, P. A. Holmans, A. Boland, V. Damotte, S. J. van der Lee, M. R. Costa, T. Kuulasmaa, Q. Yang, I. de Rojas, J. C. Bis, A. Yaqub, I. Prokic, J. Chapuis, S. Ahmad, V. Giedraitis, D. Aarsland, P. Garcia-Gonzalez, C. Abdelnour, E. Alarcon-Martin, D. Alcolea, M. Alegret, I. Alvarez, V. Alvarez, N. J. Armstrong, A. Tsolaki, C. Antunez, I. Appollonio, M. Arcaro, S. Archetti, A. A. Pastor, B. Arosio, L. Athanasiu, H. Bailly, N. Banaj, M. Baquero, S. Barral, A. Beiser, A. B. Pastor, J. E. Below, P. Benchek, L. Benussi, C. Berr, C. Besse, V. Bessi, G. Binetti, A. Bizarro, R. Blesa, M. Boada, E. Boerwinkle, B. Borroni, S. Boschi, P. Bossu, G. Brathen, J. Bressler, C. Bresner, H. Brodaty, K. J. Brookes, L. I. Brusco, D. Buiza-Rueda, K. Burger, V. Burholt, W. S. Bush, M. Calero, L. B. Cantwell, G. Chene, J. Chung, M. L. Cuccaro, A. Carracedo, R. Cecchetti, L. Cervera-Carles, C. Charbonnier, H. H. Chen, C. Chillotti, S. Ciccone, J. Claassen, C. Clark, E. Conti, A. Corma-Gomez, E. Costantini, C. Custodero, D. Daian, M. C. Dalmasso, A. Daniele, E. Dardiotis, J. F. Dartigues, P. P. de Deyn, K. de Paiva Lopes, L. D. de Witte, S. Debette, J. Deckert, T. Del Ser, N. Denning, A. DeStefano, M. Dichgans, J. Diehl-Schmid, M. Diez-Fairen, P. D. Rossi, S. Djurovic, E. Duron, E. Duzel, C. Dufouil, G. Eiriksdottir, S. Engelborghs, V. Escott-Price, A. Espinosa, M. Ewers, K. M. Faber, T. Fabrizio, S. F. Nielsen, D. W. Fardo, L. Farotti, C. Fenoglio, M. Fernandez-Fuertes, R. Ferrari, C. B. Ferreira, E. Ferri, B. Fin, P. Fischer, T. Fladby, K. Fliessbach, B. Fongang, M. Fornage, J. Fortea, T. M. Foroud, S. Fostinelli, N. C. Fox, E. Franco-Macias, M. J. Bullido, A. Frank-Garcia, L. Froelich, B. Fulton-Howard, D. Galimberti, J. M. Garcia-Alberca, P. Garcia-Gonzalez, S. Garcia-Madrona, G. Garcia-Ribas, R. Ghidoni, I. Giegling, G. Giorgio, A. M. Goate, O. Goldhardt, D. Gomez-Fonseca, A. Gonzalez-Perez, C. Graff, G. Grande, E. Green, T. Grimmer, E. Grunblatt, M. Grunin, V. Gudnason, T. Guetta-Baranes, A. Haapasalo, G. Hadjigeorgiou, J. L. Haines, K. L. Hamilton-Nelson, H. Hampel, O. Hanon, J. Hardy, A. M. Hartmann, L. Hausner, J. Harwood, S. Heilmann-Heimbach, S. Helisalmi, M. T. Heneka, I. Hernandez, M. J. Herrmann, P. Hoffmann, C. Holmes, H. Holstege, R. H. Vilas, M. Hulsman, J. Humphrey, G. J. Biessels, X. Jian, C. Johansson, G. R. Jun, Y. Kastumata, J. Kauwe, P. G. Kehoe, L. Kilander, A. K. Stahlbom, M. Kivipelto, A. Koivisto, J. Kornhuber, M. H. Kosmidis, W. A. Kukull, P. P. Kuksa, B. W. Kunkle, A. B. Kuzma, C. Lage, E. J. Laukka, L. Launer, A. Lauria, C. Y. Lee, J. Lehtisalo, O. Lerch, A. Lleo, W. Longstreth, Jr., O. Lopez, A. L. de Munain, S. Love, M. Lowemark, L. Luckcuck, K. L. Lunetta, Y. Ma, J. Macias, C. A. MacLeod, W. Maier, F. Mangialasche, M. Spallazzi, M. Marquie, R. Marshall, E. R. Martin, A. M. Montes, C. M. Rodriguez, C. Masullo, R. Mayeux, S. Mead, P. Mecocci, M. Medina, A. Meggy, S. Mehrabian, S. Mendoza, M. Menendez-Gonzalez, P. Mir, S. Moebus, M. Mol, L. Molina-Porcel, L. Montrreal, L.

Morelli, F. Moreno, K. Morgan, T. Mosley, M. M. Nothen, C. Muchnik, S. Mukherjee, B. Nacmias, T. Ngandu, G. Nicolas, B. G. Nordestgaard, R. Olaso, A. Orellana, M. Orsini, G. Ortega, A. Padovani, C. Paolo, G. Papenberg, L. Parnetti, F. Pasquier, P. Pastor, G. Peloso, A. Perez-Cordon, J. Perez-Tur, P. Pericard, O. Peters, Y. A. L. Pijnenburg, J. A. Pineda, G. Pinol-Ripoll, C. Pisanu, T. Polak, J. Popp, D. Posthuma, J. Priller, R. Puerta, O. Quenez, I. Quintela, J. Q. Thomassen, A. Rabano, I. Rainero, F. Rajabli, I. Ramakers, L. M. Real, M. J. T. Reinders, C. Reitz, D. Reyes-Dumeyer, P. Ridge, S. Riedel-Heller, P. Riederer, N. Roberto, E. Rodriguez-Rodriguez, A. Rongve, I. R. Allende, M. Rosende-Roca, J. L. Royo, E. Rubino, D. Rujescu, M. E. Saez, P. Sakka, I. Saltvedt, A. Sanabria, M. B. Sanchez-Arjona, F. Sanchez-Garcia, P. S. Juan, R. Sanchez-Valle, S. B. Sando, C. Sarnowski, C. L. Satizabal, M. Scamosci, N. Scarmeas, E. Scarpini, P. Scheltens, N. Scherbaum, M. Scherer, M. Schmid, A. Schneider, J. M. Schott, G. Selbaek, D. Seripa, M. Serrano, J. Sha, A. A. Shadrin, O. Skrobot, S. Slifer, G. J. L. Snijders, H. Soininen, V. Solfrizzi, A. Solomon, Y. Song, S. Sorbi, O. Sotolongo-Grau, G. Spalletta, A. Spottke, A. Squassina, E. Stordal, J. P. Tartan, L. Tarraga, N. Tesi, A. Thalamuthu, T. Thomas, G. Tosto, L. Traykov, L. Tremolizzo, A. Tybjaerg-Hansen, A. Uitterlinden, A. Ullgren, I. Ulstein, S. Valero, O. Valladares, C. Van Broeckhoven, J. Vance, B. N. Vardarajan, A. van der Lugt, J. Van Dongen, J. van Rooij, J. van Swieten, R. Vandenberghe, F. Verhey, J. S. Vidal, J. Vogelgsang, M. Vyhnalek, M. Wagner, D. Wallon, L. S. Wang, R. Wang, L. Weinhold, J. Wiltfang, G. Windle, B. Woods, M. Yannakoulia, H. Zare, Y. Zhao, X. Zhang, C. Zhu, M. Zulaica, EADB, GR@ACE, DEGESCO, EADI, GERAD, Demgene, FinnGen, ADGC, CHARGE, L. A. Farrer, B. M. Psaty, M. Ghanbari, T. Raj, P. Sachdev, K. Mather, F. Jessen, M. A. Ikram, A. de Mendonca, J. Hort, M. Tsolaki, M. A. Pericak-Vance, P. Amouyel, J. Williams, R. Frikke-Schmidt, J. Clarimon, J. F. Deleuze, G. Rossi, S. Seshadri, O. A. Andreassen, M. Ingelsson, M. Hiltunen, K. Sleegers, G. D. Schellenberg, C. M. van Duijn, R. Sims, W. M. van der Flier, A. Ruiz, A. Ramirez, and J. C. Lambert. 2022. New insights into the genetic etiology of Alzheimer's disease and related dementias. *Nature Genetics* 54(4):412-436.

Bhat, R., E. P. Crowe, A. Bitto, M. Moh, C. D. Katsetos, F. U. Garcia, F. B. Johnson, J. Q. Trojanowski, C. Sell, and C. Torres. 2012. Astrocyte senescence as a component of Alzheimer's disease. *PLoS ONE* 7(9):e45069.

Bhattarai, P., T. Iniyan Gunasekaran, M. E. Belloy, D. Reyes-Dumeyer, D. Jülich, H. Tayran, E. Yilmaz, D. Flaherty, B. Turgutalp, G. Sukumar, C. Alba, E. Martinez McGrath, D. N. Hupalo, D. Bacikova, Y. Le Guen, R. Lantigua, M. Medrano, D. Rivera, P. Recio, T. Nuriel, N. Ertekin-Taner, A. F. Teich, D. W. Dickson, S. Holley, M. Greicius, C. L. Dalgard, M. Zody, R. Mayeux, C. Kizil, and B. N. Vardarajanet. 2024. Rare genetic variation in fibronectin 1 (*FN1*) protects against APOEε4 in Alzheimer's disease. *Acta Neuropathologica* 147(1):70.

Biomarker Network. 2024. *Health and Retirement Study (HRS)*. https://gero.usc.edu/cbph/network/studies-with-biomarkers/the-health-and-retirement-study-hrs/ (accessed August 16, 2024).

Bohnen, N. I., D. S. Djang, K. Herholz, Y. Anzai, and S. Minoshima. 2012. Effectiveness and safety of 18F-FDG PET in the evaluation of dementia: A review of the recent literature. *Journal of Nuclear Medicine* 53(1):59-71.

Bowles, K. R., M. C. Silva, K. Whitney, T. Bertucci, J. E. Berlind, J. D. Lai, J. C. Garza, N. C. Boles, S. Mahali, K. H. Strang, J. A. Marsh, C. Chen, D. A. Pugh, Y. Liu, R. E. Gordon, S. K. Goderie, R. Chowdhury, S. Lotz, K. Lane, J. F. Crary, S. J. Haggarty, C. M. Karch, J. K. Ichida, A. M. Goate, and S. Temple. 2021. *ELAVL4*, splicing, and glutamatergic dysfunction precede neuron loss in *MAPT* mutation cerebral organoids. *Cell* 184(17):4547-4563, e4517.

Bryant, A. G., M. Hu, B. C. Carlyle, S. E. Arnold, M. P. Frosch, S. Das, B. T. Hyman, and R. E. Bennett. 2020. Cerebrovascular senescence is associated with tau pathology in Alzheimer's disease. *Frontiers in Neurology* 11:575953.

Bufill, E., R. Ribosa-Nogué, and R. Blesa. 2020. The therapeutic potential of epigenetic modifications in Alzheimer's disease. In *Alzheimer's disease: Drug discovery.* Edited by X. Huang. Brisbane, Australia: Exon Publications.

Bussian, T. J., A. Aziz, C. F. Meyer, B. L. Swenson, J. M. van Deursen, and D. J. Baker. 2018. Clearance of senescent glial cells prevents tau-dependent pathology and cognitive decline. *Nature* 562(7728):578-582.

Cacace, R., K. Sleegers, and C. Van Broeckhoven. 2016. Molecular genetics of early-onset Alzheimer's disease revisited. *Alzheimer's & Dementia* 12(6):733-748.

Cai, W., K. Zhang, P. Li, L. Zhu, J. Xu, B. Yang, X. Hu, Z. Lu, and J. Chen. 2017. Dysfunction of the neurovascular unit in ischemic stroke and neurodegenerative diseases: An aging effect. *Ageing Research Reviews* 34:77-87.

Cao, W., and H. Zheng. 2018. Peripheral immune system in aging and Alzheimer's disease. *Molecular Neurodegeneration* 13(1):51.

Carter, A. C., H. Y. Chang, G. Church, A. Dombkowski, J. R. Ecker, E. Gil, P. G. Giresi, H. Greely, W. J. Greenleaf, N. Hacohen, C. He, D. Hill, J. Ko, I. Kohane, A. Kundaje, M. Palmer, M. P. Snyder, J. Tung, U. Urban, M. Vidal, and W. Wong. 2017. Challenges and recommendations for epigenomics in precision health. *Nature Biotechnology* 35(12):1128-1132.

Cavaliere, F., and S. Gülöksüz. 2022. Shedding light on the etiology of neurodegenerative diseases and dementia: The exposome paradigm. *NPJ Mental Health Research* 1(1):20.

Cavalli, G., and E. Heard. 2019. Advances in epigenetics link genetics to the environment and disease. *Nature* 571(7766):489-499.

Cetin, S., D. Knez, S. Gobec, J. Kos and A. Pišlar. 2022. Cell models for Alzheimer's and Parkinson's disease: At the interface of biology and drug discovery. *Biomedicine & Pharmacotherapy* 149:112924.

Chakraborty, D., V. Felzen, C. Hiebel, E. Sturner, N. Perumal, C. Manicam, E. Sehn, F. Grus, U. Wolfrum, and C. Behl. 2019. Enhanced autophagic-lysosomal activity and increased BAG3-mediated selective macroautophagy as adaptive response of neuronal cells to chronic oxidative stress. *Redox Biology* 24:101181.

Chen, C., and J. M. Zissimopoulos. 2018. Racial and ethnic differences in trends in dementia prevalence and risk factors in the United States. *Alzheimer's & Dementia (N Y)* 4:510-520.

Chen, X. and D. M. Holtzman. 2022. Emerging roles of innate and adaptive immunity in Alzheimer's disease. *Immunity* 55(12):2236-2254.

Cheng, H., M. Wang, J. L. Li, N. J. Cairns, and X. Han. 2013. Specific changes of sulfatide levels in individuals with pre-clinical Alzheimer's disease: An early event in disease pathogenesis. *Journal of Neurochemistry* 127(6):733-738.

Chia, R., M. S. Sabir, S. Bandres-Ciga, S. Saez-Atienzar, R. H. Reynolds, E. Gustavsson, R. L. Walton, S. Ahmed, C. Viollet, J. Ding, M. B. Makarious, M. Diez-Fairen, M. K. Portley, Z. Shah, Y. Abramzon, D. G. Hernandez, C. Blauwendraat, D. J. Stone, J. Eicher, L. Parkkinen, O. Ansorge, L. Clark, L. S. Honig, K. Marder, A. Lemstra, P. St George-Hyslop, E. Londos, K. Morgan, T. Lashley, T. T. Warner, Z. Jaunmuktane, D. Galasko, I. Santana, P. J. Tienari, L. Myllykangas, M. Oinas, N. J. Cairns, J. C. Morris, G. M. Halliday, V. M. Van Deerlin, J. Q. Trojanowski, M. Grassano, A. Calvo, G. Mora, A. Canosa, G. Floris, R. C. Bohannan, F. Brett, Z. Gan-Or, J. T. Geiger, A. Moore, P. May, R. Kruger, D. S. Goldstein, G. Lopez, N. Tayebi, E. Sidransky, American Genome Center, L. Norcliffe-Kaufmann, J. A. Palma, H. Kaufmann, V. G. Shakkottai, M. Perkins, K. L. Newell, T. Gasser, C. Schulte, F. Landi, E. Salvi, D. Cusi, E. Masliah, R. C. Kim, C. A. Caraway, E. S. Monuki, M. Brunetti, T. M. Dawson, L. S. Rosenthal, M. S. Albert, O. Pletnikova, J. C. Troncoso, M. E. Flanagan, Q. Mao, E. H. Bigio, E. Rodriguez-Rodriguez, J. Infante, C. Lage, I. Gonzalez-Aramburu, P. Sanchez-Juan, B. Ghetti, J. Keith, S. E. Black, M. Masellis, E. Rogaeva, C. Duyckaerts, A. Brice, S. Lesage, G. Xiromerisiou, M. J. Barrett, B. S. Tilley,

S. Gentleman, G. Logroscino, G. E. Serrano, T. G. Beach, I. G. McKeith, A. J. Thomas, J. Attems, C. M. Morris, L. Palmer, S. Love, C. Troakes, S. Al-Sarraj, A. K. Hodges, D. Aarsland, G. Klein, S. M. Kaiser, R. Woltjer, P. Pastor, L. M. Bekris, J. B. Leverenz, L. M. Besser, A. Kuzma, A. E. Renton, A. Goate, D. A. Bennett, C. R. Scherzer, H. R. Morris, R. Ferrari, D. Albani, S. Pickering-Brown, K. Faber, W. A. Kukull, E. Morenas-Rodriguez, A. Lleó, J. Fortea, D. Alcolea, J. Clarimon, M. A. Nalls, L. Ferrucci, S. M. Resnick, T. Tanaka, T. M. Foroud, N. R. Graff-Radford, Z. K. Wszolek, T. Ferman, B. F. Boeve, J. A. Hardy, E. J. Topol, A. Torkamani, A. B. Singleton, M. Ryten, D. W. Dickson, A. Chio, O. A. Ross, J. R. Gibbs, C. L. Dalgard, B. J. Traynor, and S. W. Scholz. 2021. Genome sequencing analysis identifies new loci associated with Lewy body dementia and provides insights into its genetic architecture. *Nature Genetics* 53(3):294-303.

Chow, H.-M., M. Shi, A. Cheng, Y. Gao, G. Chen, X. Song, R. W. L. So, J. Zhang, and K. Herrup. 2019. Age-related hyperinsulinemia leads to insulin resistance in neurons and cell-cycle-induced senescence. *Nature Neuroscience* 22(11):1806-1819.

Ciani, M., C. Bonvicini, C. Scassellati, M. Carrara, C. Maj, S. Fostinelli, G. Binetti, R. Ghidoni, and L. Benussi. 2019. The missing heritability of sporadic frontotemporal dementia: New insights from rare variants in neurodegenerative candidate genes. *International Journal of Molecular Science* 20(16):E3903.

Claassen, J., D. H. J. Thijssen, R. B. Panerai, and F. M. Faraci. 2021. Regulation of cerebral blood flow in humans: Physiology and clinical implications of autoregulation. *Physiological Reviews* 101(4):1487-1559.

Clark, K., Y. Y. Leung, W. P. Lee, B. Voight, and L. S. Wang. 2022. Polygenic risk scores in Alzheimer's disease genetics: Methodology, applications, inclusion, and diversity. *Journal of Alzheimer's Disease* 89(1):1-12.

Cocean, A. M., and D. C. Vodnar. 2024. Exploring the gut-brain axis: Potential therapeutic impact of psychobiotics on mental health. *Progress in Neuro-Psychopharmacology & Biological Psychiatry* 134:111073.

Collins, H. M., and S. Greenfield. 2024. Rodent models of Alzheimer's disease: Past misconceptions and future prospects. *International Journal of Molecular Science* 25(11):6222.

Columbia University. 2024. *NIH Award Creates Columbia-Led Exposomics Coordinating Center.* https://www.publichealth.columbia.edu/news/nih-award-creates-columbia-led-exposomics-coordinating-center (accessed November 11, 2024).

Corriveau, R. A., F. Bosetti, M. Emr, J. T. Gladman, J. I. Koenig, C. S. Moy, K. Pahigiannis, S. P. Waddy, and W. Koroshetz. 2016. The science of vascular contributions to cognitive impairment and dementia (VCID): A framework for advancing research priorities in the cerebro-vascular biology of cognitive decline. *Cellular and Molecular Neurobiology* 36(2):281-288.

Crimmins, E. M. 2020. Social hallmarks of aging: Suggestions for geroscience research. *Ageing Research Review* 63:101136.

Cruts, M., I. Gijselinck, J. van der Zee, S. Engelborghs, H. Wils, D. Pirici, R. Rademakers, R. Vandenberghe, B. Dermaut, J.-J. Martin, C. van Duijn, K. Peeters, R. Sciot, P. Santens, T. De Pooter, M. Mattheijssens, M. Van den Broeck, I. Cuijt, K. l. Vennekens, P. P. De Deyn, S. Kumar-Singh, and C. Van Broeckhoven. 2006. Null mutations in progranulin cause ubiquitin-positive frontotemporal dementia linked to chromosome 17q21. *Nature* 442(7105):920-924.

Cummings, J., A. M. Leisgang Osse, and J. Kinney. 2023a. Geroscience and Alzheimer's disease drug development. *Journal of Prevention of Alzheimer's Disease* 10(4):620-632.

Cummings, J., Y. Zhou, G. Lee, K. Zhong, J. Fonseca, and F. Cheng. 2023b. Alzheimer's disease drug development pipeline: 2023. *Alzheimer's & Dementia (N Y)* 9(2):e12385.

Cutler, R. G., J. Kelly, K. Storie, W. A. Pedersen, A. Tammara, K. Hatanpaa, J. C. Troncoso, and M. P. Mattson. 2004. Involvement of oxidative stress-induced abnormalities in ceramide and cholesterol metabolism in brain aging and Alzheimer's disease. *Proceedings of the National Academy of Sciences USA* 101(7):2070-2075.

de Galan, B. E. 2024. Diabetes and brain disorders, a new role for insulin? *Neuroscience and Biobehavioral Review* 163:105775.

De Jager, P. L., G. Srivastava, K. Lunnon, J. Burgess, L. C. Schalkwyk, L. Yu, M. L. Eaton, B. T. Keenan, J. Ernst, C. McCabe, A. Tang, T. Raj, J. Replogle, W. Brodeur, S. Gabriel, H. S. Chai, C. Younkin, S. G. Younkin, F. Zou, M. Szyf, C. B. Epstein, J. A. Schneider, B. E. Bernstein, A. Meissner, N. Ertekin-Taner, L. B. Chibnik, M. Kellis, J. Mill, and D. A. Bennett. 2014. Alzheimer's disease: Early alterations in brain DNA methylation at *ANK1*, *BIN1*, *RHBDF2* and other loci. *Nature Neuroscience* 17(9):1156-1163.

de la Monte, S. M., T. Luong, T. R. Neely, D. Robinson, and J. R. Wands. 2000. Mitochondrial DNA damage as a mechanism of cell loss in Alzheimer's disease. *Laboratory Investigation* 80(8):1323-1335.

De Strooper, B., and E. Karran. 2016. The cellular phase of Alzheimer's disease. *Cell* 164(4):603-615.

de Vries, L. E., I. Huitinga, H. W. Kessels, D. F. Swaab, and J. Verhaagen. 2024. The concept of resilience to Alzheimer's disease: Current definitions and cellular and molecular mechanisms. *Molecular Neurodegeneration* 19(1):33.

Dehkordi, S. K., J. Walker, E. Sah, E. Bennett, F. Atrian, B. Frost, B. Woost, R. E. Bennett, T. C. Orr, Y. Zhou, P. S. Andhey, M. Colonna, P. H. Sudmant, P. Xu, M. Wang, B. Zhang, H. Zare, and M. E. Orr. 2021. Profiling senescent cells in human brains reveals neurons with *CDKN2D*/p19 and tau neuropathology. *Nature Aging* 1(12):1107-1116.

Deng, Z., P. Sheehan, S. Chen, and Z. Yue. 2017. Is amyotrophic lateral sclerosis/frontotemporal dementia an autophagy disease? *Molecular Neurodegeneration* 12(1):90.

Drzezga, A., N. Lautenschlager, H. Siebner, M. Riemenschneider, F. Willoch, S. Minoshima, M. Schwaiger, and A. Kurz. 2003. Cerebral metabolic changes accompanying conversion of mild cognitive impairment into Alzheimer's disease: A PET follow-up study. *European Journal of Nuclear Medicine and Molecular Imaging* 30(8):1104-1113.

Du, Y., W. Deng, Z. Wang, M. Ning, W. Zhang, Y. Zhou, E. H. Lo, and C. Xing. 2017. Differential subnetwork of chemokines/cytokines in human, mouse, and rat brain cells after oxygen-glucose deprivation. *Journal of Cerebral Blood Flow and Metabolism* 37(4):1425-1434.

Duelli, R., and W. Kuschinsky. 2001. Brain glucose transporters: Relationship to local energy demand. *News in Physiological Sciences* 16:71-76.

Duffy, S. S., B. A. Keating, C. J. Perera, and G. Moalem-Taylor. 2018. The role of regulatory T-cells in nervous system pathologies. *Journal of Neuroscience Research* 96(6):951-968.

Dunn, A. R., K. M. S. O'Connell, and C. C. Kaczorowski. 2019. Gene-by-environment interactions in Alzheimer's disease and Parkinson's disease. *Neuroscience & Biobehavioral Reviews* 103:73-80.

Durso, D. F., G. Silveira-Nunes, M. M. Coelho, G. C. Camatta, L. H. Ventura, L. S. Nascimento, F. Caixeta, E. H. M. Cunha, A. Castelo-Branco, D. M. Fonseca, T. U. Maioli, A. Teixeira-Carvalho, C. Sala, M. J. Bacalini, P. Garagnani, C. Nardini, C. Franceschi, and A. M. C. Faria. 2022. Living in endemic area for infectious diseases accelerates epigenetic age. *Mechanisms of Ageing and Development* 207:111713.

Dutta, M., K. M. Weigel, K. T. Patten, A. E. Valenzuela, C. Wallis, K. J. Bein, A. S. Wexler, P. J. Lein, and J. Y. Cui. 2022. Chronic exposure to ambient traffic-related air pollution (TRAP) alters gut microbial abundance and bile acid metabolism in a transgenic rat model of Alzheimer's disease. *Toxicology Report* 9:432-444.

Favier, A., G. Rocher, A. K. Larsen, R. Delangle, C. Uzan, M. Sabbah, M. Castela, A. Duval, C. Mehats, and G. Canlorbe. 2021. MicroRNA as epigenetic modifiers in endometrial cancer: A systematic review. *Cancers (Basel)* 13(5):1137.

Ferrari, R., D. G. Hernandez, M. A. Nalls, J. D. Rohrer, A. Ramasamy, J. B. Kwok, C. Dobson-Stone, W. S. Brooks, P. R. Schofield, G. M. Halliday, J. R. Hodges, O. Piguet, L. Bartley, E. Thompson, E. Haan, I. Hernandez, A. Ruiz, M. Boada, B. Borroni, A. Padovani, C. Cruchaga, N. J. Cairns, L. Benussi, G. Binetti, R. Ghidoni, G. Forloni, D. Galimberti, C. Fenoglio, M. Serpente, E. Scarpini, J. Clarimon, A. Lleo, R. Blesa, M. L. Waldo, K. Nilsson, C. Nilsson, I. R. Mackenzie, G. Y. Hsiung, D. M. Mann, J. Grafman, C. M. Morris, J. Attems, T. D. Griffiths, I. G. McKeith, A. J. Thomas, P. Pietrini, E. D. Huey, E. M. Wassermann, A. Baborie, E. Jaros, M. C. Tierney, P. Pastor, C. Razquin, S. Ortega-Cubero, E. Alonso, R. Perneczky, J. Diehl-Schmid, P. Alexopoulos, A. Kurz, I. Rainero, E. Rubino, L. Pinessi, E. Rogaeva, P. St George-Hyslop, G. Rossi, F. Tagliavini, G. Giaccone, J. B. Rowe, J. C. Schlachetzki, J. Uphill, J. Collinge, S. Mead, A. Danek, V. M. Van Deerlin, M. Grossman, J. Q. Trojanowski, J. van der Zee, W. Deschamps, T. Van Langenhove, M. Cruts, C. Van Broeckhoven, S. F. Cappa, I. Le Ber, D. Hannequin, V. Golfier, M. Vercelletto, A. Brice, B. Nacmias, S. Sorbi, S. Bagnoli, I. Piaceri, J. E. Nielsen, L. E. Hjermind, M. Riemenschneider, M. Mayhaus, B. Ibach, G. Gasparoni, S. Pichler, W. Gu, M. N. Rossor, N. C. Fox, J. D. Warren, M. G. Spillantini, H. R. Morris, P. Rizzu, P. Heutink, J. S. Snowden, S. Rollinson, A. Richardson, A. Gerhard, A. C. Bruni, R. Maletta, F. Frangipane, C. Cupidi, L. Bernardi, M. Anfossi, M. Gallo, M. E. Conidi, N. Smirne, R. Rademakers, M. Baker, D. W. Dickson, N. R. Graff-Radford, R. C. Petersen, D. Knopman, K. A. Josephs, B. F. Boeve, J. E. Parisi, W. W. Seeley, B. L. Miller, A. M. Karydas, H. Rosen, J. C. van Swieten, E. G. Dopper, H. Seelaar, Y. A. Pijnenburg, P. Scheltens, G. Logroscino, R. Capozzo, V. Novelli, A. A. Puca, M. Franceschi, A. Postiglione, G. Milan, P. Sorrentino, M. Kristiansen, H. H. Chiang, C. Graff, F. Pasquier, A. Rollin, V. Deramecourt, F. Lebert, D. Kapogiannis, L. Ferrucci, S. Pickering-Brown, A. B. Singleton, J. Hardy, and P. Momeni. 2014. Frontotemporal dementia and its subtypes: A genome-wide association study. *Lancet Neurology* 13(7):686-699.

Fillit, H. M., B. Vellas, and Y. Hara. 2023. Editorial: The state of Alzheimer's research and the path forward. *Journal of the Prevention of Alzheimer's Disease* 10(4):617-619.

Finch, C. E., and A. M. Kulminski. 2019. The Alzheimer's disease exposome. *Alzheimer's & Dementia* 15(9):1123-1132.

FNIH (Foundation for the National Institutes of Health). 2024. *AMP Parkinson's Disease and related disorders*. https://fnih.org/our-programs/accelerating-medicines-partnership-amp/parkinsons-disease-and-related-disorders/ (accessed October 23, 2024).

Fortea, J., S. H. Zaman, S. Hartley, M. S. Rafii, E. Head, and M. Carmona-Iragui. 2021. Alzheimer's disease associated with Down syndrome: A genetic form of dementia. *Lancet Neurology* 20(11):930-942.

Fortea, J., J. Pegueroles, D. Alcolea, O. Belbin, O. Dols-Icardo, L. Vaqué-Alcázar, L. Videla, J. Domingo Gispert, M. Suárez-Calvet, S. C. Johnson, R. Sperling, A. Bejanin, A. Lleó, and V. Montal. 2024. *APOE4* homozygosity represents a distinct genetic form of Alzheimer's disease. *Nature Medicine* 30(5):1284-1291.

Franceschi, C., and J. Campisi. 2014. Chronic inflammation (inflammaging) and its potential contribution to age-associated diseases. *Journals of Gerontology: Series A, Biological Sciences and Medical Sciences* 69(Suppl 1):S4-S9.

Gan, L., M. R. Cookson, L. Petrucelli, and A. R. La Spada. 2018. Converging pathways in neurodegeneration, from genetics to mechanisms. *Nature Neuroscience* 21(10):1300-1309.

Gao, C., J. Jiang, Y. Tan, and S. Chen. 2023. Microglia in neurodegenerative diseases: Mechanism and potential therapeutic targets. *Signal Transduction and Targeted Therapy* 8: 359.

Gao, X., Q. Chen, H. Yao, J. Tan, Z. Liu, Y. Zhou, and Z. Zou. 2022. Epigenetics in Alzheimer's disease. *Frontiers in Aging and Neuroscience* 14:911635.

Gate, D., E. Tapp, O. Leventhal, M. Shahid, T. J. Nonninger, A. C. Yang, K. Strmpfl, M. Unger, T. Fehlmann, H. Oh, D. Channappa, V. Henderson, A. Keller, L. Aigner, G. Galasko, M. Davis, K. Poston, and T. Wyss-Coray. 2021. CD4+ T cells contribute to neurodegeneration in Lewy body dementia. *Science* 374(6569):868-874.

Gatz, M., C. Reynolds, L. Fratiglioni, B. Johansson, J. Mortimer, S. Berg, A. Fiske, and N. Petdersen. 2006. Role of genes and environments for explaining Alzheimer's disease. *Archives of General Psychiatry* 63(2):168-174.

Gendelman, H. E., and S. H. Appel. 2011. Neuroprotective activities of regulatory T cells. *Trends in Molecular Medicine* 17(12):687-688.

Genin, E., D. Hannequin, D. Wallon, K. Sleegers, M. Hiltunen, O. Combarros, M. J. Bullido, S. Engelborghs, P. De Deyn, C. Berr, F. Pasquier, B. Dubois, G. Tognoni, N. Fiévet, N. Brouwers, K. Bettens, B. Arosio, E. Coto, M. Del Zompo, I. Mateo, J. Epelbaum, A. Frank-Garcia, S. Helisalmi, E. Porcellini, A. Pilotto, P. Forti, R. Ferri, E. Scarpini, G. Siciliano, V. Solfrizzi, S. Sorbi, G. Spalletta, F. Valdivieso, S. Vepsäläinen, V. Alvarez, P. Bosco, M. Mancuso, F. Panza, B. Nacmias, P. Bossù, O. Hanon, P. Piccardi, G. Annoni, D. Seripa, D. Galimberti, F. Licastro, H. Soininen, J. F. Dartigues, M. I. Kamboh, C. Van Broeckhoven, J. C. Lambert, P. Amouyel, and D. Campion D. 2011. APOE and Alzheimer disease: A major gene with semi-dominant inheritance. *Molecular Psychiatry* 16(9):903-907.

Gifre-Renom, L., M. Daems, A. Luttun, and E. A. V. Jones. 2022. Organ-specific endothelial cell differentiation and impact of microenvironmental cues on endothelial heterogeneity. *International Journal of Molecular Science* 23(3):1477.

Golpich, M., E. Amini, Z. Mohamed, R. Azman Ali, N. Mohamed Ibrahim, and A. Ahmadiani. 2017. Mitochondrial dysfunction and biogenesis in neurodegenerative diseases: Pathogenesis and treatment. *CNS Neuroscience and Therapy* 23(1):5-22.

Gonzales, M. M., V. R. Garbarino, E. Pollet, J. P. Palavicini, D. L. Kellogg, Jr., E. Kraig, and M. E. Orr. 2022. Biological aging processes underlying cognitive decline and neurodegenerative disease. *Journal of Clinical Investigation* 132(10):e158453.

Gonzalez, H. M., W. Tarraf, A. M. Stickel, A. Morlett, K. A. Gonzalez, A. R. Ramos, T. Rundek, L. C. Gallo, G. A. Talavera, M. L. Daviglus, R. B. Lipton, C. Isasi, M. Lamar, D. Zeng, and C. DeCarli. 2024. Glycemic control, cognitive aging, and impairment among diverse Hispanic/Latino individuals: Study of Latinos—Investigation of neurocognitive aging (Hispanic Community Health Study/Study of Latinos). *Diabetes Care* 47(7):1152-1161.

Goodenowe, D. B., L. L. Cook, J. Liu, Y. Lu, D. A. Jayasinghe, P. W. Ahiahonu, D. Heath, Y. Yamazaki, J. Flax, K. F. Krenitsky, D. L. Sparks, A. Lerner, R. P. Friedland, T. Kudo, K. Kamino, T. Morihara, M. Takeda, and P. L. Wood. 2007. Peripheral ethanolamine plasmalogen deficiency: A logical causative factor in Alzheimer's disease and dementia. *Journal of Lipid Research* 48(11):2485-2498.

Gorelick, P. B., A. Scuteri, S. E. Black, C. Decarli, S. M. Greenberg, C. Iadecola, L. J. Launer, S. Laurent, O. L. Lopez, D. Nyenhuis, R. C. Petersen, J. A. Schneider, C. Tzourio, D. K. Arnett, D. A. Bennett, H. C. Chui, R. T. Higashida, R. Lindquist, P. M. Nilsson, G. C. Roman, F. W. Sellke, S. Seshadri, American Heart Association Stroke Council, Council on Epidemiology and Prevention, Council on Cardiovascular Nursing, Council on Cardiovascular Radiology and Intervention, and Council on Cardiovascular Surgery and Anesthesia. 2011. Vascular contributions to cognitive impairment and dementia: A statement for healthcare professionals from the American Heart Association/American Stroke Association. *Stroke* 42(9):2672-2713.

Gorgoulis, V., P. D. Adams, A. Alimonti, D. C. Bennett, O. Bischof, C. Bishop, J. Campisi, M. Collado, K. Evangelou, G. Ferbeyre, J. Gil, E. Hara, V. Krizhanovsky, D. Jurk, A. B. Maier, M. Narita, L. Niedernhofer, J. F. Passos, P. D. Robbins, C. A. Schmitt, J. Sedivy, K. Vougas, T. von Zglinicki, D. Zhou, M. Serrano, and M. Demaria. 2019. Cellular senescence: Defining a path forward. *Cell* 179(4):813-827.

Greaves, C. V., and J. D. Rohrer. 2019. An update on genetic frontotemporal dementia. *Journal of Neurology* 266(8):2075-2086.

Greve, H. J., A. L. Dunbar, C. G. Lombo, C. Ahmed, M. Thang, E. J. Messenger, C. L. Mumaw, J. A. Johnson, U. P. Kodavanti, A. L. Oblak, and M. L. Block. 2023. The bidirectional lung brain-axis of amyloid-beta pathology: Ozone dysregulates the peri-plaque microenvironment. *Brain* 146(3):991-1005.

Grodstein, F., B. Lemos, L. Yu, A. Iatrou, P. L. De Jager, and D. A. Bennett. 2020. Characteristics of epigenetic clocks across blood and brain tissue in older women and men. *Frontiers in Neuroscience* 14:555307.

Guan, P. P., and P. Wang. 2023. The involvement of post-translational modifications in regulating the development and progression of Alzheimer's disease. *Molecular Neurobiology* 60(7):3617-3632.

Guerreiro, R., A. Wojtas, J. Bras, M. Carrasquillo, E. Rogaeva, E. Majounie, C. Cruchaga, C. Sassi, J. S. Kauwe, S. Younkin, L. Hazrati, J. Collinge, J. Pocock, T. Lashley, J. Williams, J. C. Lambert, P. Amouyel, A. Goate, R. Rademakers, K. Morgan, J. Powell, P. St George-Hyslop, A. Singleton, J. Hardy, and the Alzheimer Genetic Analysis Group. 2013. TREM2 variants in Alzheimer's disease. *New England Journal of Medicine* 368(2):117-127.

Guerreiro, R., E. Gibbons, M. Tabuas-Pereira, C. Kun-Rodrigues, G. C. Santo, and J. Bras. 2020. Genetic architecture of common non-Alzheimer's disease dementias. *Neurobiology of Disease* 142:104946.

Guo, P., W. Gong, Y. Li, L. Liu, R. Yan, Y. Wang, Y. Zhang, and Z. Yuan. 2022. Pinpointing novel risk loci for Lewy body dementia and the shared genetic etiology with Alzheimer's disease and Parkinson's disease: A large-scale multi-trait association analysis. *BMC Medicine* 20(1):214.

Hamamoto, R., M. Komatsu, K. Takasawa, K. Asada, and S. Kaneko. 2020. Epigenetics analysis and integrated analysis of multiomics data, including epigenetic data, using artificial intelligence in the era of precision medicine. *Biomolecules* 10(1):62.

Hampel, H., A. Vergallo, G. Perry, S. Lista, and the Alzheimer Precision Medicine Initiative. 2019. The Alzheimer's Precision Medicine Initiative. *Journal of Alzheimer's Disease* 68(1):1-24.

Hampel, H., F. Caraci, A. C. Cuello, G. Caruso, R. Nistico, M. Corbo, F. Baldacci, N. Toschi, F. Garaci, P. A. Chiesa, S. R. Verdooner, L. Akman-Anderson, F. Hernandez, J. Avila, E. Emanuele, P. L. Valenzuela, A. Lucia, M. Watling, B. P. Imbimbo, A. Vergallo, and S. Lista. 2020. A path toward precision medicine for neuroinflammatory mechanisms in Alzheimer's disease. *Frontiers in Immunology* 11:456.

Han, X. 2010. Multi-dimensional mass spectrometry-based shotgun lipidomics and the altered lipids at the mild cognitive impairment stage of Alzheimer's disease. *Biochimica et Biophysica Acta* 1801(8):774-783.

Han, X., A. M. Fagan, H. Cheng, J. C. Morris, C. Xiong, and D. M. Holtzman. 2003. Cerebrospinal fluid sulfatide is decreased in subjects with incipient dementia. *Annals of Neurology* 54(1):115-119.

Han, X., D. M. Holtzman, D. W. McKeel, Jr., J. Kelley, and J. C. Morris. 2002. Substantial sulfatide deficiency and ceramide elevation in very early Alzheimer's disease: Potential role in disease pathogenesis. *Journal of Neurochemistry* 82(4):809-818.

Hara, Y., N. McKeehan, and H. M. Fillit. 2019. Translating the biology of aging into novel therapeutics for Alzheimer disease. *Neurology* 92(2):84-93.

Hargrove-Grimes, P., L. A. Low, and D. A. Tagle. 2021. Microphysiological systems: What it takes for community adoption. *Experimental Biology and Medicine* (Maywood) 246(12):1435-1446.

Harman, D. 1956. Aging: A theory based on free radical and radiation chemistry. *Journal of Gerontology* 11(3):298-300.

Harrison, J. R., S. Mistry, N. Muskett, and V. Escott-Price. 2020. From polygenic scores to precision medicine in Alzheimer's disease: A systematic review. *Journal of Alzheimer's Disease* 74:1271-1283.

Hernán, M. A. 2018. The C-word: Scientific euphemisms do not improve causal inference from observational data. *American Journal of Public Health* 108(5):616-619.

HHS (U.S. Department of Health and Human Services). 2012. Making the case for public private partnerships for NAPA. https://aspe.hhs.gov/sites/default/files/aspe-files/cmtach121.pdf (accessed October 18, 2024).

Ho, K. M., D. J. Morgan, M. Johnstone, and C. Edibam. 2023. Biological age is superior to chronological age in predicting hospital mortality of the critically ill. *Internal Emergency Medicine* 18(7):2019-2028.

Hooten, N., N. L. Pacheco, J. T. Smith, and M. K. Evans. 2022. The accelerated aging phenotype: The role of race and social determinants of health on aging. *Ageing Research Review* 73:101536.

Horvath, S., and A. J. Levine. 2015. HIV-1 infection accelerates age according to the epigenetic clock. *Journal of Infectious Diseases* 212(10):1563-1573.

Hu, Y. B., E. B. Dammer, R. J. Ren, and G. Wang. 2015. The endosomal-lysosomal system: From acidification and cargo sorting to neurodegeneration. *Translational Neurodegeneration* 4:18.

Huang, A. R., D. L. Roth, T. Cidav, S. E. Chung, H. Amjad, R. J. Thorpe, Jr., C. M. Boyd, and T. K. M. Cudjoe. 2023. Social isolation and 9-year dementia risk in community-dwelling Medicare beneficiaries in the United States. *Journal of the American Geriatric Society* 71(3):765-773.

Huq, A. J., P. Fransquet, S. M. Laws, J. Ryan, R. Sebra, C. L. Masters, I. M. Winship, P. A. James, and P. Lacaze. 2019. Genetic resilience to Alzheimer's disease in *APOE* ε4 homozygotes: A systematic review. *Alzheimer's & Dementia* 15(12):1612-1623.

Hurst, C., D. A. Pugh, M. H. Abreha, D. M. Duong, E. B. Dammer, D. A. Bennett, J. H. Herskowitz, and N. T. Seyfried. 2023. Integrated proteomics to understand the role of neuritin (NRN1) as a mediator of cognitive resilience to Alzheimer's disease. *Molecular & Cellular Proteomics* 22(5):100542.

Ikram, M. A., A. Bersano, R. Manso-Calderón, J.-P. Jia, H. Schmidt, L. Middleton, B. Nacmias, S. Siddiqi, and H. H. H. Adams. 2017. Genetics of vascular dementia—review from the ICVD working group. *BMC Medicine* 15(1):48.

Irizarry, M. C. 2003. A turn of the sulfatide in Alzheimer's disease. *Annals of Neurology* 54(1):7-8.

Italiani, P., I. Puxeddu, S. Napoletano, E. Scala, D. Melillo, S. Manocchio, A. Angiolillo, P. Migliorini, D. Boraschi, E. Vitale, and A. Di Costanzo. 2018. Circulating levels of IL-1 family cytokines and receptors in Alzheimer's disease: New markers of disease progression? *Journal of Neuroinflammation* 15(1):342.

Itzhaki, R. F. 2021. Overwhelming evidence for a major role for herpes simplex virus type 1 (HSV1) in Alzheimer's disease (AD); underwhelming evidence against. *Vaccines (Basel)* 9(6):679.

Iwata, A., K. Nagata, H. Hatsuta, H. Takuma, M. Bundo, K. Iwamoto, A. Tamaoka, S. Murayama, T. Saido, and S. Tsuji. 2014. Altered CpG methylation in sporadic Alzheimer's disease is associated with APP and MAPT dysregulation. *Human Molecular Genetics* 23(3):648-656.

Jabbari, E., J. Woodside, M. M. X. Tan, M. Shoai, A. Pittman, R. Ferrari, K. Y. Mok, D. Zhang, R. H. Reynolds, R. de Silva, M. J. Grimm, G. Respondek, U. Muller, S. Al-Sarraj, S. M. Gentleman, A. J. Lees, T. T. Warner, J. Hardy, T. Revesz, G. U. Hoglinger, J. L. Holton, M. Ryten, and H. R. Morris. 2018. Variation at the TRIM11 locus modifies progressive supranuclear palsy phenotype. *Annals of Neurology* 84(4):485-496.

Janbek, J., T. M. Laursen, N. Frimodt-Møller, M. Magyari, J. G. Haas, R. Lathe, and G. Waldemar. 2023. Hospital-diagnosed infections, autoimmune diseases, and subsequent dementia incidence. *JAMA Network Open* 6(9):e2332635.

Jayaraj, R. L., E. A. Rodriguez, Y. Wang, and M. L. Block. 2017. Outdoor ambient air pollution and neurodegenerative diseases: The neuroinflammation hypothesis. *Current Environmental Health Reports* 4(2):166-179.

Jazwinski, S. M., and S. Kim. 2019. Examination of the dimensions of biological age. *Frontiers in Genetics* 10:263.

Jellinger, K. A. 2022. Recent update on the heterogeneity of the Alzheimer's disease spectrum. *Journal of Neural Transmission (Vienna)* 129(1):1-24.

Jellinger, K. A., and A. D. Korczyn. 2018. Are dementia with Lewy bodies and Parkinson's disease dementia the same disease? *BMC Medicine* 16(1):34.

Jia, L., F. Li, C. Wei, M. Zhu, Q. Qu, W. Qin, Y. Tang, L. Shen, Y. Wang, L. Shen, H. Li, D. Peng, L. Tan, B. Luo, Q. Guo, M. Tang, Y. Du, J. Zhang, J. Zhang, J. Lyu, Y. Li, A. Zhou, F. Wang, C. Chu, H. Song, L. Wu, X. Zuo, Y. Han, J. Liang, Q. Wang, H. Jin, W. Wang, Y. Lü, F. Li, Y. Zhou, W. Zhang, Z. Liao, Q. Qiu, Y. Li, C. Kong, Y. Li, H. Jiao, J. Lu, and J. Jia. 2021. Prediction of Alzheimer's disease using multi-variants from a chinese genome-wide association study. *Brain* 144(3):924-937.

Jones, L., D. Harold, and J. Williams. 2010. Genetic evidence for the involvement of lipid metabolism in Alzheimer's disease. *Biochimica et Biophysica Acta* 1801(8):754-761.

Jonsson, T., H. Stefansson, S. Steinberg, I. Jonsdottir, P. V. Jonsson, J. Snaedal, S. Bjornsson, J. Huttenlocher, A. I. Levey, J. J. Lah, D. Rujescu, H. Hampel, I. Giegling, O. A. Andreassen, K. Engedal, I. Ulstein, S. Djurovic, C. Ibrahim-Verbaas, A. Hofman, M. A. Ikram, C. M. van Duijn, U. Thorsteinsdottir, A. Kong, and K. Stefansson. 2013. Variant of TREM2 associated with the risk of Alzheimer's disease. *New England Journal of Medicine* 368(2):107-116.

Kalia, V., D. W. Belsky, A. A. Baccarelli, and G. W. Miller. 2022. An exposomic framework to uncover environmental drivers of aging. *Exposome* 2(1):osac002.

Kapasi, A., C. DeCarli, and J. A. Schneider. 2017. Impact of multiple pathologies on the threshold for clinically overt dementia. *Acta Neuropathologica* 134(2):171-186.

Kashyap, S. N., N. R. Boyle, and E. D. Roberson. 2023. Preclinical interventions in mouse models of frontotemporal dementia due to progranulin mutations. *Neurotherapeutics* 20(1):140-153.

Kato, T., Y. Inui, A. Nakamura, and K. Ito. 2016. Brain fluorodeoxyglucose (FDG) PET in dementia. *Ageing Research Reviews* 30:73-84.

Katzman, R., R. Terry, R. DeTeresa, T. Brown, P. Davies, P. Fuld, X. Renbing, and A. Peck. 1988. Clinical, pathological, and neurochemical changes in dementia: A subgroup with preserved mental status and numerous neocortical plaques. *Annals of Neurology* 23(2):138-144.

Kelley, M. 2023. *NIH strategic planning process overview.* Presentation at Committee on Research Priorities for Preventing and Treating Alzheimer's Disease and Related Dementias. Meeting 1, Virtual. October 2, 2024.

Kim, S. H., K. W. Oh, H. K. Jin, and J. S. Bae. 2018. Immune inflammatory modulation as a potential therapeutic strategy of stem cell therapy for ALS and neurodegenerative diseases. *BMB Reports* 51(11):545-546.

Kim, K., X. Wang, E. Ragonnaud, M. Bodogai, T. Illouz, M. DeLuca, R. A. McDevitt, F. Gusev, E. Okun, E. Rogaev, and A. Biragyn. 2021. Therapeutic B-cell depletion reverses progression of Alzheimer's disease. *Nature Communications* 12:2185.

Kind, A. J. 2023. Establishing national social exposome Alzheimer's disease and related dementias (ADRD) infrastructure. *Alzheimer's & Dementia* 19(S22): e077828.

Kind, I. 2024. *Panelist Remarks.* Committee on Research Priorities for Preventing and Treating Alzheimer's Disease and Related Dementias Public Workshop, Hybrid. January 16–17, 2024.

Klocke, C., and P. Lein. 2019. *Environmental exposures during early life influence adult disease risk*. https://www.openaccessgovernment.org/environmental-exposures-adult-disease-risk/75696/ (accessed August 16, 2024).

Knopman, D. S., H. Amieva, R. C. Petersen, G. Chetelat, D. M. Holtzman, B. T. Hyman, R. A. Nixon, and D. T. Jones. 2021. Alzheimer disease. *Nature Reviews Disease Primers* 7(1):33.

Kremer, I. 2024. *Panelist Remarks*. Committee on Research Priorities for Preventing and Treating Alzheimer's Disease and Related Dementias Public Workshop, Hybrid. January 16–17, 2024.

Krishnan, K. J., T. E. Ratnaike, H. L. De Gruyter, E. Jaros, and D. M. Turnbull. 2012. Mitochondrial DNA deletions cause the biochemical defect observed in Alzheimer's disease. *Neurobiology and Aging* 33(9):2210-2214.

Lamar, M., K. N. Kershaw, S. E. Leurgans, R. R. Mukherjee, B. S. Lange-Maia, D. X. Marquez, and L. L. Barnes. 2023. Neighborhood-level social vulnerability and individual-level cognitive and motor functioning over time in older non-Latino Black and Latino adults. *Frontiers of Human Neuroscience* 17:1125906.

Lamb, B. 2024. *Panelist Remarks*. Committee on Research Priorities for Preventing and Treating Alzheimer's Disease and Related Dementias Public Workshop, Hybrid. January 16–17, 2024.

Lambert, J. C., A. Ramirez, B. Grenier-Boley, and C. Bellenguez. 2023. Step by step: Towards a better understanding of the genetic architecture of Alzheimer's disease. *Molecular Psychiatry* 28:2716-2727.

Landau, S. M., D. Harvey, C. M. Madison, E. M. Reiman, N. L. Foster, P. S. Aisen, R. C. Petersen, L. M. Shaw, J. Q. Trojanowski, C. R. Jack, Jr., M. W. Weiner, and W. J. Jagust. 2010. Comparing predictors of conversion and decline in mild cognitive impairment. *Neurology* 20(75):230-238.

Lawlor, D. A., K. Tilling, and G. Davey Smith. 2016. Triangulation in aetiological epidemiology. *International Journal of Epidemiology* 45(6):1866-1886.

Lee, J. H., D. S. Yang, C. N. Goulbourne, E. Im, P. Stavrides, A. Pensalfini, H. Chan, C. Bouchet-Marquis, C. Bleiwas, M. J. Berg, C. Huo, J. Peddy, M. Pawlik, E. Levy, M. Rao, M. Staufenbiel, and R. A. Nixon. 2022. Faulty autolysosome acidification in Alzheimer's disease mouse models induces autophagic build-up of Aβ in neurons, yielding senile plaques. *Nature Neuroscience* 25(6):688-701.

Lefevre-Arbogast, S., J. Chaker, F. Mercier, R. Barouki, X. Coumoul, G. W. Miller, A. David, and C. Samieri. 2024. Assessing the contribution of the chemical exposome to neurodegenerative disease. *Nature Neuroscience* 27(5):812-821.

Lehmann, D., A. Elshorbagy, and M. Hurley. 2023. Many paths to Alzheimer's disease: A unifying hypothesis integrating biological, chemical and physical risk factors. *Journal of Alzheimer's Disease* 95(4):1371-1382.

Liddelow, S. A., K. A. Guttenplan, L. E. Clarke, F. C. Bennett, C. J. Bohlen, L. Schirmer, M. L. Bennett, A. E. Munch, W. S. Chung, T. C. Peterson, D. K. Wilton, A. Frouin, B. A. Napier, N. Panicker, M. Kumar, M. S. Buckwalter, D. H. Rowitch, V. L. Dawson, T. M. Dawson, B. Stevens, and B. A. Barres. 2017. Neurotoxic reactive astrocytes are induced by activated microglia. *Nature* 541(7638):481-487.

Lim, Y., V. M. Kehm, E. B. Lee, J. H. Soper, C. Li, J. Q. Trojanowski, and V. M. Lee. 2011. Alpha-syn suppression reverses synaptic and memory defects in a mouse model of dementia with Lewy bodies. *Journal of Neuroscience* 31(27):10076-10087.

Lima, T., T. Y. Li, A. Mottis, and J. Auwerx. 2022. Pleiotropic effects of mitochondria in aging. *Nature Aging* 2(3):199-213.

Lin, Y. F., L. Y. Wang, C. S. Chen, C. C. Li, and Y. H. Hsiao. 2021. Cellular senescence as a driver of cognitive decline triggered by chronic unpredictable stress. *Neurobiology Stress* 15:100341.

Lin, P. B., A. P. Tsai, D. Soni, A. Lee-Gosselin, M. Moutinho, S. S. Puntambekar, G. E. Landreth, B. T. Lamb, and A. L. Oblak. 2023. *INPP5D* deficiency attenuates amyloid pathology in a mouse model of Alzheimer's disease. *Alzheimer's & Dementia* 19(6):2528-2537.

Lindbohm, J. V., N. Mars, P. N. Sipilä, A. Singh-Manoux, H. Runz; FinnGen; G. Livingston, S. Seshadri, R. Xavier, A. D. Hingorani, S. Ripatti, and M. Kivimäki. 2022. Immune system-wide Mendelian randomization and triangulation analyses support autoimmunity as a modifiable component in dementia-causing diseases. *Nature Aging* 2(10):956-972.

Liu, F., J. Xu, L. Guo, W. Qin, M. Liang, G. Schumann, and C. Yu. 2023a. Environmental neuroscience linking exposome to brain structure and function underlying cognition and behavior. *Molecular Psychiatry* 28(1):17-27.

Liu, N., X. Jiang, and H. Li. 2023b. The viral hypothesis in Alzheimer's disease: SARS-CoV-2 on the cusp. *Frontiers in Aging and Neuroscience* 15:1129640.

Livingston, G., J. Huntley, K. Y. Liu, S. G. Costafreda, G. Selbæk, S. Alladi, D. Ames, S. Banerjee, A. Burns, C. Brayne, N. C. Fox, C. P. Ferri, L. N. Gitlin, R. Howard, H. C. Kales, M. Kivimäki, E. B. Larson, N. Nakasujja, K. Rockwood, Q. Samus, K. Shirai, A. Singh-Manoux, L. S. Schneider, S. Walsh, Y. Yao, A. Sommerlad, and N. Mukadam. 2024. Dementia prevention, intervention, and care: 2024 Report of the Lancet Standing Commission. *Lancet* 404(10452):572-628.

Loeffler, D. A. 2019. Influence of normal aging on brain autophagy: A complex scenario. *Frontiers in Aging and Neuroscience* 11:49.

López-Otín, C., M. A. Blasco, L. Partridge, M. Serrano, and G. Kroemer. 2023. Hallmarks of aging: An expanding universe. *Cell* 186(2):243-278.

Lourida, I., E. Hannon, T. J. Littlejohns, K. M. Langa, E. Hypponen, E. Kuzma, and D. J. Llewellyn. 2019. Association of lifestyle and genetic risk with incidence of dementia. *JAMA* 322(5):430-437.

Lutshumba, J., B. Nikolajczyk, and A. Bachstetter. 2021. Dysregulation of systemic immunity in aging and dementia. *Frontiers in Cellular Neuroscience* 15:652111.

Magen, I., and M. F. Chesselet. 2011. Mouse models of cognitive deficits due to alpha-synuclein pathology. *Journal of Parkinson's Disease* 1(3):217-227.

Maloney, B., and D. Lahiri. 2016. Epigenetics of dementia: Understanding the disease as a transformation rather than a state. *Lancet* 15(7):760-774.

Manzoni, C., D. A. Kia, R. Ferrari, G. Leonenko, B. Costa, V. Saba, E. Jabbari, M. M. Tan, D. Albani, V. Alvarez, I. Alvarez, O. A. Andreassen, A. Angiolillo, A. Arighi, M. Baker, L. Benussi, V. Bessi, G. Binetti, D. J. Blackburn, M. Boada, B. F. Boeve, S. Borrego-Ecija, B. Borroni, G. Brathen, W. S. Brooks, A. C. Bruni, P. Caroppo, S. Bandres-Ciga, J. Clarimon, R. Colao, C. Cruchaga, A. Danek, S. C. de Boer, I. de Rojas, A. di Costanzo, D. W. Dickson, J. Diehl-Schmid, C. Dobson-Stone, O. Dols-Icardo, A. Donizetti, E. Dopper, E. Durante, C. Ferrari, G. Forloni, F. Frangipane, L. Fratiglioni, M. G. Kramberger, D. Galimberti, M. Gallucci, P. Garcia-Gonzalez, R. Ghidoni, G. Giaccone, C. Graff, N. R. Graff-Radford, J. Grafman, G. M. Halliday, D. G. Hernandez, L. E. Hjermind, J. R. Hodges, G. Holloway, E. D. Huey, I. Illan-Gala, K. A. Josephs, D. S. Knopman, M. Kristiansen, J. B. Kwok, I. Leber, H. L. Leonard, I. Libri, A. Lleo, I. R. Mackenzie, G. K. Madhan, R. Maletta, M. Marquie, A. Maver, M. Menendez-Gonzalez, G. Milan, B. L. Miller, C. M. Morris, H. R. Morris, B. Nacmias, J. Newton, J. E. Nielsen, N. Nilsson, V. Novelli, A. Padovani, S. Pal, F. Pasquier, P. Pastor, R. Perneczky, B. Peterlin, R. C. Petersen, O. Piguet, Y. A. Pijnenburg, A. A. Puca, R. Rademakers, I. Rainero, L. M. Reus, A. M. Richardson, M. Riemenschneider, E. Rogaeva, B. Rogelj, S. Rollinson, H. Rosen, G. Rossi, J. B. Rowe, E. Rubino, A. Ruiz, E. Salvi, R. Sanchez-Valle, S. B. Sando, A. F. Santillo, J. A. Saxon, J. C. Schlachetzki, S. W. Scholz, H. Seelaar, W. W. Seeley, M. Serpente, S. Sorbi, S. Sordon, P. St George-Hyslop, J. C. Thompson, C. Van Broeckhoven, V. M. Van Deerlin, S. J. Van der Lee, J. Van Swieten, F. Tagliavini, J. van der Zee, A. Veronesi, E. Vitale, M. L.

Waldo, J. S. Yokoyama, M. A. Nalls, P. Momeni, A. B. Singleton, J. Hardy, and V. Escott-Price. 2024. Genome-wide analyses reveal a potential role for the MAPT, MOBP, and APOE loci in sporadic frontotemporal dementia. *American Journal of Human Genetics* 111(7):1316-1329.

Marlies Oosthoek, L. V., A. de Wilde, B. Bongers, D. Antwi-Berko, P. Scheltens, P. van Bokhoven, E. G. B. Vijverberg, and C. E. Teunissen. 2024. Utilization of fluid-based biomarkers as endpoints in disease-modifying clinical trials for Alzheimer's disease: A systematic review. *Alzheimer's Research & Therapy* 16:93.

Marquez, F., W. Tarraf, A. M. Stickel, K. A. Gonzalez, F. D. Testai, J. Cai, L. C. Gallo, G. A. Talavera, M. L. Daviglus, S. Wassertheil-Smoller, C. DeCarli, N. Schneiderman, and H. M. Gonzalez. 2024. Hypertension, cognitive decline, and mild cognitive impairment among diverse Hispanics/Latinos: Study of Latinos—Investigation of Neurocognitive Aging Results (SOL-INCA). *Journal of Alzheimer's Disease* 97(3):1449-1461.

Marsit, C. J. 2015. Influence of environmental exposure on human epigenetic regulation. *Journal of Experimental Biology* 218(Pt 1):71-79.

Martinez-Feduchi, P., P. Jin, and B. Yao. 2024. Epigenetic modifications of DNA and RNA in Alzheimer's disease. *Frontiers in Molecular Neuroscience* 17:1398026.

Matthay, E. C., E. Hagan, L. M. Gottlieb, M. L. Tan, D. Vlahov, N. E. Adler, and M. M. Glymour. 2020. Alternative causal inference methods in population health research: Evaluating tradeoffs and triangulating evidence. *SSM Population Health* 10:100526.

Mayne, K., J. A. White, C. E. McMurran, F. J. Rivera, and A. G. de la Fuente. 2020. Aging and neurodegenerative disease: Is the adaptive immune system a friend or foe? *Frontiers in Aging Neuroscience* 12:572090.

Mehta, R. I., and R. I. Mehta. 2023. The vascular-immune hypothesis of Alzheimer's disease. *Biomedicines* 11(2):408.

Mei, Z., G. Liu, B. Zhao, Z. He, and S. Gu. 2023. Emerging roles of epigenetics in lead-induced neurotoxicity. *Environment International* 181:108253.

Melcher, E. M., L. Vilen, A. Pfaff, S. Lim, A. DeWitt, W. R. Powell, B. B. Bendlin, and A. J. H. Kind. 2024. Deriving life-course residential histories in brain bank cohorts: A feasibility study. *Alzheimer's & Dementia* 20(5):3219-3227.

Mensikova, K., R. Matej, C. Colosimo, R. Rosales, L. Tuckova, J. Ehrmann, D. Hrabos, K. Kolarikova, R. Vodicka, R. Vrtel, M. Prochazka, M. Nevrly, M. Kaiserova, S. Kurcova, P. Otruba, and P. Kanovsky. 2022. Lewy body disease or diseases with Lewy bodies? *NPJ Parkinsons Disease* 8(1):3.

Mez, J., J. Chung, G. Jun, J. Kriegel, A. P. Bourlas, R. Sherva, M. W. Logue, L. L. Barnes, D. A. Bennett, J. D. Buxbaum, G. S. Byrd, P. K. Crane, N. Ertekin-Taner, D. Evans, M. D. Fallin, T. Foroud, A. Goate, N. R. Graff-Radford, K. S. Hall, M. I. Kamboh, W. A. Kukull, E. B. Larson, J. J. Manly, J. L. Haines, R. Mayeux, M. A. Pericak-Vance, G. D. Schellenberg, K. L. Lunetta, and L. A. Farrer. 2017. Two novel loci, *COBL* and *SLC10A2*, for Alzheimer's disease in African Americans. *Alzheimer's & Dementia* 13(2):119-129.

Mielke, M. 2024. Sex and gender differences in Alzheimer's disease and Alzheimer's disease related dementias. Commissioned Paper for the Committee on Research Priorities for Preventing and Treating Alzheimer's Disease and Related Dementias.

Migliore, L., and F. Coppedè. 2022. Gene–environment interactions in Alzheimer disease: The emerging role of epigenetics. *Nature Reviews Neurology* 18:643-660.

Miller, G. 2024. Presentation at Committee on Research Priorities for Preventing and Treating Alzheimer's Disease and Related Dementias Public Workshop, Hybrid. January 16–17, 2024.

Miller, M. B., A. Y. Huang, J. Kim, Z. Zhou, S. L. Kirkham, E. A. Maury, J. S. Ziegenfuss, H. C. Reed, J. E. Neil, L. Rento, S. C. Ryu, C. C. Ma, L. J. Luquette, H. M. Ames, D. H. Oakley, M. P. Frosch, B. T. Hyman, M. A. Lodato, E. A. Lee, and C. A. Walsh. 2022. Somatic genomic changes in single Alzheimer's disease neurons. *Nature* 604(7907):714-722.

Miyashita, A., A. Koike, G. Jun, L. S. Wang, S. Takahashi, E. Matsubara, T. Kawarabayashi, M. Shoji, N. Tomita, H. Arai, T. Asada, Y. Harigaya, M. Ikeda, M. Amari, H. Hanyu, S. Higuchi, T. Ikeuchi, M. Nishizawa, M. Suga, Y. Kawase, H. Akatsu, K. Kosaka, T. Yamamoto, M. Imagawa, T. Hamaguchi, M. Yamada, T. Morihara, M. Takeda, T. Takao, K. Nakata, Y. Fujisawa, K. Sasaki, K. Watanabe, K. Nakashima, K. Urakami, T. Ooya, M. Takahashi, T. Yuzuriha, K. Serikawa, S. Yoshimoto, R. Nakagawa, J. W. Kim, C. S. Ki, H. H. Won, D. L. Na, S. W. Seo, I. Mook-Jung, P. St George-Hyslop, R. Mayeux, J. L. Haines, M. A. Pericak-Vance, M. Yoshida, N. Nishida, K. Tokunaga, K. Yamamoto, S. Tsuji, I. Kanazawa, Y. Ihara, G. D. Schellenberg, L. A. Farrer, and R. Kuwano. 2013. *SORL1* is genetically associated with late-onset Alzheimer's disease in Japanese, Koreans and Caucasians. *PLoS ONE* 8(4):e58618.

Miyashita, A., M. Kikuchi, N. Hara, and T. Ikeuchi. 2023. Genetics of Alzheimer's disease: An East Asian perspective. *Journal of Human Genetics* 68(3):115-124.

MODEL-AD. 2024. *MODEL-AD*. https://www.model-ad.org/ (accessed August 22, 2024).

Morawe, T., C. Hiebel, A. Kern, and C. Behl. 2012. Protein homeostasis, aging and Alzheimer's disease. *Molecular Neurobiology* 46(1):41-54.

Musi, N., J. M. Valentine, K. R. Sickora, E. Baeuerle, C. S. Thompson, Q. Shen, and M. E. Orr. 2018. Tau protein aggregation is associated with cellular senescence in the brain. *Aging Cell* 17(6):e12840.

NASEM (National Academies of Sciences, Engineering, and Medicine). 2018. *Future directions for the demography of aging: Proceedings of a workshop.* Edited by M. K. Majmundar and M. D. Hayward. Washington, DC: The National Academies Press.

NASEM. 2020a. *Environmental neuroscience: Advancing the understanding of how chemical exposures impact brain health and disease: Proceedings of a workshop.* Edited by C. Stroud, S. M. Posey Norris and L. Bain. Washington, DC: The National Academies Press.

NASEM. 2020b. *Integrating the science of aging and environmental health research: Proceedings of a workshop—in brief.* Edited by K. Sawyer, F. Sharples and R. Poole. Washington, DC: The National Academies Press.

NASEM. 2023. *Nonhuman primate models in biomedical research: State of the science and future needs.* Edited by O. C. Yost, A. Downey and K. S. Ramos. Washington, DC: The National Academies Press.

NASEM. 2024. *Preventing and treating Alzheimer's disease and related dementias: Promising research and opportunities to accelerate progress: Proceedings of a workshop—in brief.* Edited by A. Downey and O. Yost. Washington, DC: The National Academies Press.

Nativio, R., G. Donahue, A. Berson, Y. Lan, A. Amlie-Wolf, F. Tuzer, J. B. Toledo, S. J. Gosai, B. D. Gregory, C. Torres, J. Q. Trojanowski, L. S. Wang, F. B. Johnson, N. M. Bonini, and S. L. Berger. 2018. Dysregulation of the epigenetic landscape of normal aging in Alzheimer's disease. *Nature Neuroscience* 21(4):497-505.

Nativio, R., Y. Lan, G. Donahue, S. Sidoli, A. Berson, A. R. Srinivasan, O. Shcherbakova, A. Amlie-Wolf, J. Nie, X. Cui, C. He, L. S. Wang, B. A. Garcia, J. Q. Trojanowski, N. M. Bonini, and S. L. Berger. 2020. An integrated multi-omics approach identifies epigenetic alterations associated with Alzheimer's disease. *Nature Genetics* 52(10):1024-1035.

Naudi, A., R. Cabre, M. Jove, V. Ayala, H. Gonzalo, M. Portero-Otin, I. Ferrer, and R. Pamplona. 2015. Lipidomics of human brain aging and Alzheimer's disease pathology. *International Review of Neurobiology* 122:133-189.

Neuner, S. M., M. Telpoukhovskaia, V. Menon, K. M. S. O'Connell, T. J. Hohman, and C. C. Kaczorowski. 2022. Translational approaches to understanding resilience to Alzheimer's disease. *Trends in neurosciences* 45(5):369–383.

NIA (National Insitute on Aging). 2016. *Decoding the molecular ties between vascular disease and Alzheimer's.* https://www.nia.nih.gov/news/decoding-molecular-ties-between-vascular-disease-and-alzheimers (accessed October 17, 2024).

NIA. 2019. *NIH-funded translational research centers to speed, diversify Alzheimer's drug discovery.* https://www.nia.nih.gov/news/nih-funded-translational-research-centers-speed-diversify-alzheimers-drug-discovery#:~:text=To%20help%20meet%20the%20urgent,over%20the%20next%20five%20years (accessed October 18, 2024).

NIA. 2020. *Understanding the role of the exposome in brain aging, Alzheimer's disease (AD) and AD-related dementias (ADRD).* Baltimore, MD: NIA.

NIA. 2022a. *Microphysiological systems to advance precision medicine for Alzheimer's disease (AD) and AD-related dementias (ADRD) treatment and prevention.* Baltimore, MD: NIA.

NIA. 2022b. *Accelerating Medicines Partnership program for Alzheimer's Disease (AMP AD 2.0).* https://www.nia.nih.gov/research/amp-ad-second-iteration (accessed August 19, 2024).

NIA. 2023a. *Exploring the role of the exposome in aging and age-related diseases.* https://www.nia.nih.gov/exposome (accessed August 16, 2024).

NIA. 2023b. *Research enterprise.* https://www.nia.nih.gov/report-2019-2020-scientific-advances-prevention-treatment-and-care-dementia/research-enterprise (accessed August 22, 2024).

NIA. 2023c. *TREAT-AD centers: Open source tools to reinvigorate Alzheimer's drug discovery.* https://www.nia.nih.gov/research/blog/2023/12/treat-ad-centers-open-source-tools-reinvigorate-alzheimers-drug-discovery (accessed August 19, 2024).

NIA. 2023d. *Fiscal year 2024 budget.* https://www.nia.nih.gov/about/budget/fiscal-year-2024-budget (accessed August 22, 2024).

NIA. 2024a. *Alzheimer Biomarkers Consortium—Down Syndrome* (ABC-DS). https://www.nia.nih.gov/research/abc-ds (accessed August 23, 2024).

NIA. 2024b. *Alzheimer's disease sequencing project consortia.* https://www.nia.nih.gov/research/dn/alzheimers-disease-sequencing-project-consortia (accessed August 22, 2024).

NIA. 2024c. *Successful Trajectories of Aging: Reserve and Resilience in Rats (STARRRS).* https://www.nia.nih.gov/research/labs/about-irp/successful-trajectories-of-aging-reserve-and-resilience-in-rats#:~:text=About%20STARRRS,-Aging%20in%20humans&text=In%20contrast%2C%20other%20people%20experience,of%20neurocognitive%20aging%20in%20rats (accessed October 23, 2024).

NIA. 2024d. *Accelerating Medicines Partnership Program for Alzheimer's Disease (AMP AD).* https://www.nia.nih.gov/research/amp-ad (accessed August 22, 2024).

NIA. 2024e. *2024 NIH Alzheimer's Research Summit: Building a precision medicine research enterprise.* https://www.nia.nih.gov/2024-alzheimers-summit (accessed October 25, 2024).

NIA. 2024f. *Fiscal year 2025 budget.* https://www.nia.nih.gov/about/budget/fiscal-year-2025-budget (accessed August 22, 2024).

NIH (National Insitutes of Health). 2015. *Consideration of sex as a biological variable in NIH-funded research.* https://grants.nih.gov/grants/guide/notice-files/not-od-15-102.html (accessed October 23, 2024).

NIH. 2019. *New NIH-funded translational research centers to speed, diversify Alzheimer's drug discovery.* https://www.nih.gov/news-events/news-releases/new-nih-funded-translational-research-centers-speed-diversify-alzheimers-drug-discovery (accessed August 22, 2024).

NIH. 2023. *Center for exposome research coordination to accelerate precision environmental health.* https://grants.nih.gov/grants/guide/rfa-files/RFA-ES-23-010.html (accessed August 16, 2024).

NIH. 2024. *Celluar Senescence Network (SenNet).* https://commonfund.nih.gov/senescence (accessed August 19, 2024).

Nikolac Perkovic, M., A. Videtic Paska, M. Konjevod, K. Kouter, D. Svob Strac, G. Nedic Erjavec, and N. Pivac. 2021. Epigenetics of Alzheimer's disease. *Biomolecules* 11(2):195.

NINDS (National Institute of Neurological Disorders and Stroke). 2024a. *The neural exposome*. https://www.ninds.nih.gov/current-research/research-funded-ninds/translational-research/onetox-neural-exposome-and-toxicology-programs/neural-exposome (accessed August 16, 2024).

NINDS. 2024b. *Accelerating Medicines Partnership® for Amyotrophic Lateral Sclerosis (AMP® ALS)*. https://www.ninds.nih.gov/current-research/focus-disorders/amyotrophic-lateral-sclerosis/accelerating-medicines-partnershipr-amyotrophic-lateral-sclerosis-ampr-als (accessed October 24, 2024).

Nixon, R. A. 2013. The role of autophagy in neurodegenerative disease. *Nature Medicine* 19(8):983-997.

Nixon, R. A. 2020. The aging lysosome: An essential catalyst for late-onset neurodegenerative diseases. *Biochimica et Biophysica Acta Proteins & Proteomics* 1868(9):140443.

Noche, J. A., H. Radhakrishnan, M. F. Ubele, K. Boaz, J. L. Mefford, E. D. Jones, H. Y. van Rooyen, J. A. Perpich, K. McCarty, B. Meacham, J. Smiley, S. A. Bembenek Bailey, L. G. Puskas, D. K. Powell, L. Sordo, M. J. Phelan, C. M. Norris, E. Head, and C. E. L. Stark. 2024. Age-related brain atrophy and the positive effects of behavioral enrichment in middle-aged beagles. *Journal of Neuroscience* 44(20):e2366232024.

Oblak, A. L., S. Forner, P. R. Territo, M. Sasner, G. W. Carter, G. R. Howell, S. J. Sukoff-Rizzo, B. A. Logsdon, L. M. Mangravite, A. Mortazavi, D. Baglietto-Vargas, K. N. Green, G. R. MacGregor, M. A. Wood, A. J. Tenner, F. M. LaFerla, B. T. Lamb, and the MODEL-AD and Consortium. 2020. Model organism development and evaluation for late-onset Alzheimer's disease: MODEL-AD. *Alzheimer's & Dementia (N Y)* 6(1):e12110.

Ogrodnik, M., Y. Zhu, L. G. P. Langhi, T. Tchkonia, P. Kruger, E. Fielder, S. Victorelli, R. A. Ruswhandi, N. Giorgadze, T. Pirtskhalava, O. Podgorni, G. Enikolopov, K. O. Johnson, M. Xu, C. Inman, A. K. Palmer, M. Schafer, M. Weigl, Y. Ikeno, T. C. Burns, J. F. Passos, T. von Zglinicki, J. L. Kirkland, and D. Jurk. 2019. Obesity-induced cellular senescence drives anxiety and impairs neurogenesis. *Cell Metabolism* 29(5):1061-1077.e8.

Oppenheim, H. A., J. Lucero, and A. Guyot. 2013. Exposure to vehicle emissions results in altered blood brain barrier permeability and expression of matrix metalloproteinases and tight junction proteins in mice. *Particle and Fibre Toxicology* 10:62.

Orme, T., R. Guerreiro, and J. Bras. 2018. The genetics of dementia with Lewy bodies: Current understanding and future directions. *Current Neurology and Neuroscience Reports* 18:67.

Owaki, A., A. Tanaka, K. Furuhashi, Y. Watanabe, E. Koshi-Ito, T. Imaizumi, and S. Maruyama. 2024. Prognosis of microscopic polyangiitis is well predictable in the first 2 weeks of treatment. *Clinical Experiments in Nephrology* 28(7):701-706.

Pacholko, A., and C. Iadecola. 2024. Hypertension, neurodegeneration, and cognitive decline. *Hypertension* 81(5):991-1007.

Padmanabhan, P., and J. Gotz. 2023. Clinical relevance of animal models in aging-related dementia research. *Nature Aging* 3(5):481-493.

PAHO/WHO (Pan American Health Organization/World Health Organization). 2024. *Healthy aging*. https://www.paho.org/en/healthy-aging (accessed August 16, 2024).

Parrish, M. C., Y. J. Tan, K. V. Grimes, and D. Mochly-Rosen. 2019. Surviving in the valley of death: Opportunities and challenges in translating academic drug discoveries. *Annual Review of Pharmacology and Toxicology* 59:405-421.

Paşca, S. 2019. Assembling human brain organoids. *Science* 363(6423):126-127.

Patrick, K. L., S. L. Bell, C. G. Weindel, and R. O. Watson. 2019. Exploring the "multiple-hit hypothesis" of neurodegenerative disease: Bacterial infection comes up to bat. *Frontiers in Cellular and Infection Microbiology* 9:138.

Patten, K. T., and P. J. Lein. 2019. Gene-environment interactions determine risk for dementia: The influence of lifestyle on genetic risk for dementia. *Annals of Translational Medicine* 7(Suppl 8):S322.

Paulson, H. L., and I. Igo. 2011. Genetics of dementia. *Seminal Neurology* 31(5):449-460.

Pearl, J. 2009. *Causality: Models, Reasoning, and Inference.* Cambridge, UK: Cambridge University Press.

Peleg, S., C. Feller, A. G. Ladurner, and A. Imhof. 2016. The metabolic impact on histone acetylation and transcription in ageing. *Trends in Biochemical Sciences* 41(8):700-711.

Pellegrini, C., C. Pirazzini, C. Sala, L. Sambati, I. Yusipov, A. Kalyakulina, F. Ravaioli, K. M. Kwiatkowska, D. F. Durso, M. Ivanchenko, D. Monti, R. Lodi, C. Franceschi, P. Cortelli, P. Garagnani, and M. G. Bacalini. 2021. A meta-analysis of brain DNA methylation across sex, age, and Alzheimer's disease points for accelerated epigenetic aging in neuro-degeneration. *Frontiers in Aging Neuroscience* 13:639428.

Pericak-Vance, M. 2024. *Alzheimer's Disease Sequencing Project (ADSP).* Presentation at Committee on Research Priorities for Preventing and Treating Alzheimer's Disease and Related Dementias Public Workshop, Hybrid. January 16–17, 2024.

Peters, R., N. Ee, J. Peters, A. Booth, I. Mudway, and K. J. Anstey. 2019. Air pollution and dementia: A systematic review. *Journal of Alzheimer's Disease* 70(S1):S145-S163.

Pham, T. N. M., N. Perumal, C. Manicam, M. Basoglu, S. Eimer, D. C. Fuhrmann, C. U. Pietrzik, A. M. Clement, H. Korschgen, J. Schepers, and C. Behl. 2023. Adaptive responses of neuronal cells to chronic endoplasmic reticulum (ER) stress. *Redox Biology* 67:102943.

Pilling, L. C., R. Joehanes, D. Melzer, L. W. Harries, W. Henley, J. Dupuis, H. Lin, M. Mitchell, D. Hernandez, S. X. Ying, K. L. Lunetta, E. J. Benjamin, A. Singleton, D. Levy, P. Munson, J. M. Murabito, and L. Ferrucci. 2015. Gene expression markers of age-related inflammation in two human cohorts. *Experimental Gerontology* 70:37-45.

Powell, W. R., W. R. Buckingham, J. L. Larson, L. Vilen, M. Yu, M. S. Salamat, B. B. Bendlin, R. A. Rissman, and A. J. H. Kind. 2020. Association of neighborhood-level disadvantage with Alzheimer disease neuropathology. *JAMA Network Open* 3(6):e207559.

Quach, A., M. E. Levine, T. Tanaka, A. T. Lu, B. H. Chen, L. Ferrucci, B. Ritz, S. Bandinelli, M. L. Neuhouser, J. M. Beasley, L. Snetselaar, R. B. Wallace, P. S. Tsao, D. Absher, T. L. Assimes, J. D. Stewart, Y. Li, L. Hou, A. A. Baccarelli, E. A. Whitsel, and S. Horvath. 2017. Epigenetic clock analysis of diet, exercise, education, and lifestyle factors. *Aging* 9(2):419-446.

Rabinovici, G. D., M. C. Carrillo, M. Forman, S. DeSanti, D. S. Miller, N. Kozauer, R. C. Petersen, C. Randolph, D. S. Knopman, E. E. Smith, M. Isaac, N. Mattsson, L. J. Bain, J. A. Hendrix, and J. R. Sims. 2017. Multiple comorbid neuropathologies in the setting of Alzheimer's disease neuropathology and implications for drug development. *Alzheimer's & Dementia (N Y)* 3(1):83-91.

Ramesh, M., P. Gopinath, and T. Govindaraju. 2019. Role of post-translational modifications in Alzheimer's disease. *ChemBioChem* 21(8):1052-1079.

Raulin, A.-C., S. V. Doss, Z. A. Trottier, T. C. Ikezu, G Bu, and C.-C. Liu. 2022. ApoE in Alzheimer's disease: Pathophysiology and therapeutic strategies. *Molecular Neurodegeneration* 17(1):72.

Reitz, C., G. Jun, A. Naj, R. Rajbhandary, B. N. Vardarajan, L.-S. Wang, O. Valladares, C.-F. Lin, E. B. Larson, N. R. Graff-Radford, D. Evans, P. L. De Jager, P. K. Crane, J. D. Buxbaum, J. R. Murrell, T. Raj, N. Ertekin-Taner, M. Logue, C. T. Baldwin, R. C. Green, L. L. Barnes, L. B. Cantwell, M. D. Fallin, R. C. P. Go, P. Griffith, T. O. Obisesan, J. J. Manly, K. L. Lunetta, M. I. Kamboh, O. L. Lopez, D. A. Bennett, H. Hendrie, K. S. Hall, A. M. Goate, G. S. Byrd, W. A. Kukull, T. M. Foroud, J. L. Haines, L. A. Farrer, M. A. Pericak-Vance, G. D. Schellenberg, R. Mayeux, and Alzheimer Disease Genetics Consortium. 2013. Variants in the ATP-binding cassette transporter (*ABCA7*), Apolipoprotein E ε4, and the risk of late-onset Alzheimer disease in African Americans. JAMA 309(14):1483-1492.

Reitz, C., M. A. Pericak-Vance, T. Foroud, and R. Mayeux. 2023. A global view of the genetic basis of Alzheimer's disease. *Nature Reviews Neurology* 19(5):261-277.

Reuben, A., L. S. Richmond-Rakerd, B. Milne, D. Shah, A. Pearson, S. Hogan, D. Ireland, R. Keenan, A. R. Knodt, T. Melzer, R. Poulton, S. Ramrakha, E. T. Whitman, A. R. Hariri, T. E. Moffitt, and A. Caspi. 2024. Dementia, dementia's risk factors and premorbid brain structure are concentrated in disadvantaged areas: National register and birth-cohort geographic analyses. *Alzheimer's & Dementia* 20(5):3167-3178.

Roberson, E. D. 2012. Mouse models of frontotemporal dementia. *Annals of Neurology* 72(6):837-849.

Robinson, J. L., H. Richardson, S. X. Xie, E. Suh, V. M. Van Deerlin, B. Alfaro, N. Loh, M. Porras-Paniagua, J. J. Nirschl, D. Wolk, V. M. Lee, E. B. Lee, and J. Q. Trojanowski. 2021. The development and convergence of co-pathologies in Alzheimer's disease. *Brain* 144(3):953-962.

Rongve, A., A. Witoelar, A. Ruiz, L. Athanasiu, C. Abdelnour, J. Clarimon, S. Heilmann-Heimbach, I. Hernández, S. Moreno-Grau, I. de Rojas, E. Morenas-Rodríguez, T. Fladby, S. B. Sando, G. Bråthen, F. Blanc, O. Bousiges, A. W. Lemstra, I. van Steenoven, E. Londos, I. S. Almdahl, L. Pålhaugen, J. A. Eriksen, S. Djurovic, E. Stordal, I. Saltvedt, I. D. Ulstein, F. Bettella, R. S. Desikan, A. V. Idland, M. Toft, L. Pihlstrøm, J. Snaedal, L. Tárraga, M. Boada, A. Lleó, H. Stefánsson, K. Stefánsson, A. Ramírez, D. Aarsland, and O. A. Andreassen. 2019. *GBA* and *APOE* ε4 associate with sporadic dementia with Lewy bodies in European genome wide association study. *Scientific Reports* 9(1):7013.

Rozek, L. S., D. C. Dolinoy, M. A. Sartor, and G. S. Omenn. 2014. Epigenetics: Relevance and implications for public health. *Annual Review of Public Health* 35:105-122.

Rubinsztein, D. C., G. Marino, and G. Kroemer. 2011. Autophagy and aging. *Cell* 146(5):682-695.

Ryu, J. K., and J. G. McLarnon. 2009. A leaky blood-brain barrier, fibrinogen infiltration and microglial reactivity in inflamed Alzheimer's disease brain. *Journal of Cellular and Molecular Medicine* 13(9A):2911-2925.

Safarlou, C. W., K. R. Jongsma, R. Vermeulen, and A. L. Bredenoord. 2023. The ethical aspects of exposome research: A systematic review. *Exposome* 3(1):osad004.

Salter, M. W., and B. Stevens. 2017. Microglia emerge as central players in brain disease. *Nature Medicine* 23(9):1018-1027.

Sampson, T. R., J. W. Debelius, T. Thron, S. Janssen, G. G. Shastri, Z. E. Ilhan, C. Challis, C. E. Schretter, S. Rocha, V. Gradinaru, M. F. Chesselet, A. Keshavarzian, K. M. Shannon, R. Krajmalnik-Brown, P. Wittung-Stafshede, R. Knight, and S. K. Mazmanian. 2016. Gut microbiota regulate motor deficits and neuroinflammation in a model of Parkinson's disease. *Cell* 167(6):1469-1480 e1412.

Sander, M., J. Brown, K. Lunnon, and C. Ballard. 2023. Characterising the D409V/WT mouse as a novel model of Lewy body dementia. *Alzheimer's & Dementia* 19(S12).

Scheltens, P., B. De Strooper, M. Kivipelto, H. Holstege, G. Chételat, C. E. Teunissen, J. Cummings, and W. M. van der Flier. 2021. Alzheimer's disease. *Lancet* 397(10284):1577-1590.

Schrott, R., A. Song, and C. Ladd-Acosta. 2022. Epigenetics as a biomarker for early-life environmental exposure. *Current Environmental Health Reports* 9:604-624.

Schumacher, B., J. Pothof, J. Vijg, and J. H. J. Hoeijmakers. 2021. The central role of DNA damage in the ageing process. *Nature* 592(7856):695-703.

Scrivo, A., M. Bourdenx, O. Pampliega, and A. M. Cuervo. 2018. Selective autophagy as a potential therapeutic target for neurodegenerative disorders. *Lancet Neurology* 17(9):802-815.

SenNet Consortium. 2022. NIH SenNet consortium to map senescent cells throughout the human lifespan to understand physiological health. *Nature Aging* 2(12):1090-1100.

Seok, J., H. S. Warren, A. G. Cuenca, M. N. Mindrinos, H. V. Baker, W. Xu, D. R. Richards, G. P. McDonald-Smith, H. Gao, L. Hennessy, C. C. Finnerty, C. M. Lopez, S. Honari, E. E. Moore, J. P. Minei, J. Cuschieri, P. E. Bankey, J. L. Johnson, J. Sperry, A. B. Nathens, T. R. Billiar, M. A. West, M. G. Jeschke, M. B. Klein, R. L. Gamelli, N. S. Gibran, B. H. Brownstein, C. Miller-Graziano, S. E. Calvano, P. H. Mason, J. P. Cobb, L. G. Rahme, S. F. Lowry, R. V. Maier, L. L. Moldawer, D. N. Herndon, R. W. Davis, W. Xiao, R. G. Tompkins, and the Inflammation and Host Response to Injury, Large Scale Collaborative Research Program. 2013. Genomic responses in mouse models poorly mimic human inflammatory diseases. *Proceedings of the National Academy of Sciences USA* 110(9):3507-3512.

Shen, Q., K. T. Patten, A. Valenzuela, P. J. Lein, and A. Y. Taha. 2022. Probing changes in brain esterified oxylipin concentrations during the early stages of pathogenesis in Alzheimer's disease transgenic rats. *Neuroscience Letters* 791:136921.

Shi, L., K. Steenland, H. Li, P. Liu, Y. Zhang, R. H. Lyles, W. J. Requia, S. D. Ilango, H. H. Chang, T. Wingo, R. J. Weber, and J. Schwartz. 2021. A national cohort study (2000-2018) of long-term air pollution exposure and incident dementia in older adults in the United States. *Nature Communication* 12(1):6754.

Shigemizu, D., R. Mitsumori, S. Akiyama, A. Miyashita, T. Morizono, S. Higaki, Y. Asanomi, N. Hara, G. Tamiya, K. Kinoshita, T. Ikeuchi, S. Niida, and K. Ozaki. 2021. Ethnic and trans-ethnic genome-wide association studies identify new loci influencing Japanese Alzheimer's disease risk. *Translational Psychiatry* 11(1):151.

Shih, R. A., H. Hu, M. G. Weisskopf, and B. S. Schwartz. 2007. Cumulative lead dose and cognitive function in adults: A review of studies that measured both blood lead and bone lead. *Environmental Health Perspectives* 115(3):483-492.

Shireby, G. L., J. P. Davies, P. T. Francis, J. Burrage, E. M. Walker, G. W. A. Neilson, A. Dahir, A. J. Thomas, S. Love, R. G. Smith, K. Lunnon, M. Kumari, L. C. Schalkwyk, K. Morgan, K. Brookes, E. Hannon, and J. Mill. 2020. Recalibrating the epigenetic clock: Implications for assessing biological age in the human cortex. *Brain* 143(12):3763-3775.

Sierra, F. 2016. The emergence of geroscience as an interdisciplinary approach to the enhancement of health span and life span. *Cold Spring Harbor Perspectives in Medicine* 6(4):a025163.

Sierra, F., A. Caspi, R. H. Fortinsky, L. Haynes, G. J. Lithgow, T. E. Moffitt, S. J. Olshansky, D. Perry, E. Verdin, and G. A. Kuchel. 2021. Moving geroscience from the bench to clinical care and health policy. *Journal of the American Geriatric Society* 69(9):2455-2463.

Silberstein, M., N. Nesbit, J. Cai, and P. H. Lee. 2021. Pathway analysis for genome-wide genetic variation data: Analytic principles, latest developments, and new opportunities. *Journal of Genetics and Genomics* 48(3):173-183.

Sims, R., M. Hill, and J. Williams. 2020. The multiplex model of the genetics of Alzheimer's disease. *Nature Neuroscience* 23(3):311-322.

Sinclair, D., A. J. Canty, J. M. Ziebell, A. Woodhouse, J. M. Collins, S. Perry, E. Roccati, M. Kuruvilla, J. Leung, R. Atkinson, J. C. Vickers, A. L. Cook, and A. E. King. 2024. Experimental laboratory models as tools for understanding modifiable dementia risk. *Alzheimer's & Dementia* 20(6):4260-4289.

Sipilä, P. N., N. Heikkila, J. V. Lindbohm, C. Hakulinen, J. Vahtera, M. Elovainio, S. Suominen, A. Vaananen, A. Koskinen, S. T. Nyberg, J. Pentti, T. E. Strandberg, and M. Kivimaki. 2021. Hospital-treated infectious diseases and the risk of dementia: A large, multicohort, observational study with a replication cohort. *Lancet Infectious Diseases* 21(11):1557-1567.

Siroux, V., L. Agier, and R. Slama. 2016. The exposome concept: A challenge and a potential driver for environmental health research. *European Respiratory Review* 25(140):124-129.

Slanzi, A., G. Iannoto, B. Rossi, E. Zenaro, and G. Constantin. 2020. In vitro models of neurodegenerative diseases. *Frontiers in Cell and Developmental Biology* 8:328.

Smith, M. 2024. *Panelist Remarks.* Committee on Research Priorities for Preventing and Treating Alzheimer's Disease and Related Dementias Public Workshop, Hybrid. January 16–17, 2024.

Steele, O. G., A. C. Stuart, L. Minkley, K. Shaw, O. Bonnar, S. Anderle, A. C. Penn, J. Rusted, L. Serpell, C. Hall, and S. King. 2022. A multi-hit hypothesis for an *APOE4*-dependent pathophysiological state. *European Journal of Neuroscience* 56(9):5476-5515.

Stephan, B. C. M., L. Cochrane, A. H. Kafadar, J. Brain, E. Burton, B. Myers, C. Brayne, A. Naheed, K. J. Anstey, A. W. Ashor, and M. Siervo. 2024. Population attributable fractions of modifiable risk factors for dementia: A systematic review and meta-analysis. *Lancet Healthy Longevity* 5(6):e406-e421.

Stern, Y., C. A. Barnes, C. Grady, R. N. Jones, and N. Raz. 2019. Brain reserve, cognitive reserve, compensation, and maintenance: Operationalization, validity, and mechanisms of cognitive resilience. *Neurobiology and Aging* 83:124-129.

Stern, Y., M. Albert, C. A. Barnes, R. Cabeza, A. Pascual-Leone, and P. R. Rapp. 2023. A framework for concepts of reserve and resilience in aging. *Neurobiology and Aging* 124:100-103.

Stites, S. D., S. Midgett, D. Mechanic-Hamilton, M. Zuelsdorff, C. M. Glover, D. X. Marquez, J. E. Balls-Berry, M. L. Streitz, G. Babulal, J. F. Trani, J. N. Henderson, L. L. Barnes, J. Karlawish, and D. A. Wolk. 2022. Establishing a framework for gathering structural and social determinants of health in Alzheimer's disease research centers. *Gerontologist* 62(5):694-703.

Streit, W. J., and Q. S. Xue. 2014. Human CNS immune senescence and neurodegeneration. *Current Opinion in Immunology* 29:93-96.

Stylianou, M., B. Zaaimi, A. Thomas, J. P. Taylor, and F. E. N. LeBeau. 2020. Early disruption of cortical sleep-related oscillations in a mouse model of dementia with Lewy bodies (DLB) expressing human mutant (A30P) alpha-synuclein. *Frontiers in Neuroscience* 14:579867.

Sukoff Rizzo, S. J., G. Homanics, D. J. Schaeffer, L. Schaeffer, J. E. Park, J. Oluoch, T. Zhang, A. Haber, N. T. Seyfried, B. Paten, A. Greenwood, T. Murai, S. H. Choi, H. Huhe, J. Kofler, P. L. Strick, G. W. Carter, and A. C. Silva. 2023. Bridging the rodent to human translational gap: Marmosets as model systems for the study of Alzheimer's disease. *Alzheimer's & Dementia (N Y)* 9(3):e12417.

Sun, J. K., D. Wu, G. C. Wong, T. M. Lau, M. Yang, R. P. Hart, K. M. Kwan, H. Y. E. Chan, and H. M. Chow. 2023. Chronic alcohol metabolism results in DNA repair infidelity and cell cycle-induced senescence in neurons. *Aging Cell* 22(2):e13772.

Swardfager, W., K. Lanctot, L. Rothenburg, A. Wong, J. Cappell, and N. Herrmann. 2010. A meta-analysis of cytokines in Alzheimer's disease. *Biological Psychiatry* 68(10):930-941.

Swerdlow, R. H., and S. M. Khan. 2004. A "mitochondrial cascade hypothesis" for sporadic Alzheimer's disease. *Medical Hypotheses* 63(1):8-20.

Swerdlow, R. H., S. Koppel, I. Weidling, C. Hayley, Y. Ji, and H. M. Wilkins. 2017. Mitochondria, cybrids, aging, and Alzheimer's disease. In *Progress in molecular biology and translational science.* Edited by P. H. Reddy. Vol. 146. Cambridge, MA: Academic Press. Pp. 259-302.

Taha, A. 2024. *Panelist Remarks.* Committee on Research Priorities for Preventing and Treating Alzheimer's Disease and Related Dementias Public Workshop, Hybrid. January 16–17, 2024.

Tamiz, A. P., W. J. Koroshetz, N. T. Dhruv, and D. A. Jett. 2022. A focus on the neural exposome. *Neuron* 110(8):1286-1289.

Tejera, D., D. Mercan, J. M. Sanchez-Caro, M. Hanan, D. Greenberg, H. Soreq, E. Latz, D. Golenbock, and M. T. Heneka. 2019. Systemic inflammation impairs microglial Aβ clearance through NLRP3 inflammasome. *EMBO Journal* 38(17):e101064.

Terron, H. M., S. J. Parikh, S. O. Abdul-Hay, T. Sahara, D. Kang, D. W. Dickson, P. Saftig, F. M. LaFerla, S. Lane, and M. A. Leissring. 2024. Prominent tauopathy and intracellular beta-amyloid accumulation triggered by genetic deletion of cathepsin D: Implications for Alzheimer disease pathogenesis. *Alzheimer's Research & Therapy* 16(1):70.

Theurey, P., and P. Pizzo. 2018. The aging mitochondria. *Genes (Basel)* 9(1):22.

Thurmond, V. A. 2001. The point of triangulation. *Journal of Nursing Scholarship* 33(3):253-258.

Tijms, B. M., E. M. Vromen, O. Mjaavatten, H. Holstege, L. M. Reus, S. van der Lee, K. E. J. Wesenhagen, L. Lorenzini, L. Vermunt, V. Venkatraghavan, N. Tesi, J. Tomassen, A. den Braber, J. Goossens, E. Vanmechelen, F. Barkhof, Y. A. L. Pijnenburg, W. M. van der Flier, C. E. Teunissen, F. S. Berven, and P. J. Visser. 2024. Cerebrospinal fluid proteomics in patients with Alzheimer's disease reveals five molecular subtypes with distinct genetic risk profiles. *Nature Aging* 4(1):33-47.

Traxler, L., J. R. Herdy, D. Stefanoni, S. Eichhorner, S. Pelucchi, A. Szucs, A. Santagostino, Y. Kim, R. K. Agarwal, J. C. M. Schlachetzki, C. K. Glass, J. Lagerwall, D. Galasko, F. H. Gage, A. D'Alessandro, and J. Mertens. 2022. Warburg-like metabolic transformation underlies neuronal degeneration in sporadic Alzheimer's disease. *Cell Metabolism* 34(9):1248-1263, e1246.

Traxler, L., R. Lucciola, J. R. Herdy, J. R. Jones, J. Mertens, and F. H. Gage. 2023. Neural cell state shifts and fate loss in ageing and age-related diseases. *Nature Reviews Neurology* 19(7):434-443.

TREAT-AD (TaRget Enablement to Accelerate Therapy Development for Alzheimer's Disease). 2024. *Two centers, one mission.* https://treatad.org/about/ (accessed October 18, 2024).

Trotter, M. B., T. D. Stephens, J. P. McGrath, and M. L. Steinhilb. 2017. The *Drosophila* model system to study tau action. *Methods in Cell Biology* 141:259-286.

Uemura, M. T., T. Maki, M. Ihara, V. M. Y. Lee, and J. Q. Trojanowski. 2020. Brain microvascular pericytes in vascular cognitive impairment and dementia. *Frontiers in Aging Neuroscience* 12:80.

Van Deerlin, V. M., P. M. Sleiman, M. Martinez-Lage, A. Chen-Plotkin, L. S. Wang, N. R. Graff-Radford, D. W. Dickson, R. Rademakers, B. F. Boeve, M. Grossman, S. E. Arnold, D. M. Mann, S. M. Pickering-Brown, H. Seelaar, P. Heutink, J. C. van Swieten, J. R. Murrell, B. Ghetti, S. Spina, J. Grafman, J. Hodges, M. G. Spillantini, S. Gilman, A. P. Lieberman, J. A. Kaye, R. L. Woltjer, E. H. Bigio, M. Mesulam, S. Al-Sarraj, C. Troakes, R. N. Rosenberg, C. L. White, 3rd, I. Ferrer, A. Llado, M. Neumann, H. A. Kretzschmar, C. M. Hulette, K. A. Welsh-Bohmer, B. L. Miller, A. Alzualde, A. Lopez de Munain, A. C. McKee, M. Gearing, A. I. Levey, J. J. Lah, J. Hardy, J. D. Rohrer, T. Lashley, I. R. Mackenzie, H. H. Feldman, R. L. Hamilton, S. T. Dekosky, J. van der Zee, S. Kumar-Singh, C. Van Broeckhoven, R. Mayeux, J. P. Vonsattel, J. C. Troncoso, J. J. Kril, J. B. Kwok, G. M. Halliday, T. D. Bird, P. G. Ince, P. J. Shaw, N. J. Cairns, J. C. Morris, C. A. McLean, C. DeCarli, W. G. Ellis, S. H. Freeman, M. P. Frosch, J. H. Growdon, D. P. Perl, M. Sano, D. A. Bennett, J. A. Schneider, T. G. Beach, E. M. Reiman, B. K. Woodruff, J. Cummings, H. V. Vinters, C. A. Miller, H. C. Chui, I. Alafuzoff, P. Hartikainen, D. Seilhean, D. Galasko, E. Masliah, C. W. Cotman, M. T. Tunon, M. C. Martinez, D. G. Munoz, S. L. Carroll, D. Marson, P. F. Riederer, N. Bogdanovic, G. D. Schellenberg, H. Hakonarson, J. Q. Trojanowski, and V. M. Lee. 2010. Common variants at 7p21 are associated with frontotemporal lobar degeneration with TDP-43 inclusions. *Nature Genetics* 42(3):234-239.

van Oijen, M., J. C. Witteman, A. Hofman, P. J. Koudstaal, and M. M. Breteler. 2005. Fibrinogen is associated with an increased risk of Alzheimer's disease and vascular dementia. *Stroke* 36(12):2637-2641.

Vasic, V., K. Barth, and M. H. H. Schmidt. 2019. Neurodegeneration and neuro-regeneration—Alzheimer's disease and stem cell therapy. *International Journal of Molecular Sciences* 20(17):4272.

Vandereyken, K., A. Sifrim, B. Thienpont, and T. Voet. 2023. Methods and applications for single-cell and spatial multi-omics. *Nature Reviews Genetics* 24(8):494-515.

Vermeulen, R., E. L. Schymanski, A. L. Barabasi, and G. W. Miller. 2020. The exposome and health: Where chemistry meets biology. *Science* 367(6476):392-396.

Vestin, E., G. Bostrom, J. Olsson, F. Elgh, L. Lind, L. Kilander, H. Lovheim, and B. Weidung. 2024. Herpes simplex viral infection doubles the risk of dementia in a contemporary cohort of older adults: A prospective study. *Journal of Alzheimer's Disease* 97(4):1841-1850.

Viggars, A. P., S. B. Wharton, J. E. Simpson, F. E. Matthews, C. Brayne, G. M. Savva, C. Garwood, D. Drew, P. J. Shaw, and P. G. Ince. 2011. Alterations in the blood brain barrier in ageing cerebral cortex in relationship to Alzheimer-type pathology: A study in the MRC-CFAS population neuropathology cohort. *Neuroscience Letters* 505(1):25-30.

Vineis, P., O. Robinson, M. Chadeau-Hyam, A. Dehghan, I. Mudway, and S. Dagnino. 2020. What is new in the exposome? *Environment International* 143:105887.

Walsemann, K., N. Hair, M. Farina, P. Tyagi, H. Jackson, and J. Ailshire. 2023. State-level desegregation in the U.S. South and mid-life cognitive function among Black and White adults. *Social Science and Medicine* 338(116319).

Wang, Z. and G. Chen. 2023. Immune regulation in neurovascular units after traumatic brain injury. *Neurobiology of Disease* 179:106060.

Wang, X., H. J. He, X. Xiong, S. Zhou, W. W. Wang, L. Feng, R. Han, and C. L. Xie. 2021. NAD+ in Alzheimer's disease: Molecular mechanisms and systematic therapeutic evidence obtained in vivo. *Frontiers in Cell and Developmental Biology* 9:668491.

Wang, C., S. Zong, X. Cui, X. Wang, S. Wu, L. Wang, Y. Liu, and Z. Lu. 2023. The effects of microglia-associated neuroinflammation on Alzheimer's disease. *Frontiers of Immunology* 14:1117172.

Ward-Caviness, C. K., J. C. Nwanaji-Enwerem, K. Wolf, S. Wahl, E. Colicino, L. Trevisi, I. Kloog, A. C. Just, P. Vokonas, J. Cyrys, C. Gieger, J. Schwartz, A. A. Baccarelli, A. Schneider, and A. Peters. 2016. Long-term exposure to air pollution is associated with biological aging. *Oncotarget* 15(7):74510-74525.

Watanabe, C., T. Imaizumi, H. Kawai, K. Suda, Y. Honma, M. Ichihashi, M. Ema, and K.-i. Mizutani. 2020. Aging of the vascular system and neural diseases. *Frontiers in Aging Neuroscience* 12:557384.

WHO (World Health Organization). 2022. *Ageing and health.* https://www.who.int/news-room/fact-sheets/detail/ageing-and-health (accessed August 16, 2024).

Wild, C. P. 2005. Complementing the genome with an "exposome": The outstanding challenge of environmental exposure measurement in molecular epidemiology. *Cancer Epidemiology, Biomarkers and Prevention* 14(8):1847-1850.

Wilker, E. H., M. Osman, and M. G. Weisskopf. 2023. Ambient air pollution and clinical dementia: Systematic review and meta-analysis. *BMJ* 381:e071620.

Wilkins, H. M., and R. H. Swerdlow. 2021. Mitochondrial links between brain aging and Alzheimer's disease. *Translational Neurodegeneration* 10(1):33.

Wilson, R. S., J. A. Schneider, J. L. Bienias, S. E. Arnold, D. A. Evans, and D. A. Bennett. 2003. Depressive symptoms, clinical AD, and cortical plaques and tangles in older persons. *Neurology* 61(8):1102-1107.

Wilson, R., S. Arnold, J. Schneider, J. Kelly, Y. Tang, and D. A. Bennett. 2006. Chronic psychological distress and risk of Alzheimer's disease in old age. *Neuroepidemiology* 27(3):143-153.

Wilson, R. S., S. E. Arnold, J. A. Schneider, Y. Li, and D. A. Bennett. 2007a. Chronic distress, age-related neuropathology, and late-life dementia. *Psychosomatic Medicine* 69(1):47-53.

Wilson, R. S., K. Krueger, S. Arnold, J. Schneider, J. Kelly, L. Barnes, Y. Tang, and D. Bennet. 2007b. Loneliness and risk of Alzheimer's disease. *Archives of General Psychiatry* 64(2):234-240.

Xu, P., M. Wang, W. M. Song, Q. Wang, G. C. Yuan, P. H. Sudmant, H. Zare, Z. Tu, M. E. Orr, and B. Zhang. 2022. The landscape of human tissue and cell type specific expression and co-regulation of senescence genes. *Molecular Neurodegeneration* 17(1):5.

Yamanaka, S. 2012. Induced pluripotent stem cells: Past, present, and future. *Cell Stem Cell* 10(6):678-684.

Yan, X., Y. Hu, B. Wang, S. Wang, and X. Zhang. 2020. Metabolic dysregulation contributes to the progression of Alzheimer's disease. *Frontiers in Neuroscience* 14:530219.

Yang, W., X. Chen, S. Li, and X. J. Li. 2021. Genetically modified large animal models for investigating neurodegenerative diseases. *Cell & Bioscience* 11(1):218.

Yin, F., R. Banerjee, B. Thomas, P. Zhou, L. Qian, T. Jia, X. Ma, Y. Ma, C. Iadecola, M. F. Beal, C. Nathan, and A. Ding. 2010. Exaggerated inflammation, impaired host defense, and neuropathology in progranulin-deficient mice. *Journal of Experimental Medicine* 207(1):117-128.

Yousefzadeh, M. J., J. E. Wilkinson, B. Hughes, N. Gadela, W. C. Ladiges, N. Vo, L. J. Niedernhofer, D. M. Huffman, and P. D. Robbins. 2020. Heterochronic parabiosis regulates the extent of cellular senescence in multiple tissues. *GeroScience* 42(3):951-961.

Yousefzadeh, M. J., R. R. Flores, Y. Zhu, Z. C. Schmiechen, R. W. Brooks, C. E. Trussoni, Y. Cui, L. Angelini, K. A. Lee, S. J. McGowan, A. L. Burrack, D. Wang, Q. Dong, A. Lu, T. Sano, R. D. O'Kelly, C. A. McGuckian, J. I. Kato, M. P. Bank, E. A. Wade, S. P. S. Pillai, J. Klug, W. C. Ladiges, C. E. Burd, S. E. Lewis, N. F. LaRusso, N. V. Vo, Y. Wang, E. E. Kelley, J. Huard, I. M. Stromnes, P. D. Robbins, and L. J. Niedernhofer. 2021. An aged immune system drives senescence and ageing of solid organs. *Nature* 594(7861):100-105.

Yu, L., L. B. Chibnik, G. P. Srivastava, N. Pochet, J. Yang, J. Xu, J. Kozubek, N. Obholzer, S. E. Leurgans, J. A. Schneider, A. Meissner, P. L. De Jager, and D. A. Bennett. 2015. Association of brain DNA methylation in SORL1, ABCA7, HLA-DRB5, SLC24A4, and BIN1 with pathological diagnosis of Alzheimer's disease. *JAMA Neurology* 72(1):15-24.

Zammit, A. R., D. A. Bennett, and A. S. Buchman. 2023. From theory to practice: Translating the concept of cognitive resilience to novel therapeutic targets that maintain cognition in aging adults. *Frontiers in Aging and Neuroscience* 15:1303912.

Zhang, B., and V. N. Gladyshev. 2020. How can aging be reversed? Exploring rejuvenation from a damage-based perspective. *Advances in Genetics (Hoboken)* 1(1):e10025.

Zhang, B., C. Gaiteri, L. G. Bodea, Z. Wang, J. McElwee, A. A. Podtelezhnikov, C. Zhang, T. Xie, L. Tran, R. Dobrin, E. Fluder, B. Clurman, S. Melquist, M. Narayanan, C. Suver, H. Shah, M. Mahajan, T. Gillis, J. Mysore, M. E. MacDonald, J. R. Lamb, D. A. Bennett, C. Molony, D. J. Stone, V. Gudnason, A. J. Myers, E. E. Schadt, H. Neumann, J. Zhu, and V. Emilsson. 2013. Integrated systems approach identifies genetic nodes and networks in late-onset Alzheimer's disease. *Cell* 153(3):707-720.

Zhang, B., J. Weuve, K. M. Langa, J. D'Souza, A. Szpiro, J. Faul, C. Mendes de Leon, J. Gao, J. D. Kaufman, L. Sheppard, J. Lee, L. C. Kobayashi, R. Hirth, and S. D. Adar. 2023a. Comparison of particulate air pollution from different emission sources and incident dementia in the U.S. *JAMA Internal Medicine* 183(10):1080-1089.

Zhang, L., T. M. Flagan, S. Häkkinen, S. A. Chu, J. A. Brown, A. J. Lee, L. Pasquini, M. L. Mandelli, M. L. Gorno-Tempini, V. E. Sturm, J. S. Yokoyama, B. S. Appleby, Y. Cobigo, B. C. Dickerson, K. Domoto-Reilly, D. H. Geschwind, N. Ghoshal, N. R. Graff-Radford, M. Grossman, G. R. Hsiung, E. D. Huey, K. Kantarci, A. Lario Lago, I. Litvan, I. R. Mackenzie, M. F. Mendez, C. U. Onyike, E. M. Ramos, E. D. Roberson, M. C. Tartaglia, A. W. Toga, S. Weintraub, Z. K. Wszolek, L. K. Forsberg, H. W. Heuer, B. F. Boeve, A. L. Boxer, H. J. Rosen, B. L. Miller, W. W. Seeley, S. E. Lee and ARTFL/LEFFTDS/ALLFTD Consortia. 2023b. Network Connectivity Alterations across the MAPT Mutation Clinical Spectrum. *Annals of Neurology* 94(4):632-646.

Zhang, L., F. Xu, Y. Yang, L. Yang, Q. Wu, H. Sun, Z. An, J. Li, H. Wu, J. Song, and W. Wu. 2024. PM$_{2.5}$ exposure upregulates pro-inflammatory protein expression in human microglial cells via oxidant stress and TLR4/NF-κB pathway. *Ecotoxicology and Environmental Safety* 277:116386.

Zhang, M., and Z. Bian. 2021. Alzheimer's disease and microRNA-132: A widespread pathological factor and potential therapeutic target. *Frontiers in Neuroscience* 15:687973.

Zhang, M., A. B. Ganz, S. Rohde, A. J. M. Rozemuller, N. B. Bank, M. J. T. Reinders, P. Scheltens, M. Hulsman, J. J. M. Hoozemans, and H. Holstege. 2023e. Resilience and resistance to the accumulation of amyloid plaques and neurofibrillary tangles in centenarians: An age-continuous perspective. *Alzheimer's & Dementia* 19(7):2831-2841.

Zhang, P., Y. Kishimoto, I. Grammatikakis, K. Gottimukkala, R. G. Cutler, S. Zhang, K. Abdelmohsen, V. A. Bohr, J. Misra Sen, M. Gorospe, and M. P. Mattson. 2019. Senolytic therapy alleviates Aβ-associated oligodendrocyte progenitor cell senescence and cognitive deficits in an Alzheimer's disease model. *Nature Neuroscience* 22(5):719-728.

Zhang, W., D. Xiao, Q. Mao, and H. Xia. 2023c. Role of neuroinflammation in neurodegeneration development. *Signal Transduction and Targeted Therapy* 8(1):267.

Zhang, Z. Y., D. S. Harischandra, R. Wang, S. Ghaisas, J. Y. Zhao, T. P. McMonagle, G. Zhu, K. D. Lacuarta, J. Song, J. Q. Trojanowski, H. Xu, V. M. Lee, and X. Yang. 2023d. TRIM11 protects against tauopathies and is down-regulated in Alzheimer's disease. *Science* 381(6656):eadd6696.

Zheng, Y., L. Bonfili, T. Wei, and A. M. Eleuteri. 2023. Understanding the gut–brain axis and its therapeutic implications for neurodegenerative disorders. *Nutrients* 15(21):4631.

4

Development and Evaluation of Interventions for the Prevention and Treatment of AD/ADRD

The committee was charged with reviewing and synthesizing the most promising areas of research into preventing and treating Alzheimer's disease and related dementias (AD/ADRD), including nonpharmacological interventions (NPIs) and pharmacological interventions, and combinations thereof. To address this aspect of its task, the committee relied on input from a variety of sources. These included information and perspectives shared during a public workshop and findings from a scoping review of existing systematic reviews of the evidence on pharmacological agents and NPIs, supplemented with targeted literature searches of interventions not captured in the recent systematic reviews examined by the committee.

The committee was encouraged by the diversity of preventive and therapeutic interventions that are being evaluated for effectiveness against AD/ADRD, representing a notable expansion of intervention targets that reflects the growing understanding of the complex and multifactorial pathways that contribute to AD/ADRD (see Chapter 3). This expansion in candidate interventions demonstrates the value of the investments in basic and translational science that have been made over the last decade. Still, there is much additional work to be accomplished. There remains considerable uncertainty about steps that can be taken to prevent and slow the progression of AD/ADRD and about the optimal timing and strategy for intervening to maintain brain health. As a result, the substantial scientific advances in AD/ADRD research in recent years have not translated into a widespread perception of progress among the public and policy makers. This arises in part from a failure to effectively communicate important achievements to audiences outside of the scientific community. Communication efforts aimed at sharing progress on dementia prevention and treatment with the public need to be programmatically enabled and use formats accessible to the public (e.g., social media). The perceptions of stalled progress also underscores an urgent need for more rapid development of interventions to prevent or cure AD/ADRD, as well as treatments that substantially enhance the lives of people living with these diseases and those of their families, care partners, and caregivers.

This chapter presents the committee's assessment of the evidence on interventions to prevent and treat AD/ADRD and opportunities to accelerate progress. The chapter begins with a discussion of a framework that lays out the multiple dimensions for consideration in the pursuit of prevention and treatment strategies. It then highlights interventions that have promise for preventing, delaying, slowing, halting, or reversing AD/ADRD. This is followed by a discussion of strategies for improving clinical trials to accelerate the development of interventions that are safe and effective for the vastly heterogeneous populations at risk for and living with AD/ADRD and that have the potential to reduce the societal impact of these diseases. The chapter ends with a discussion of opportunities to advance a precision medicine approach to ensure people are getting the right combination of interventions at the right time based on their specific characteristics and stage in both the life-course and the brain health continuum.

A FRAMEWORK FOR CONSIDERING
PREVENTION AND TREATMENT STRATEGIES

In considering opportunities and potential strategies for preventing and treating AD/ADRD, multiple dimensions need to be considered, including

- type of intervention (pharmacological versus nonpharmacological)
- target of intervention,
- life-course timing,
- balance of benefits and harms,
- level of intervention (population versus individual levels), and
- potential public health effects.

Type of Intervention

Interventions for preventing or treating AD/ADRD may be pharmacological, nonpharmacological, or a combination of both. NPIs represent a diverse collection of intervention strategies (Li et al., 2023), many of which target modifiable risk factors for dementia (Livingston et al., 2024). Included within this broad category are interventions focused on behavior (e.g., diet, use of vitamins and other supplements, exercise, stress management, art-based therapies, mind–body–spirit connection approaches), cognitive stimulation and training, preserved and/or improved hearing, education, and social interactions.

Quite different in form but also falling within the NPI category are neuromodulation procedures—both invasive and noninvasive—including deep brain stimulation, transcranial pulse stimulation, repetitive transcranial magnetic stimulation, and ultrasound (Leinenga et al., 2024). Each type of NPI can be implemented alone (single-component interventions), or multiple NPIs may be combined as part of a multimodal intervention. The Finnish Geriatric Intervention Study to Prevent Cognitive Impairment and Disability (FINGER), which evaluated a combination of diet, exercise, cognitive training, and socialization, is an example of a multimodal NPI (Ngandu et al., 2015). In some studies, the same NPI will be used for all participants, while personalized risk-reduction trials may tailor interventions to the specific risks and preferences of each participant (Yaffe et al., 2024).

Pharmacological agents being evaluated for AD/ADRD include both novel therapeutics and repurposed drugs (i.e., drugs originally approved for an indication other than AD or related dementias) (Thunell et al., 2021). Therapeutics can be in the form of small-molecule drugs or biologics, such as monoclonal antibody infusions and vaccines. The Translational Research and Clinical Interventions category of the Common Alzheimer's Disease Research Ontology (CADRO) provides a standardized mechanism for categorizing targets for therapeutics.[1] Of note, many of the targets are not specific to AD or a related dementia but rather represent more conserved pathways or resilience mechanisms. Like NPIs, pharmacological agents can be used alone or in combination (e.g., anti-amyloid therapy plus a therapeutic targeting a different mechanistic pathway).

Target of Intervention

While interventions commonly target aspects of disease, in the case of AD/ADRD there are also opportunities for interventions to increase an individual's resilience, by building cognitive reserve or enhancing the brain's ability to adapt to neuropathological changes and thereby enhance and/or preserve its function. Resilience-focused strategies have received

---

[1] CADRO lists the following potential targets for drug discovery and development: amyloid beta; tau; apolipoprotein E (APOE), lipids, and lipoprotein receptors; neurotransmitter receptors; or several pathways including neurogenesis; inflammation; oxidative stress; cell death; proteostasis/proteinopathies; metabolism and bioenergetics; vasculature; growth factors and hormones; synaptic plasticity/neuroprotection; gut–brain axis; circadian rhythm; epigenetic regulators; multitarget; unknown target; and other. CADRO is available at https://iadrp.nia.nih.gov/about/cadro (accessed April 16, 2024).

less attention in clinical intervention research but have the benefit of being agnostic to pathology classification, an important consideration given the predominance of mixed forms of dementia. Interventions that (1) promote early-life cognitive development, (2) promote brain health through improved vascular health, (3) reduce brain insults including head injury, stroke, and pathology based on proteins aggregates, or (4) enhance plasticity and reorganization after injury or within the context of disease (i.e., rehabilitation) may all reduce dementia burden. Within each of these categories there are many different intervention approaches. For example, stroke prevention would entail distinct interventions from head injury prevention.

Life-Course Timing

The question of life-course timing as it relates to the prevention and treatment of AD/ADRD is important because although cognitive development is most marked in early life, it continues across the life course, and brain injuries may occur at any age (WHO, 2022). Our understanding of brain plasticity and adaptability in adults is still unfolding, with important progress in recent decades in areas such as stroke recovery. Major opportunities for prevention of AD/ADRD are likely to present from early childhood through old age, but the timing of interventions can significantly shape who will potentially benefit (e.g., current cohorts of older adults will not benefit from childhood interventions) and the time delay before a payoff in terms of dementia prevention.

Much of the emphasis on opportunities for prevention, such as those based on the population attributable fraction popularized in the Lancet Commission report (Livingston et al., 2020, 2024), frames the fraction of cases preventable as a static number. However, the potential for prevention that might be achieved by targeting any specific preventive strategy will vary over time. It should also be acknowledged that preventive strategies that make people healthier means they will live longer, and even as more is understood regarding healthy aging and cognitive decline, age remains one of the strongest risk factors for AD/ADRD.

Balance of Benefits and Harms

The balancing of benefits and harms is integral to considering intervention strategies. While benefits and harms are often thought of in terms of health effects, a broader scope can include other considerations such as financial risk and exposure to stigma. Some interventions are desirable for benefits outside of their potential effect on AD/ADRD (e.g., hypertension management strategies or smoking reduction), or at least are unlikely to have adverse consequences beyond opportunity costs (e.g., brain games). Others have uncertain or, in such cases as monoclonal antibody-based immunotherapies, known potential for harm. The potential for harm is especially important when considering scaling an intervention to a large number of individuals. If a serious adverse event occurs in only 1 percent of individuals, treating 6 million individuals with Alzheimer's disease (AD) will lead to 60,000 such adverse events. The potential for harm is even greater if a treatment with the same rate of adverse events was applied to the nearly 50 million people estimated to be living with preclinical disease (i.e., people with AD pathology but who remain asymptomatic) (Brookmeyer and Abdalla, 2018; NASEM, 2021). Measuring the various benefits and costs (e.g., earnings, hope, medical costs, pain, risk of death) associated with a treatment will support decision making about its use by people living with AD/ADRD and their families.

These harms and benefits can be understood as components of the meaningful value provided by an intervention. Quantifying the value provided by these multiple considerations allows for a more comprehensive understanding of the meaningful benefit that can be offered by an intervention at a societal level (Neumann et al., 2022). For example, a disease modifying therapy that delays cognitive and functional decline at early stages of disease would likely also support greater workforce productivity from both persons living with the disease and their intended caregivers, increased social enjoyment, and reduced time requiring long-term support and services and would provide hope. However, the same therapy may also impose high out-of-pocket costs for patients and families, impose high costs on payers, lead to suffering via treatment administration or side effects, and, if the disease modifying therapy leads to increased risk of treatment-related death, shorten lifespan. Such approaches as dynamic microsimulation modeling can be used to assess the effect of these complex variables to estimate the meaningful benefit of an intervention.

Level of Intervention

Interventions for preventing and treating AD/ADRD can be categorized as targeting an individual or an entire population. Individual-level interventions require individuals to pursue specific behaviors (e.g., engaging in cognitive training), lifestyle changes, or medical treatments, whereas population-level interventions change the context in which individuals live to create a healthier environment or to reduce known determinants of AD/ADRD risk. Such categorization of interventions mirrors the individual- and system- or structural-level components that have a cumulative effect on AD/ADRD outcomes over the life course (see Figure 1-5). Personalized approaches can be used to adapt intervention strategies to reflect variations across individuals and help to overcome some of the barriers that might otherwise hinder adoption and adherence. While pharmacological agents are inherently individual-level interventions, many NPIs can be implemented at the population level, such as through public health initiatives and policy changes.

Population-level interventions ultimately work via changes at an individual level, but they can be implemented at scale. For example, tobacco taxes or indoor smoking bans are population-level interventions geared to ultimately affect individual behaviors, such as those achieved with smoking cessation counseling. Population-level interventions focus on contextual changes, such as public health campaigns to raise awareness of hypertension management for AD/ADRD prevention. Research on health equity has emphasized the greater potential for population-level interventions to narrow equity gaps because individuals who are systematically disadvantaged are less able to take advantage of individual-level programs or behavior modification interventions.

Public Health Impacts

All proposed interventions should be evaluated against their potential to reduce the incidence and prevalence of AD/ADRD, as well as inequalities. This entails considering the feasibility of delivering proposed interventions to all individuals at risk and any differential effects of an intervention across diverse population groups. For many interventions, there may be an interaction with an individual's level of risk, in which case it may be necessary to consider whether those at higher risk are likely to get more, the same, or less benefit. Understanding this interaction effect is important for targeting interventions most effectively—and cost-effectively.

CURRENT STATE OF EVIDENCE ON INTERVENTIONS FOR PREVENTING AND TREATING AD/ADRD

The committee's assessment of the state of evidence on interventions for preventing and treating AD/ADRD was informed, in part, by an analysis of recent systematic reviews that evaluated pharmacological, nonpharmacological, and combination interventions for AD/ADRD. The methods used in the scoping review and descriptive summaries of included systematic reviews can be found in Appendix A. While this approach was useful for developing an overarching view of the landscape of intervention research, it was also subject to biases and limitations. These include the potential for a compounding of biases from individual systematic reviews (e.g., accumulation of publication and selection biases), variation in the quality of the included reviews, variation in the quality of primary literature included in those systematic reviews, overlap in the primary studies included, and the inclusion of outdated information (Ballard and Montgomery, 2017). Additionally, because a limited number of systematic reviews were selected for the scoping review and given the potential lag between publication of primary studies and the conduct of systematic reviews synthesizing the body of evidence, the failure to identify a systematic review for a given intervention or population may not indicate a lack of primary evidence. This represents an important limitation when using a scoping review of existing systematic reviews for a gap analysis. To the extent possible, the review protocol sought to directly address some of these limitations. For these reasons, the committee chose to not make any conclusion on the effectiveness of a given intervention but rather to summarize major findings of relevance and indicate existing research gaps and future needs. Therefore, the committee used this analysis to identify gaps in the research landscape but relied on additional sources of information to guide its identification of promising interventions.

The scoping review captured research on a wide range of NPIs and pharmacological interventions, including some that are well-established as well as more cutting-edge approaches for which there is emerging clinical evidence, such as gene therapy. NPIs reviewed included lifestyle approaches but also more invasive modalities such as brain stimulation. The 65 articles reviewed illustrate a highly active research field that is focused on improving the lives of people living with AD/ADRD. However, this review revealed several critical research gaps in the landscape that impede the generation of the evidence required to develop effective and clinically meaningful interventions for people living with these conditions.

First, the scoping review found a paucity of evidence from studies evaluating population-level interventions. The absence of this evidence could be, in part, caused by limitations of the literature search methodology. However, further evaluation suggests that the effects of population-level interventions, which are often assessed using natural experiments, are rarely comprehensively evaluated, in part because of inadequate data infrastructure (see Chapter 5) (Kind, 2024). Concerted efforts to evaluate population-level interventions are needed to understand the observed decline in dementia prevalence and incidence in some high-income countries and to identify the key contributing factors so the same successes can be achieved in all populations.

Relatedly, very few systematic reviews were identified in the scoping review that assessed combination interventions (e.g., two or more interventions, including at least one pharmacological intervention) as the primary objective of the review. As described previously in this report, combination approaches may be able to target multiple mechanisms simultaneously or sequentially, potentially leading to more effective treatments. The combined use of memantine and cholinesterase inhibitors represents the most commonly studied combination therapy identified in the scoping review, but many other combinations have been assessed (Kabir et al., 2020). The development of anti-amyloid monoclonal antibodies, as well as the demonstrated potential of multimodal approaches targeting modifiable risk factors, has invigorated interest in combination approaches that can be applied prior to or early in the disease trajectory. Several trials are underway to evaluate anti-amyloid antibodies in combination with other agents such as anti-tau agents and antisenescence agents (Cummings et al., 2024), and a trial evaluating the combination of a multidomain lifestyle intervention and metformin (an antidiabetes drug) was recently initiated (Barbera et al., 2023).

Clinical research on combination therapies is operationally complex. Carrying out this research requires access to appropriate clinical trial infrastructure that is capable of delivering multiple therapies acting on different biological pathways across multiple trial centers and conducting factorial design studies. Such research also necessitates the building of cooperative partnerships that enable collaboration between participating companies with candidates available for codevelopment, as well as the necessary philanthropic, federal, and academic partners. Agreements regarding study management, data sharing, investigational new drug possessorship, and new drug application filing responsibilities need to be worked out. Demonstrating the additive or synergistic efficacy and safety of components in combination therapies is more complicated than the evaluation of monotherapies and may require the use of factorial study designs that employ larger sample sizes, which results in increased costs. Additionally, the perceived costs and time requirements to comply with FDA regulatory requirements specific to combination therapies, such as long treatment exposure time and large number of participants, add an additional layer of difficulty (Salloway et al., 2020). The thorough examination of different combination approaches and the quantification of the relative effects of each intervention is essential to optimizing more personalized and effective intervention strategies.

Conclusion 4-1: Combinatorial interventions hold promise for addressing the multifactorial nature of dementia by simultaneously addressing multiple pathways and mechanisms.

Conclusion 4-2: The exploration of combination intervention approaches is limited by operational complexities that necessitate partnership building and access to appropriate clinical trial infrastructure, in addition to complicated and costly study designs. The evaluation of combinatorial interventions that include one or more nonpharmacological approaches is further limited by deficiencies in the rigor of study designs and the required time investment for both investigators and participants.

The most apparent gap identified in the scoping review was the paucity of evidence specific to related dementias. The majority of articles in the review included participant populations living with mild cognitive impairment (MCI) or AD or included a broad participant population iving with dementia. In the latter case, the inclusion and exclusion criteria for dementia varied by study and in many cases related dementias were specifically excluded, whereas in other cases no reference was made to the specific dementia types. Where multiple types of dementia were explicitly included in the study, often insightful subgroup analyses were not possible owing to a lack of individual data or because of significant methodological limitations of the included primary research. Just one systematic review dedicated to assessing pharmacological interventions for frontotemporal dementia (FTD) was identified and included in the scoping review.

Evidence for Lewy body dementia (LBD) and vascular dementia was similarly sparse. No reviews were found that specifically examined mixed etiology dementia. Predictably, exclusions of specific types of dementia were more prevalent in the literature for pharmacological interventions. The absence of evidence for related dementias was compounded by the limited and poor quality of the primary evidence, particularly for LBD and FTD. Juxtaposed against the many systematic reviews of well-designed randomized controlled trials (RCTs) of interventions for AD, the included systematic reviews for LBD and FTD primarily pulled from case reports and uncontrolled trial designs. There are only so many ways the authors can state that more well-designed trials are needed to advance therapies to treat these understudied conditions.

The scoping review was designed to capture a wide range of outcomes and was not restricted to outcomes associated with cognitive function. Cognitive and neuropsychiatric outcomes were most widely reported by the studies included in the scoping review. Functional outcomes and assessments of quality of life and overall well-being, which may be most important to people living with dementia, were rarely reported. In cases where these outcomes were reported, in nearly all cases they were included as secondary outcomes and the studies often lacked sufficient power to reliably detect an effect. Relatedly, in some cases, cognitive outcomes may be secondary outcomes of interest for interventions primarily focused on other health conditions, such as improving cardiovascular health, as was the case for the SPRINT MIND clinical trial.

It is important to note that this assessment represents a snapshot of the state of the evidence at the time of the review and does not take into account the most recently published primary studies, which would not have been included in systematic reviews. Additionally, the scoping review was not designed to capture information regarding the demographics (e.g., race, ethnicity, socioeconomic status) of the research participants included in the primary studies for each of the systematic reviews. However, this does not imply the absence of a gap related to evidence for diverse populations and, as discussed later in this chapter and in Chapter 5, the committee notes that there is a vital need for greater inclusiveness and representativeness in AD/ADRD research.

Promising Interventions for Prevention and Treatment of AD/ADRD

Consideration of Different Endpoints

In considering which interventions under study for preventing and/or treating AD/ADRD show promise, the committee identified the following three categories of interventions based on different endpoints of relevance. Of note, these are not mutually exclusive, and some interventions will fall into more than one of the categories.

Interventions that show promise in improving quality of life and function in daily activities of living This category includes interventions that are not specific to pathologic processes underlying AD/ADRD but may improve overall well-being, quality of life, and the ability to function more independently, which are important outcomes for people living with AD/ADRD. Examples of interventions in this category include art and music therapy, as well as some medications that treat neuropsychiatric symptoms of dementia. Some promising interventions, such as physical activity, may fit in this category and one or both categories that follow, and the evidence for such interventions is discussed in the sections below. Interventions that fit only in this category are generally considered *care interventions*, which are excluded from the committee's charge and are therefore not a primary focus of this report. While not reviewed in depth in this report, interventions that specifically address neuropsychiatric symptoms may make a huge difference for people living with AD/ADRD and their care networks, even if they do not affect biological pathways thought to underlie the disease causing dementia. Such interventions merit priority and rigorous research alongside interventions targeting the biological mechanisms of AD/ADRD. Moreover, the links between treatment of neuropsychiatric symptoms and trajectories of cognitive decline remain inadequately explored and warrant further investigation. Treatment for depression, for example, is not only important to improving quality of life, but may also impact cognitive outcomes (Livingston et al., 2024), though evidence has been mixed and further studies are needed to draw firm conclusions (NASEM, 2017).

Interventions that may have some effect on the prevention of neurodegenerative diseases or the building of brain resilience This category includes those interventions that address known risk factors for the development of AD/ADRD and that may prevent the development of brain pathology or enhance the brain's ability to adapt to neuropathological changes and maintain cognitive function (e.g., through cognitive reserve or neuroplasticity). In many cases, the mechanisms of action for such interventions are not well understood but are likely not specific to a single form of dementia. Examples of interventions that fit in this category (discussed further below) include those targeting social isolation, sensory impairment (e.g., hearing aids), and exposure to neurotoxicants. While it can be challenging to generate strong evidence demonstrating prevention or enhanced resilience, an example of evidence for such interventions is improvement in, or maintenance of, cognition independent of neuropathologic burden (Leng and Yaffe, 2024). Importantly, such interventions are often low cost, relatively safe, may have other health benefits, and could be combined with future therapies specifically targeting neurodegeneration.

Interventions that show promise in slowing neurodegeneration or represent an exciting research area for further exploration of its potential for slowing neurodegeneration   This category includes interventions aimed specifically at slowing or halting the accumulation of neuropathologies and the loss of neurons and synapses in individuals already experiencing neurodegeneration. Many of the promising interventions in this category are relatively new or underexplored and have emerged from recent basic and translational research on mechanistic pathways contributing to AD/ADRD (see Chapter 3). As a result, evidence from large phase 3 efficacy trials may not yet be available, but evidence of promise may come from preclinical research or mechanistic studies. While many emerging pharmacological agents fall into this category, some NPIs also show promise for slowing neurodegeneration.

The sections below discuss the pharmacological interventions and NPIs that the committee believes hold promise for preventing or treating AD/ADRD. For each intervention, the evidence related to each applicable category above is discussed.

Promising NPIs

NPIs can affect any of the three categories of endpoints discussed above. They generally are not targeted to a specific pathology but affect cognition and resilience through other mechanisms.

Cognitive interventions   Cognitive function interventions include several approaches—cognitive training, cognitive rehabilitation, and cognitive stimulation—that target different domains to promote cognitive enhancement and maintenance. These approaches have been applied to a variety of psychiatric and neurodegenerative conditions with the goal of improving cognitive and functional outcomes in these contexts. Cognitive training is intended to strengthen specific cognitive functions through repetitive practice of a defined task or exercise with the goal to achieve generalizing effects beyond the trained task, while cognitive rehabilitation seeks to improve or maintain the cognitive ability to perform everyday tasks and can include compensatory strategies that can be modified at an individual level. Cognitive stimulation includes general engagement-oriented interventions that are intended to broadly enhance cognitive or social functions (e.g., reminiscence therapy) (He et al., 2019; Vemuri et al., 2016). Cognitive training and stimulation may provide a neuroprotective effect by promoting neuroplasticity and the building of cognitive reserve (Park and Bischof, 2013). Importantly, these interventions appear to carry few risks beyond opportunity costs, and can be easily combined with other interventions (see section on multimodal approaches). The effectiveness of these approaches in preventing or slowing cognitive and functional decline associated with AD/ADRD and whether these approaches have broader benefits to overall well-being among older adults have been subjects of extensive research; however, the findings are highly variable.

The ACTIVE study, the first large-scale, randomized trial to evaluate the effect of cognitive training interventions in community-dwelling older adults without significant cognitive impairment found evidence that these interventions may preserve the cognitive abilities necessary to maintain functional competence and to cope with functional impairments even after a long duration (up to 10 years for some intervention groups) (Rebok et al., 2014; Tennstedt and Unverzagt, 2013). Additionally, some evidence was found for reduced risk of dementia over 10 years among participants randomized to a speed-processing cognitive training intervention as compared to untreated controls (Edwards et al., 2017). However, limited high-quality experimental evidence is available to conclude that cognitive training interventions are effective in preventing or slowing cognitive decline in individuals living with MCI (Bahar-Fuchs et al., 2019; Basak et al., 2020; Gates et al., 2019).

Beyond the ACTIVE study, computerized cognitive training approaches have been found to be associated with improvements in global cognition in older, cognitively healthy adults (Bonnechère and Klass, 2023; Gates et al., 2020; Hu et al., 2021; Zhang et al., 2019a) and with improvements to verbal, visual, and working memory in people living with MCI (Chan et al., 2024). Additionally, the use of such immersive modalities as virtual reality technologies benefit global cognition and subdomains of executive functions in people living with MCI (Kim et al., 2019; Papaioannou et al., 2022; Zhong et al., 2021). Cognitive stimulation activities have demonstrated improvements in quality of life and well-being in several observational studies and experimental trials (Gomez-Soria et al., 2023; Tulliani et al., 2022; Vemuri et al., 2016), and cognitive rehabilitation interventions have been linked to improved daily function in people living with mild-to-moderate cognitive impairment due to dementia (Clare et al., 2019). Importantly, although some of the effects summarized here offer some promise, the evidence for commercially available cognitive interventions remains equivocal (Nguyen et al., 2022). Further research is needed to elucidate the mechanisms underlying the function of cognitive interventions and to evaluate their efficacy over time.

Interventions to promote social interaction and reduce social isolation and loneliness Loneliness and social isolation are a growing public health concern owing to accumulating evidence linking these conditions to an increased risk of all-cause mortality (NASEM, 2020; Yu et al., 2023) and other health conditions. Social isolation—"the objective state of having few social relationships or infrequent social contact with others" (NASEM, 2020)—is distinct from loneliness, which is a subjective or perceived feeling of isolation. Of relevance to this report, both are associated with increased risk of dementia (Elovainio et al., 2022; Salinas et al., 2022; Sutin et al., 2020). The mechanisms by which loneliness and social isolation increase dementia risk are not well understood and remain a focus of ongoing study (Guarnera et al., 2023), but loneliness has been linked to several early cognitive and neuroanatomical markers of vulnerability (Salinas et al., 2022).

In observational studies, social activity and social support provide benefit for some measures of cognitive function for community-dwelling adults without AD/ADRD (Baptista et al., 2024), and social contact and engagement have been found to be protective for dementia (Joshi et al., 2024; Livingston et al., 2024). Social interactions may function in part to build cognitive reserve, which confers resilience even in the presence of brain pathologies (Xu et al., 2019). As a result, there is significant interest in interventions to promote social interaction and reduce social isolation and loneliness. Such interventions come in many forms, from in-person facilitator-led group discussions or activities (Kelly et al., 2017) to the use of web-based social networking sites (Baptista et al., 2024).

While some programs focus on creating opportunities for social engagement among older adults, others have been designed with the goal of creating opportunities for nonfamilial intergenerational engagement (Krzeczkowska et al., 2021; Petersen, 2023). The Experience Corp program, for example, trains older adults to volunteer as mentors for children in neighborhood elementary schools during the academic year, which not only addresses the social engagement needs of the adults but has the added potential benefit of improving the academic performance of children in underserved areas. An RCT of the

Baltimore Experience Corps program showed the program led to improved cognitive function, particularly for those with impaired executive function at baseline, as well as physical and social activity (Carlson, 2021; Carlson et al., 2008). Ongoing evaluations seek to determine whether these short-term effects translate to longer-term benefits in reducing risk for dementia. Innovative technologies, such as interactive social robots, are also providing new ways to increase social engagement and potentially reduce social isolation and loneliness in older adults (Baptista et al., 2024; Joshi et al., 2024).

Despite the promise suggested by observational studies and the Experience Corp program, recent reviews show that the results from intervention trials have generally been mixed with regards to the effects on cognitive function and social measures (e.g., loneliness, social identification, perceived social support) in people with and without AD/ADRD (Baptista et al., 2024; Joshi et al., 2024). This may stem, in part, from the heterogeneity of the interventions and outcome measures evaluated in the studies included in the reviews. There is, however, evidence suggesting that interventions to address social isolation and loneliness can improve quality of life in people living with AD/ADRD (Joshi et al., 2024).

While there is currently limited high-quality research on interventions to address social isolation and loneliness, this is an important area for future research and has the potential to offer benefit at the population level. The question of whether earlier and better interventions can not only improve quality of life but also maintain or improve cognition remains unanswered and should be a priority going forward. Given the heterogeneity of existing interventions, future trials would benefit from efforts to determine the specific aspects of social relationships that are needed to benefit cognitive function.

Physical activity interventions   Physical activity (e.g., aerobic exercise, mind–body exercise, strength and resistance training) practiced alone or in combination with other nonpharmacological and pharmacological approaches has been the subject of substantial research and public interest as a potentially effective strategy for preventing and treating cognitive decline associated with AD/ADRD, as well as for improving functional outcomes and the management of common neuropsychiatric symptoms. Physical activity has been hypothesized to reduce the risk of dementia and the development of neuropathologies through both direct (e.g., improved brain vasculature and blood flow and a reduction in inflammation and amyloid beta production) and indirect pathways (e.g., improved cardiovascular health) (De la Rosa et al., 2020; Iso-Markku et al., 2022). The effect of physical activity on the prevention of dementia, specifically AD and all-cause dementia, has been well demonstrated in the recent literature (De la Rosa et al., 2020; Guure et al., 2017; Iso-Markku et al., 2022; López-Ortiz et al., 2023; Zhang et al., 2023).

One umbrella review of published meta-analyses estimated a 30–40 percent reduction in risk of incident AD with regular physical activity as compared to inactivity (López-Ortiz et al., 2023). While a protective effect is relatively well documented, much less is known regarding the specific physical activity type, intensity, duration, and frequency that affords optimal protective benefits and how these factors may vary across individuals and dementia types. For example, there may be sex differences in optimal design of physical activity interventions. Several studies have shown that the cognitive gains from aerobic training are greater for older women as compared to older men (Mielke, 2024). Generally, though, moderate- and high-intensity exercise, as opposed to low-intensity exercise, has been demonstrated to be more effective in reducing risk for incident AD (Zhang et al., 2023).

Beyond promising evidence on the potential for prevention, evidence for the effect of physical activity on improvement of cognitive function in people already living with dementia remains less clear. Improvements in cognitive function associated with physical activity as measured by various cognitive assessments have been described in multiple studies across various types of dementia (De la Rosa et al., 2020; Groot et al., 2016; López-Ortiz et al., 2023). However, evidence for the beneficial effect of physical activity on improved cognitive function in people living with one or more types of dementia is not universally demonstrated (Brasure et al., 2017), and methodological limitations common to the study of nonpharmacological approaches limit the ability to make conclusions on causality and level of effect.

As with prevention, it is likely that the effect of physical activity on improvements in cognitive function is moderated by the type, intensity, and duration of the activity (Karamacoska et al., 2023) and more research is needed to systematically assess these components. Aerobic exercise has been linked to greater cognitive benefits in populations living with MCI, vascular dementia (Ahn and Kim, 2023; Zheng et al., 2016), AD (De la Rosa et al., 2020; Morris et al., 2017), and all-cause dementia (Groot et al., 2016) as compared to nonaerobic types of physical activity. The recently published EXERT trial, however, found that a stretching, balance, and range-of-motion exercise program was equally effective at slowing cognitive decline in participants with MCI as moderate-intensity aerobic training (Baker et al., 2022).

Physical activity may also be effective as a strategy for managing neuropsychiatric symptoms common to dementia, such as disturbed sleep and depression (Ahn and Kim, 2023; Cai et al., 2023; Wilfling et al., 2023), and for improving such physical functions as balance, gait function and speed, and muscular strength (Cai et al., 2023; Connors et al., 2018; López-Ortiz et al., 2023), which may translate to greater overall well-being and independence regardless of cognitive status. As one of many known, modifiable risk factors, physical activity has been explored in combination with other NPIs (e.g., diet, cognitive training), as will be discussed in the next section.

These findings indicate that physical activity may be promising in the prevention of cognitive decline, and some evidence suggests that physical activity also provides a cognitive benefit for people living with related dementias. Critically, in both cases, insufficient evidence is available to confirm which activity types, intensities, and durations of activity are most efficacious to achieve a meaningful benefit and how these factors may change to achieve optimal benefit based on the characteristics of the intended user (e.g., age, comorbidities, health, and physical status).

Multicomponent lifestyle approaches The highly complex and multifactorial nature of AD/ADRD and the high prevalence of mixed pathologies—which may result from common and pathology-specific mechanisms—suggest that targeting a single pathology or mechanism is unlikely to be sufficient for preventing or treating AD/ADRD on a large scale. There is increasing interest in understanding how multimodal interventions, which combine multiple therapeutic strategies, can simultaneously or sequentially target multiple modifiable risk factors and mechanisms underlying dementia (Barbera et al., 2023). Multimodal lifestyle interventions, which often include combinations of physical activity and exercise programs, diet and nutritional modifications, cognitive training approaches, social stimulation, and management of vascular and metabolic risk factors, have shown promise in both preventing and potentially slowing cognitive decline associated with various types of dementia (Thunborg et al., 2021), as well as contributing to improved physical and mental health, function, and well-being. The evidence remains unclear regarding how multimodal interventions may function to improve cognition or build cognitive reserve or resilience. However, it is likely that the targeting of multiple risk factors through multiple domains acts on various mechanisms and pathways, such as vascular pathways, inflammatory-immune mediated responses, insulin signaling, and mechanisms related to biological aging, both in isolation and synergistically (Barbera et al., 2023; Song et al., 2022).

Demonstrating the effect of individual lifestyle interventions (e.g., diet, cognitive training, exercise) has been challenging. In contrast, recent assessments of multimodal lifestyle interventions have expanded understanding of the potential of lifestyle approaches to slow or improve cognitive decline in cognitively healthy populations at risk for dementia (Ngandu et al., 2015; Yaffe et al., 2024) and to slow cognitive decline in individuals living with AD/ADRD (McMaster et al., 2020; Meng et al., 2022; Salzman et al., 2022), in addition to providing broader functional and quality-of-life benefits. The FINGER study, for example, demonstrated a 25 percent greater improvement in global cognition and significantly decreased risk of cognitive decline in cognitively healthy, older participants as compared to controls (Ngandu et al., 2015). Cognitive benefits from lifestyle approaches have been observed among higher-risk *APOE4* carriers (Solomon et al., 2018). Importantly, multimodal lifestyle interventions may reduce the risk of functional decline (Kulmala et al., 2019). Other research has demonstrated that the combination of computerized cognitive training and physical exercise interventions has more pronounced effects on cognition in both healthy older adults and those with MCI as compared to either intervention alone (Gavelin et al., 2021).

One of the most promising aspects of these multimodal approaches is the potential to tailor interventions to an individual's personal risk factors and preferences, which may improve adherence and provide greater individual benefits. The Systematic Multi-Domain Alzheimer Risk Reduction Trial (SMARRT) applied this approach to its intervention group, allowing participants (cognitively healthy older adults at high risk for dementia) to select and set personalized risk-reduction goals based on their personal risk profile, preferences, and priorities for risk reduction. The findings of this 24-month trial indicated that this participant-driven, tailored multimodal approach has modest effects on improved cognitive function, risk composite scores, and quality of life and, importantly, was well received by participants (Yaffe et al., 2024).

Further interrogation of new combinations of interventions and deeper examination of specific individual characteristics (e.g., *APOE* genotype; comorbidities) may result in more precise and effective approaches for preventing disease and slowing cognitive decline. Efforts to evaluate the combined use of pharmacological interventions (disease modifying interventions for conditions that share risk factors with AD/ADRD) in conjunction with traditional lifestyle approaches to prevent dementia in high-risk populations are now underway. For example, the MET-FINGER study will apply the FINGER 2.0 multimodal intervention approach in combination with metformin in high-risk older adult participants with the *APOE4* allele (Barbera et al., 2023).

Ultimately, multimodal interventions are likely feasible, tailorable to individual risk factors and preferences, and compatible with disease modifying therapies, suggesting that these approaches offer promise in the prevention and treatment of AD/ADRD. In future explorations, multimodal lifestyle interventions could be designed to be dynamic, allowing not only personalization but adjustment of thresholds, as in increasing physical activity intensity, over time.

Interventions to address sensory impairment   Hearing and vision problems are common conditions affecting older adults. Although the mechanisms are not yet well understood, these sensory impairments are thought to not only co-occur with, but also contribute to, cognitive decline and dementia (Livingston et al., 2024) and may have some relationship with cardio-vascular disease risk factors (Baiduc et al., 2023). As effective interventions to treat hearing and vision loss are widely available, there is great interest in understanding the effects those interventions may have on cognitive function, AD/ADRD risk, and quality of life for people living with MCI or dementia.

Hearing loss has been identified as a significant modifiable risk fac-tor for developing dementia (Livingston et al., 2020, 2024). Associations between hearing loss and cognitive decline have been reported in numerous studies (Jayakody et al., 2018; Ray et al., 2018), although other studies have failed to find an association and questions remain regarding the causal nature of this association (Asakawa et al., 2024). Hearing loss is also linked to volume loss in specific brain regions (Armstrong et al., 2019; Llano et al., 2021). In contrast to many other AD/ADRD risk factors, a relatively simple and accessible intervention for hearing loss is available in the form of hearing aids, which have so far demonstrated very low risk levels for users. Observational studies have reported that use of hearing aids protects against dementia in people experiencing hearing loss and other risk factors (Livingston et al., 2024), suggesting this is a promising intervention for pre-venting AD/ADRD. Results from controlled intervention studies, however, have been mixed as to whether hearing aids maintain or improve cognitive function in people without preexistent dementia (Sanders et al., 2021). The signal was greatest for the executive-function cognitive domain, but study limitations precluded definitive conclusions. In older adults with cognitive impairment, there is some evidence that hearing aid use can improve quality of life and dementia-related behavioral symptoms but has little apparent effect on cognitive outcomes in this population (Dawes et al., 2019; Mamo et al., 2018).

This is an important area for additional research with the potential to help millions at risk for cognitive decline and dementia, and many questions remain that should be answerable with current science. For example, could better hearing aids have a greater effect? Is some form of cognitive or other training required to realize the benefits of improved hearing? Given the limited availability of high-quality evidence, it will be important for future research to address the methodological limitations (e.g., small study size, lack of control groups, problems with consistent hearing aid use) that have impeded efforts to assess the beneficial effects of hearing aid use on cognitive function (Asakawa et al., 2024; Dawes et al., 2019). Such research may inform future recommendations regard-ing screening for hearing loss in older adults (U.S. Preventive Services Task Force, 2021) and prompt further investment in the development of more accessible and low-cost assessment methods to screen for hearing impairment (Lelo de Larrea-Mancera et al., 2022). Today, Medicare does not cover the cost of hearing aids. If they are or could be made to be effective in maintaining or improving cognition, and could be made affordable through better insurance coverage, these devices could make a significant difference in quality of life and could improve cognitive health on a population basis.

Vision impairment has also been identified as a risk factor for cognitive decline and dementia (Cao et al., 2023; Ehrlich et al., 2022; Livingston et al., 2024). As most cases of vision impairment are treatable with two cost-effective interventions—eyeglasses or contacts, and cataract surgery—the modifiable nature of this risk factor makes it an attractive target for intervention studies aimed at identifying strategies to slow cognitive decline and prevent dementia. While research is still ongoing, there is a small but growing evidence base suggesting the cognitive benefits of cataract surgery for older adults. Cataract surgery is associated with reduced risk for MCI (Miyata et al., 2018), and a number of studies (primarily observational) examining the effects of cataract surgery have observed beneficial effects on cognitive function in cognitively healthy adults (Pellegrini et al., 2020) and people living with MCI (Yoshida et al., 2024), although one RCT showed no improvement in performance on neuropsychological tests in cognitively healthy adults after surgery (Anstey et al., 2006).

While many studies evaluating cognitive effects have relatively short follow-up periods, one observational study with a control group found that cataract surgery slowed the rate of cognitive decline over a period of more than 10 years as measured using a test of episodic memory (Maharani et al., 2018). Additionally, surgery has been shown to reverse cataract-induced neuroanatomical changes (Lin et al., 2018). While the committee did not find evidence of cognitive benefits for people living with dementia (Yoshida et al., 2024), cataract surgery may improve quality of life and neuropsychiatric symptoms (Dawes et al., 2019).

The evidence base for the use of eyeglasses or contacts on AD/ADRD risk is extremely sparse, making it difficult to draw conclusions. One study found a correlation between wearing reading glasses and cognitive function, although the linkage was no longer significant after adjusting for education (Spierer et al., 2016).

As with hearing aids, the evidence base for interventions to address vision impairment is hampered by methodological limitations of existing studies. Future research should include adequate control groups and follow-up periods and address problems with cognitive tests, such as vision dependency and practice effects (Fukuoka et al., 2016).

Promising Pharmacological Interventions

The following promising pharmacological interventions are aimed at preventing or slowing neurodegeneration. With few exceptions (e.g., anti-amyloid antibodies), most are still in early phases of clinical research and efficacy data from large phase 3 or 4 clinical trials are not yet available.

Anti-amyloid treatments The recent approval of two anti-amyloid monoclonal antibody therapies—lecanemab and donanemab—for early, symptomatic AD has generated much interest regarding the effectiveness of these therapies in slowing cognitive decline. While these approved anti-amyloid therapies are not a panacea, they represent two more tools than what previously existed for use in the treatment of AD. Much remains to be learned about how these anti-amyloid therapies can be implemented for maximum benefit and limited harm.

The clinical benefits and potential harms of anti-amyloid therapies have been well described in the literature. A phase 3 trial of lecanemab, which binds to amyloid beta-soluble protofibrils, demonstrated a reduction in brain amyloid levels and slowed clinical decline in select groups of participants living with early AD after 18 months. The study findings indicated modest improvements in cognitive and functional measures compared to placebo but were accompanied by risk of serious adverse events, particularly for carriers of two copies the *APOE4* allele (van Dyck et al., 2023). Of note, a posthoc analysis suggested that the cognitive benefits of lecanemab may differ by gender with women potentially receiving less benefit (Mielke, 2024), but this requires further investigation in studies designed to detect such differences.

In clinical trials, donanemab, which removes amyloid plaques via microglial-mediated clearance, was also found to improve cognition and functional measures in participants with early AD after 76 weeks as compared to placebo (Mintun et al., 2021). As with lecanemab, adverse effects associated with amyloid-related imaging abnormalities were reported (Mintun et al., 2021; van Dyck et al., 2023). Top-line results from these trials indicated that the greatest clinical benefit was found in those participants presenting with the earliest levels of cognitive impairment. The donanemab trials, for example, found a 60 percent slowing of disease severity following treatment in those living with MCI as measured by the Integrated Alzheimer's Disease Rating Scale (iADRS); a 40 percent decline in iADRS was observed across the total study population (AlzForum, 2024a).

These results and other questions raised from prior trials (e.g., differences across *APOE4* status, sex, prevalence of adverse effects, long-term effects) open new opportunities to assess how these therapies can be used most effectively to slow and possibly prevent AD neuropathology and cognitive decline. Two trials, the AHEAD Study (lecanemab) and TRAIL-BLAZER-Alz-3 (donanemab), are now in the process of evaluating the effect of these therapies on the prevention of disease progression in people at high risk of AD, as measured by time to clinical progression (AHEAD Study, 2024; Pugh, 2023). The phase 3 TRAILBLAZER-Alz-3 prevention trial enrolled cognitively unimpaired individuals who are considered to be at high risk for clinical AD, as determined by elevated plasma p-tau217 (AlzForum, 2024a). Similarly, the AHEAD Study enrolled cognitively unimpaired individuals with elevated brain amyloid (Rafii et al., 2023). The findings from these studies and others will provide critical evidence on the optimization of timing, dosing, and safety, as well as greater insights into target populations for maximum benefit in prevention and treatment of AD.

While initial evaluations of anti-amyloid therapies have occurred in people diagnosed with AD (with or without clinical symptoms), the safety and efficacy of these therapies in the context of mixed etiology dementia is of great interest given the prevalence of co-occurring pathologies. NIH posted a request for applications in 2024 to support the evaluation of anti-amyloid therapies in people with a clinical diagnosis of LBD who also exhibit evidence of AD brain pathology (NIH, 2024).

As discussed earlier in this chapter, there is also interest in combination interventions that involve the administration of other therapeutics, including anti-tau therapies, to patients alongside amyloid-lowering therapies (Cummings et al., 2024). Such studies may aid in understanding which molecular drivers are additive to amyloid lowering in terms of reducing or reversing symptoms. The combination of anti-amyloid antibodies with focused ultrasound to transiently open the blood–brain barrier is also being investigated as a means of enhancing delivery of the therapeutics to the brain (Rezai et al., 2024).

Importantly, the long-term effects of anti-amyloid therapies need to be evaluated and can be accomplished through the long-term follow-up of those patients who received treatment. Such assessments will help elucidate how the removal of amyloid from the brain affects clinical symptoms and disease progression over time and whether these represent meaningful therapeutic benefits. Additionally, long-term follow-up will help to understand the safety of these treatments (e.g., whether changes in brain volume have any negative effect) (Alves et al., 2023) and the effects of amyloid removal on the development of other neuropathologies, such as the progression of tau pathologies.

Immunomodulatory agents   There is a substantial body of evidence suggesting that neuroinflammation and immune dysfunction play key roles in the etiologic cascade that leads to neurodegeneration and AD/ADRD, as discussed in Chapter 3. Neuroinflammation may result from a number of different mechanisms, such as the activation of microglia to a pro-inflammatory phenotype (Tejera et al., 2019; Wang et al., 2023) and the secretion of proinflammatory mediators by accumulating senescent cells, which may lead to tissue infiltration of immune cells, chronic inflammation, and tissue damage (Islam et al., 2023; Riessland and Orr, 2023). These processes are thought to be characteristics of immunosenescence, a gradual deterioration and dysfunction of immune function with aging that is also believed to contribute to neurodegenerative diseases, such as AD/ADRD (Bowirrat, 2022; Liu et al., 2023; Rommer et al., 2022; Zhao et al., 2020).

With the growing awareness of the role of inflammation in AD/ADRD has come interest in anti-inflammatory interventions as a means to prevent or slow neurodegeneration. The challenge for such therapies is to ameliorate detrimental inflammatory responses without impairing immune responses critical to the clearance of pathogenic protein aggregates. While data from clinical trials of nonsteroidal anti-inflammatory drugs such as aspirin have been disappointing in light of the epidemiological evidence suggesting a protective effect (ADAPT Research Group, 2013; Meyer et al., 2019), a multitude of other anti-inflammatory agents are under investigation and show promise in preclinical and early clinical research. For example, senolytics—compounds that selectively clear senescent cells that accumulate with age (Riessland and Orr, 2023)—may reduce inflammation associated with the senescence-associated secretory phenotype (see Chapter 3). Senolytic compounds under evaluation in phase 2 clinical trials include a combination of dasatinib (a tyrosine kinase inhibitor approved by FDA for the treatment of leukemia) and quercetin (a flavonoid with anti-inflammatory properties) (Cummings et al., 2024; Riessland and Orr, 2023). Data from a phase 1 feasibility trial showed that treatment of adults with early-stage AD with a combination of dasatinib and quercetin was well tolerated, and promising results from an exploratory analysis indicated the potential reduction of inflammatory markers (Gonzales et al., 2023) consistent with responses observed in preclinical studies (Zhang et al., 2019b).

Given the current absence of approved treatments for Lewy body dementia, there is considerable interest in neflamapimod, "an oral drug targeting the effects of neuroinflammation on the molecular mechanisms underlying degeneration of cholinergic degeneration in the basal forebrain" (Prins et al., 2024, p. 549). Results from a phase 2a trial were promising, with greater cognitive benefits observed for those without AD copathology, and the drug is now in phase 2b trials. Glucagon-like peptide-1 (GLP-1) agonists, discussed below, may also exert anti-inflammatory effects. Other novel therapies for AD that target inflammation and are currently being evaluated in clinical trials are described by Cummings and colleagues (2023a, 2024).

In addition to dysregulated inflammatory responses, other dysfunctions of the immune system accompany immunosenescence. While the myriad changes that occur with immunosenescence are complex and not fully under-stood, in relation to AD/ADRD, a key dysfunction is impaired chemotaxis (cell movement in response to a chemical stimulus) and phagocytic function of microglia in the brain and peripheral macrophages (Liu et al., 2023; Rawji et al., 2016; Zhao et al., 2020). Such changes are thought to impair the clear-ance of abnormal protein aggregates. Thus, paradoxically, while some thera-peutic strategies for AD/ADRD involve dampening elements of the immune system (inflammation), others are aimed at stimulating an immune response to enhance immune-mediated clearance of protein aggregates (Cummings et al., 2023b). One example of such immunostimulants under investigation in clinical trials for AD/ADRD is sargramostim, a recombinant form of a cytokine known to stimulate the development of phagocytosis by cells of the innate immune system (currently in phase 2 trials) (Cummings et al., 2023a,b; Van Eldik et al., 2016). Preclinical studies using AD mouse models showed that treatment with sargramostim activated microglia, reduced AD pathology by more than 50 percent, and rescued cognitive function (Kiyota et al., 2018). Exploratory analyses from the phase 1 trial were encouraging, showing evidence of cognitive benefit for the treated group and reduced markers of neurodegeneration (Potter et al., 2021a).

A different immunostimulatory approach being evaluated for AD/ADRD is the use of a vaccine adjuvant, protollin, which is a combination of bacterial outer membrane proteins and lipopolysaccharide. While vac-cines usually contain a pathogen-specific component, the response to which is nonspecifically enhanced by the adjuvant, in this case the adjuvant is administered on its own to stimulate cells of the innate immune system, which will recognize the bacterial cell components. Researchers hope that the activated innate immune cells will move from the cervical lymph nodes to the brain and clear protein aggregates, such as amyloid beta (Valiukas et al., 2022). Following preclinical studies showing that protollin was effective in stimulating amyloid removal (Frenkel et al., 2008), a phase 1 clinical trial was initiated in 2021.

Importantly, both sargramostim and protollin are already approved by FDA for other uses and thus represent opportunities for drug repurpos-ing. Moreover, because inflammation and immunosenescence are thought to be common underlying neurodegenerative mechanisms, the potential application of these immune-modulating therapies is not limited to AD and may extend to related dementias, offering promise of disease-agnostic approaches that can prevent or slow neurodegeneration. There is still much that is not well understood regarding the function of the immune systems and inflammation, however, and enhanced understanding of the timing and context of immune system modulation, as well as the contribution of spe-cific mechanisms to disease states, will be critically important to knowing how and when to intervene safely using immunomodulatory agents.

Tau antisense oligonucleotides   Like anti-amyloid antibodies, antisense oligonucleotides (ASOs) are biologic therapeutics targeted to specific proteins implicated in the development of AD/ADRD. Whereas antibody-based therapeutics directly bind the protein of interest, ASOs target the protein by altering its gene expression. ASOs are synthetic oligonucleotides (or analogs of oligonucleotides) generally 12 to 30 nucleotides in length that bind to RNA (messenger RNAs that encode proteins or noncoding RNAs) (Bennett et al., 2019). RNA binding by ASOs can promote degradation of the bound RNA molecule, modulate the processing of the RNA through splicing and polyadenylation, or otherwise affect the translation of mRNA into protein, such as by disrupting RNA structures that block translation (Bennett et al., 2019; Silva et al., 2020). An advantageous feature of ASOs is the ability to directly translate genetic discoveries into drug discovery programs (Bennett et al., 2019).

ASOs are emerging as a class of therapeutics with great potential to treat neurodegenerative diseases. In 2016, an ASO was approved by FDA for the treatment of spinal muscular atrophy (FDA, 2016), and, in 2023, FDA granted accelerated approval to an ASO used to treat amyotrophic lateral sclerosis (FDA, 2023). The AD/ADRD clinical trials pipeline currently includes tau-targeted ASOs that are in phase 1 and 2 clinical trials (Cummings et al., 2024). Tauopathy is a feature of several neurodegenerative diseases, including AD and FTD. It is hoped that tau-targeted ASOs may slow or halt neurodegeneration by preventing the aggregation of hyperphosphorylated tau into neurofibrillary tangles—believed to be a key driver of neuronal loss—and the spreading of tau across neural networks (seeding). Encouraging data from a phase 1b trial showed that treatment of participants living with mild AD with a tau-targeted ASO was well tolerated and reduced cerebrospinal fluid (CSF) total tau concentration in a dose-dependent manner, achieving a mean reduction from baseline levels of more than 50 percent at 24 weeks after the last dose (Mummery et al., 2023). Brain tau levels were also reduced by the treatment as measured by tau-PET (Edwards et al., 2023).

Although data demonstrating the effects of anti-tau ASOs on cognitive outcomes in humans are not yet available, treatment of mice carrying a human tau gene rescued nest-building performance, a functional task that is deficient in mouse models of tauopathy and considered to be reflective of social behavior and cognitive function (DeVos et al., 2017). The prospect of a treatment to slow neurodegeneration caused by tauopathy associated with AD/ADRD is exciting; however, approval of such a treatment would require consideration of barriers to implementation, such as high cost of treatment and health care system delivery of a drug administered via an invasive procedure (recurring lumbar puncture).

Gene and cell therapy interventions Gene and cell therapies represent increasingly active areas of intervention research for dementia, especially in AD. Gene therapy may show promise in the future based on recent advances in other neurodegenerative diseases, as in FDA approval of a gene therapy for spinal muscular atrophy (FDA, 2019a; Lennon et al., 2021; Sun and Roy, 2021). The development of gene therapies for dementia are exciting as these approaches are designed to prevent the development of neuropathologies and to slow or halt cognitive decline by precisely targeting the underlying mechanisms contributing to disease. Much of this research remains in preclinical stages, where the focus is on the development of vectors and well-validated targets. Potential targets being explored for AD gene therapies include amyloid pathway intermediates and the modulation of enzymes, tau protein downregulation, *APOE4* downregulation and *APOE2* upregulation, neurotrophin expression, and inflammatory cytokine alteration (Lennon et al., 2021). Gene therapies are also being pursued for related dementias. For example, one gene therapy target in FTD is the progranulin gene, mutation in which contributes to approximately 22 percent of familial FTD cases (Sevigny et al., 2024).

Preclinical studies using animal models have yielded some promising results from gene therapy candidates for improvements in the cognitive domains of memory and learning (Lennon et al., 2021; Tedeschi et al., 2021) and in the reduction of accumulated amyloid beta and tau (Loera-Valencia et al., 2018). However, the few early-stage clinical trials completed thus far, targeting the regulation of neurotrophic factors, have demonstrated mixed effects (Tedeschi et al., 2021) and suggest the need for further work on the development of effective delivery modalities (Lennon et al., 2021), along with continued identification of new vectors and therapeutic targets (Chen et al., 2020a). Preclinical studies and interim results from an early-phase clinical trial show that a gene therapy delivering the granulin gene using an adeno-associated virus vector was generally safe and well tolerated and could increase progranulin levels in vivo (Sevigny et al., 2024). Longer follow-up and additional studies are needed to assess the duration of effects and the clinical (e.g., cognitive, behavioral) benefits of treatment.

Cell therapies involve the use of living cells (e.g., stem cells, immune system cells) to prevent or treat diseases. At present, there are no FDA-approved cell therapies for the treatment of neurodegenerative diseases, but a variety of different cell therapies are under investigation in both preclinical and clinical studies (Chan et al., 2021; Cummings et al., 2023b). Cell types and anticipated mechanisms of action for investigational cell therapies vary (Kwak et al., 2018; Temple, 2023). Some stem cell therapies have been aimed at direct replacement of neuronal cells lost during neurodegeneration (Chen et al., 2023a). While this may be a viable therapeutic approach for some neurodegenerative diseases, such as replacing dopaminergic neurons lost in Parkinson's disease (Cha et al., 2023), a cell replacement strategy is more complex for diseases such as AD that feature a multiplicity of affected phenotypes and the loss of multiple distinct neuronal cell types (Goldman, 2016; Kwak et al., 2018; Loera-Valencia et al., 2018).

Alternative strategies to cell replacement that are of growing interest include modulating inflammation and stimulating neurogenesis and tissue regeneration, particularly in the hippocampal region of the brain (Kwak et al., 2018). Cell therapies using mesenchymal stem cells (MSCs, also known as medicinal signaling cells) have shown promise for these nonreplacement strategies (Chan et al., 2021). Most cell therapies being evaluated in clinical trials for treatment of AD use MSCs (Chan et al., 2021). While labeled as stem cells owing to their multipotential capacities, the use of MSCs in cell therapies is primarily focused on their ability to migrate to sites of injury or inflammation within the body and to modulate immune responses and stimulate tissue regeneration through their secretion of bioactive factors and via cell–cell interactions (Caplan, 2017; Chan et al., 2021; Jimenez-Puerta et al., 2020; Kwak et al., 2018).

One MSC-based cell therapy was given fast-track status by FDA in July 2024 for the treatment of mild AD following a successful phase 2a trial that achieved its primary safety and secondary efficacy endpoints, showing preliminary evidence of slowing cognitive and functional decline (Ciccone, 2024). While there has been some encouraging evidence for cell-based therapies, ongoing studies are needed to better elucidate mechanisms of action, to understand the duration of any beneficial effects, and to address such concerns as tumorigenesis and immune rejection of grafted cells (Chan et al., 2021; Chen et al., 2023a; Goldman, 2016). Scalability of cell-based therapies also needs to be considered.

While gene and cell therapies represent exciting avenues for research, evaluation of their safety and effectiveness for treating AD/ADRD is still underway, and it is unlikely that these therapies will be available for broad clinical use in the very near future.

Interventions targeting synaptic dysfunction Synaptic dysfunction is a primary correlate of cognitive impairment in progressive neurodegenerative diseases. Synaptic impairment is thought to occur early in the neurodegenerative process across a range of pathologies and may result from a complex combination of pathologic mechanisms including toxic amyloid beta and tau oligomers (Gutierrez and Limon, 2022; Li and Selkoe, 2020); overactive glial cells (Yu et al., 2024); mitochondrial dysfunction (Morton et al., 2021); abnormal accumulation of alpha-synuclein (Trudler et al., 2021); and genetic mutations (Gelon et al., 2022). The development of therapeutics to enhance synaptic plasticity or confer synaptic neuroprotection represents an increasingly active area of early-phase drug development for AD (Cummings et al., 2023b).

At present, there are multiple phase 2 and 3 trials of novel agents in progress for various unique drug targets related to synaptic dysfunction, some of which have demonstrated promise in enhancing synaptic function in early to moderate AD (Cummings et al., 2023b, 2024). Phase 2a clinical testing of a first-in-class small-molecule compound that targets a p75 neurotrophin receptor, for example, demonstrated potential efficacy in slowing AD pathology in participants with mild to moderate AD, as measured by CSF biomarkers amyloid beta40 and amyloid beta42; however, no change was observed in cognitive testing (Shanks et al., 2024). CT1812, a sigma-2 receptor antagonist that interferes with amyloid beta oligomer binding to neurons and thereby prevents synaptotoxicity, demonstrated promise in transgenic mouse models. A recent pilot study found no significant change from baseline as indicated by FDG-PET, clinical cognitive scales, or CSF biomarkers, but volumetric MRI illustrated "a trend towards tissue preservation" in the CT1812 treatment group (van Dyck et al., 2024). As of June 2023, CT1812 has advanced to a phase 2 trial that is being run by the Alzheimer's Clinical Trials Consortium and will evaluate the safety and efficacy of different dosages as compared to placebo in participants with MCI or mild AD (AlzForum, 2024b).

Unlike anti-amyloid therapies currently on the market, these small-molecule drug therapies are administered orally and, thus, may be more accessible and require less costly clinical infrastructure. Additional, longer clinical trials for interventions targeting synaptic dysfunction will be required to monitor the safety of these compounds and to evaluate efficacy in larger study populations. In addition to further development and evaluation of agents targeting synaptic functions, parallel efforts are needed to identify and validate biomarkers and outcomes for synaptic function that can be used in clinical research to accurately measure target engagement and response (see later section on Identifying biomarkers for demonstrating target engagement and measuring treatment response).

Antidiabetic treatments Shared pathophysiological mechanisms underlying both type 2 diabetes (T2D) and dementia, specifically AD, have led to growing interest in the use of antidiabetic treatments, such as glucagon-like peptide-1 receptor agonists (GLP-1RA) and metformin, to prevent AD in high-risk groups and to slow cognitive decline in those living with AD (Michailidis et al., 2022; Muñoz-Jiménez et al., 2020). Shared metabolic impairments, such as insulin resistance, impaired glucose metabolism, mitochondrial dysfunction, oxidative stress, and inflammation, mean that T2D and neurodegenerative diseases are closely linked, and individuals with T2D are at high risk of developing a neurodegenerative disease (Carvalho and Moreira, 2023). The growing prevalence of chronic metabolic disorders in the United States indicates the need to evaluate antidiabetic treatments as strategies to both prevent incident dementia in people with T2D and to slow decline in people living with dementia with and without a T2D comorbidity.

Metformin, a commonly prescribed and extensively studied drug for treating high blood sugar associated with T2D, has shown some benefit in reducing the risk of incident cognitive decline and dementia in participants with T2D (Michailidis et al., 2022; Zhang et al., 2022). However, overall evidence for its protective effects on cognition remain mixed and necessitate further study (Luchsinger et al., 2017; Michailidis et al., 2022; Weinstein et al., 2019). GLP-1 receptor antagonists are newer T2D treatments that have shown early promise in improving cognitive function and memory and decreasing amyloid beta deposition and tau hyperphosphorylation in people living with dementia, although this research remains in preclinical and early clinical stages (Michailidis et al., 2022; Wang et al., 2022a). These drugs may also provide neuroprotective effects in cognitively healthy people living with diabetes (Hölscher, 2022; Nørgaard et al., 2022).

The approval of dual GLP-1/GIP receptor agonists for the treatment of T2D in 2022 has spurred even greater excitement about the potential benefits of these drugs for dementia and many other chronic diseases and health conditions, including prediabetes and obesity. These dual agonist treatments, which are more effective in crossing the blood–brain barrier, have demonstrated superior protective effects in preclinical and clinical studies as compared with single-receptor antagonists in study populations with diabetes as well as in study populations with AD and other neuro-degenerative diseases such as Parkinson's disease (Hölscher, 2022).

Promising Interventions That May Be Pharmacologic, Nonpharmacologic, or a Combination

Management of hypertension and other interventions that target vascular health   Risk factors associated with overall cardiovascular health, includ-ing hypertension, hypercholesterolemia, and metabolic disease, are also strongly associated with an increased risk of vascular dementia, AD, and mixed etiology dementia involving vascular pathologies. Risks of vascular dementia from these comorbid conditions may be higher for females than males (Mielke, 2024). Epidemiological research suggests that control of these overlapping risk factors may present opportunities to prevent the development of these highly prevalent neuropathologies in high-risk popu-lations, while also simultaneously improving cardiovascular health.

Hypertension is a well-established risk factor for cerebrovascular disease, which is itself a major contributor to vascular dementia and AD. Hyperten-sion in midlife has been associated with increased risk of dementia later in life

(Peters et al., 2019; Sierra, 2020). The damage associated with hypertension develops insidiously over the life course, beginning with arteriolar narrowing and microvascular changes that may develop into more significant cerebrovascular disease and an increased risk of cognitive impairment. The direct management of hypertension using antihypertensive agents (e.g., angiotensin II receptor blockers, angiotensin-converting enzyme inhibitors, calcium channel blockers) in midlife and later has been extensively explored as a strategy for the prevention of dementia, and many observational studies have suggested that the use of antihypertensive agents has a beneficial effect on the prevention of dementia (Olmastroni et al., 2022; Petek et al., 2023; Sierra, 2020). However, results from large randomized trials have been inconsistent (Forette et al., 2002; Peters et al., 2008; SPRINT MIND Investigators, 2019), and the lack of conclusive evidence of effect from these trials may be in part attributable to the variation in blood pressure target levels and the assessment of cognitive outcomes (SPRINT MIND Investigators, 2019).

A 2021 Cochrane review concluded that there is insufficient evidence available from these trials to make a conclusion on the effect of hypertensive treatment on dementia or to inform clinical guidelines for the use of these agents to prevent dementia. Elucidating the efficacy of antihypertension interventions will likely require long-term follow-up of participants beginning in midlife and employing cognition as a primary rather than secondary outcome measure (Cunningham et al., 2021). Such efforts need to consider sex-specific differences in antihypertensive prescribing practices for males and females and potential effects on sex differences in cerebrovascular pathology and AD/ADRD (Mielke, 2024).

Chronically high levels of low-density lipoprotein (LDL) and total cholesterol in midlife, which are associated with poor cardiovascular health, have been linked to the occurrence of dementia in late life, specifically AD and vascular dementia. Hypercholesterolemia in late life does not appear to be associated with the development of AD. However, the underlying mechanisms associated with cholesterol and neurodegeneration are complex and likely involve multiple mediating factors (e.g., genetics; life stage; presence of comorbidities) (Loera-Valencia et al., 2018). As with antihypertensive agents, the protective effects of lipid-lowering medications (e.g., statins) described in observational trials (Chu et al., 2018; Olmastroni et al., 2022) have not been mirrored by results from recent RCTs. However, these trials primarily assessed the use of statins in late life in participants at risk of dementia (McGuinness et al., 2016). Understanding the control of hypercholesterolemia and dyslipidemia beginning in midlife, when its detrimental effects to brain health are thought to be most pervasive (Anstey et al., 2017), may provide new insights into the potential use of statins and or the identification of novel targets that could advance midlife preventive strategies for dementia in certain populations.

NPIs that can be broadly categorized as healthy lifestyle interventions (e.g., diet designed to reduce hypertension, physical exercise) have been assessed for their ability to prevent AD/ADRD through the targeting of modifiable risk factors that are shared with vascular health. Such interventions are discussed earlier in this chapter in the context of physical activity and multimodal NPIs.

Autophagy and mitophagy inducers   Analyses of AD/ADRD risk genes and drug targets have pointed to the key role played by impaired autophagy caused by dysfunction in the endosomal–lysosomal system in forms of dementia characterized by proteiopathies (Bellenguez et al., 2022; Caberlotto and Nguyen, 2014; Deng et al., 2017; Nixon and Rubinsztein, 2024). Autophagy is a highly conserved cellular process by which damaged proteins and organelles are delivered to lysosomes for degradation, thereby helping to maintain protein and overall cellular homeostasis (Klionsky and Emr, 2000). Mitophagy is a special case of autophagy involving the removal of excess or damaged mitochondria by encapsulation of the mitochondria in autophagosomes, which then fuse with lysosomes to create the phagocytic vacuoles in which the mitochondria are digested and degraded (Yang et al., 2024). Lysosomal dysfunction (e.g., caused by inadequate lysosomal acidification) and impaired autophagy are shared characteristics of aging and multiple neurodegenerative diseases (Nixon, 2020), as discussed in more detail in Chapter 3.

Neurons are unable to dilute cellular waste products through cell division and are therefore vulnerable to breakdowns in autophagy (Nixon, 2020), which leads to the buildup and aggregation of misfolded proteins and the accumulation of damaged mitochondria (Yang et al., 2024). There is consequently great interest in the induction of autophagy (including mitophagy) as a therapeutic strategy for AD/ADRD (Corasaniti et al., 2024; Djajadikerta et al., 2020; Eshraghi et al., 2022; Wang et al., 2021; Yang et al., 2024). Such strategies are supported by the observation that autophagy hyperactivation through genetic modification significantly decreased the accumulation of amyloid and prevented cognitive decline in AD mouse models (Rocchi et al., 2017). Importantly, autophagy induction strategies have the potential to affect multiple proteinopathies simultaneously, an advantage over single-target therapies such as monoclonal antibodies, given that mixed pathologies are found in most older people living with dementia.

Autophagy/mitophagy inducers being evaluated for effects on AD/ADRD include both small-molecule drugs and plant-derived phytochemicals, some of which are marketed and sold as dietary supplements or nutraceuticals. Several phytochemicals have shown encouraging effects on autophagy and mitophagy function in preclinical studies, both in vitro and in vivo, but with few exceptions, clinical data have yet to be generated

(Yang et al., 2024). One notable phytochemical autophagy inducer for which some clinical trial data are available is resveratrol, a polyphenolic compound found in a number of different plants but perhaps best known as a contributor to the health benefits of grapes and red wine. While effects on some biomarker trajectories were observed, larger trials are needed to evaluate changes in clinical outcomes (Jin et al., 2023; Moussa et al., 2017; Turner et al., 2015; Zhu et al., 2018). Rapamycin is another promising autophagy inducer being evaluated in phase 2 trials (Cummings et al., 2023a,b, 2024). A preclinical study showed that rapamycin induced autophagy and reduced amyloid beta levels and plaques (Chen et al., 2019).

Of note, autophagy inducers are often pleiotropic and drugs under investigation for other mechanisms of action may also exert effects on autophagy pathways, as is the case for metformin (discussed above) (Corasaniti et al., 2024; Yang et al., 2024). This yields opportunities for drug repurposing (Eshraghi et al., 2022). An important focus for future research is to elucidate the pathways by which these pleiotropic compounds exert their effects on AD/ADRD and the implications for such factors as dose and timing of treatment (Majumder et al., 2011).

Interventions to increase slow-wave sleep   Sleep has a complex, bidirectional relationship with AD/ADRD pathology and may be associated with the clearance of neurotoxic byproducts from the brain. Sleep architecture changes over the life course, with the time spent in slow-wave sleep (e.g., deep sleep) decreasing and becoming fragmented over time. For women, hormonal changes during the pre-, peri- and postmenopausal states have been shown to affect sleep (Mielke, 2024). Sleep–wake disorders are common in dementia and may play a role in worsening or accelerated cognitive and functional impairment through a variety of mechanisms, such as the accumulation of amyloid beta and tau (Wang and Holtzman, 2020). Increasing slow-wave sleep and sleep quality more broadly through the reduction of sleep disturbances has been of interest in interventions for AD/ADRD, but medications such as benzodiazepines and anticholinergics may not be effective or safe for longer-term use in older adults (Ferreira et al., 2021; Gerlach et al., 2018; Taylor-Rowan et al., 2021).

Orexin, a neuropeptide that plays a role in the regulation of multiple physiological processes, including the sleep–wake cycle (Sun et al., 2022), has been associated with increased nighttime wakefulness and sleep latency and decreased sleep efficiency in AD (Wang and Holtzman, 2020). Dysregulation of the orexinergic system may be associated with worsening cognitive decline (Liguori et al., 2014). Emerging research suggests treatments inhibiting orexin, such as dual orexin receptor antagonists, may have some effect on the improvement of sleep quality in preclinical studies (Duncan et al., 2019; Zhou and Tang, 2022) and in limited clinical studies in older adults with insomnia (Zammit et al., 2020) and in people living with MCI or mild AD (Blackman et al., 2021). However, little is known regarding the cognitive or functional effects of orexin inhibitors. In one RCT involving people living with MCI, suvorexant, a dual orexin receptor antagonist, was found to significantly increase total sleep time and sleep efficiency as compared to placebo. However, these effects were not significant when assessed in participants living with mild AD (Blackman et al., 2021).

Bringing Interventions for Preventing AD/ADRD to Scale: Public Health and Policy Opportunities

The promising interventions discussed in the preceding sections, both pharmacological and nonpharmacological, are targeted to the individual level. Most NPIs and some pharmacologic interventions (e.g., medications for hypertension) focus on modifiable risk factors. A challenge, however, is that implementing such interventions often requires significant personal motivation, which has been a limiting factor in the success of such strategies as increasing physical activity. Moreover, some risk and protective factors for dementia originate from, and can only be addressed at, societal levels (Livingston et al., 2024). Examples include access to higher education (Xu et al., 2019)— as well as structural factors that perpetuate social disadvantage for some groups and exposure to such environmental contaminants as air pollution (Livingston et al., 2024). Often there are interactions among these factors that compound AD/ADRD risk. For example, socially disadvantaged groups are more likely to live in areas where there is greater exposure to environmental pollutants (Fairburn et al., 2019; Hauptman et al., 2023) and less opportunity for physical activity and social interaction (Finlay et al., 2022), which may contribute to increased risk for conditions that contribute to cardiovascular disease (e.g., hypertension, diabetes).

Targeting causative upstream social and environmental modifiers can thus have a broader and more significant effect on reducing AD burden than modifying proximal individual-level risk factors (Paul et al., 2019). This argues for increased attention to public health and policy population-level interventions to bring dementia prevention to scale. Examples of such interventions include public health campaigns to raise awareness of the importance of reducing cardiovascular disease risk for AD/ADRD prevention, programs to address nutritional deficiencies, neighborhood revitalization initiatives, programs such as Experience Corps that foster intergenerational exchange (AARP, 2024), and standard-setting policy actions to reduce environmental exposures. Additional important policies target social determinants of health, such as lifelong educational activities, food security, financial vulnerability, healthy housing access, workplace safety, retirement policies, and opportunities for older adults to continue to meaningfully engage in community activities. Importantly, beyond the reduced risk of dementia and benefits to overall health, prevention strategies may delay dementia onset to later in life, resulting in an expansion in the number of healthy years of life and a compression in the amount of time living with disease (Livingston et al., 2024).

In some cases, efforts to implement such population-level strategies are already underway in the context of other public health threats or social needs and could be additionally framed as potential strategies preventing AD/ADRD. Although the mechanisms are not always well understood, the decline in age-specific dementia incidence in high-income countries such as the United States suggests that some approaches have already yielded success (Farina et al., 2022; Wolters et al., 2020). Improved understanding of the contributors to the observed decrease in dementia incidence, quantifying the role of changes in cardiovascular risk profiles and educational attainment for example, may open opportunities to accelerate prevention efforts and to better use public health investments not specifically targeted to AD/ADRD (e.g., initiatives aimed at improving cardiovascular health). Importantly, such efforts can be pursued now even in the absence of a complete understanding of the underlying biological mechanisms that mediate the effects of public health strategies. However, motivating the implementation of population-level interventions, particularly those with far-reaching consequences such as policy changes will require a robust evidence base. For example, compelling evidence causally linking specific environmental pollutants to increased incidence and/or earlier onset of AD/ADRD (and other neurodegenerative diseases) will likely be needed to persuade policy and law makers to change standards and to identify pollutant sources that can be controlled by regulation (Kilian and Kitazawa, 2018). There is generally a lack of evidence on the social and environmental exposures to target to enhance resilience and prevent the development and progression of AD/ADRD pathology.

As noted earlier, there is a paucity of data on the effectiveness of population-level strategies from intervention studies, likely caused, in part, by the challenges of rigorously studying these strategies. Going forward, there are new research opportunities to incorporate blood-based biomarkers into studies investigating population-level interventions. This will allow for the stratification of results based on the presence of pathological changes and permit the evaluation of an intervention's effect on the risk of developing symptoms.

Conclusion 4-3: A holistic approach to dementia prevention, involving policies that foster quality education, health-promoting environments, and overall health improvement, is crucial and goes beyond the research-focused institutes. This is particularly true for low-income residents, where prevention potential is high. These populations often grapple with resource, infrastructure, and funding challenges. Concurrently, research dedicated to public health initiatives aimed at monitoring success of dementia prevention is essential.

OPPORTUNITIES TO IMPROVE CLINICAL TRIALS FOR AD/ADRD

Improving Representativeness and External Validity Through Inclusive Clinical Trials

AD/ADRD is observed across all demographics. Therefore, any study aiming to better understand, prevent, or treat AD/ADRD should recruit and retain as diverse a population as possible. Limiting a study sample to a single demographic increases the likelihood that any effect observed represents an artifact of that sample instead of a feature of the disease; such design problems result in selection bias. From a scientific and clinical perspective, to fully understand and mitigate the complex and heterogeneous mechanisms underlying AD/ADRD pathology, it is necessary to design clinical trials that include diverse participant populations. For example, unexplained observations that could shed light on AD/ADRD etiology include the higher prevalence of AD/ADRD among African American and Hispanic individuals, and yet, these groups are consistently underrepresented in both AD/ADRD observational studies and randomized clinical trials (ADNI, 2012; Faison et al., 2007; Raman et al., 2022). In aducanumab trials, for example, only 3.2 percent of trial participants were of Hispanic/Latino background while a mere 0.6 percent of participants were African American (ICER, 2021). The lack of diversity across trials that are modeling disease progression or assessing the efficacy of interventions can result in biased or inaccurate findings that have low external validity, or generalizability, and can further exacerbate existing disparities in AD/ADRD health outcomes. Beyond race and ethnicity, other aspects of diversity that need to be better represented in clinical trial populations include sex and geography (e.g., rural, suburban, and urban), as well as socioeconomic status and social phenotypes.

One strategy to improve the applicability of AD/ADRD trial data to more heterogeneous populations is to modify the exclusion criteria used when recruiting trial participants. In many cases, researchers have relied on arbitrary exclusion criteria carried over from previous similar studies with very little to no justification for continued use (FDA, 2018; Indorewalla et al., 2021). Moreover, studies have shown that differential exclusion criteria based on race and ethnicity have been one significant barrier to entry for minority populations in AD/ADRD clinical trials (Raman et al., 2021). The screening criteria for trial participation, particularly among trials examining monoclonal antibodies, are also very restrictive when it comes to prioritizing patients with high levels of amyloid deposits in their brain, and this requirement often results in the exclusion of people with less observable pathology (Reardon, 2023).

Although there are reasonable rationales for excluding people with comorbidities, such as diabetes and hypertension, and mixed pathologies from some trials, ultimately these are also critical elements of diversity needed to evaluate the potential of interventions for real-world effectiveness. Careful consideration will be needed to address such deficiencies and to incorporate participant populations that are multidimensionally diverse into future trial designs.

Trial participants are also often excluded from studies if they are already participating in other clinical trials (Myles et al., 2014). While such exclusions may be justified, strategies need to be explored to maximize the involvement of these (presumably highly engaged) participants once they become eligible. One such strategy may involve the creation of a database of eligible volunteers that can be used to track current involvement in clinical trials in real time so they can be notified of opportunities once their participation ends. Similar challenges arise with the exclusion of individuals who lack a care partner or caregiver or those who are excluded due to surpassing arbitrary age cutoffs (Mitchell et al., 2024). Thus, there is a need to rethink the exclusion criteria currently being employed in AD/ADRD clinical trials to ensure that researchers are not inadvertently excluding individuals who could both benefit from and contribute to the success of any given trial.

Efforts to increase recruitment of representative clinical trial participants would benefit from mechanisms that encourage a seamless transition from AD/ADRD diagnosis to trial recruitment. As such, trained primary care providers could play an important role in recruitment by informing patients of available study opportunities or by requesting their consent to be notified about future AD/ADRD research initiatives. Another approach could involve presenting an option to receive trial information and invitations to contribute to research at the time of Medicare or retirement benefits enrollment (Cummings, 2024). Mechanisms to enroll clinical trial participants from existing longitudinal observational studies may also help improve representativeness and external validity, particularly as cohorts become more diverse, although such practices need to be carefully orchestrated to ensure there is no risk to the integrity of the cohort study. A notable example comes from ALLFTD, a longitudinal study designed to help researchers better understand the natural history of frontotemporal lobar degeneration (both sporadic and autosomal-dominant forms) through the collection of clinical, neuropsychological, neuroimaging, and biofluid data (Boeve et al., 2020). Not only was the study designed to inform future clinical trials, but study participants may also be recruited into trials that evaluate potential disease modifying therapies or other interventions.

Providing research participants with increased ownership and decision making when it comes to choosing which studies they would like to participate in, instead of relying on study sites to make these decisions, can be another means to improve clinical trial recruitment and potentially the diversity of participants (Smith, 2024). Providing persons living with AD/ADRD and their caregivers and care partners with plenty of opportunities to ask questions, reiterating important trial details throughout the entirety of their involvement, as well as clearly communicating the risks and benefits of participation, are all strategies that can help people feel more empowered to make informed decisions and reduce some of the uncertainties and anxieties surrounding clinical trial enrollment (Connell et al., 2001; Indorewalla et al., 2021; Yancey et al., 2006).

To be successful in recruiting diverse study populations, it is important for AD/ADRD researchers to build long-term reciprocal relationships with communities, particularly those that have been traditionally excluded from research studies. Making use of community-based participatory research approaches can help with relationship building (NASEM, 2024). Researchers can also form working relationships with community-based primary care providers in order to receive referrals of patients who meet their study criteria (Heller et al., 2014; Indorewalla et al., 2021). Other opportunities to better engage with diverse communities include embedding trial sites within community settings (i.e., decentralized trials) and including people from those communities in the trial leadership. This could be done, for example, by partnering with federally qualified health centers and community health resource centers.

NIH has invested in developing and testing approaches to build community collaborations as a means of increasing participation in clinical research by diverse and underrepresented populations (NIA, n.d.). Funded efforts have included several research collaborations focused on testing approaches for, and building research partnerships with, priority populations. For example, the NIA-funded Engaging Communities of Hispanics/Latinos for Aging Research Network assesses barriers to research participation and builds collaborations between health centers, community-based organizations, residents, and researchers within Hispanic and Latinx populations in three large metropolitan areas (ECHAR, 2024).

Decentralized trials can use a hub-and-spoke model to allow the centralization of some core infrastructure while reducing barriers to trial participation by enabling data and sample collection at the embedded sites in diverse communities (Cummings, 2024). The Alzheimer's Clinical Trials Consortium, for example, uses this model to encourage collaboration between the "hub," which consists of leadership with extensive expertise in AD/ADRD research methods, and the "spokes," which include site recruitment and engagement teams operating on the ground, with the ultimate goal of enhancing community partnerships and increasing the participation of underserved populations in AD/ADRD clinical trials (Raman et al., 2022). Some aspects of participant screening (e.g., blood collection and testing), for example, could be conducted at community sites near residential areas and those who pass screening could then be referred on to trial sites.

Going one step further, trials are increasingly moving the interface with participants, including data and sample collection, to participants' homes, which may address barriers to access for underrepresented participant populations. Digital health technologies are making such approaches more feasible. For example, a recent study demonstrated the feasibility of using a smartphone app to collect data on cognition, speech and language, and motor function in participants living with FTD (Taylor et al., 2023). However, such tools require careful evaluation for reliability and appropriate contexts of use given that people living with AD/ADRD may increasingly struggle with some data collection tasks as their disease progresses. Remote data collection also has the potential to reduce the level of effort required for caregivers or care partners who otherwise may have had to accompany the study participant to trial sites since the availability of a care giver or care partner is a common condition of participation for safety reasons.

In addition to collaborating with community members to advance AD/ADRD research goals, investigators can also encourage the sharing of participant experiences in past clinical trials through targeted education efforts in order to mitigate fears surrounding trial participation and promote the potential benefits (Clement et al., 2019; Indorewalla et al., 2021). By using these strategies and prioritizing inclusivity when designing clinical trials, researchers can better capture the heterogeneity of AD/ADRD disease mechanisms and develop interventions that can benefit more diverse populations.

Conclusion 4-4: The elimination of barriers to increasing clinical trial accessibility and reducing disparities in research participation decreases selection bias, improves the efficiency of clinical trials, and enhances the external validity and generalizability of trial results.

Improving the Evaluation of Interventions

Numerous factors contribute to the complexity related to assessing the effects of interventions and understanding the observed variability in intervention effects over time and in diverse populations. Population heterogeneity (e.g., genetic and epigenetic differences, comorbidities, sex and gender differences) needs to be considered and may be better understood by stratifying results by population group, such as by gender or genetic risk. The routine provision of sex/gender-disaggregated results from clinical trials, for example, is important for understanding differences in the efficacy of interventions and may help to guide precision medicine approaches. Other contributing factors include the different measures and instruments currently used to assess outcomes and the challenges related to the complexity of interventions and the contexts in which they are implemented. Given these complexities, the ability to better integrate different data—genetic variants, biomarkers, and clinical endpoints, including both short- and long-term outcomes—will enable improvements in the evaluation of interventions.

As discussed earlier in this chapter, the evaluation of interventions needs to consider not just efficacy, but also other benefits (e.g., reduced costs of care, ability to continue working or living independently) and harms. Cost-effectiveness studies and the incorporation of pharmacoeconomic outcomes (e.g., episodes of hospitalization or other acute care) into late-stage clinical trials can help to generate data needed to understand the balance of benefits and harms for a given intervention (Fillit et al., 2010). However, novel frameworks are needed that move beyond traditional health economics measures of health care costs and quality of life. One such framework, the Value Flower, developed by the 2018 International Society for Pharmacoeconomics and Outcomes Research (ISPOR) Special Task Force on US Value Assessments (Neumann et al., 2022), can guide new measures and data collection to quantify often overlooked elements of value, such as productivity, adherence-improving factors, reduction in uncertainty, real option value, value of hope, and scientific spillovers, among others.

Measuring Responses to Interventions

A notable gap related to assessing AD/ADRD interventions is the lack of consensus on what success looks like. Depending on the disease state of the population under study (e.g., preclinical, symptomatic, late-stage disease) and the objective of the intervention (prevention versus treatment), efficacy can be measured in different ways and commonly relies on the use of measures related to cognitive and functional outcomes, as well as changes in markers of pathobiology. For preventive strategies, risk-reduction outcomes as measured, for example, by risk scores that quantify risk and protective factors, provide a means of evaluating the intervention in the absence of clinical symptomology. Such approaches are particularly relevant for trials of NPIs targeting modifiable risk factors (Deckers et al., 2021; Hall et al., 2024; Yaffe et al., 2024).

A well-recognized challenge in evaluating AD/ADRD interventions is the variability in measures and instruments used to assess cognitive and functional status of study participants. Moreover, cognitive impairment exists on a spectrum and can be modifiable in real time, thus challenging the ability to report or measure cognitive change, especially when study subjects may be slightly impaired compared to those who are at more advanced stages of cognitive decline. Neuropsychological assessments (e.g., Mini-Mental State Examination, Montreal Cognitive Assessment) are advantageous in that they do not require lengthy assessments by specialized clinicians and provide a numerical measure of cognitive function, but such tests have well-known limitations (Ritchie et al., 2015), as discussed in Chapter 2. Additionally, the multiplicity of test batteries that are used across AD/ADRD intervention studies complicates efforts to compare different study results in meta-analyses and impedes pooled analyses (NASEM, 2017).

Functional outcomes are often identified as measures of intervention effectiveness that are important to people living with AD/ADRD and their caregivers and care partners. However, similar to cognitive measures, there is variability in the ways that functional outcomes are assessed, and instruments such as the Instrumental Activities of Daily Living scale rely on reporting by study participants or their caregivers or care partners, which is subject to bias (Ritchie et al., 2015). Moreover, tools used to evaluate functional change in later dementia stages may not be sensitive enough to detect more subtle changes in function that may be observed in earlier stages of AD/ADRD (FDA, 2024a; NIA, 2024).

For related dementias, a notable challenge with the evaluation of interventions in clinical trials is the lack of validated, disease-specific outcome measures. For example, primary end points used in LBD trials are often AD-centric, using such scales as the AD Assessment Scale–Cognitive Subscale and the AD Cooperative Study–Clinical Global Impression of Change to measure cognitive function (Goldman et al., 2020). Moreover, the over-emphasis on cognitive endpoints in clinical trials has contributed to the paucity of trials capturing other core or supportive features of LBD, such as visual hallucinations, REM sleep behavior disorder, autonomic symptoms, or motor signs of parkinsonism (Goldman et al., 2020). Improving clinical trials for related dementias will require the validation of outcomes in the target population.

For interventions that require regulatory approval (e.g., drugs and biologics), FDA historically has required demonstration of clinically meaningful effects. For interventions tested after the onset of dementia, this generally has entailed reporting on outcomes for both cognitive and functional measures, since small changes in cognitive outcomes measured with existing test batteries are not inherently considered to be clinically meaningful (FDA, 2024a). However, the shift in intervention strategies to initiate therapies at the earliest stages of disease, even prior to the development of any clinical symptoms, has necessitated reconsideration of approaches to evaluate interventions and to show clinically meaningful benefit. In early disease stages, clinical changes may be subtle and challenging to capture using tools developed for evaluating interventions in later-stage patients (Boxer and Sperling, 2023). Recognizing this need, FDA has developed guidance on drug development for the treatment of early AD (prior to onset of clinical dementia) that builds on a staging system for the disease. The most recent version of the FDA's draft guidance was released in March 2024 (FDA, 2024a). Similar guidelines are not available for other forms of dementia.

One evaluation approach for studies in early disease stages is to extend clinical trial durations to allow a time-to-event analysis for which time to a clinically meaningful event (cognition and/or function) can be compared between treatment groups. This could, for example, entail the evaluation of time required for conversion from preclinical to symptomatic disease or, for study populations that are already symptomatic, conversion from MCI to clinical dementia. It is important to keep in mind, however, that such clinical progression is not inevitable in the absence of intervention (Ritchie et al., 2015) and could require trials to have remarkably long follow-up periods in cases where onset of clinical symptoms may not be expected for years or even decades. For instance, even in studies enrolling only high-risk populations, evaluation of the preventive effects of anti-amyloid antibodies requires more than 4 years of follow-up owing to the variation in the rates at which individuals identified as having preclinical disease begin to show signs of cognitive decline. Long follow-up periods that extend the length of clinical trials can add substantially to the cost. Therefore, careful balancing of cost and length need to be considered during the design phase.

When clinically meaningful benefit of an intervention is demonstrated based on changes in cognitive measures relative to the comparison group, a stronger case can be made when there is evidence of benefit across multiple neuropsychological tests and when there are concomitant changes in characteristic pathophysiologic features (FDA, 2024a). FDA has indicated that it will consider surrogate endpoints that are "reasonably likely to predict clinical benefit" for the purposes of accelerated approval but emphasized the need for postapproval trials to "verify and describe clinical benefit" (FDA, 2024a, p. 6). This approach was used in the approval of two anti-amyloid antibody-based therapies for AD, aducanumab and lecanemab, with a biomarker—reduction in brain amyloid beta as measured by PET—serving as a surrogate endpoint for prediction of clinical benefit. This approach, while controversial (particularly as related to aducanumab approval), demonstrates the importance of the selection of appropriate surrogate endpoints, which will depend on the disease stage of study participants at the time of trial initiation and the mechanism of action for the intervention (FDA, 2024a). Such decisions by study sponsors are also likely to be influenced by current guidance from regulatory authorities (Yu et al., 2022).

Identifying biomarkers for demonstrating target engagement and measuring treatment response As discussed in Chapter 2, biomarkers can serve multiple purposes in the context of AD/ADRD research. In addition to being used for clinical diagnosis (diagnostic biomarkers), determination of clinical trial eligibility (screening biomarkers), and guiding treatment decisions (prognostic biomarkers), biomarkers can also be used to demonstrate target engagement and to assess the response to an intervention (response biomarkers) (Cummings, 2019; Hampel et al., 2019). Given that large, long-duration studies may be needed to demonstrate that a disease-modifying therapy is engaging the intended target and modifying disease progression, biomarkers can play an important role in phase 2 clinical trials to demonstrate proof of concept prior to initiating trials intended to demonstrate clinical benefit (Cummings, 2019; Cummings et al., 2018). Without the ability to demonstrate target engagement, it can be challenging to know why a trial failed.

A notable impediment to drug development is the lack of biomarkers that could be used to demonstrate target engagement for many of the mechanistic pathways that might be targetable to prevent or treat AD/ADRD. Such biomarkers may need to be developed in conjunction with a candidate therapy to more readily establish clinical efficacy (Cummings, 2019). As noted in the preceding section, biomarkers may also be important intermediate or surrogate endpoints for phase 3 clinical trials testing the efficacy of an intervention in study populations that have not yet developed signs of AD/ADRD or who are in early stages (e.g., preclinical). Even when trials in academic settings are not intended to support regulatory approval of an intervention, the 5-year grant cycle may necessitate intermediate outcomes that can be measured before clinical endpoints may be reasonably expected.

While amyloid-PET is a frequently used response biomarker that has already been incorporated into regulatory approval processes for AD evaluation and treatments, the identification of additional response biomarkers is an active area of investigation. For AD, brain tau levels as measured by PET are also being evaluated as a response biomarker, but the evidence from past clinical trials of anti-amyloid antibody treatments regarding the ability of tau-PET to reflect clinically meaningful intervention effects has been mixed (Aisen et al., 2021; Boxer and Sperling, 2023). Also under development is a PET tracer for synaptic loss, which is not AD specific and may be more easily linked to meaningful cognitive and functional outcomes than biomarkers for other pathologic features such as plaques and tangles (Gregory et al., 2022; Márquez and Yassa, 2019). Disease-nonspecific biomarkers that closely correlate with clinical outcomes may be particularly beneficial for the study of mixed forms of dementia (Toledo et al., 2023).

Given the logistical difficulty and significant cost of PET scans, there is great interest in fluid-phase biomarkers of intervention response (Boxer and Sperling, 2023). CSF biomarker levels are reflective of pathophysiologic processes in the central nervous system (Abdelmoaty et al., 2023), and CSF levels of amyloid beta and phosphorylated tau (p-tau)[2] have been monitored in trials of anti-amyloid treatments (Cummings, 2019). However, collection of CSF poses its own logistical challenges. Blood-based biomarkers, which would be less invasive, have the potential to be useful tools for measuring intervention responses. Plasma levels of p-tau have been shown to be sensitive to the effects of anti-amyloid antibody treatments, although reductions in plasma p-tau181 and p-tau217 have been observed in clinical trials following treatment even in the absence of observed clinical benefit (Boxer and Sperling, 2023), indicating a need for further investigation of the ability of these biomarkers to predict clinically meaningful change during clinical trials. Such discrepancies also reinforce the need to study endpoints of disease over extended periods in ways that more realistically capture the clinical progression of study participants.

As is the case for diagnostic biomarkers (discussed in Chapter 2), the identification of response biomarkers for LBD, FTD, and other related dementias lags behind the progress made for AD, and this represents an area of unmet need (Abdelmoaty et al., 2023; Del Campo et al., 2022). While useful for LBD diagnostic purposes, alpha-synuclein seed amplification assays are not currently well suited for predicting or tracking disease progression (Vijiaratnam and Foltynie, 2023). It is therefore not clear whether they will be useful as measures of treatment response. In the absence of disease-specific response markers, biomarkers of neurodegeneration, which would be expected to change in response to disease-modifying therapies, may be of use in the evaluation of interventions for AD/ADRD. CSF total tau, atrophy on MRI, fluorodeoxyglucose (FDG) PET (which measures brain metabolic activity), neurofilament light chain (NfL), neurogranin, and visinin-like protein-1 (VILIP-1) are all potential biomarkers of neurodegeneration; as they are not specific to AD, they may be useful for evaluating interventions for related dementias (Abdelmoaty et al., 2023; Boxer et al., 2020; Cummings, 2019). Given that inflammation is a common shared feature of AD/ADRD (as discussed in Chapter 3), inflammatory markers are also being investigated as potential response biomarkers (Abdelmoaty et al., 2023). This approach could be broadened to consider other metrics of accelerated or premature aging (López-Otín et al., 2023).

While not required for use in clinical trials to evaluate the effects of interventions, qualification of response biomarkers through established FDA processes could help to accelerate the development of effective interventions

---

[2] Tau, a microtubule-associated protein that plays an important role in intracellular transportation is thought to become hyperphosphorylated during the formation of neurofibrillary tangles, resulting in p-tau (Cummings, 2019).

for AD/ADRD (Cummings, 2019). A biomarker that has been qualified for a specific context of use can be relied upon to have a specific interpretation (FDA, 2020a,b), thus reducing the uncertainty that is currently involved in interpreting biomarker results from clinical trials.

While useful as intermediate outcomes and for early-response monitoring, a key issue with biomarkers is the lack of a direct link to functional or quality-of-life outcomes. The ideal measure would be one that can link interventions to cognitive changes. Further efforts are needed to better integrate molecular and clinical biomarkers.

Conclusion 4-5: The lack of validated mechanistic biomarkers, beyond amyloid and tau, that can confirm that a pathway has been engaged by an intervention is compounded by the lack of markers that can act as a surrogate endpoint for assessing the efficacy of an intervention and limit the capacity of clinical trials to rapidly evaluate interventions.

Importance of person-centered outcomes The effectiveness of an intervention should be considered and defined in relation to what is important to those living with (or at risk for) the disease (DiBenedetti et al., 2020; Paulsen, 2024). While changes in biomarker levels thought to reflect changes in the underlying disease pathology have been used as a primary measure of successful treatment (e.g., as with anti-amyloid therapies), such outcomes may not necessarily correlate with the goal of actually helping people living with AD/ADRD along with their family members and care partners. Furthermore, many neuropsychological tests that are currently employed to assess disease severity may not accurately capture the priorities of people living with the disease, particularly regarding emotional and psychological effects (Hartry et al., 2018; NIA, 2024).

An analysis conducted by Harding and colleagues (2020) of over 350 outcome measurement instruments used in dementia research demonstrated that none of these tools had sufficient face validity to adequately capture the needs and priorities of people living with dementia and their care partners and caregivers. For this reason, having a thorough understanding of what matters most to people living with AD/ADRD can inform the development of interventions that better address their quality of life and well-being (Jessen et al., 2022).

The use of qualitative or ethnographic studies to obtain narratives from people living with AD/ADRD is one way to highlight individual experiences with these diseases and to uncover the treatment outcomes they value most (Saunders et al., 2021). According to one of the few qualitative studies that have examined patient-centered outcomes for AD, improving cognitive changes characterized by worsening memory and forgetfulness was the most important outcome for study participants, followed by stopping or slowing the progression of the disease, and improving the ability to function on a day-to-day basis (DiBenedetti et al., 2020). Moreover, the emotional and social effects of AD, including increased feelings of frustration and stress, along with decreased outgoingness, was reported by most participants to be the most detrimental (DiBenedetti et al., 2020). Another study uncovered that, along with cognitive and functional outcomes, additional priorities for people living with AD include the desire to maintain their quality of life along with their identity and personality, recognizing the effect of mental health, and maintaining a healthy patient–caregiver relationship (Jessen et al., 2022; Tochel et al., 2019). In addition, the ability to remain at home or in community settings instead of receiving care at an in-patient institution could also improve disease trajectory and reduce economic costs at the individual or family levels and for society at large.

The push to have more representation from those with lived experience in determining dementia research priorities and outcomes has been rapidly growing in recent years, both from patient-advocacy groups and from the scientific community. Bechard and colleagues (2022), for example, found that almost all researchers surveyed advocated for the value of people with lived experience contributing to dementia research. However, the support for including the views of those living with AD/ADRD conceptually has not been translated adequately into practice because of a lack of prioritization along with a range of methodological challenges that accompany the engagement of this specific population in research (ASPE, 2017).

There have been active efforts internationally to overcome some of these challenges and better incorporate the voices of those with lived experience into AD/ADRD research. Alzheimer's Europe, along with other government and charitable organizations, have emphasized the right of people living with AD/ADRD and caregivers and care partners to be included in dementia research (Alzheimer Society of Ireland, 2017; Gove et al., 2018; Miah et al., 2019). Moreover, the UK's National Institute for Health and Care Research has provided guidance to researchers on engaging patients and the public in their research, including guidance related to coproducing a research project with members of the public along with payment for research participation (NIHR, 2019). Thus, codesign approaches and funding requirements are mechanisms that can better ensure the inclusion of outcomes that matter to those most affected.

Given the cognitive impairment resulting from AD/ADRD, people living with these diseases can struggle to articulate what really matters to them. For this reason, research tools used to engage individuals living with AD/ADRD need to be employed at different stages of disease and address the diversity of unique perspectives and experiences. The use of study partners could be one way to help people living with AD/ADRD monitor and report on various cognitive, functional, and emotional outcomes to ensure that the wide breadth of the experiences of this population is fully captured. To enhance the benefits of using study partners in research, sponsors and investigators should work toward addressing the barriers for their participation and properly compensate them for their labor (Largent and Lynch, 2017). Caution is needed, however, when it comes to relying on subjective observations as primary data points; for example, men and women may report differently about a spouse suffering from cognitive decline (Stites et al., 2023). The efforts to prioritize person-centered outcomes should therefore have these considerations at the forefront to ensure that the voices of people living with AD/ADRD are incorporated in research that is both rigorous and representative of those most affected.

Evaluating longitudinal outcomes   Outcome measurement in dementia research can be challenging when conducting multiple or long-term assessments. Many neuropsychological tests measuring memory, for example, do not work well when used repeatedly, particularly over shorter time intervals (Lim et al., 2022). Using the same measurements numerous times over an extended period can result in unwanted noise and impair the assessment's ability to accurately capture the desired construct. Moreover, the repeated use of the same instruments can result in improved performance owing to practice effects, thereby compromising the ability to effectively measure disease trajectory (Calamia et al., 2012; Duff et al., 2017; Lim et al., 2022)—although lack of a practice effect could be interpreted as an indicator of a cognitive issue (Öhman et al., 2021). The use of novel digital assessment tools can help overcome some of these challenges. Mobile devices, for example, can potentially provide more robust and reliable information over long-term application compared to traditional assessments (Öhman et al., 2021; Sliwinski et al., 2018). In addition, computerized or algorithm-based measures that can automatically generate alternative items or forms can help reduce the effect of practice or version effects (Miller and Barr, 2017; Öhman et al., 2021), while artificial intelligence methods can also be employed to better analyze cognitive data (Laske et al., 2015).

Given the long-term course of AD/ADRD and the numerous challenges associated with running clinical trials over an extended time period, researchers often have very little knowledge of what happens after a trial ends, including the degree to which participants continue to adhere to interventions. This knowledge gap is a persistent issue that extends to intervention approaches for many health conditions (NIH, 2021) and impedes efforts to understand how long-term maintenance affects outcomes such as the prevention or delay of disease onset. Generally, the more complex or demanding an intervention is, the harder it is for participants to consistently adhere to the regimen (Coley et al., 2019). Moreover, conducting research with people living with AD/ADRD presents an additional layer of complexity given that cognitive status moderates adherence; thus, individuals with more advanced cognitive impairment will likely have more difficulty adhering to an intervention (Smith et al., 2017).

There have been numerous past efforts to characterize and improve patient adherence to AD/ADRD interventions. Tullo and colleagues (2023), for example, examined the effect of personal and demographic factors such as age, gender, cognitive ability, and personality, along with the influence of the spacing and consistency of training sessions, on adherence to a cognitive training regimen among adult participants. The study found that none of these variables reliably predicted compliance with cognitive training exercises, suggesting the limited and inconsistent role of individual difference factors in modulating adherence. Turunen and colleagues (2019) similarly investigated the long-term adherence of older adults to computerized cognitive training and found that familiarity with computers, having a spouse or roommate, better memory performance, and a positive outlook toward the study predicted an increased likelihood of beginning the training regimen; however, only previous computer use was associated with higher completion rates of the cognitive training exercises. Other studies have pointed toward building agency and encouraging participant engagement as critical components of intervention design (Yaffe et al., 2024). Furthermore, incorporating motivational features into the intervention to build self-efficacy (Jaeggi et al., 2023), increasing gamification (Koivisto and Malik, 2021), and capitalizing on a patient's existing support system by having caregivers and care partners send personalized reminders and conduct regular check-ins can also be very beneficial for intervention adherence.

Given the limited follow-up period of many traditional clinical trials, it can be expected that additional data regarding long-term outcomes from interventions may be generated after the intervention has been implemented in real-world settings. Consequently, establishing systems to collect evidence on interventions that have been implemented in community and/or health care settings can help assess their real-world effectiveness in addition to their external validity. For example, the Alzheimer's Network for Treatment and Diagnostics (ALZ-NET), a voluntary health care provider-enrolled network established in 2021 and led by the Alzheimer's Association, is an initiative that will collect real-world data from clinical practice into a registry (Alzheimer's Network, 2024; Carillo, 2024; NIA, 2022). This initiative will generate data to further evaluate the usage, effectiveness, and safety of FDA-approved therapies for AD. Registries and other real-world data collection platforms have the potential to significantly enhance the ability to evaluate interventions longitudinally and to elucidate the effects of such factors as social determinants of health and polypharmacy on intervention effectiveness. Partnership with advocacy organizations has the potential to improve such real-world data collection platforms developed in the future, but realizing their potential will require overcoming numerous barriers to collecting and using real-world evidence, including siloed data sources, need for data harmonization, and privacy and data security concerns (NIA, 2022).

For decades, patient registries, which systematically collect and store uniform data on patients with a specific disease, condition, or procedure, have informed public health priorities, programs, and spending, as well as basic science and clinical and social science research (AHRQ, 2014). In the United States, cancer and kidney disease registries and, more recently, vaccination registries have been particularly effective along these dimensions. Despite the potential value of registries, it is only recently that registries focused on AD/ADRD were established. The dementia registries that do exist differ in their goals, the populations represented, the types of data collected and/or linked to, their geographical coverage, and how they are funded and sustained.

Recent and ongoing advances in AD/ADRD prevention, diagnosis, and treatment further underscore the importance of dementia registry data. Scientific advances are reshaping prevention strategies. Technological innovations are changing interactions with medical care. The health care system is exploring improved care delivery methods, and ongoing research is deepening insights into how social determinants of health affect dementia risk. New AD treatments are entering the market. With linkages to other datasets, a population-based dementia registry can support efforts to monitor these changes and assess, for example, who has access to new therapies and conduct postmarket surveillance to establish the effectiveness and safety of these treatments in real-world settings. The Swedish Dementia Registry (SveDem), which was initiated in 2007 and covers most of Sweden, is an example of a population-based registry that is informing researchers, policy makers, patients, and the public about current dementia treatment and care in Sweden. SveDem's annual reports provide knowledge about diagnostics, medical treatment, and community and social support (Religa et al., 2015).

Monitoring Safety Outcomes

Adverse event monitoring is a critical part of the evaluation of novel and investigational therapies and extends beyond the clinical trial phase of research into postmarket surveillance. Adverse events can take myriad forms, both physical and psychological. Examples of adverse events associated with AD/ADRD treatments include gastrointestinal ulceration and bleeding, cardiovascular conditions such as severe sinus bradycardia, worsening neuropsychological symptoms, and in some extreme cases can lead to hospitalization and death (Khoury et al., 2018; Ruangritchankul et al., 2021). Current FDA-approved anti-amyloid antibody therapies for AD can result in adverse events that can be detected through magnetic resonance imaging (MRI) in the form of amyloid-related imaging abnormalities

(ARIA) (Withington and Turner, 2022). The imaging abnormalities have been linked to microhemorrhages (ARIA-H) and the leakage of fluid from blood vessels in the brain, which causes the collection of the fluid in the interstitial spaces and localized edema (ARIA-E). ARIA risk increases with drug dose, thus raising the potential for a tradeoff between safety and efficacy that needs to be considered in development of dosing regimens (Boxer and Sperling, 2023). In most cases ARIA is asymptomatic, but for some patients it can have serious health effects and in rare cases is fatal (Solopova et al., 2023; Sperling et al., 2011; Withington and Turner, 2022). As referenced later in the chapter, risk of ARIA is known to be increased among those with the *APOE4* allele, a group that is also at higher risk for AD (Sperling et al., 2011). These combined factors complicate the assessment of risks and benefits in the use of current anti-amyloid therapies.

Mitigating the harms associated with potentially life-threatening adverse events requires effective mechanisms to carefully monitor and address their effects. Biomarkers such as liver function, muscle enzymes, and electrocardiograms can play a key role in indicating drug toxicity and have been used in the development of disease-modifying therapies for AD/ADRD (Cummings, 2019). The use of MRI to monitor the presence of ARIA has also been essential to monitoring safety outcomes for treatment with anti-amyloid therapies (Cummings, 2019). Scheduling multiple MRIs in regular intervals during the first month of drug exposure along with subsequent monitoring if ARIA symptoms are detected is one strategy employed to prioritize safety, both in clinical care and throughout the course of a trial (Cummings and Kinney, 2022). In addition, researchers and care providers can use blood tests and physical examination, along with future markers and direct reports from patients, to evaluate the safety and tolerability of AD/ADRD medication (Cummings et al., 2018).

Beyond the physiological adverse effects that can accompany pharmacologic treatments, there are additional safety considerations related to patient privacy and the stigma surrounding an AD/ADRD diagnosis (see Chapter 2). The need to maintain participant privacy and confidentiality in AD/ADRD research is especially prominent with the increased use of mobile applications in combination with artificial intelligence and machine learning approaches to report and monitor clinical symptoms and other pertinent health information. Without proper regulation, the use of these digital tools could lead to individuals having their data sold or misused and could even result in discrimination by insurance companies and employers (Anthes, 2020; Piendel et al., 2023). A review of 83 mobile health applications for neuropsychiatric conditions, including AD and dementia, found a significant lack of policies protecting patient privacy along with deficient HIPPA regulations regarding use of the data (Minen et al., 2021; Piendel et al., 2023). Thus, the continued use of these technologies to aid research efforts needs to be accompanied by increased guardrails around their use to ensure that the privacy of patients and research participants is not compromised.

Understanding the Effects of Multicomponent Interventions

There is increasing interest in multimodal and combination interventions that have the ability to simultaneously or sequentially target multiple etiologies or risk factors and thereby prevent or delay the onset of dementia. In previous studies, a factorial study design has been used to elucidate the value of a multicomponent intervention over a single-component intervention for enhancing treatment outcomes (NASEM, 2017). However, there is an urgent need to also identify strategies that help determine which components or combinations of components contribute to notable benefits, whether that be maintaining overall brain health or slowing the progression of disease. A multiphase optimization strategy may be useful for this purpose when designing and implementing an intervention (Strayhorn et al., 2024).

When evaluating the effect of a multicomponent intervention using traditional methods, such as a two-arm RCT, the efficacy of each individual component is not estimated empirically (Strayhorn et al., 2024). Since the intervention components are combined as a package and evaluated together in these trials, this creates notable limitations when attempting to modify the interventions to make them more scalable, affordable, and efficient. A multiphase optimization strategy, however, enables researchers to assess the contributions of individual intervention components by allowing them to identify from a set of components the combination that best demonstrates effectiveness, affordability, scalability, and efficiency (Collins, 2018; Strayhorn et al., 2024). This strategy employs multiple phases of research, beginning with an optimization phase during which components are assessed individually and in combination and decisions are made about which combination to move forward. Then, in a subsequent evaluation stage, their combined efficacy is assessed, typically in a RCT. Thus, by using similar innovative decision-making strategies, AD/ADRD researchers can better understand the interactions between different components of a multimodal intervention, and be better equipped to tailor intervention approaches to meet the needs of a diverse population.

Accelerating Decision Making Within the Clinical Trial Pipeline

In the last 20 years, only three drugs—aducanumab, lecanemab, and donanemab—have been approved by FDA for the treatment of AD (Cummings et al., 2023a; FDA, 2024b), and the modest clinical benefits of these drugs are accompanied by risk for serious adverse effects. There are currently no drugs specifically approved for the treatment of LBD (MacDonald et al., 2022), FTD (Khoury et al., 2021), limbic-predominant age-related TDP-43 encephalopathy (LATE) (Nag et al., 2020), or vascular dementia (Alzheimer's Association, 2024), beyond those for managing symptoms. While there has been some promising evidence for nonpharmacological approaches to preventing dementia (NASEM, 2017), much of the evidence from clinical trials on NPIs has been negative or mixed, making it difficult to draw definitive conclusions. The prospect of waiting additional decades to develop safe, effective preventive and therapeutic interventions for AD/ADRD is untenable given the human and economic costs associated with these devastating diseases. To accelerate this timeline, mechanisms such as those discussed in the following sections are needed to facilitate the timely, successive progression of interventions through the clinical trial pipeline, maximally leveraging the results from earlier trials.

Prespecifying Go/No-Go Criteria

The incorporation of prespecified, go/no-go criteria into the clinical trials pipeline provides one means of accelerating decision making regarding interventions that should be advanced into subsequent trials. The incorporation of interim analyses into trial timelines for highest-priority outcomes, when appropriate, can improve efficiency. While safety and tolerability have traditionally been used as go/no-go criteria in early-phase clinical trials (Stallard et al., 2001), a growing repertoire of biomarkers that can be used to evaluate short-term intervention effects, such as target engagement, pharmacodynamics, and effects predictive of clinical benefit, may additionally be used to inform go/no-go decisions and over time begin to reduce the number of negative phase 3 clinical trials (Boxer and Sperling, 2023; Cummings, 2019). This further underscores the critical importance of continued biomarker discovery for improved clinical outcomes and the acceleration of progress in the prevention and treatment of AD/ADRD. However, a consideration in the use of go/no-go criteria to stop trials (particularly in early-stage phase 1b and 2 trials) early is the tradeoff between improving efficiency and loss of opportunities to learn about the biology of AD/ADRD, which is a fundamental element of NIH-funded AD/ADRD clinical research. Thus, use of go/no-go criteria, may not be appropriate in all trials.

Implementing Innovative Clinical Trial Designs

Although expansion of the portfolio of novel strategies for prevention and treatment of AD/ADRD is encouraging and should remain a priority, evaluating the safety and efficacy of this growing number of interventions will require an increase in the efficiency and speed of clinical trials. The expense and time required for traditional clinical research approaches that entail successive testing of single interventions in a single study population serve as major impediments to the identification of effective interventions for AD/ADRD. Similar challenges experienced in the field of oncology led to the implementation of innovative clinical trial designs, such as platform trials (see Box 4-1) and the use of master protocols to increase efficiency (Boxer and Sperling, 2023). Such approaches may also be useful in the AD/ADRD field.

Master trial protocols enable the evaluation of multiple interventions in more than one target population within the same overall trial structure. Thus, a single protocol can be used to answer multiple research questions (Aisen et al., 2021; Woodcock and LaVange, 2017), thereby helping to achieve efficiencies in trial infrastructure, regulatory interactions, and data standardization (Boxer and Sperling, 2023). Master protocols are applicable to multiple trial types, including umbrella, basket, and platform trials (see Figures 4-1 and 4-2). These and other examples of innovative trial designs with the potential to accelerate the evaluation of interventions for preventing and treating AD/ADRD are described in Table 4-1. Importantly, basket trials have the potential to reduce siloing in AD/ADRD clinical research by incorporating multiple target populations into a single trial. A consideration related to the implementation of innovative trial designs for the evaluation of experimental pharmacological agents is the potential impact on processes and timelines for FDA approval (Brooks, 2024). Increased adoption of innovative trial designs by investigators will depend in part on the degree to which they are embraced by federal research funders and regulators.

In addition to novel clinical trial designs, enrichment strategies also have the potential to increase the efficiency of clinical trials. Enrichment involves the selection of a study population based on prospectively defined patient (or individual) characteristics to increase the likelihood of detecting an intervention effect (FDA, 2019b). Enrichment strategies also help to support precision medicine by targeting and tailoring interventions to those patients who would be expected to benefit from them based on results from subtyping (endotyping or phenotyping) using clinical or multiomics data, as discussed further later in this chapter. An important consideration for enrichment designs is whether the strategy could be used in practice to identify people to whom the intervention should be targeted and its potential usefulness in a broader population. FDA defines three categories of enrichment strategies:

- Strategies to decrease variability—The selection of study participants whose baseline measurements of a disease phenotype or a biomarker reflecting a disease fall within a narrow range can decrease variability and thereby increase study power.

BOX 4-1
Accelerated Decision Making in a Platform Trial:
Lessons from I-SPY and Breast Cancer

The I-SPY 2 clinical trial was one of the first platform trials and employed an innovative research paradigm to enhance the development of neoadjuvant therapy for locally advanced breast cancer (QLHC, 2024). This novel paradigm differs from traditional clinical trial methods in its ability to test multiple therapeutic agents adaptively, thereby reducing the amount of time and the number of participants needed to carry out a study and improving trial efficiency (Esserman, 2024; QLHC, 2024). In addition, the adaptive trial design allows the use of early data from one group of patients to predict the response of subsequent patient groups and inform the assignment of participants to study arms, thus minimizing the exposure of study participants to therapies that do not work for them (FNIH, 2023; QLHC, 2024; Wang and Yee, 2019).

The I-SPY 2 trial model uses clinical biomarkers to classify a patient's breast cancer into 1 of 10 molecular subtypes and then assigns that patient to a study arm using adaptive randomization. The primary endpoint is the pathologic complete response (pCR) or the complete elimination of the tumor in the breast and lymph nodes at the time of surgery, which follows treatment (Wang and Yee, 2019). Using statistical methods appropriate for a Bayesian adaptive design (Potter et al., 2021b), the predictive probabilities of each therapeutic agent are updated in real time based on the patient's tumor subtype, the treatment received, and notable biomarker outcomes such pCR or MRI tumor volume (QLHC, 2024). A therapeutic agent under evaluation would be considered a success if it reaches a predetermined level of efficacy in one or more tumor subtypes; alternatively, its use may be discontinued if the predictive probability of success falls below a set threshold across subtypes (QLHC, 2024; Wang and Yee, 2019). This approach not only enables the assessment of multiple therapies simultaneously, but it also better mirrors how cancer patients receive clinical care in the real world (Esserman, 2024). Thus, researchers have an opportunity to use innovative clinical trials to inform care and, in turn, better use real-world data to optimize clinical trial design.

I-SPY 2 employs a master protocol that allows multiple agents to enter and leave the trial without having to stop enrollment or resubmit the entire study protocol for regulatory review (QLHC, 2024). Investigators are also aiming to receive accelerated approval for agents with optimal pCR rates, emphasizing the need for FDA collaboration (Esserman, 2024). In addition to unique regulatory considerations, the facilitation of

continued

BOX 4-1 Continued

data sharing among researchers across all sectors is another hallmark of this study. Study investigators have made data from the trial publicly available to researchers under the condition that those who use the data in their studies put their own results back into the open-access platform (Esserman, 2024). In this way, researchers working in this space are not hindered unnecessarily by data availability concerns and can instead focus their efforts on developing effective therapies for breast cancer patients.

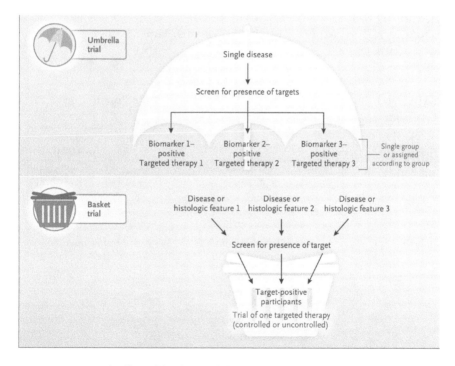

FIGURE 4-1 Umbrella and basket trial designs.
SOURCE: Woodcock and LaVange, 2017. Copyright © Reprinted with permission from Massachusetts Medical Society.

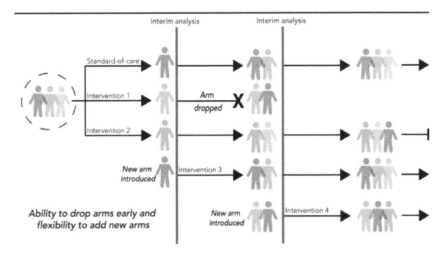

FIGURE 4-2 Schematic of a platform trial design.
SOURCE: Park et al., 2020. CC BY-NC-ND 4.0. https://creativecommons.org/licenses/by-nc-nd/4.0/.

TABLE 4-1 Innovative Clinical Trial Designs with the Potential to Accelerate Evaluation of AD/ADRD Interventions

Trial Design	Description	Illustrative Example of Application to AD/ADRD
Basket trials	Trials are designed for testing a single intervention in multiple populations (e.g., people with different disease types or subtypes) (Boxer and Sperling, 2023; Woodcock and LaVange, 2017).	A trial for a tau-targeted intervention in participants with AD or related dementia types characterized by tau pathology
Umbrella trials	Trials are designed to study multiple interventions (or combination interventions) in a single clinical population (e.g., people with the same disease). The use of a single placebo group increases the likelihood of participants receiving an intervention under study (Boxer and Sperling, 2023; Woodcock and LaVange, 2017).	A trial testing multiple different combinations of NPIs and anti-amyloid therapies in an AD population

TABLE 4-1 Continued

Trial Design	Description	Illustrative Example of Application to AD/ADRD
Platform trials	Trials are designed to study multiple interventions for a single disease type in an open-ended manner with new interventions entering the trial as others leave it, based on a specified decision algorithm (Woodcock and LaVange, 2017). This design allows interventions to be tested in parallel instead of sequentially. *Adaptive platform trials* allow the addition of new study arms or individual arms to be halted based on an interim analysis indicating a lack of efficacy (Aisen et al., 2021).	A trial testing multiple anti-amyloid antibodies in an AD population with study arms halted as some antibodies are found to be ineffective and new arms started as new antibodies are ready for testing in clinical trials.
Seamless trials	Trials may facilitate expediency by consolidating clinical phases of drug development into a single, continuously amended protocol, thus eliminating gaps between phased trials (Hobbs et al., 2019).	Different doses of an investigational new drug for FTD are evaluated in a phase 2A trial that then transitions into a phase 2B trial with the selected dose without pausing or stopping the trial.
Phase 0 exploratory microdosing trials	Exploratory clinical trials evaluate subtherapeutic doses of novel drugs in first-in-human studies (Burt et al., 2020).	A new drug targeting a signaling pathway thought to be involved in AD is tested at subtherapeutic doses for safety, tolerability, and pharmacokinetics.
Pragmatic trials	The primary purpose of these trials is providing information to decision makers on the balance of benefits, burdens, and risks of an intervention implemented at the individual or population level (Califf and Sugarman, 2015). *Embedded pragmatic clinical trials* are often conducted in care delivery settings, thus serving to bridge clinical care and research (NIH Collaboratory, n.d.).	A trial of one or more NPIs implemented in a clinical practice setting and using electronic health records data to guide participant recruitment and for outcome monitoring.
N-of-1 trials	Personalized or single-subject clinical trials often use multiple-time-period, active-comparator crossover designs that allow randomization and masking and can provide answers about the optimal intervention for an individual (Davidson et al., 2021).	Evaluation of a treatment for sleep disorders in an individual living with LBD where the participant receives the treatment or placebo in random order over the specified treatment periods.

NOTE: AD = Alzheimer's disease; AD/ADRD = Alzheimer's disease and related dementias; FTD = frontotemporal dementia; LBD = Lewy body dementia; NPI = nonpharmacological intervention.

- Prognostic enrichment strategies—The selection of study participants who are more likely to have a disease-related endpoint or significant worsening of a condition can result in greater between-group differences in absolute effect.
- Predictive enrichment strategies—The selection of study participants with a greater likelihood of responding to an intervention (based on physiologic/disease characteristics or a biomarker related to the mechanism of action) than other patients or people with the same condition can result in larger effect sizes and reduce the required size of the study population needed to detect an effect (FDA, 2019b).

Conclusion 4-6: The sequential and individual testing of interventions that characterizes the current clinical trial landscape impedes the rapid identification of effective interventions to prevent and treat AD/ADRD.

Leveraging Public–Private Partnerships

Government, private, philanthropic, and academic organizations all play major roles in accelerating the translation of scientific advances into clinical diagnostics and interventions for AD/ADRD and contribute complementary resources and expertise. While private industry is active in the development and evaluation of pharmacological agents, other kinds of interventions and certain trial designs may be less appealing to industry owing to financial risk or the lack of financial incentives. This may be the case, for example, with many NPIs, repurposed drugs, combination interventions, and even prevention trials, which are generally of long duration and require large study populations, evaluating novel pharmacological agents (Boxer and Sperling, 2023). Funding from public and philanthropic entities and other resources, such as academic consortia, can help to incentivize industry engagement by decreasing perceived financial risks, which is particularly important for smaller companies with more limited resources, and providing access to unique patient populations and valuable scientific expertise (Boxer and Sperling, 2023).

Notable examples of academic consortia that have partnered with industry to evaluate novel AD/ADRD interventions include the Dominantly Inherited Alzheimer's Network Trials Unit, the Alzheimer's Prevention Initiative, and the Alzheimer's Clinical Trials Consortium. In addition to providing platforms for testing interventions, such consortia can help to ensure that data and samples from clinical trials are made available to other researchers (e.g., through data commons and biobanks), and that even negative trial results are published, all of which are recognized challenges when trials are solely industry sponsored (Boxer and Sperling, 2023). Academic researchers involved with such consortia can also gain valuable experience with large trials, thus helping to train and expand the clinical research workforce. However, industry engagement may depend on how trials conducted by such consortia fit into the overall development program and timeline for drug candidates and whether the studies will be supportive for regulatory submission and approval (NASEM, 2024). Joint steering committees featuring leadership from academic and industry partners can be helpful for ensuring the needs of all partners are considered and met (Irizarry, 2024).

In addition to hosting clinical trial consortia, academic medical centers are also increasingly engaging with private partners in biomarker discovery. As noted earlier in this chapter, biomarkers are likely to play an increasingly important role in accelerating decision making within the clinical trial pipeline and reducing the number of failed efficacy trials. Much of current biomarker identification is being undertaken using discovery-based platforms, but ultimately biomarkers may form the basis for companion diagnostic assays that can help to identify which patients are likely to benefit from particular therapies or to be at increased risk of adverse side effects (Arafah et al., 2023). Academic researchers may be less familiar with FDA requirements for candidate biomarkers used in therapeutic decision making and may benefit from industry diagnostic partnerships, ideally early in the drug development process so that regulatory, legal, quality, and commercial considerations are factored into early clinical studies (Silva et al., 2018).

Reconfiguring Funding Models

Innovative funding models have the potential to overcome current barriers that impede timely progression of candidate interventions through the clinical trials pipeline. For example, in response to a gap/opportunity identified at the 2021 Alzheimer's Research Summit, NIH initiated a new funding opportunity with the goal of streamlining and supporting seamless transitions in the early-stage evaluation of promising novel pharmacological interventions for AD/ADRD (NIH, 2023). The funding opportunity, released in 2023, bundles funding for early-stage clinical trials and thereby facilitates timely, successive progression from phase 1 to phase 1b/2a trials for drug candidates that meet prespecified, go/no-go safety and tolerability criteria.

Minimizing Barriers to Data Access and Usability

A final factor with the potential to accelerate decision making within the clinical trial pipeline and advance the prevention and treatment of AD/ADRD is the minimization of barriers to data access and usability so trials can evolve in real time and new insights can be gained from cross-study analyses. For example, data access is critical to conducting rigorous meta-analyses, which can help to overcome the limitations of single clinical trials, including a lack of adequate power to detect intervention effects in the many subpopulations of interest (NASEM, 2024). However, inadequate budgeting within studies and a fragmented national data infrastructure creates significant challenges to data sharing efforts. Data are currently distributed across many different systems, which can impede the conduct of collaborative and integrative research.

In 2022, NIH held a workshop on real-world data infrastructure that supports research and clinical trials for AD/ADRD. Gaps and opportunities identified during the NIH workshop overlapped with opportunities shared with the committee during its public information-gathering workshop, including the need to (1) develop common data elements (CDEs) or harmonize data to improve interoperability and the ability to aggregate or pool data, (2) improve data access, and (3) protect privacy and confidentiality through data de-identification approaches. While harmonization and the development of CDEs has been a major focus area for NIA and NINDS, further efforts to standardize CDEs across AD/ADRD research resources are needed to maximize data sharing and interoperability (Hao et al., 2024), as discussed further in Chapter 5. As noted during the NIH workshop, data infrastructures also "must serve and include the communities who would most benefit from the treatments, innovations, and ideas that emerge from that infrastructure" (NIA, 2022, p. 1).

Recognizing the critical importance of data sharing, NIH issued a final data management and sharing policy that went into effect in January 2023.[3] Under the policy, recipients are required to submit data management and sharing plans and to comply with those plans following NIH approval. While such requirements help to ensure the availability of data from NIH-funded trials, they do not address the underlying barriers (e.g., cost burden to investigators) at a study level, inadequacies of the existing data infrastructure, availability of tools (e.g., artificial intelligence/machine learning approaches) for enhancing data usability, or access to data from trials funded by other sponsors (see Chapter 5).

Learning from Clinical Trial Failures

Given the considerable investment of resources (monetary and other) required for clinical trials, a failure at phase 2 often results in the discontinuation of further evaluation of the intervention under study. However, this approach limits what can be learned from the study and the potential returns that can still be gained from the investment. Each clinical trial, even

---

[3] https://grants.nih.gov/grants/guide/notice-files/NOT-OD-21-013.html (accessed May 21, 2024).

those that have not yielded hoped-for results, has the potential to provide valuable insights into disease mechanisms and avenues for future research. A negative clinical trial does not necessarily mean that the intervention under study was ineffective. For example, the follow-up period may have been insufficient to detect a difference between intervention and control arms, the trial may have failed to reach adequate therapeutic doses in affected regions of the central nervous system (Boxer and Sperling, 2023), or population heterogeneity may not have been adequately accounted for in the selection of the study population. The latter is a challenge for diseases such as AD/ADRD characterized by substantial heterogeneity despite similarity in clinical symptoms. Therefore, it is important to understand why a clinical trial might have failed and to use that knowledge to inform future trials; however, the publication of failed trial results is not standard practice.

Opportunities to learn from clinical trial failures include confirmatory trials, as well as subgroup analyses to understand if an intervention worked for some subpopulation of the study participants and if so, why. For example, a phase 2 RCT testing an inhibitor of 11-beta-hydroxysteroid dehydrogenase 1 (11β-HSD1)—an enzyme involved in the conversion of inert cortisone to active cortisol, which, when elevated in CSF, has been linked to cognitive decline—failed to find any cognitive benefit for AD patients with mild to moderate symptoms (Seckl, 2024). However, subgroup analysis suggested that the inhibitor may slow cognitive decline in patients with higher levels of p-tau181 who are at elevated risk of disease progression. The negative trial was unpublished, highlighting the challenges that arise when data from industry-sponsored trials are not accessible. Thus, there is a need to address disincentives that prevent companies from making data available that can enable learning from trial failures (Boxer and Sperling, 2023). It should be noted, however, that post hoc subgroup analyses can be misleading for various reasons (e.g., the analysis may not be adequately powered owing to smaller subgroup sizes, or there may be issues related to randomization). Consequently, it may be better to test new hypotheses based on subgroup analyses in phase 2 rather than phase 3 trials (Cummings, 2018).

Additionally, as described in Chapter 3, well-designed trials that employ specific and validated target engagement and measures can provide important information about a hypothesized mechanism of action, regardless of the success of the primary clinical endpoint in early drug discovery trials (Mohs and Greig, 2017). This means that failure of phase 2 candidates still provides valuable data about the targeted mechanism of action, which can then be used to refine research earlier in the therapeutic pipeline and future trials. However, the testing and measurement of specific mechanistic hypotheses in addition to the primary clinical endpoint is not routinely applied in drug discovery trials despite the potential return on investment.

Drug discovery trials, including those funded by NIH, would benefit from including measures for mechanistic hypothesis in addition to primary clinical endpoints in early-stage trials to accelerate future therapeutics development regardless of trial success.

In addition to informing future clinical trials, trial failures may present opportunities for reverse translation, whereby knowledge and experiences obtained through the study are used to guide new approaches to basic and preclinical research (Cummings et al., 2018). Observations of variability in intervention response can lead to new testable hypotheses regarding mechanisms of action, which may in turn help to identify new intervention targets that can be tested in future clinical trials. In this way, research is transformed from a linear to a continuous, cyclical process (Shakhnovich, 2018).

Conclusion 4-7: A deeper understanding of why clinical trials fail can provide critically important information that can inform the design of future clinical trials and present opportunities to guide new inquiries in basic and translational research.

ADVANCING A PRECISION MEDICINE APPROACH TO AD/ADRD PREVENTION AND TREATMENT

Despite similarity in clinical features, it is increasingly clear that the multifactorial nature of AD/ADRD means that the underlying disease processes vary widely across individuals, featuring differences at multiple levels, including genetics, transcriptomics, proteomics, lipidomics, epigenetics, metabolomics, and biochemistry, thus revealing perturbations in many biological pathways including but not limited to myelination, innate immunity, mitochondrial, vascular, and synaptic transmission (Allen et al., 2018; Barupal et al., 2019; Batra et al., 2024; Carrasquillo et al., 2017; Conway et al., 2018; Higginbotham et al., 2020; Johnson et al., 2022; McKenzie et al., 2017; Mostafavi et al., 2018; Mukherjee et al., 2020; Oatman et al., 2023; Strickland et al., 2020; Toledo et al., 2017; Yang et al., 2020). Further, studies focusing on cell-specific molecular perturbations demonstrated involvement in AD/ADRD of all brain cell types and identified many cell subtypes associated with risk or other endophenotypes of AD/ADRD, such as pathology or cognition (Cain et al., 2023; Green et al., 2024; İş et al., 2024; McKenzie et al., 2018; Min et al., 2023; Patel et al., 2022; Patrick et al., 2020; Wang et al., 2020). Given this complex and heterogeneous disease etiology, several groups have begun to propose molecular subtypes for AD/ADRD to facilitate discovery of treatments and biomarkers in a precision medicine framework (Chen et al., 2023b; Higginbotham et al., 2023; Hou et al., 2024; Iturria-Medina et al., 2022; Lian et al., 2023; Neff et al., 2021; Wan et al., 2020).

The multifactorial complexity, heterogeneity, and individuality in AD/ADRD pose a significant challenge to developing and selecting effective prevention and treatment strategies because responses to interventions can be highly variable. An intervention that is beneficial for one subset of the population may be ineffective or even harmful in other subgroups (Hampel et al., 2020; Neff et al., 2021; Sarkar et al., 2024). Precision medicine approaches, which often use genomic and other biomarker information to target and tailor interventions, are precisely suited to addressing the challenge of heterogeneity.

Accordingly, advancing precision medicine in AD/ADRD research has been a notable area of emphasis for NIH in recent years. The theme of the 2024 NIH Alzheimer's Research Summit was "Building a Precision Medicine Research Enterprise."[4] Other recent meetings and workshops have focused on enabling precision medicine through open science[5] and precision medicine approaches to combination therapies for preventing and treating AD/ADRD.[6]

Although precision medicine has been envisioned since the sequencing of the human genome, technological advances are providing the opportunity to bring the vision to fruition (Hampel et al., 2019). Multiomics methods, along with the data integration and predictive capabilities of artificial intelligence (Geifman et al., 2018; Vrahatis et al., 2023), are enabling the identification of disease subtypes and improved population risk stratification, while digital health technologies (e.g., wearables, sensors) allow individual-specific health information to guide precision intervention approaches in combination with more disease-specific data (Mohler et al., 2015). With these advances, it is possible to envision a not-so-distant future wherein individual-level profiling using multiomics (e.g., genomic, transcriptomics, proteomic, epigenetic, metabolomic), biomarkers, exposomes, digital health technology, and clinical data guides precision prevention and treatment approaches to optimize brain health over the life course (Hampel et al., 2022).

Despite their potential to better address complex, multifactorial diseases, precision medicine approaches have not yet been fully integrated into the development and evaluation (e.g., clinical trials) of interventions for AD/ADRD. This may in part stem from the incomplete understanding of the biological basis for AD/ADRD, as precision approaches are grounded

---

[4] More information on the 2024 NIH Alzheimer's Research Summit is available at https://www.nia.nih.gov/2024-alzheimers-summit (accessed October 20, 2024).

[5] For more information see https://www.alz.org/alzheimers-precision-medicine/overview.asp (accessed October 20, 2024).

[6] For more information see https://www.nia.nih.gov/research/dn/workshops/precision-medicine-approaches-developing-combination-therapies-treatment-and (accessed October 20, 2024).

in the disease biology. Continued investment in basic and translational science that leads to the identification of different disease subtypes and an understanding of differences across population groups (e.g., sex/gender, genetic ancestry, ethnoracial) will be pivotal to the rollout of precision medicine approaches. Indeed, research on intersectionality highlights that individuals live with multiple identities (e.g., gender, race, sexual orientation), each of which may be associated with distinct sources of disadvantage or resilience. These intersectional identities may synergistically influence response to interventions and treatments and thus should be considered as the field evolves in efforts to design inclusive studies and target and tailor interventions. Moreover, to prevent further exacerbation of disparities, precision medicine research needs to examine how social determinants of health may support or undermine precision health interventions (Hekler et al., 2020). Finally, molecular studies in AD/ADRD that are essential for a precision medicine approach are relatively rare in populations traditionally understudied in research despite having a higher AD risk, such as African Americans and Latin Americans with few exceptions (Hohman et al., 2016; Jin et al., 2015; Logue et al., 2014; N'Songo et al., 2017; Reddy et al., 2022, 2024; Reitz et al., 2013).

Precision medicine, which aims to diagnose and treat the right patient with the right therapy at the right time, is a broad and multifaceted field that is evolving at a rapid pace. In keeping with its charge, the committee focused its assessment of the application of precision medicine to AD/ADRD on research opportunities. While beyond the scope of this report, the committee recognizes that there are barriers that will need to be addressed in the translation of precision medicine approaches to AD/ADRD from research to real-world implementation. One example is the lack of clinician and public understanding of the scientific foundations of precision medicine. Training for primary care providers and education of the public will be important to advance precision medicine approaches to AD/ADRD prevention and treatment. Trained community health workers and patient navigators may be well positioned to bridge the gap between clinicians, patients, and research participants (Ramos et al., 2019a).

The sections below highlight opportunities to better use precision medicine approaches in developing and evaluating interventions for preventing and treating AD/ADRD.

Population Stratification

Too often clinical trial designs assume that diseases to which interventions are targeted are the same for all participants (Reitz, 2016). Observation of subpopulation responses indicates this is not the case (Yip et al., 2016) and repeatedly emphasizes the highly individualized character of many chronic illnesses. AD/ADRD are a heterogeneous group of diseases caused by myriad pathophysiologic mechanisms (Allen et al., 2018; Barupal et al., 2019; Batra et al., 2024; Carrasquillo et al., 2017; Conway et al., 2018; Higginbotham et al., 2020; Oatman et al., 2023; Johnson et al., 2022; McKenzie et al., 2017; Mostafavi et al., 2018; Mukherjee et al., 2020; Strickland et al., 2020; Toledo et al., 2017; Yang et al., 2020). This heterogeneity suggests a need for stratification when evaluating interventions for prevention and treatment. Improving the success rate of AD/ADRD clinical trials is contingent on determining the right target population for each intervention study (Boxer and Sperling, 2023) and the use of tailored interventions that are provided at the appropriate time and using an optimized regimen.

Precision medicine approaches target interventions to specific populations or even individuals based on a set of characteristics that determine the likely effectiveness of a given approach for that person or subpopulation (Sarkar et al., 2024). This approach requires:

- the identification of criteria and factors that are appropriate for use in population stratification to optimally define differences across large and heterogenous populations, and
- the ability to screen individuals for those specific factors in order to target and tailor interventions in ways that optimize clinical outcomes.

This strategy has been effective in oncology (Lazar et al., 2010) (see Box 4-2) but is in its infancy for the prevention and treatment of AD/ADRD.

As shown in Figure 4-3, stratification to a subgroup level represents a first step in the transition from the one-size-fits-all model to a precision-based model. The stratification process can then be extended further to the personalization of intervention approaches based on an individual's unique biological makeup and other factors such as lifestyle, family history, and preference. Importantly, a precision medicine approach does not imply the need to develop different therapies for each individual. Rather, therapies will be designed around subgroups of individuals who share certain characteristics, such as genetic risk or biomarkers, and are likely to benefit from the same intervention. Application of available interventions (e.g., treatment plans) can then be refined and tailored based on further stratification of patients into additional subgroup clusters, and in some cases, even to the individual level. As a simple, illustrative example, a cardiovascular exercise intervention could be modified from walking to swimming for individuals living with AD/ADRD who have balance issues.

Myriad characteristics can be used to stratify populations, including clinical disease stage and phenotype, genetics (e.g., *APOE* status, antioxidant

---

BOX 4-2
Precision Medicine Advances in
Breast, Lung, and Other Cancers

Precision medicine for breast cancer involves testing to individualize interventions and treatment approaches. Testing often involves the evaluation of inherited risk, which has been estimated to be up to 10 percent of all breast cancer cases (Rizzolo et al., 2011). This type of evaluation is exemplified by testing for gene mutations in BRCA1 and BRCA2 and other genes, such as PALB2. Additional testing is also used to identify molecular targets for treatment or to predict drug responsiveness to treatment. In the first case, testing can help determine if drugs targeting specific targets, such as the HER2 protein, may be effective (Sun et al., 2021), and in the second case to determine if the patient can convert inactive drugs to their active forms, as seen with the popular agent tamoxifen (Dahabreh et al., 2010).

Transformational changes in the treatment of lung cancer have been realized with drugs targeting PD-1 receptor status for patients amenable to immune checkpoint therapy (Chen et al., 2020b; Jain et al., 2018). PD-1 is one of the best-characterized checkpoint proteins that when bound by its ligand PD-L1 or PD-L2 suppresses T-cell activation and allows cancer cells to escape the body's intrinsic ability to fight the disease. In recent years, multiple lines of anti-PD-1 drugs have been developed. Patients with melanoma, renal cell carcinoma, non-small cell lung cancer, and some hematological cancers have all been found to respond positively to this type of treatment (Chen et al., 2020b).

---

genes)—including mitochondrial genes (e.g., *TOMM22* and others)—other multiomics measures (e.g., transcriptome, proteome, metabolome), neuroimaging results (e.g., amyloid-PET), and other biological markers, as well as lifestyle factors, socioeconomic status, past exposures, and personality features (Sarkar et al., 2024). Advances in biomarkers enable stratification by copathology, which will be important as more therapies with specific pathological targets become available (Gibson et al., 2023; Toledo et al., 2023).

An ongoing problem with AD/ADRD clinical trials to date is the failure to adequately stratify populations. Studies may stratify participants based on a single genetic factor such as *APOE* status or neuropathology but not take into account other important contributing factors. An increasingly common precision medicine approach applied in AD/ADRD clinical trials is the use of enrichment designs (described earlier in this chapter)

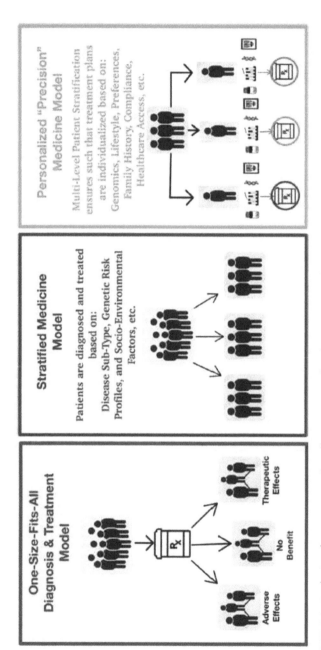

FIGURE 4-3 Evolution from one-size-fits-all to a personalized precision medicine model.
SOURCE: Sarkar et al., 2024. Copyright© and reprinted with permission from Elsevier.

that limit recruitment based on biomarker or other screening results to better target AD/ADRD interventions to at-risk populations. For example, the Anti-Amyloid Treatment in Asymptomatic Alzheimer's Disease (A4) trial screened potential participants and selected at-risk individuals for the trial population based on evidence of brain amyloid accumulation on PET imaging and cognitive status (Sperling et al., 2014). Following a subgroup analysis for the FINGER prevention trial that showed that the beneficial cognitive effects of the multicomponent intervention were enhanced among *APOE4* carriers (Solomon et al., 2018), a subsequent trial evaluating the FINGER multidomain lifestyle intervention in combination with metformin, a diabetes drug, was enriched for *APOE4* carriers (Barbera et al., 2024). The Systematic Multi-Domain Alzheimer Risk Reduction Trial (SMARRT) included only participants with two or more dementia risk factors (Yaffe et al., 2024). While there are clear advantages to enrichment approaches to clinical trials, a tradeoff worth noting is the potential impact on the generalizability of the findings to a broader population (FDA, 2019b), which needs to be factored into decision making. Additionally, targeted trials utilizing stratification carry biases that need to be managed in the statistical analyses. Appropriate trial design is thus critical to successful execution of targeted clinical trials.

With recent advances in high-throughput multiomics approaches (e.g., genomics, proteomics, transcriptomics, metabolomics), progress is being made in the identification of different disease subtypes based on molecular markers that can be linked to specific underlying disease pathways and that may guide more effective stratification and intervention targeting strategies going forward (Arafah et al., 2023; Hampel et al., 2022; Harrison et al., 2020; Higginbotham et al., 2023; Iturria-Medina et al., 2022; Neff et al., 2021; Tijms et al., 2024; Wan et al., 2020). Bioinformatics approaches are enabling the identification of groups or modules of related molecular and biological functions (e.g., lipid metabolism, immune response, synaptic processes, myelination, mitochondrial, vascular) that may be altered (elevated or depressed) in AD/ADRD and their linkage to different subtypes (Higginbotham et al., 2023; Iturria-Medina et al., 2022; Johnson et al., 2022; Mostafavi et al., 2018; Neff et al., 2021; Tijms et al., 2024; Wan et al., 2020). These clusters of related molecular functions hint at specific pathophysiologic mechanisms that may give rise to different disease subtypes (as well as neuroprotective mechanisms in the case of resilience-associated subtypes).

While there has been some alignment in subtype identification across different omics approaches (e.g., proteomic versus transcriptomic versus metabolomic), differences have also been identified, emphasizing the value of complementary approaches that can yield different insights (Allen et al., 2018; Batra et al., 2024; Higginbotham et al., 2023; Johnson et al., 2022;

Wang et al., 2022b). Subtyping is also being pursued using data other than those generated with multiomics methods. For example, functional MRI has been used to identify subtypes displaying different patterns of impairment in functional connectivity within the brain (Chen et al, 2023b). As research advancing subtype discovery progresses, it will be important to integrate findings from different omic approaches and with other relevant data (e.g., clinical, cognitive, genetic risk, imaging, neuropathology) collected from research participants whose samples were used in subtyping (Allen et al., 2018; Campbell et al., 2022; Carrasquillo et al., 2015; Iturria-Medina et al., 2022; Reddy et al., 2021, 2024). These integrated findings may enhance understanding of subtypes and better guide stratification efforts.

Multiomic methods for subtyping are commonly carried out on brain tissue samples (Higginbotham et al., 2023; Iturria-Medina et al., 2022; Neff et al., 2021, Wan et al., 2020). Realizing the diagnostic and therapeutic potential of these methods will require understanding how subtypes identified in biofluid samples (e.g., CSF, plasma) reflect those identified in brain tissue (Higginbotham et al., 2023; Iturria-Medina et al., 2022; Tijms et al., 2024). Tijms and colleagues (2024) recently identified five distinct AD subtypes using mass spectrometry-based proteomic analysis of CSF. Each identified subtype featured a distinct genetic risk profile and was linked to a specific molecular process. Multiplexed blood-based biomarker panels based on the proteomics profiles are now being developed to increase the feasibility of subtyping individuals as part of a stratification and targeted treatment approach (Tijms et al., 2024).

As has been the case in oncology (see Box 4-1), the ability to subtype individuals based on distinct biological mechanisms will likely be key to effective prevention and treatment of AD/ADRD and requires continued investment in multiomics studies and advancing neuroimaging capabilities and the identification of diverse fluid-based biomarkers that can be developed into multiplexed panels. As with other areas of research, subtyping studies have primarily been conducted using samples from populations with limited diversity (Higginbotham et al., 2023) and have focused on AD. Thus, the expansion to diverse populations and related dementias should be a focus of future research (Reddy et al., 2024; Seifar et al., 2024), as should prospective studies that investigate whether an individual's subtype changes with aging and disease progression from preclinical to MCI to clinical dementia (Iturria-Medina et al., 2022; Neff et al., 2021). The implications of mixed dementias for subtype-based population stratification and precision medicine approaches also need to be investigated (Boxer and Sperling, 2023).

Conclusion 4-8: Stratifying populations in a meaningful way using precision medicine approaches and applying this level of resolution to the prevention and treatment of AD/ADRD will require investment in exploratory research, neuroimaging and multiomics approaches, and computational tools and analytics to elucidate determinants of AD/ADRD risk and variability of response to interventions in diverse populations.

Precision Approaches to AD/ADRD Prevention and Treatment

Precision prevention and treatment approaches are specifically designed to address the issue of molecular and clinical heterogeneity by identifying a person's specific pattern of risk factors and/or underlying pathophysiologic processes and selecting a preventive or therapeutic intervention strategy that is likely to provide benefit. While much effort has gone into understanding genetic risk, precision approaches for AD/ADRD would benefit from a better understanding of underlying environmental factors and gene–environment interactions (discussed in Chapter 3) (Reitz, 2016), as well as integration of these data to guide clinical interventions. This will enable the consideration of potential interaction between an intervention and the individual level of risk—for instance, whether those at higher genetic risk for AD are likely to get more, the same, or less benefit from an intervention (Deckers et al., 2021; Hall et al., 2024; Lourida et al., 2019; Solomon et al., 2018). Different interventions may interact with an individual's risk in different ways, and understanding interaction effects is critical for targeting interventions most effectively and cost-effectively.

Large and complex datasets are being generated using a combination of multiomics approaches, clinical assessments, and, increasingly, digital technologies. As such, the development of such computational tools and analytics as sophisticated multivariate methods and artificial intelligence/machine learning that can integrate datasets and extract patterns has become an important area for investment to advance precision medicine for AD/ADRD, as discussed further in Chapter 5. The application of such tools and methods to determine optimal approaches for stratifying populations, matching identified subgroups to interventions, and guiding the life-course timing of those interventions is a major research priority.

Precision Brain Health Approach to AD/ADRD Prevention

While many interventions for AD/ADRD have focused on midlife and late-life deficits, a precision brain health approach to AD/ADRD prevention should consider opportunities for personalized interventions implemented at earlier ages as part of a life-course approach to brain health optimization and resilience. Precision prevention approaches are predictive and rely on the ability to screen populations to identify those with increased susceptibility (Ramos et al., 2019b). This enables a transition from generic risk-reduction strategies to personalized interventions focused on specific risk factors (Arafah et al., 2023).

Given the many factors that contribute to AD/ADRD risk (as discussed in Chapter 3) and the identification of distinct disease subtypes, as well as the limited success observed with single-component prevention trials, multifactorial prevention strategies designed based on risk profiles are increasingly being pursued (Gregory et al., 2022). While results from earlier trials of multicomponent risk-reduction interventions for AD/ADRD have been mixed (Rosenberg et al., 2020), the recent success of randomized trials such as SMARRT underscores the potential of a more tailored approach to simultaneously targeting multiple contributors to AD/ADRD (Yaffe et al., 2024). The design of SMARRT included enrichment for a higher-risk population and employing codesigned preventive strategies personalized to the participants' specific risk factors (e.g., physical inactivity, poor sleep, social isolation, smoking behavior).

The integration of SMARRT with the health care delivery system was another important aspect of the trial that facilitated a personalized approach. The increased integration of clinical trials with health care delivery systems, which enables data collection on individual health profiles from electronic health records, was recommended previously as a priority for advancing dementia prevention (NASEM, 2017). Importantly, SMARRT included management of chronic conditions known to contribute to AD/ADRD risk (e.g., hypertension, diabetes), highlighting opportunities to better integrate personalized AD/ADRD, cardiovascular, and metabolic disease prevention. More collaborative approaches to intervention research are needed so prevention research for overlapping public health priorities is not hampered by existing—and often funding-related—silos.

Although personalized approaches to implementing interventions and shared decision making can help patients feel more empowered in their care and, in some cases, improve treatment adherence (Montori et al., 2023; Simmons et al., 2010; Umar et al., 2012), it is also important to recognize that individuals may at times be reluctant or unable to express their preferences and may not always choose the treatment strategy that is best supported by evidence-based guidelines (Say and Thomson, 2003). For this reason, the successful implementation of a multicomponent intervention not only requires an understanding of how different components perform, both individually and together, but also needs to factor in how patient preferences and attitudes can affect treatment outcomes.

The ecosystem in which an individual lives, studies, and works (i.e., social determinants of health) may enable or hamper their ability to take the actions necessary to prevent disease. This contextual component may contribute to the observed variation in effect when the same intervention is implemented in diverse populations (e.g., low versus high education, low versus high socioeconomic status, those with or without a supportive family and/or social network). This variation can arise as a result of differences in uptake, adherence, and/or efficacy (Rebok et al., 2023). For instance, a person with very constrained financial resources living in a dangerous neighborhood may have limited ability to increase physical activity as part of a lifestyle-focused preventive intervention given the lack of safe places to walk or exercise in their surroundings. For this reason, the design of personalized prevention strategies needs to account for social determinants of health, including structural factors.

With the recent approval of pharmacological agents targeting underlying disease pathways for AD and the expectation that more may come to the market in the near future, it is likely that precision prevention approaches for AD/ADRD will increasingly feature multicomponent interventions that include both pharmacological agents and NPIs, particularly for people at heightened risk based on genetic markers and/or family history. As pharmacological agents may have more targeted mechanisms of action as compared to NPIs, precision approaches to combination interventions will need to be guided by an analysis of an individual's biological makeup, including, optimally, genetic risk factors and multiomics perturbations that have been linked to specific disease pathways or susceptibility. A combination approach to precision prevention that follows a brain health optimization framework could involve sequential interventions such that relatively low-risk NPIs are implemented earlier in the life course. Monitoring of those at high risk (e.g., members of families in which AD or a related dementia is prevalent) could begin decades before typical age of onset of clinical symptoms to enable identification of early pathophysiologic changes that may trigger the use of pharmacological agents to complement NPIs. By monitoring for early signs of preclinical disease, initiation of pharmacological therapies could prevent overt and potentially irreversible cognitive change.

Precision Approaches to AD/ADRD Treatment

While prevention is the ultimate goal for AD/ADRD intervention research, effective treatments remain a priority given the millions of people living with cognitive impairment and clinical dementia in the United States and globally. Considering the vast heterogeneity of AD/ADRD, the predominance of mixed pathologies, and the co-occurrence with other diseases that may contribute to or exacerbate these neurodegenerative conditions, targeting and tailoring of treatment will likely be necessary (Devi, 2023). Precision treatment approaches can predict and guide the selection of therapies that maximize benefits to individuals while minimizing toxicity and adverse events. Informed by genetics, molecular make-up derived from multiomics, biomarkers, and other individual-level information, precision treatment approaches targeting the specifics of the disease at a patient-level (drivers of disease and/or downstream consequences) can change the shape of the curve for mortality and/or severity of illness.

Given the multiple and interdependent disease pathways that contribute to AD/ADRD, advancing precision treatment approaches will require continued efforts to deconstruct AD/ADRD into distinct biological subtypes (or endophenotypes) so appropriate therapies can be selected (Hampel et al., 2017). An intervention that is effective for one subtype may not provide benefit for another (Devi, 2023). Moreover, different subtypes may progress at different rates, with implications for the timing of intervention approaches in a personalized management strategy (Geifman et al., 2018). Ongoing efforts employing multiomics approaches to identify subtypes (Higginbotham et al., 2023; Iturria-Medina et al., 2022; Neff et al., 2021), like the work by Tijms and colleagues (2024) described earlier, are helping to set the stage for precision treatment approaches. Each of the AD subtypes identified by their laboratory featured a distinct genetic risk profile and was linked to a specific molecular process (neuronal hyperplasticity, innate immune activation, RNA dysregulation, choroid plexus dysfunction, blood–brain barrier impairment). Different subtypes, which are continuing to be uncovered in this rapidly moving field, may benefit from treatments that target specific perturbed pathways in each individual as part of a precision medicine approach (Tijms et al., 2024). Where multiple pathways are engaged, potentially resulting in a mix of pathologic features, combination drug therapies may be needed to target each independently or in a coordinated manner. Combination therapies may be administered simultaneously or in sequence. In the case of sequential administration, optimum sequencing needs to be determined (Boxer and Sperling, 2023). Although there has been significant emphasis on the development of novel therapies for AD/ADRD, the ability to subtype individuals may alternatively enable an individualized drug repurposing approach whereby existing FDA-approved drugs are matched to an individual based on integrated multiomics data (Fang et al., 2020).

As noted earlier, there is increasing interest in leveraging artificial intelligence/machine learning methods to facilitate precision medicine approaches to treatment. Such methods use patient-level data (e.g., clinical and demographic information) and predictive models of disease progression under various treatment options to make personalized treatment recommendations (Hu et al., 2023; Liu et al., 2022). One recent study showed that a neural network was effective at predicting the most beneficial dementia treatment (acetylcholinesterase inhibitors and memantine) as measured by decline in cognitive test scores (Liu et al., 2022). While requiring further validation and evaluation in real-world settings, such methods may also have utility in personalizing treatments with disease modifying therapies for AD/ADRD as more such treatments become available.

Precision Approaches to Addressing Safety Considerations

Although NPIs may generally have lower risk profiles, many drugs can have adverse effects. Such risks are common across diseases requiring drug treatment, but acceptability could differ for AD/ADRD depending on disease stage. For example, there may be less tolerance for risks during the preclinical stage when there is no apparent effect on cognitive function, and it is unclear whether the individual may go on to develop clinical symptoms.

For treatments that have known serious adverse effects (e.g., anti-amyloid antibody therapies), a personalized approach to treatment needs to include the consideration of the risk–benefit ratio, which may be affected by age, biomarker status, and other risk factors (Boxer and Sperling, 2023). It is also important to consider the timing of treatment initiation, balancing the risks from starting early versus waiting too long when the treatment may no longer be optimally effective.

In precision medicine approaches for cancer, companion diagnostic tests are used to match patients with specific therapies that are likely to provide benefit and can include components for identifying safety and tolerability concerns. Such testing may also be part of a precision medicine approach to AD/ADRD. Biomarkers that can predict who is at risk for developing more severe forms of ARIA or other adverse events that may be associated with future FDA-approved drugs could enable analogous testing to identify individuals in whom existing therapies are contraindicated, thus supporting a more personalized approach to treatment (Arafah et al., 2023). This is already being done to some degree with *APOE4* testing (Cummings and Kinney, 2022). *APOE4* carriers—and particularly people with two copies of the allele—are more likely to develop severe ARIA (Loomis et al., 2024), affecting the risk–benefit tradeoff for treatment with anti-amyloid therapies, although effects of pretreatment on amyloid burden and presence of vascular pathology (e.g., infarcts) need to be better understood, as do differences in risk among non-White populations. Appropriate use recommendations for anti-amyloid therapies include a recommendation for *APOE* genotyping (Blasco and Roberts, 2023). When such genotyping is conducted, genetic counseling is generally recommended. Given the paucity of skilled genetic counselors, this role may fall to treating clinicians (e.g., geriatricians, neurologists), highlighting the importance of equipping health care providers with resources needed to understand and counsel patients about safety considerations when implementing precision approaches to assessing and mitigating safety concerns.

RESEARCH PRIORITIES

Accelerating the evaluation of interventions for AD/ADRD and advancing precision approaches to ensure that individuals receive the right combination of interventions at the right times are critical to reducing the individual and societal impact of these diseases. NIH has made major research investments and created essential infrastructure to improve the clinical trial pipeline for AD/ADRD and advance precision medicine approaches. These investments have included the creation of programs and resources for improving the inclusivity of clinical research, collaborative research programs to identify and de-risk promising therapeutic targets, the creation of public–private partnerships to centralize essential resources and expertise for innovative clinical trial approaches (e.g., Alzheimer's Prevention Initiative, Alzheimer's Clinical Trials Consortium), and support for well-designed clinical trials of pharmacological and nonpharmacological approaches. The committee identified five research priorities that align with and build upon this broad foundation of NIH investments. These research priorities are listed in Table 4-2 and include key scientific questions and near-term research opportunities that would advance progress on the research priorities.

TABLE 4-2 Committee-Identified Research Priorities Related to Catalyzing Advances in Interventions for the Prevention and Treatment of AD/ADRD Spanning from Precision Medicine to Public Health Strategies

Research Priority	Key Scientific Questions	Near-Term Research Opportunities to Address Key Scientific Questions
4-1: Integrate innovative approaches and novel tools into the planning, design, and execution of studies to accelerate the identification of effective interventions.	• What outcomes and biomarkers can be used to assess the interactive effects of mixed pathologies (e.g., vascular, alpha-synuclein, TDP-43, and AD pathology)? • What biological markers can be used to show that the intended pathway is engaged and the therapy is having the expected effect? • How can trial design be improved to determine whether late-stage trial failures are the result of ineffective interventions versus limitations in trial designs or execution? • How can trials be designed to incorporate and test innovative methodologies in ways that do not pose risks to the primary objective of the trial and the timely execution of clinical research? • What innovative approaches can be used to increase the value of observational studies to inform prevention, including short- and long-term effects? • Can risk profiles based on biomarker testing of asymptomatic individuals decrease required sample sizes and accelerate trials?	• Incorporate innovative substudies into ongoing clinical trials to pilot novel approaches (e.g., new biomarkers as secondary outcomes, digital tools for remote data collection). • Create mechanisms to share successes and failures from innovative operational trial design aspects. • Optimize proof-of-concept trials with informative biomarkers and outcomes. • Identify and evaluate causal evidence on the role of past and ongoing public health initiatives, clinical care changes, and policy changes on AD/ADRD prevention at a population level (e.g., trial emulations using real-world data). • Use existing data (e.g., electronic health data) to identify subpopulations. • Use platform randomized trials to evaluate multiple interventions in parallel. • Conduct long-term follow-up of early- and midlife prevention strategies using networked data infrastructure. • Develop and use social determinants of health metrics in clinical research.

TABLE 4-2 Continued

Research Priority	Key Scientific Questions	Near-Term Research Opportunities to Address Key Scientific Questions
4-2: Advance the development and evaluation of combination therapies (including pharmacological and nonpharmacological approaches) to better address the multifactorial nature of AD/ADRD.	• Which combinations of interventions (drug combinations and combinations of drugs and nonpharmacological interventions [NPIs]) will work synergistically to prevent AD/ADRD or slow its clinical progression? • What are the long-term effects of combination interventions? • How does the sequencing of interventions affect their combined effectiveness and safety? • How do different combinations of interventions interact, and how can their effects be maximized? • Can combination interventions targeting multiple mechanistic pathways improve the effectiveness of treatment for people with mixed pathologies? • For combination trials that include NPIs, how can the trial be designed with adequate blinding and appropriate control groups? What are the relevant endpoints?	• Explore and understand the independent and/or synergistic mechanisms of multidomain interventions and combination therapies.

continued

TABLE 4-2 Continued

Research Priority	Key Scientific Questions	Near-Term Research Opportunities to Address Key Scientific Questions
4-3: Evaluate precision medicine approaches for the prevention and treatment of AD/ADRD to better identify interventions likely to benefit specific groups of individuals.	• Can an understanding of the exposome guide population stratification to facilitate precision approaches to AD/ADRD interventions? • What criteria and molecular or multiomics factors and biomarkers are appropriate for use in (1) identifying subtypes and endophenotypes and (2) stratifying populations at a population and an individual level? • Does giving people more agency in how they implement interventions (e.g., personalized approaches to NPIs) affect trial outcomes?	• Integrate findings from multiomic approaches and other modalities to characterize AD/ADRD subtypes that can be used to identify commonalities and stratify across different subtypes. • Use innovative research designs (e.g., platform trials, personalized interventions) that support precision medicine approaches. • Conduct intervention trials that include study populations living with multiple pathologies. • Invest in longer-term studies of postintervention outcomes in diverse populations, including in populations with different comorbidities and levels of adherence. • Conduct follow-up studies of individuals treated with anti-amyloid antibodies to better understand the effects of copathologies on patient symptoms and to identify key targets to include in combination interventions. • Collaborate with safety registries to evaluate safety outcomes from real-world evidence.

TABLE 4-2 Continued

Research Priority	Key Scientific Questions	Near-Term Research Opportunities to Address Key Scientific Questions
4-4: Advance the adoption of standardized outcomes for assessing interventions that are sensitive, person-centered, clinically meaningful, and reflect the priorities of those at risk for or living with AD/ADRD.	• What outcomes matter most for people living with AD/ADRD and their caregivers and care partners? • How do intermediate outcomes such as biomarkers and risk scores translate to outcomes that are clinically meaningful? • What metrics are most important for assessing quality of life, well-being, and functional outcomes in diverse populations? • What are the continued clinical and biological outcomes in those who received an intervention? • How can study designs incorporate research questions around maximizing adherence to interventions?	• Develop and validate intermediate outcomes, including biomarkers and risk scores, that are robustly linked to cognitive, functional, or quality-of-life outcomes. • Use metrics that can be personalized for desired individual outcomes. • Conduct ethnographic and other similar studies to identify person-centered outcomes for use in clinical research. • Engage clinicians (e.g., primary care providers, geriatricians) and people living with AD/ADRD in the identification of clinically meaningful outcomes for use in clinical research. • Evaluate factors that influence adherence to interventions and how it affects outcomes.

continued

TABLE 4-2 Continued

Research Priority	Key Scientific Questions	Near-Term Research Opportunities to Address Key Scientific Questions
4-5: Evaluate the causal effects of public health approaches on overall dementia incidence and incidence in understudied and/or disproportionately affected populations.	• What is the potential effect of a population approach (e.g., modifying exposure to an adverse environmental or social factor or behavior) on dementia incidence and inequalities relative to a precision medicine or high-risk individual-level approach (i.e., targeting risk reduction in individuals with the highest level of an adverse risk factor)? • Considering mediating mechanisms and spillover effects, what are the most effective strategies for population interventions to reduce dementia incidence? • What interventions can be most easily scaled to reduce risk of dementia at a population level in the near and medium term?	• Estimate population-attributable fractions associated with identified risk factors for all-cause dementia risk, dementia subtypes, and on social inequalities in dementia risk. • Compare plausible population-attributable fractions for AD/ADRD cases prevented associated with high-risk/precision medicine versus population approaches. • Evaluate the evidence for causality of known risk factors with high population prevalence, with specificity regarding dose, duration, timing (age), and other possible sources of heterogeneity in exposure effects. • Evaluate whether there are important distinct determinants of dementia that are common in groups historically underrepresented in AD/ADRD research (e.g., Black, Latino, Asian, or Indigenous populations; rural populations; and individuals from low socioeconomic backgrounds) and may be targets for public health approaches. • Evaluate how specific policies or interventions that can be scaled to large populations influence dementia risk overall and inequalities in dementia risk.

TABLE 4-2 Continued

Research Priority	Key Scientific Questions	Near-Term Research Opportunities to Address Key Scientific Questions
4-5: Continued		• Evaluate how changes in existing policies shaping social and environmental determinants of health (e.g., policies shaping food security, economic security, healthy housing access, educational experiences across the life course, safe working conditions, retirement policies, violence exposure, air pollution and other environmental toxins, and community climate resilience) influence biomarkers associated with AD/ADRD risk and clinical AD/ADRD. • Contrast the near- and medium-term impact of clinical care strategies (e.g., hypertension treatment, access to amyloid-targeting therapies, or management of comorbid conditions and infectious diseases) versus behavior change strategies (e.g., dietary or physical activity interventions) versus policy interventions (e.g., changes in retirement age or clean air and water standards). • Incorporate estimates of spillover effects of modifying risk factors and of prevented dementia cases on family and other social network members.

REFERENCES

AARP. 2024. *AARP Foundation Experience Corps.* https://www.aarp.org/volunteer/programs/experience-corps/?intcmp=AE-VOL-PROG-C1R1 (accessed October 18, 2024).

Abdelmoaty, M. M., E. Lu, R. Kadry, E. G. Foster, S. Bhattarai, R. L. Mosley, and H. E. Gendelman. 2023. Clinical biomarkers for Lewy body diseases. *Cell & Bioscience* 13(1):209.

ADAPT Research Group. 2013. Results of a follow-up study to the randomized Alzheimer's Disease Anti-inflammatory Prevention Trial (ADAPT). *Alzheimer's & Dementia* 9(6):714-723.

ADNI (Alzheimer's Disease Neuroimaging Initiative). 2012. *Menu of demographics tables.* https://adni.loni.usc.edu/wp-content/uploads/2012/08/ADNI_Enroll_Demographics.pdf (accessed August 19, 2024).

AHEAD Study. 2024. *AHEAD Study.* https://www.aheadstudy.org/ (accessed August 19, 2024).

Ahn, J., and M. Kim. 2023. Effects of exercise therapy on global cognitive function and, depression in older adults with mild cognitive impairment: A systematic review and meta-analysis. *Archives of Gerontology and Geriatrics* 106:104855.

AHRQ (Agency for Healthcare Research and Quality). 2014. AHRQ methods for effective health care. In *Registries for evaluating patient outcomes: A user's guide.* Edited by R. E. Gliklich, N. A. Dreyer, and M. B. Leavy. Rockville, MD: Agency for Healthcare Research and Quality.

Aisen, P. S., R. J. Bateman, M. Carrillo, R. Doody, K. Johnson, J. R. Sims, R. Sperling, and B. Vellas. 2021. Platform trials to expedite drug development in Alzheimer's disease: A report from the EU/US CTAD Task Force. *Journal of the Prevention of Alzheimer's Disease* 8(3):306-312.

Allen, M., X. Wang, J. D. Burgess, J. Watzlawik, D. J. Serie, C. S. Younkin, T. Nguyen, K. G. Malphrus, S. Lincoln, M. M. Carrasquillo, C. Ho, P. Chakrabarty, S. Strickland, M. E. Murray, V. Swarup, D. H. Geschwind, N. T. Seyfried, E. B. Dammer, J. J. Lah, A. I. Levey, T. E. Golde, C. Funk, H. Li, N. D. Price, R. C. Petersen, N. R. Graff-Radford, S. G. Younkin, D. W. Dickson, J. R. Crook, Y. W. Asmann, and N. Ertekin-Taner. 2018. Conserved brain myelination networks are altered in Alzheimer's and other neurodegenerative diseases. *Alzheimer's & Dementia* 14(3):352-366.

Alves, F., P. Kalinowski, and S. Ayton. 2023. Accelerated brain volume loss caused by anti-β-amyloid drugs: A systematic review and meta-analysis. *Neurology* 100(20):e2114-e2124.

AlzForum. 2024a. *Donanemab.* https://www.alzforum.org/therapeutics/donanemab (accessed August 19, 2024).

AlzForum. 2024b. *Ct1812.* https://www.alzforum.org/therapeutics/ct1812 (accessed October 29, 2024).

Alzheimer Society of Ireland. 2017. *Human rights and dementia.* https://alzheimer.ie/creating-change/policy-on-dementia-in-ireland/human-rights-and-dementia/ (accessed August 20, 2024).

Alzheimer's Association. 2024. *Vascular dementia.* https://www.alz.org/alzheimers-dementia/what-is-dementia/types-of-dementia/vascular-dementia (accessed August 20, 2024).

Alzheimer's Network. 2024. *Alzheimer's network for treatment and diagnostics (ALZ-NET).* https://www.alz-net.org/ (accessed August 20, 2024).

Anstey, K. J., S. R. Lord, M. Hennessy, P. Mitchell, K. Mill, and C. von Sanden. 2006. The effect of cataract surgery on neuropsychological test performance: A randomized controlled trial. *Journal of the International Neuropsychological Society* 12(5):632-639.

Anstey, K. J., K. Ashby-Mitchell, and R. Peters. 2017. Updating the evidence on the association between serum cholesterol and risk of late-life dementia: Review and meta-analysis. *Journal of Alzheimer's Disease* 56(1):215-228.

Anthes, E. 2020. Alexa, do I have Covid-19? *Nature* 586(7827):22-25.

Arafah, A., S. Khatoon, I. Rasool, A. Khan, M. A. Rather, K. A. Abujabal, Y. A. H. Faqih, H. Rashid, S. M. Rashid, S. Bilal Ahmad, A. Alexiou, and M. U. Rehman. 2023. The future of precision medicine in the cure of Alzheimer's disease. *Biomedicines* 11(2):335.

Armstrong, N. M., Y. An, J. Doshi, G. Erus, L. Ferrucci, C. Davatzikos, J. A. Deal, F. R. Lin, and S. M. Resnick. 2019. Association of midlife hearing impairment with late-life temporal lobe volume loss. *JAMA Otolaryngology—Head & Neck Surgery* 145(9):794-802.

Asakawa, T., Y. Yang, Z. Xiao, Y. Shi, W. Qin, Z. Hong, and D. Ding. 2024. Stumbling blocks in the investigation of the relationship between age-related hearing loss and cognitive impairment. *Perspectives on Psychological Science* 19(1):137-150.

ASPE (Office of Assistant Secretary for Planning and Evaluation Department of Health and Human Services). 2017. *Challenges in involving people with dementia as study participants in research on care and services.* https://aspe.hhs.gov/reports/challenges-involving-people-dementia-study-participants-research-care-services-0 (accessed August 20, 2024).

Bahar-Fuchs, A., A. Martyr, A. M. Y. Goh, J. Sabates, and L. Clare. 2019. Cognitive training for people with mild to moderate dementia. *Cochrane Database of Systematic Reviews* 3(3):CD013069.

Baiduc, R. R., J. W. Sun, C. M. Berry, M. Anderson, and E. A. Vance. 2023. Relationship of cardiovascular disease risk and hearing loss in a clinical population. *Scientific Reports* 13(1):1642.

Baker, L. D., C. W. Cotman, R. Thomas, S. Jin, A. H. Shadyab, J. Pa, R. A. Rissman, J. B. Brewer, J. Zhang, Y. Jung, A. Z. LaCroix, K. Messer, and H. H. Feldman. 2022. Topline results of EXERT: Can exercise slow cognitive decline in MCI? *Alzheimer's & Dementia* 18(S11):e069700.

Ballard, M., and P. Montgomery. 2017. Risk of bias in overviews of reviews: A scoping review of methodological guidance and four-item checklist. *Research Synthesis Methods* 8(1):92-108.

Baptista, C., A. R. Silva, M. P. Lima, and R. M. Afonso. 2024. Evaluating the cognitive effects of interventions to reduce social isolation and loneliness in older adults: A systematic review. *Aging & Mental Health* 28(12):1767-1776.

Barbera, M., D. Perera, A. Matton, F. Mangialasche, A. Rosenberg, L. Middleton, T. Ngandu, A. Solomon, and M. Kivipelto. 2023. Multimodal precision prevention—a new direction in Alzheimer's disease. *Journal of Prevention of Alzheimer's Disease* 10(4):718-728.

Barbera, M., J. Lehtisalo, D. Perera, M. Aspö, M. Cross, C. A. De Jager Loots, E. Falaschetti, N. Friel, J. A. Luchsinger, H. M. Gavelin, M. Peltonen, G. Price, A. S. Neely, C. Thunborg, J. Tuomilehto, F. Mangialasche, L. Middleton, T. Ngandu, A. Solomon, M. Kivipelto, S. A. Adeleke, C. Arvidsson, I. Barton, M. Bas, K. Cosby, J. Crispin, L. Dunn, M. Durkina, O. Elebring, J. Ford, P. Giannakopoulou, H. Gilkes, H. Graham, G. Hagman, R. Hall, H. Hallinder, A. Haqqee, M. Hartmanis, K. Hemiö, Z. Istvánfyová, D. Kafetsouli, K. Lakey, S. Lehtimäki, L. Lindström, P. MacDonald, A. Mäkelä, S. McGinn-Summers, C. Meius, A. Mirza, C. Oesterling, J. Ojala, A. Olawale, I. Ramanath, H.-M. Roitto, B. Sahib, S. Singh, M. Sundell, S. Taylor, D. Tharumaratnam, K. Uusimäki, J. Vaarala, H. Voutilainen, J. Åsander, the MET-FINGER study team. 2024. A multimodal precision-prevention approach combining lifestyle intervention with metformin repurposing to prevent cognitive impairment and disability: The MET-FINGER randomised controlled trial protocol. *Alzheimer's Research & Therapy* 16(1):23.

Barupal, D. K., R. Baillie, S. Fan, A. J. Saykin, P. J. Meikle, M. Arnold, K. Nho, O. Fiehn, R. Kaddurah-Daouk, and C. Alzheimer Disease Metabolomics. 2019. Sets of coregulated serum lipids are associated with Alzheimer's disease pathophysiology. *Alzheimer's Dementia (Amsterdam, Netherlands)* 11:619-627.

Basak, C., S. Qin, and M. A. O'Connell. 2020. Differential effects of cognitive training modules in healthy aging and mild cognitive impairment: A comprehensive meta-analysis of randomized controlled trials. *Psychology and Aging* 35(2):220-249.

Batra, R., J. Krumsiek, X. Wang, M. Allen, C. Blach, G. Kastenmuller, M. Arnold, N. Ertekin-Taner, R. Kaddurah-Daouk, and Alzheimer's Disease Metabolomics. Consortium 2024. Comparative brain metabolomics reveals shared and distinct metabolic alterations in Alzheimer's disease and progressive supranuclear palsy. *Alzheimer's & Dementia* 20(12):8294-8307.

Bechard, L. E., K. S. McGilton, L. E. Middleton, H. Chertkow, S. Sivananthan, and J. Bethell. 2022. Engaging people with lived experience of dementia in research: Perspectives from a multi-disciplinary research network. *Canadian Geriatrics Journal* 25(3):254-261.

Bellenguez, C., F. Kucukali, I. E. Jansen, L. Kleineidam, S. Moreno-Grau, N. Amin, A. C. Naj, R. Campos-Martin, B. Grenier-Boley, V. Andrade, P. A. Holmans, A. Boland, V. Damotte, S. J. van der Lee, M. R. Costa, T. Kuulasmaa, Q. Yang, I. de Rojas, J. C. Bis, A. Yaqub, I. Prokic, J. Chapuis, S. Ahmad, V. Giedraitis, D. Aarsland, P. Garcia-Gonzalez, C. Abdelnour, E. Alarcon-Martin, D. Alcolea, M. Alegret, I. Alvarez, V. Alvarez, N. J. Armstrong, A. Tsolaki, C. Antunez, I. Appollonio, M. Arcaro, S. Archetti, A. A. Pastor, B. Arosio, L. Athanasiu, H. Bailly, N. Banaj, M. Baquero, S. Barral, A. Beiser, A. B. Pastor, J. E. Below, P. Benchek, L. Benussi, C. Berr, C. Besse, V. Bessi, G. Binetti, A. Bizarro, R. Blesa, M. Boada, E. Boerwinkle, B. Borroni, S. Boschi, P. Bossu, G. Brathen, J. Bressler, C. Bresner, H. Brodaty, K. J. Brookes, L. I. Brusco, D. Buiza-Rueda, K. Burger, V. Burholt, W. S. Bush, M. Calero, L. B. Cantwell, G. Chene, J. Chung, M. L. Cuccaro, A. Carracedo, R. Cecchetti, L. Cervera-Carles, C. Charbonnier, H. H. Chen, C. Chillotti, S. Ciccone, J. Claassen, C. Clark, E. Conti, A. Corma-Gomez, E. Costantini, C. Custodero, D. Daian, M. C. Dalmasso, A. Daniele, E. Dardiotis, J. F. Dartigues, P. P. de Deyn, K. de Paiva Lopes, L. D. de Witte, S. Debette, J. Deckert, T. Del Ser, N. Denning, A. DeStefano, M. Dichgans, J. Diehl-Schmid, M. Diez-Fairen, P. D. Rossi, S. Djurovic, E. Duron, E. Duzel, C. Dufouil, G. Eiriksdottir, S. Engelborghs, V. Escott-Price, A. Espinosa, M. Ewers, K. M. Faber, T. Fabrizio, S. F. Nielsen, D. W. Fardo, L. Farotti, C. Fenoglio, M. Fernandez-Fuertes, R. Ferrari, C. B. Ferreira, E. Ferri, B. Fin, P. Fischer, T. Fladby, K. Fliessbach, B. Fongang, M. Fornage, J. Fortea, T. M. Foroud, S. Fostinelli, N. C. Fox, E. Franco-Macias, M. J. Bullido, A. Frank-Garcia, L. Froelich, B. Fulton-Howard, D. Galimberti, J. M. Garcia-Alberca, P. Garcia-Gonzalez, S. Garcia-Madrona, G. Garcia-Ribas, R. Ghidoni, I. Giegling, G. Giorgio, A. M. Goate, O. Goldhardt, D. Gomez-Fonseca, A. Gonzalez-Perez, C. Graff, G. Grande, E. Green, T. Grimmer, E. Grunblatt, M. Grunin, V. Gudnason, T. Guetta-Baranes, A. Haapasalo, G. Hadjigeorgiou, J. L. Haines, K. L. Hamilton-Nelson, H. Hampel, O. Hanon, J. Hardy, A. M. Hartmann, L. Hausner, J. Harwood, S. Heilmann-Heimbach, S. Helisalmi, M. T. Heneka, I. Hernandez, M. J. Herrmann, P. Hoffmann, C. Holmes, H. Holstege, R. H. Vilas, M. Hulsman, J. Humphrey, G. J. Biessels, X. Jian, C. Johansson, G. R. Jun, Y. Kastumata, J. Kauwe, P. G. Kehoe, L. Kilander, A. K. Stahlbom, M. Kivipelto, A. Koivisto, J. Kornhuber, M. H. Kosmidis, W. A. Kukull, P. P. Kuksa, B. W. Kunkle, A. B. Kuzma, C. Lage, E. J. Laukka, L. Launer, A. Lauria, C. Y. Lee, J. Lehtisalo, O. Lerch, A. Lleo, W. Longstreth, Jr., O. Lopez, A. L. de Munain, S. Love, M. Lowemark, L. Luckcuck, K. L. Lunetta, Y. Ma, J. Macias, C. A. MacLeod, W. Maier, F. Mangialasche, M. Spallazzi, M. Marquie, R. Marshall, E. R. Martin, A. M. Montes, C. M. Rodriguez, C. Masullo, R. Mayeux, S. Mead, P. Mecocci, M. Medina, A. Meggy, S. Mehrabian, S. Mendoza, M. Menendez-Gonzalez, P. Mir, S. Moebus, M. Mol, L. Molina-Porcel, L. Montrreal, L. Morelli, F. Moreno, K. Morgan, T. Mosley, M. M. Nothen, C. Muchnik, S. Mukherjee, B. Nacmias, T. Ngandu, G. Nicolas, B. G. Nordestgaard, R. Olaso, A. Orellana, M. Orsini, G. Ortega, A. Padovani, C. Paolo, G. Papenberg, L. Parnetti, F. Pasquier, P. Pastor, G. Peloso, A. Perez-Cordon, J. Perez-Tur, P. Pericard, O. Peters, Y. A. L. Pijnenburg, J. A.

Pineda, G. Pinol-Ripoll, C. Pisanu, T. Polak, J. Popp, D. Posthuma, J. Priller, R. Puerta, O. Quenez, I. Quintela, J. Q. Thomassen, A. Rabano, I. Rainero, F. Rajabli, I. Ramakers, L. M. Real, M. J. T. Reinders, C. Reitz, D. Reyes-Dumeyer, P. Ridge, S. Riedel-Heller, P. Riederer, N. Roberto, E. Rodriguez-Rodriguez, A. Rongve, I. R. Allende, M. Rosende-Roca, J. L. Royo, E. Rubino, D. Rujescu, M. E. Saez, P. Sakka, I. Saltvedt, A. Sanabria, M. B. Sanchez-Arjona, F. Sanchez-Garcia, P. S. Juan, R. Sanchez-Valle, S. B. Sando, C. Sarnowski, C. L. Satizabal, M. Scamosci, N. Scarmeas, E. Scarpini, P. Scheltens, N. Scherbaum, M. Scherer, M. Schmid, A. Schneider, J. M. Schott, G. Selbaek, D. Seripa, M. Serrano, J. Sha, A. A. Shadrin, O. Skrobot, S. Slifer, G. J. L. Snijders, H. Soininen, V. Solfrizzi, A. Solomon, Y. Song, S. Sorbi, O. Sotolongo-Grau, G. Spalletta, A. Spottke, A. Squassina, E. Stordal, J. P. Tartan, L. Tarraga, N. Tesi, A. Thalamuthu, T. Thomas, G. Tosto, L. Traykov, L. Tremolizzo, A. Tybjaerg-Hansen, A. Uitterlinden, A. Ullgren, I. Ulstein, S. Valero, O. Valladares, C. V. Broeckhoven, J. Vance, B. N. Vardarajan, A. van der Lugt, J. V. Dongen, J. van Rooij, J. van Swieten, R. Vandenberghe, F. Verhey, J. S. Vidal, J. Vogelsang, M. Vyhnalek, M. Wagner, D. Wallon, L. S. Wang, R. Wang, L. Weinhold, J. Wiltfang, G. Windle, B. Woods, M. Yannakoulia, H. Zare, Y. Zhao, X. Zhang, C. Zhu, M. Zulaica, EADB, GR@ACE, DEGESCO, EADI, GERAD, Demgene, FinnGen, ADGC, CHARGE, L. A. Farrer, B. M. Psaty, M. Ghanbari, T. Raj, P. Sachdev, K. Mather, F. Jessen, M. A. Ikram, A. de Mendonca, J. Hort, M. Tsolaki, M. A. Pericak-Vance, P. Amouyel, J. Williams, R. Frikke-Schmidt, J. Clarimon, J. F. Deleuze, G. Rossi, S. Seshadri, O. A. Andreassen, M. Ingelsson, M. Hiltunen, K. Sleegers, G. D. Schellenberg, C. M. van Duijn, R. Sims, W. M. van der Flier, A. Ruiz, A. Ramirez, and J. C. Lambert. 2022. New insights into the genetic etiology of Alzheimer's disease and related dementias. *Nature Genetics* 54(4):412-436.

Bennett, C. F., A. R. Krainer, and D. W. Cleveland. 2019. Antisense oligonucleotide therapies for neurodegenerative diseases. *Annual Review of Neuroscience* 42:385-406.

Blackman, J., M. Swirski, J. Clynes, S. Harding, Y. Leng, and E. Coulthard. 2021. Pharmacological and non-pharmacological interventions to enhance sleep in mild cognitive impairment and mild Alzheimer's disease: A systematic review. *Journal of Sleep Research* 30(4):e13229.

Blasco, D., and J. S. Roberts. 2023. Implications of emerging uses of genetic testing for Alzheimer's disease. *Journal of Prevention of Alzheimer's Disease* 10(3):359-361.

Boeve, B., A. Boxer, H. Rosen, L. Forsberg, H. Heuer, D. Brushaber, B. Appleby, J. Biernacka, Y. Bordelon, H. Botha, P. Brannelly, B. Dickerson, S. Dickinson, D. Dickson, K. Domoto-Reilly, K. Faber, A. Fagan, J. Fields, A. Fishman, T. Foroud, D. Galasko, R. Gavrilova, T. Gendron, D. Geschwind, N. Ghoshal, J. Goldman, J. Graff-Radford, N. Graff-Radford, I. Grant, M. Grossman, G.-Y. Hsiung, E. Huang, E. Huey, D. Irwin, D. Jones, K. Kantarci, A. Karydas, D. Kaufer, D. Knopman, J. Kramer, W. Kremers, J. Kornak, W. Kukull, E. Lagone, I. Litvan, P. Ljubenkov, D. Lucente, I. R. A. Mackenzie, M. Manoochehri, J. Masdeu, S. McGinnis, M. Mendez, B. Miller, T. Miyagawa, K. Nelson, C. Onyike, A. Pantelyat, B. Pascual, R. Pearlman, L. Petrucelli, R. Rademakers, E. M. Ramos, K. Rankin, K. Rascovsky, J. Rexach, A. Ritter, E. Roberson, J. R. Martinez, M. Sabbagh, D. Salmon, R. Savica, W. Seeley, A. Staffaroni, J. Syrjanen, C. Tartaglia, N. Tatton, J. Taylor, A. Toga, S. Weintraub, D. Wheaton, B. Wong, and Z. Wszolek. 2020. The ARTFL LEFFTDS fronto-temporal lobar degeneration (ALLFTD) protocol: Preliminary data and future plans (2081). *Neurology* 94(15Suppl).

Bonnechère, B., and M. Klass. 2023. Cognitive computerized training for older adults and patients with neurological disorders: Do the amount and training modality count? An umbrella meta-regression analysis. *Games for Health Journal* 12(2):100-117.

Bowirrat, A. 2022. Immunosenescence and aging: Neuroinflammation is a prominent feature of Alzheimer's disease and is a likely contributor to neurodegenerative disease pathogenesis. *Journal of Personalized Medicine* 12(11):1817.

Boxer, A. L., and R. Sperling. 2023. Accelerating Alzheimer's therapeutic development: The past and future of clinical trials. *Cell* 186(22):4757-4772.

Boxer, A. L., M. Gold, H. Feldman, B. F. Boeve, S. L.-J. Dickinson, H. Fillit, C. Ho, R. Paul, R. Pearlman, M. Sutherland, A. Verma, S. P. Arneric, B. M. Alexander, B. C. Dickerson, E. R. Dorsey, M. Grossman, E. D. Huey, M. C. Irizarry, W. J. Marks, M. Masellis, F. McFarland, D. Niehoff, C. U. Onyike, S. Paganoni, M. A. Panzara, K. Rockwood, J. D. Rohrer, H. Rosen, R. N. Schuck, H. D. Soares, and N. Tatton. 2020. New directions in clinical trials for frontotemporal lobar degeneration: Methods and outcome measures. *Alzheimer's & Dementia* 16(1):131-143.

Brasure, M., P. Desai, H. Davila, V. A. Nelson, C. Calvert, E. Jutkowitz, M. Butler, H. A. Fink, E. Ratner, L. S. Hemmy, J. R. McCarten, T. R. Barclay, and R. L. Kane. 2017. Physical activity interventions in preventing cognitive decline and Alzheimer-type dementia. *Annals of Internal Medicine* 168(1):30-38.

Brookmeyer, R., and N. Abdalla. 2018. Estimation of lifetime risks of Alzheimer's disease dementia using biomarkers for preclinical disease. *Alzheimer's & Dementia* 14(8):981-988.

Brooks, M. 2024. *FDA delays decision on Alzheimer's hopeful donanemab.* https://www.medscape.com/viewarticle/fda-delays-decision-alzheimers-hopeful-donanemab-2024a10000i7?ecd=WNL_trdalrt_pos1_240308_etid6362693&uac=345736CV&impID=6362693 (accessed August 20, 2024).

Burt, T., G. Young, W. Lee, H. Kusuhara, O. Langer, M. Rowland, and Y. Sugiyama. 2020. Phase 0/microdosing approaches: Time for mainstream application in drug development? *Nature Reviews Drug Discovery* 19(11):801-818.

Caberlotto, L., and T. P. Nguyen. 2014. A systems biology investigation of neurodegenerative dementia reveals a pivotal role of autophagy. *BMC Systems Biology* 8:65.

Cai, H., K. Zhang, M. Wang, X. Li, F. Ran, and Y. Han. 2023. Effects of mind-body exercise on cognitive performance in middle-aged and older adults with mild cognitive impairment: A meta-analysis study. *Medicine (Baltimore)* 102(34):e34905.

Cain, A., M. Taga, C. McCabe, G. S. Green, I. Hekselman, C. C. White, D. I. Lee, P. Gaur, O. Rozenblatt-Rosen, F. Zhang, E. Yeger-Lotem, D. A. Bennett, H. S. Yang, A. Regev, V. Menon, N. Habib, and P. L. De Jager. 2023. Multicellular communities are perturbed in the aging human brain and Alzheimer's disease. *Nature Neuroscience* 26(7):1267-1280.

Calamia, M., K. Markon, and D. Tranel. 2012. Scoring higher the second time around: Meta-analyses of practice effects in neuropsychological assessment. *Clinical Neuropsychologist* 26(4):543-570.

Califf, R. M., and J. Sugarman. 2015. Exploring the ethical and regulatory issues in pragmatic clinical trials. *Clinical Trials* 12(5):436-441.

Campbell, A. S., C. C. G. Ho, M. Atık, M. Allen, S. Lincoln, K. Malphrus, T. Nguyen, S. R. Oatman, M. Corda, O. Conway, S. Strickland, R. C. Petersen, D. W. Dickson, N. R. Graff-Radford, and N. Ertekin-Taner. 2022. Clinical deep phenotyping of *ABCA7* mutation carriers. *Neurology Genetics* 8(2):e655.

Cao, G.-Y., Z.-S. Chen, S.-S. Yao, K. Wang, Z.-T. Huang, H.-X. Su, Y. Luo, C. M. De Fries, Y.-H. Hu, and B. Xu. 2023. The association between vision impairment and cognitive outcomes in older adults: A systematic review and meta-analysis. *Aging & Mental Health* 27(2):350-356.

Caplan, A. I. 2017. Mesenchymal stem cells: Time to change the name! *Stem Cells Translational Medicine* 6(6):1445-1451.

Carillo, M. 2024. *Envisioning the Future of AD/ADRD Research.* Presentation at Committee on Research Priorities for Preventing and Treating Alzheimer's Disease and Related Dementias Public Workshop, Hybrid. January 16–17, 2024.

Carlson, M. C. 2021. Productive social engagement as a vehicle to promote activity and neuro-cognitive health in later adulthood. *Archives of Clinical Neuropsychology* 36(7):1274-1278.

Carlson, M. C., J. S. Saczynski, G. W. Rebok, T. Seeman, T. A. Glass, S. McGill, J. Tielsch, K. D. Frick, J. Hill, and L. P. Fried. 2008. Exploring the effects of an "everyday" activity program on executive function and memory in older adults: Experience Corps®. *Gerontologist* 48(6):793-801.

Carrasquillo, M. M., J. E. Crook, O. Pedraza, C. S. Thomas, V. S. Pankratz, M. Allen, T. Nguyen, K. G. Malphrus, L. Ma, G. D. Bisceglio, R. O. Roberts, J. A. Lucas, G. E. Smith, R. J. Ivnik, M. M. Machulda, N. R. Graff-Radford, R. C. Petersen, S. G. Younkin, and N. Ertekin-Taner. 2015. Late-onset Alzheimer's risk variants in memory decline, incident mild cognitive impairment, and Alzheimer's disease. *Neurobiology of Aging* 36(1):60-67.

Carrasquillo, M. M., M. Allen, J. D. Burgess, X. Wang, S. L. Strickland, S. Aryal, J. Siuda, M. L. Kachadoorian, C. Medway, C. S. Younkin, A. Nair, C. Wang, P. Chanana, D. Serie, T. Nguyen, S. Lincoln, K. G. Malphrus, K. Morgan, T. E. Golde, N. D. Price, C. C. White, P. L. De Jager, D. A. Bennett, Y. W. Asmann, J. E. Crook, R. C. Petersen, N. R. Graff-Radford, D. W. Dickson, S. G. Younkin, and N. Ertekin-Taner. 2017. A candidate regulatory variant at the *TREM* gene cluster associates with decreased Alzheimer's disease risk and increased *TREMl1* and *TREM2* brain gene expression. *Alzheimer's & Dementia* 13(6):663-673.

Carvalho, C., and P. I. Moreira. 2023. Metabolic defects shared by Alzheimer's disease and diabetes: A focus on mitochondria. *Current Opinion in Neurobiology* 79:102694.

Cha, Y., T. Y. Park, P. Leblanc, and K. S. Kim. 2023. Current status and future perspectives on stem cell-based therapies for Parkinson's disease. *Journal of Movement Disorders* 16(1):22-41.

Chan, H. J., Yanshree, J. Roy, G. L. Tipoe, M. L. Fung, and L. W. Lim. 2021. Therapeutic potential of human stem cell implantation in Alzheimer's disease. *International Journal of Molecular Science* 22(18):10151.

Chan, A. T. C., R. T. F. Ip, J. Y. S. Tran, J. Y. C. Chan, and K. K. F. Tsoi. 2024. Computerized cognitive training for memory functions in mild cognitive impairment or dementia: A systematic review and meta-analysis. *NPJ Digital Medicine* 7(1):1.

Chen, J., Z. Long, Y. Li, M. Luo, S. Luo, and G. He. 2019. Alteration of the Wnt/gsk3β/β-catenin signalling pathway by rapamycin ameliorates pathology in an Alzheimer's disease model. *International Journal of Molecular Medicine* 44(1):313-323.

Chen, W., Y. Hu, and D. Ju. 2020a. Gene therapy for neurodegenerative disorders: Advances, insights and prospects. *Acta Pharmaceutica Sinica B* 10(8):1347-1359.

Chen, Y., Y. Pei, J. Luo, Z. Huang, J. Yu, and X. Meng. 2020b. Looking for the optimal PD-1/PD-L1 inhibitor in cancer treatment: A comparison in basic structure, function, and clinical practice. *Frontiers in Immunology* 11:1088.

Chen, X., S. Jiang, R. Wang, X. Bao, and Y. Li. 2023a. Neural stem cells in the treatment of Alzheimer's disease: Current status, challenges, and future prospects. *Journal of Alzheimer's Disease* 94(s1):S173-S186.

Chen, P., H. Yao, B. M. Tijms, P. Wang, D. Wang, C. Song, H. Yang, Z. Zhang, K. Zhao, Y. Qu, X. Kang, K. Du, L. Fan, T. Han, C. Yu, X. Zhang, T. Jiang, Y. Zhou, J. Lu, Y. Han, B. Liu, B. Zhou, Y. Liu, and Alzheimer's Disease Neuroimaging Initiative. 2023b. Four distinct subtypes of Alzheimer's disease based on resting-state connectivity biomarkers. *Biological Psychiatry* 93(9):759-769.

Chu, C.-S., P.-T. Tseng, B. Stubbs, T.-Y. Chen, C.-H. Tang, D.-J. Li, W.-C. Yang, Y.-W. Chen, C.-K. Wu, N. Veronese, A. F. Carvalho, B. S. Fernandes, N. Herrmann, and P.-Y. Lin. 2018. Use of statins and the risk of dementia and mild cognitive impairment: A systematic review and meta-analysis. *Scientific Reports* 8(1):5804.

Ciccone, I. 2024. FDA grants fast track designation for Longeveron's Lomecel-B in mild Alzheimer's disease. *NeurologyLive*. July 18. https://www.neurologylive.com/view/fda-grants-fast-track-designation-longeveron-lomecel-b-mild-ad. 2024.

Clare, L., A. Kudlicka, J. R. Oyebode, R. W. Jones, A. Bayer, and I. Leroi. 2019. Individual goal-oriented cognitive rehabilitation to improve everyday functioning for people with early-stage dementia: A multi-centre randomised controlled trial (the GREAT trial). *International Journal of Geriatric Psychiatry* 34(5):709-721.

Clement, C., L. E. Selman, P. G. Kehoe, B. Howden, J. A. Lane, and J. Horwood. 2019. Challenges to and facilitators of recruitment to an Alzheimer's disease clinical trial: A qualitative interview study. *Journal of Alzheimer's Disease* 69(4):1067-1075.

Coley, N., T. Ngandu, J. Lehtisalo, H. Soininen, B. Vellas, E. Richard, M. Kivipelto, S. Andrieu, E. Richard, P. van Gool, E. M. van Charante, C. Beishuizen, S. Jongstra, T. van Middelaar, L. van Wanrooij, M. Hoevenaar-Blom, H. Soininen, T. Ngandu, M. Barbera, M. Kivipelto, F. Mangiasche, S. Andrieu, N. Coley, J. Guillemont, Y. Meiller, B. van de Groep, C. Brayne, M. Kivipelto, T. Ngandu, A. Solomon, T. Laatikainen, T. Strandberg, H. Soininen, J. Tuomilehto, R. Antikainen, J. Lindström, J. Lehtisalo, S. Havulinna, R. Rauramaa, T. Hänninen, T. Ngandu, L. Bäckman, A. Stigsdotter-Neely, T. Strandberg, R. Antikainen, J. Tuomilehto, A. Jula, M. Peltonen, E. Levälahti, M. Grönholm, J. Lehtisalo, K. Hemiö, B. Vellas, S. Guyonnet, I. Carrié, L. Brigitte, C. Faisant, F. Lala, J. Delrieu, H. Villars, E. Combrouze, C. Badufle, A. Zueras, S. Andrieu, C. Cantet, C. Morin, G. A. Van Kan, C. Dupuy, Y. Rolland, C. Caillaud, P.-J. Ousset, F. Lala, B. Fougère, S. Willis, S. Belleville, B. Gilbert, F. Fontaine, J.-F. Dartigues, I. Marcet, F. Delva, A. Foubert, S. Cerda, C. Marie Noëlle, C. Costes, O. Rouaud, P. Manckoundia, V. Quipourt, S. Marilier, E. Franon, L. Bories, M.-L. Pader, M.-F. Basset, B. Lapoujade, V. Faure, M. L. Yung Tong, C. Malick-Loiseau, E. Cazaban-Campistron, F. Desclaux, C. Blatge, T. Dantoine, C. Laubarie-Mouret, I. Saulnier, J.-P. Clément, M.-A. Picat, L. Bernard-Bourzeix, S. Willebois, I. Désormais, N. Cardinaud, M. Bonnefoy, P. Livet, P. Rebaudet, C. Gédéon, C. Burdet, F. Terracol, A. Pesce, S. Roth, S. Chaillou, S. Louchart, K. Sudres, N. Lebrun, N. Barro-Belaygues, J. Touchon, K. Bennys, A. Gabelle, A. Romano, L. Touati, C. Marelli, C. Pays, P. Robert, F. Le Duff, C. Gervais, S. Gonfrier, Y. Gasnier, S. Bordes, D. Begorre, C. Carpuat, K. Khales, J.-F. Lefebvre, S. M. El Idrissi, P. Skolil, J.-P. Salles, C. Dufouil, S. Lehéricy, M. Chupin, J.-F. Mangin, A. Bouhayia, M. Allard, F. Ricolfi, D. Dubois, M. P. Bonceour Martel, F. Cotton, A. Bonafé, S. Chanalet, F. Hugon, F. Bonneville, C. Cognard, F. Chollet, P. Payoux, T. Voisin, J. Delrieu, S. Peiffer, A. Hitzel, M. Allard, M. Zanca, J. Monteil, J. Darcourt, L. Molinier, H. Derumeaux, N. Costa, C. Vincent, B. Perret, C. Vinel, P. Olivier-Abbal, S. Andrieu, C. Cantet, and N. Coley. 2019. Adherence to multidomain interventions for dementia prevention: Data from the FINGER and MAPT trials. *Alzheimer's & Dementia* 15(6):729-741.

Collins, L. M. (2018). *Optimization of behavioral, biobehavioral, and biomedical Interventions: The Multiphase Optimization Strategy (MOST)*. Springer.

Connell, C. M., B. A. Shaw, S. B. Holmes, and N. L. Foster. 2001. Caregivers' attitudes toward their family members' participation in Alzheimer disease research: Implications for recruitment and retention. *Alzheimer's Disease and Associated Disorders* 15(3):137-145.

Connors, M. H., L. Quinto, I. McKeith, H. Brodaty, L. Allan, C. Bamford, A. Thomas, J. P. Taylor, and J. T. O'Brien. 2018. Non-pharmacological interventions for Lewy body dementia: A systematic review. *Psychological Medicine* 48(11):1749-1758.

Conway, O. J., M. M. Carrasquillo, X. Wang, J. M. Bredenberg, J. S. Reddy, S. L. Strickland, C. S. Younkin, J. D. Burgess, M. Allen, S. J. Lincoln, T. Nguyen, K. G. Malphrus, A. I. Soto, R. L. Walton, B. F. Boeve, R. C. Petersen, J. A. Lucas, T. J. Ferman, W. P. Cheshire, J. A. van Gerpen, R. J. Uitti, Z. K. Wszolek, O. A. Ross, D. W. Dickson, N. R. Graff-Radford, and N. Ertekin-Taner. 2018. *ABI3* and *PLCG2* missense variants as risk factors for neurodegenerative diseases in Caucasians and African Americans. *Molecular Neurodegeneration* 13(1):53.

Corasaniti, M. T., G. Bagetta, P. Nicotera, S. Maione, P. Tonin, F. Guida, and D. Scuteri. 2024. Exploitation of autophagy inducers in the management of dementia: A systematic review. *International Journal of Molecular Science* 25(2):1264.

Cummings, J. 2018. Lessons learned from Alzheimer disease: Clinical trials with negative outcomes. *Clinical and Translational Science* 11(2):147-152.

Cummings, J. 2019. The role of biomarkers in Alzheimer's disease drug development. *Advances in Experimental Medical Biology* 1118:29-61.

Cummings, J. 2024. Presentation at the Committee on Research Priorities for Preventing and Treating Alzheimer's Disease and Related Dementias Public Workshop, Hybrid. January 16–17, 2024.

Cummings, J., and J. Kinney. 2022. Biomarkers for Alzheimer's disease: Context of use, qualification, and roadmap for clinical implementation. *Medicina (Kaunas)* 58(7):952.

Cummings, J., A. Ritter, and K. Zhong. 2018. Clinical trials for disease-modifying therapies in Alzheimer's disease: A primer, lessons learned, and a blueprint for the future. *Journal of Alzheimer's Disease* 64(s1):S3-S22.

Cummings, J., Y. Zhou, G. Lee, K. Zhong, J. Fonseca, and F. Cheng. 2023a. Alzheimer's disease drug development pipeline: 2023. *Alzheimer's & Dementia (NY)* 9(2):e12385.

Cummings, J. L., A. M. L. Osse, and J. W. Kinney. 2023b. Alzheimer's disease: Novel targets and investigational drugs for disease modification. *Drugs* 83(15):1387-1408.

Cummings, J., Y. Zhou, G. Lee, K. Zhong, J. Fonseca, and F. Cheng. 2024. Alzheimer's disease drug development pipeline: 2024. *Alzheimer's & Dementia: Translational Research & Clinical Interventions* 10(2):e12465.

Cunningham, E. L., S. A. Todd, P. Passmore, R. Bullock, and B. McGuinness. 2021. Pharmacological treatment of hypertension in people without prior cerebrovascular disease for the prevention of cognitive impairment and dementia. *Cochrane Database of Systematic Reviews* 5(5):CD004034.

Dahabreh, I., T. Terasawa, P. Castaldi, and T. A. Trikalinos. 2010. CYP2D6 testing to predict response to tamoxifen in women with breast cancer: Pharmacogenomic. *PLoS Currents* 2:RRN1176.

Davidson, K. W., M. Silverstein, K. Cheung, R. A. Paluch, and L. H. Epstein. 2021. Experimental designs to optimize treatments for individuals: Personalized N-of-1 trials. *JAMA Pediatrics* 175(4):404-409.

Dawes, P., L. Wolski, I. Himmelsbach, J. Regan, and I. Leroi. 2019. Interventions for hearing and vision impairment to improve outcomes for people with dementia: A scoping review. *International Psychogeriatrics* 31(2):203-221.

De la Rosa, A., G. Olaso-Gonzalez, C. Arc-Chagnaud, F. Millan, A. Salvador-Pascual, C. García-Lucerga, C. Blasco-Lafarga, E. Garcia-Dominguez, A. Carretero, A. G. Correas, J. Viña, and M. C. Gomez-Cabrera. 2020. Physical exercise in the prevention and treatment of Alzheimer's disease. *Journal of Sport and Health Science* 9(5):394-404.

Deckers, K., S. Köhler, T. Ngandu, R. Antikainen, T. Laatikainen, H. Soininen, T. Strandberg, F. Verhey, M. Kivipelto, and A. Solomon. 2021. Quantifying dementia prevention potential in the FINGER randomized controlled trial using the LIBRA prevention index. *Alzheimer's & Dementia* 17(7):1205-1212.

Del Campo, M., H. Zetterberg, S. Gandy, C. U. Onyike, C. Oliveira, C. Udeh-Momoh, A. Lleó, C. E. Teunissen, and Y. Pijnenburg. 2022. New developments of biofluid-based biomarkers for routine diagnosis and disease trajectories in frontotemporal dementia. *Alzheimer's & Dementia* 18(11):2292-2307.

Deng, Z., P. Sheehan, S. Chen, and Z. Yue. 2017. Is amyotrophic lateral sclerosis/frontotemporal dementia an autophagy disease? *Molecular and Neurodegeneration* 12(1):90.

Devi, G. 2023. A how-to guide for a precision medicine approach to the diagnosis and treatment of Alzheimer's disease. *Frontiers in Aging and Neuroscience* 15:1213968.

DeVos, S. L., R. L. Miller, K. M. Schoch, B. B. Holmes, C. S. Kebodeaux, A. J. Wegener, G. Chen, T. Shen, H. Tran, B. Nichols, T. A. Zanardi, H. B. Kordasiewicz, E. E. Swayze, C. F. Bennett, M. I. Diamond, and T. M. Miller. 2017. Tau reduction prevents neuronal loss and reverses pathological tau deposition and seeding in mice with tauopathy. *Science Translational Medicine* 9(374):eaag0481.

DiBenedetti, D. B., C. Slota, S. L. Wronski, G. Vradenburg, M. Comer, L. F. Callahan, J. Winfield, I. Rubino, H. B. Krasa, A. Hartry, D. Wieberg, I. N. Kremer, D. Lappin, A. D. Martin, T. Frangiosa, V. Biggar, and B. Hauber. 2020. Assessing what matters most to patients with or at risk for Alzheimer's and care partners: A qualitative study evaluating symptoms, impacts, and outcomes. *Alzheimer's Research & Therapy* 12(1):90.

Djajadikerta, A., S. Keshri, M. Pavel, R. Prestil, L. Ryan, and D. C. Rubinsztein. 2020. Autophagy induction as a therapeutic strategy for neurodegenerative diseases. *Journal of Molecular Biology* 432(8):2799-2821.

Duff, K., T. J. Atkinson, K. R. Suhrie, B. C. A. Dalley, S. Y. Schaefer, and D. B. Hammers. 2017. Short-term practice effects in mild cognitive impairment: Evaluating different methods of change. *Journal of Clinical and Experimental Neuropsychology* 39(4):396-407.

Duncan, M. J., H. Farlow, C. Tirumalaraju, D.-H. Yun, C. Wang, J. A. Howard, M. N. Sanden, B. F. O'Hara, K. J. McQuerry, and A. D. Bachstetter. 2019. Effects of the dual orexin receptor antagonist DORA-22 on sleep in XFAD mice. *Alzheimer's & Dementia: Translational Research & Clinical Interventions* 5(1):70-80.

ECHAR (Engaging Communities of Hispanics/Latinos for Aging Research). 2024. *Welcome to the ECHAR network.* https://www.echarnetwork.com/ (accessed August 19, 2024).

Edwards, A. L., J. A. Collins, C. Junge, H. Kordasiewicz, L. Mignon, S. Wu, Y. Li, L. Lin, J. DuBois, R. M. Hutchison, N. Ziogas, M. Shulman, L. Martarello, D. Graham, R. Lane, S. Budd Haeberlein, and J. Beaver. 2023. Exploratory tau biomarker results from a multiple ascending-dose study of BIIB080 in Alzheimer disease: A randomized clinical trial. *JAMA Neurology* 80(12):1344-1352.

Edwards, J. D., H. Xu, D. O. Clark, L. T. Guey, L. A. Ross, and F. W. Unverzagt. 2017. Speed of processing training results in lower risk of dementia. *Alzheimer's & Dementia: Translational Research & Clinical Interventions* 3(4):603-611.

Ehrlich, J. R., J. Goldstein, B. K. Swenor, H. Whitson, K. M. Langa, and P. Veliz. 2022. Addition of vision impairment to a life-course model of potentially modifiable dementia risk factors in the U.S. *JAMA Neurology* 79(6):623-626.

Elovainio, M., J. Lahti, M. Pirinen, L. Pulkki-Råback, A. Malmberg, J. Lipsanen, M. Virtanen, M. Kivimäki, and C. Hakulinen. 2022. Association of social isolation, loneliness and genetic risk with incidence of dementia: UK Biobank Cohort Study. *BMJ Open* 12(2):e053936.

Eshraghi, M., M. Ahmadi, S. Afshar, S. Lorzadeh, A. Adlimoghaddam, N. Rezvani Jalal, R. West, S. Dastghaib, S. Igder, S. R. N. Torshizi, A. Mahmoodzadeh, P. Mokarram, T. Madrakian, B. C. Albensi, M. J. Łos, S. Ghavami, and S. Pecic. 2022. Enhancing autophagy in Alzheimer's disease through drug repositioning. *Pharmacology & Therapeutics* 237:108171.

Esserman, L. 2024. *Panelist remarks.* Presentation at the Committee on Research Priorities for Preventing and Treating Alzheimer's Disease and Related Dementias Public Workshop, Hybrid. January 16–17, 2024.

Fairburn, J., S. A. Schüle, S. Dreger, L. Karla Hilz, and G. Bolte. 2019. Social inequalities in exposure to ambient air pollution: A systematic review in the WHO European region. *International Journal of Environmental Research and Public Health* 16(17):3127.

Faison, W. E., S. K. Schultz, J. Aerssens, J. Alvidrez, R. Anand, L. A. Farrer, L. Jarvik, J. Manly, T. McRae, G. M. Murphy, Jr., J. T. Olin, D. Regier, M. Sano, and J. E. Mintzer. 2007. Potential ethnic modifiers in the assessment and treatment of Alzheimer's disease: Challenges for the future. *International Psychogeriatrics* 19(3):539-558.

Fang, J., A. A. Pieper, R. Nussinov, G. Lee, L. Bekris, J. B. Leverenz, J. Cummings, and F. Cheng. 2020. Harnessing endophenotypes and network medicine for Alzheimer's drug repurposing. *Medical Research Reviews* 40(6):2386-2426.

Farina, M. P., Y. S. Zhang, J. K. Kim, M. D. Hayward, and E. M. Crimmins. 2022. Trends in dementia prevalence, incidence, and mortality in the United States (2000-2016). *Journal of Aging and Health* 34(1):100-108.

FDA (U.S. Food and Drug Administration). 2016. *FDA approves first drug for spinal muscular atrophy.* https://www.fda.gov/news-events/press-announcements/fda-approves-first-drug-spinal-muscular-atrophy (accessed August 19, 2024).

FDA. 2018. *Evaluating inclusion and exclusion criteria in clinical trials: Workshop report.* National Press Club: Washington, D.C.

FDA. 2019a. *FDA approves innovative gene therapy to treat pediatric patients with spinal muscular atrophy, a rare disease and leading genetic cause of infant mortality.* https://www.fda.gov/news-events/press-announcements/fda-approves-innovative-gene-therapy-treat-pediatric-patients-spinal-muscular-atrophy-rare-disease (accessed September 24, 2024).

FDA. 2019b. *Enrichment strategies for clinical trials to support approval of human drugs and biological products.* https://www.fda.gov/regulatory-information/search-fda-guidance-documents/enrichment-strategies-clinical-trials-support-approval-human-drugs-and-biological-products (accessed August 20, 2024).

FDA. 2020a. *Qualification process for drug development tools guidance for industry and FDA staff.* https://www.fda.gov/regulatory-information/search-fda-guidance-documents/qualification-process-drug-development-tools-guidance-industry-and-fda-staff (accessed August 20, 2024).

FDA. 2020b. *FDA approves first drug to image tau pathology in patients being evaluated for Alzheimer's disease.* https://www.fda.gov/news-events/press-announcements/fda-approves-first-drug-image-tau-pathology-patients-being-evaluated-alzheimers-disease (accessed August 14, 2024).

FDA. 2023. *FDA approves treatment of amyotrophic lateral sclerosis associated with a mutation in the SOD1 gene.* https://www.fda.gov/drugs/news-events-human-drugs/fda-approves-treatment-amyotrophic-lateral-sclerosis-associated-mutation-sod1-gene (accessed August 19, 2024).

FDA. 2024a. *Early Alzheimer's disease: Developing drugs for treatment.* https://www.fda.gov/regulatory-information/search-fda-guidance-documents/early-alzheimers-disease-developing-drugs-treatment (accessed August 19, 2024).

FDA. 2024b. *FDA approves treatment for adults with Alzheimer's disease.* https://www.fda.gov/drugs/news-events-human-drugs/fda-approves-treatment-adults-alzheimers-disease (accessed October 23, 2024).

Ferreira, P., A. R. Ferreira, and L. Fernandes. 2021. Use of benzodiazepines and related drugs and the risk of dementia: A review of reviews. *European Psychiatry* 64(S1):S423-S423.

Fillit, H., J. Cummings, P. Neumann, T. McLaughlin, P. Salavtore, and C. Leibman. 2010. Novel approaches to incorporating pharmacoeconomic studies into phase III clinical trials for Alzheimer's disease. *Journal of Nutrition, Health and Aging* 14(8):640-647.

Finlay, J., M. Esposito, K. M. Langa, S. Judd, and P. Clarke. 2022. Cognability: An ecological theory of neighborhoods and cognitive aging. *Social Science and Medicine* 309:115220.

FNIH (Foundation for the National Institutes of Health). 2023. *Biomarkers Consortium—I-SPY Trial-2 investigation of serial studies to predict your therapeutic response with imaging and molecular analysis: An adaptive breast cancer trial design in the setting of neoadjuvant chemotherapy.* https://fnih.org/our-programs/biomarkers-consortium-i-spy-trial-2-investigation-of-serial-studies-to-predict-your-therapeutic-response-with-imaging-and-molecular-analysis-an-adaptive-breast-cancer-trial-design-in-the-setting/ (accessed August 20, 2024).

Forette, F., M.-L. Seux, J. A. Staessen, L. Thijs, M.-R. Babarskiene, S. Babeanu, A. Bossini, R. Fagard, B. Gil-Extremera, T. Laks, Z. Kobalava, C. Sarti, J. Tuomilehto, H. Vanhanen, J. Webster, Y. Yodfat, and W. H. Birkenhäger; Systolic Hypertension in Europe Investigators. 2002. The prevention of dementia with antihypertensive treatment: New evidence from the Systolic Hypertension in Europe (Syst-Eur) Study. *Archives of Internal Medicine* 162(18):2046-2052.

Frenkel, D., L. Puckett, S. Petrovic, W. Xia, G. Chen, J. Vega, A. Dembinsky-Vaknin, J. Shen, M. Plante, D. S. Burt, and H. L. Weiner. 2008. A nasal proteosome adjuvant activates microglia and prevents amyloid deposition. *Annals of Neurology* 63(5):591-601.

Fukuoka, H., C. Sutu, and N. A. Afshari. 2016. The impact of cataract surgery on cognitive function in an aging population. *Current Opinions in Ophthalmology* 27(1):3-8.

Gates, N. J., R. W. M. Vernooij, M. Di Nisio, S. Karim, E. March, G. Martínez, and A. W. S. Rutjes. 2019. Computerised cognitive training for preventing dementia in people with mild cognitive impairment. *Cochrane Database of Systematic Reviews* 3(3):CD012279.

Gates, N. J., A. W. S. Rutjes, M. Di Nisio, S. Karim, L. Y. Chong, E. March, G. Martínez, and R. W. M. Vernooij. 2020. Computerised cognitive training for 12 or more weeks for maintaining cognitive function in cognitively healthy people in late life. *Cochrane Database of Systematic Reviews* 2(2):CD012277.

Gavelin, H. M., C. Dong, R. Minkov, A. Bahar-Fuchs, K. A. Ellis, N. T. Lautenschlager, M. L. Mellow, A. T. Wade, A. E. Smith, C. Finke, S. Krohn, and A. Lampit. 2021. Combined physical and cognitive training for older adults with and without cognitive impairment: A systematic review and network meta-analysis of randomized controlled trials. *Ageing Research Reviews* 66:101232.

Geifman, N., R. E. Kennedy, L. S. Schneider, I. Buchan, and R. D. Brinton. 2018. Data-driven identification of endophenotypes of Alzheimer's disease progression: Implications for clinical trials and therapeutic interventions. *Alzheimer's Research & Therapy* 10(1):4.

Gelon, P. A., P. A. Dutchak, and C. F. Sephton. 2022. Synaptic dysfunction in ALS and FTD: Anatomical and molecular changes provide insights into mechanisms of disease. *Frontiers in Molecular Neuroscience* 15:1000183.

Gerlach, L. B., I. R. Wiechers, and D. T. Maust. 2018. Prescription benzodiazepine use among older adults: A critical review. *Harvard Review of Psychiatry* 26(5):264-273.

Gibson, L. L., C. Abdelnour, J. Chong, C. Ballard, and D. Aarsland. 2023. Clinical trials in dementia with Lewy bodies: The evolving concept of co-pathologies, patient selection and biomarkers. *Current Opinion in Neurology* 36(4):264-275.

Goldman, S. A. 2016. Stem and progenitor cell-based therapy of the central nervous system: Hopes, hype, and wishful thinking. *Cell Stem Cell* 18(2):174-188.

Goldman, J. G., L. K. Forsberg, B. F. Boeve, M. J. Armstrong, D. J. Irwin, T. J. Ferman, D. Galasko, J. E. Galvin, D. Kaufer, J. Leverenz, C. F. Lippa, K. Marder, V. Abler, K. Biglan, M. Irizarry, B. Keller, L. Munsie, M. Nakagawa, A. Taylor, and T. Graham. 2020. Challenges and opportunities for improving the landscape for Lewy body dementia clinical trials. *Alzheimer's Research & Therapy* 12(1):137.

Gomez-Soria, I., I. Iguacel, J. N. Cuenca-Zaldivar, A. Aguilar-Latorre, P. Peralta-Marrupe, E. Latorre, and E. Calatayud. 2023. Cognitive stimulation and psychosocial results in older adults: A systematic review and meta-analysis. *Archives of Gerontology and Geriatrics* 115:105114.

Gonzales, M. M., V. R. Garbarino, T. F. Kautz, J. P. Palavicini, M. Lopez-Cruzan, S. K. Dehkordi, J. J. Mathews, H. Zare, P. Xu, B. Zhang, C. Franklin, M. Habes, S. Craft, R. C. Petersen, T. Tchkonia, J. L. Kirkland, A. Salardini, S. Seshadri, N. Musi, and M. E. Orr. 2023. Senolytic therapy in mild Alzheimer's disease: A phase 1 feasibility trial. *Nature Medicine* 29(10):2481-2488.

Gove, D., A. Diaz-Ponce, J. Georges, E. Moniz-Cook, G. Mountain, R. Chattat, and L. Øksnebjerg. 2018. Alzheimer Europe's position on involving people with dementia in research through PPI (patient and public involvement). *Aging & Mental Health* 22(6):723-729.

Green, G. S., M. Fujita, H. S. Yang, M. Taga, A. Cain, C. McCabe, N. Comandante-Lou, C. C. White, A. K. Schmidtner, L. Zeng, A. Sigalov, Y. Wang, A. Regev, H. U. Klein, V. Menon, D. A. Bennett, N. Habib, and P. L. De Jager. 2024. Cellular communities reveal trajectories of brain ageing and Alzheimer's disease. *Nature* 633(8030):634-645.

Gregory, S., S. Saunders, and C. W. Ritchie. 2022. Science disconnected: The translational gap between basic science, clinical trials, and patient care in Alzheimer's disease. *Lancet Healthy Longevity* 3(11):e797-e803.

Groot, C., A. M. Hooghiemstra, P. G. H. M. Raijmakers, B. N. M. van Berckel, P. Scheltens, E. J. A. Scherder, W. M. van der Flier, and R. Ossenkoppele. 2016. The effect of physical activity on cognitive function in patients with dementia: A meta-analysis of randomized control trials. *Ageing Research Reviews* 25:13-23.

Guarnera, J., E. Yuen, and H. Macpherson. 2023. The impact of loneliness and social isolation on cognitive aging: A narrative review. *Journal of Alzheimer's Disease Reports* 7(1):699-714.

Gutierrez, B. A., and A. Limon. 2022. Synaptic disruption by soluble oligomers in patients with Alzheimer's and Parkinson's disease. *Biomedicines* 10(7):1743.

Guure, C. B., N. A. Ibrahim, M. B. Adam, and S. M. Said. 2017. Impact of physical activity on cognitive decline, dementia, and its subtypes: Meta-analysis of prospective studies. *BioMed Research International* 2017(1):9016924.

Hall, A., M. Barbera, J. Lehtisalo, R. Antikainen, H. Huque, T. Laatikainen, T. Ngandu, H. Soininen, R. Stephen, T. Strandberg, M. Kivipelto, K. J. Anstey, and A. Solomon. 2024. The Australian National University Alzheimer's Disease Risk Index (ANU-ADRI) score as a predictor for cognitive decline and potential surrogate outcome in the FINGER lifestyle randomized controlled trial. *European Journal of Neurology* 31(5):e16238.

Hampel, H., S. E. O'Bryant, S. Durrleman, E. Younesi, K. Rojkova, V. Escott-Price, J. C. Corvol, K. Broich, B. Dubois, and S. Lista. 2017. A precision medicine initiative for Alzheimer's disease: The road ahead to biomarker-guided integrative disease modeling. *Climacteric* 20(2):107-118.

Hampel, H., A. Vergallo, G. Perry, and S. Lista; Alzheimer Precision Medicine Initiative. 2019. The Alzheimer Precision Medicine Initiative. *Journal of Alzheimer's Disease* 68(1):1-24.

Hampel, H., F. Caraci, A. C. Cuello, G. Caruso, R. Nistico, M. Corbo, F. Baldacci, N. Toschi, F. Garaci, P. A. Chiesa, S. R. Verdooner, L. Akman-Anderson, F. Hernandez, J. Avila, E. Emanuele, P. L. Valenzuela, A. Lucia, M. Watling, B. P. Imbimbo, A. Vergallo, and S. Lista. 2020. A path toward precision medicine for neuroinflammatory mechanisms in Alzheimer's disease. *Frontiers in Immunology* 11:456.

Hampel, H., R. Au, S. Mattke, W. M. van der Flier, P. Aisen, L. Apostolova, C. Chen, M. Cho, S. De Santi, P. Gao, A. Iwata, R. Kurzman, A. J. Saykin, S. Teipel, B. Vellas, A. Vergallo, H. Wang, and J. Cummings. 2022. Designing the next-generation clinical care pathway for Alzheimer's disease. *Nature Aging* 2(8):692-703.

Hao, X., R. Abeysinghe, F. Zheng, P. E. Schulz, Alzheimer's Disease Neuroimaging Initiative, and L. Cui. 2024. Mapping of Alzheimer's disease related data elements and the NIH Common Data Elements. *BMC Medical Informatics and Decision Making* 24(Suppl 3):103.

Harding, A. J. E., H. Morbey, F. Ahmed, C. Opdebeeck, R. Elvish, I. Leroi, P. R. Williamson, J. Keady, and S. T. Reilly. 2020. A core outcome set for nonpharmacological community-based interventions for people living with dementia at home: A systematic review of outcome measurement instruments. *The Gerontologist* 61(8):e435-e448.

Harrison, J. R., S. Mistry, N. Muskett, and V. Escott-Price. 2020. From polygenic scores to precision medicine in Alzheimer's disease: A systematic review. *Journal of Alzheimer's Disease* 74:1271-1283.

Hartry, A., N. V. J. Aldhouse, T. Al-Zubeidi, M. Sanon, R. G. Stefanacci, and S. L. Knight. 2018. The conceptual relevance of assessment measures in patients with mild/mild-moderate Alzheimer's disease. *Alzheimers & Dementia (Amsterdam, Netherlands)* 10:498-508.

Hauptman, M., M. L. Rogers, M. Scarpaci, B. Morin, and P. M. Vivier. 2023. Neighborhood disparities and the burden of lead poisoning. *Pediatric Research* 94(2):826-836.

He, W., M. Wang, L. Jiang, M. Li, and X. Han. 2019. Cognitive interventions for mild cognitive impairment and dementia: An overview of systematic reviews. *Complementary Therapies in Medicine* 47:102199.

Hekler, E., J. A. Tiro, C. M. Hunter, and C. Nebeker. 2020. Precision health: The role of the social and behavioral sciences in advancing the vision. *Annals of Behavioral Medicine* 54(11):805-826.

Heller, C., J. E. Balls-Berry, J. D. Nery, P. J. Erwin, D. Littleton, M. Kim, and W. P. Kuo. 2014. Strategies addressing barriers to clinical trial enrollment of underrepresented populations: A systematic review. *Contemporary Clinical Trials* 39(2):169-182.

Higginbotham, L., L. Ping, E. B. Dammer, D. M. Duong, M. Zhou, M. Gearing, C. Hurst, J. D. Glass, S. A. Factor, E. C. B. Johnson, I. Hajjar, J. J. Lah, A. I. Levey, N. T. Seyfried. 2020. Integrated proteomics reveals brain-based cerebrospinal fluid biomarkers in asymptomatic and symptomatic Alzheimer's disease. *Science Advances* 6(43):eaaz9360.

Higginbotham, L., E. K. Carter, E. B. Dammer, R. U. Haque, E. C. B. Johnson, D. M. Duong, L. Yin, P. L. De Jayer, D. A. Bennett, D. Felsky, E. S. Tio, J. J. Lah, A. I. Levey, and N. T. Seyfried. 2023. Unbiased classification of the elderly human brain proteome resolves distinct clinical and pathophysiological subtypes of cognitive impairment. *Neurobiology of Disease* 186:106286.

Hobbs, B. P., P. C. Barata, Y. Kanjanapan, C. J. Paller, J. Perlmutter, G. R. Pond, T. M. Prowell, E. H. Rubin, L. K. Seymour, N. A. Wages, T. A. Yap, D. Feltquate, E. Garrett-Mayer, W. Grossman, D. S. Hong, S. P. Ivy, L. L. Siu, S. A. Reeves, and G. L. Rosner. 2019. Seamless designs: Current practice and considerations for early-phase drug development in oncology. *Journal of the National Cancer Institute* 111(2):118-128.

Hohman, T. J., J. N. Cooke-Bailey, C. Reitz, G. Jun, A. Naj, G. W. Beecham, Z. Liu, R. M. Carney, J. M. Vance, M. L. Cuccaro, R. Rajbhandary, B. N. Vardarajan, L. S. Wang, O. Valladares, C. F. Lin, E. B. Larson, N. R. Graff-Radford, D. Evans, P. L. De Jager, P. K. Crane, J. D. Buxbaum, J. R. Murrell, T. Raj, N. Ertekin-Taner, M. W. Logue, C. T. Baldwin, R. C. Green, L. L. Barnes, L. B. Cantwell, M. D. Fallin, R. C. Go, P. Griffith, T. O. Obisesan, J. J. Manly, K. L. Lunetta, M. I. Kamboh, O. L. Lopez, D. A. Bennett, J. Hardy, H. C. Hendrie, K. S. Hall, A. M. Goate, R. Lang, G. S. Byrd, W. A. Kukull, T. M. Foroud, L. A. Farrer, E. R. Martin, M. A. Pericak-Vance, G. D. Schellenberg, R. Mayeux, J. L. Haines, and T. A. Thornton-Wells; Alzheimer Disease Genetics Consortium. 2016. Global and local ancestry in African-Americans: Implications for Alzheimer's disease risk. *Alzheimer's & Dementia* 12(3):233-243.

Hölscher, C. 2022. Protective properties of GLP-1 and associated peptide hormones in neurodegenerative disorders. *British Journal of Pharmacology* 179(4):695-714.

Hou, B., Z. Wen, J. Bao, R. Zhang, B. Tong, S. Yang, J. Wen, Y. Cui, J. H. Moore, A. J. Saykin, H. Huang, P. M. Thompson, M. D. Ritchie, C. Davatzikos, and L. Shen; Alzheimer's Disease Neuroimaging Initiative. 2024. Interpretable deep clustering survival machines for Alzheimer's disease subtype discovery. *Medical Image Analysis* 97:103231.

Hu, M., X. Wu, X. Shu, H. Hu, Q. Chen, L. Peng, and H. Feng. 2021. Effects of computerised cognitive training on cognitive impairment: A meta-analysis. *Journal of Neurology* 268(5):1680-1688.

Hu, Y., J. Huerta, N. Cordella, R. G. Mishuris, and I. C. Paschalidis. 2023. Personalized hypertension treatment recommendations by a data-driven model. *BMC Medical Informatics and Decision Making* 23(1):44.

ICER (Institute for Clinical and Economic Review). 2021. *Aducanumab for Alzheimer's disease: Effectiveness and value.* https://icer.org/wp-content/uploads/2020/10/ICER_ALZ_Final_Report_080521.pdf (accessed September 16, 2024).

Indorewalla, K. K., M. K. O'Connor, A. E. Budson, C. Guess DiTerlizzi, and J. Jackson. 2021. Modifiable barriers for recruitment and retention of older adults participants from underrepresented minorities in Alzheimer's disease research. *Journal of Alzheimer's Disease* 80(3):927-940.

Irizarry, M. 2024. *Panelist Remarks.* Presentation at the Committee on Research Priorities for Preventing and Treating Alzheimer's Disease and Related Dementias Public Workshop, Hybrid. January 16–17, 2024.

Islam, M. T., E. Tuday, S. Allen, J. Kim, D. W. Trott, W. L. Holland, A. J. Donato, and L. A. Lesniewski. 2023. Senolytic drugs, dasatinib and quercetin, attenuate adipose tissue inflammation, and ameliorate metabolic function in old age. *Aging Cell* 22(2):e13767.

İş, Ö., X. Wang, J. S. Reddy, Y. Min, E. Yilmaz, P. Bhattarai, T. Patel, J. Bergman, Z. Quicksall, M. G. Heckman, F. Q. Tutor-New, B. Can Demirdogen, L. White, S. Koga, V. Krause, Y. Inoue, T. Kanekiyo, M. I. Cosacak, N. Nelson, A. J. Lee, B. Vardarajan, R. Mayeux, N. Kouri, K. Deniz, T. Carnwath, S. R. Oatman, L. J. Lewis-Tuffin, T. Nguyen, ADNI, M. M. Carrasquillo, J. Graff-Radford, R. C. Petersen, C. R. Jack, Jr., K. Kantarci, M. E. Murray, K. Nho, A. J. Saykin, D. W. Dickson, C. Kizil, M. Allen, and N. Ertekin-Taner. 2024. Gliovascular transcriptional perturbations in Alzheimer's disease reveal molecular mechanisms of blood brain barrier dysfunction. *Nature Communications* 15(1):4758.

Iso-Markku, P., U. M. Kujala, K. Knittle, J. Polet, E. Vuoksimaa, and K. Waller. 2022. Physical activity as a protective factor for dementia and Alzheimer's disease: Systematic review, meta-analysis and quality assessment of cohort and case-control studies. *British Journal of Sports Medicine* 56(12):701-709.

Iturria-Medina, Y., Q. Adewale, A. F. Khan, S. Ducharme, P. Rosa-Neto, K. O'Donnell, V. A. Petyuk, S. Gauthier, P. L. De Jager, J. Breitner, D. A. Bennett. 2022. Unified epigenomic, transcriptomic, proteomic, and metabolomic taxonomy of Alzheimer's disease progression and heterogeneity. *Science Advances* 8(46):eabo6764.

Jaeggi, S. M., A. N. Weaver, E. Carbone, F. E. Trane, R. N. Smith-Peirce, M. Buschkuehl, C. Flueckiger, M. Carlson, J. Jonides, and E. Borella. 2023. EngAge—a metacognitive intervention to supplement working memory training: A feasibility study in older adults. *Aging Brain* 4:100083.

Jain, P., C. Jain, and V. Velcheti. 2018. Role of immune-checkpoint inhibitors in lung cancer. *Therapeutic Advances in Respiratory Disease* 12:1753465817750075.

Jayakody, D. M. P., P. L. Friedland, R. N. Martins, and H. R. Sohrabi. 2018. Impact of aging on the auditory system and related cognitive functions: A narrative review. *Frontiers in Neuroscience* 12:125.

Jessen, F., J. Georges, M. Wortmann, and S. Benham-Hermetz. 2022. What matters to patients with Alzheimer's disease and their care partners? Implications for understanding the value of future interventions. *Journal of Prevention of Alzheimer's Disease* 9(3):550-555.

Jimenez-Puerta, G. J., J. A. Marchal, E. López-Ruiz, and P. Gálvez-Martín. 2020. Role of mesenchymal stromal cells as therapeutic agents: Potential mechanisms of action and implications in their clinical use. *Journal of Clinical Medicine* 9(2):445.

Jin, S. C., M. M. Carrasquillo, B. A. Benitez, T. Skorupa, D. Carrell, D. Patel, S. Lincoln, S. Krishnan, M. Kachadoorian, C. Reitz, R. Mayeux, T. S. Wingo, J. J. Lah, A. I. Levey, J. Murrell, H. Hendrie, T. Foroud, N. R. Graff-Radford, A. M. Goate, C. Cruchaga, and N. Ertekin-Taner. 2015. TREM2 is associated with increased risk for Alzheimer's disease in African Americans. *Molecular Neurodegeneration* 10:19.

Jin, S., X. Guan, and D. Min. 2023. Evidence of clinical efficacy and pharmacological mechanisms of resveratrol in the treatment of Alzheimer's disease. *Current Alzheimer's Research* 20(8):588-602.

Johnson, E. C. B., E. K. Carter, E. B. Dammer, D. M. Duong, E. S. Gerasimov, Y. Liu, J. Liu, R. Betarbet, L. Ping, L. Yin, G. E. Serrano, T. G. Beach, J. Peng, P. L. De Jager, V. Haroutunian, B. Zhang, C. Gaiteri, D. A. Bennett, M. Gearing, T. S. Wingo, A. P. Wingo, J. J. Lah, A. I. Levey, and N. T. Seyfried. 2022. Large-scale deep multi-layer analysis of Alzheimer's disease brain reveals strong proteomic disease-related changes not observed at the RNA level. *Nature Neuroscience* 25(2):213-225.

Joshi, P., K. Hendrie, D. J. Jester, D. Dasarathy, H. Lavretsky, B. S. Ku, H. Leutwyler, J. Torous, D. V. Jeste, and R. R. Tampi. 2024. Social connections as determinants of cognitive health and as targets for social interventions in persons with or at risk of Alzheimer's disease and related disorders: A scoping review. *International Psychogeriatrics* 36(2):92-118.

Kabir, M. T., M. S. Uddin, A. A. Mamun, P. Jeandet, L. Aleya, R. A. Mansouri, G. M. Ashraf, B. Mathew, M. N. Bin-Jumah, and M. M. Abdel-Daim. 2020. Combination drug therapy for the management of Alzheimer's disease. *International Journal of Molecular Science* 21(9):3272.

Karamacoska, D., A. Butt, I. H. K. Leung, R. L. Childs, N. J. Metri, V. Uruthiran, T. Tan, A. Sabag, and G. Z. Steiner-Lim. 2023. Brain function effects of exercise interventions for cognitive decline: A systematic review and meta-analysis. *Frontiers in Neuroscience* 17:1127065.

Kelly, M. E., H. Duff, S. Kelly, J. E. McHugh Power, S. Brennan, B. A. Lawlor, and D. G. Loughrey. 2017. The impact of social activities, social networks, social support and social relationships on the cognitive functioning of healthy older adults: A systematic review. *Systematic Reviews* 6(1):259.

Khoury, R., J. Rajamanickam, and G. T. Grossberg. 2018. An update on the safety of current therapies for Alzheimer's disease: Focus on rivastigmine. *Therapeutic Advances in Drug Safety* 9(3):171-178.

Khoury, R., Y. Liu, Q. Sheheryar, and G. T. Grossberg. 2021. Pharmacotherapy for frontotemporal dementia. *CNS Drugs* 35(4):425-438.

Kilian, J., and M. Kitazawa. 2018. The emerging risk of exposure to air pollution on cognitive decline and Alzheimer's disease—evidence from epidemiological and animal studies. *Biomedical Journal* 41(3):141-162.

Kim, O., Y. Pang, and J.-H. Kim. 2019. The effectiveness of virtual reality for people with mild cognitive impairment or dementia: A meta-analysis. *BMC Psychiatry* 19(1):219.

Kind, A. 2024. *Panelist remarks.* Presentation at the Committee on Research Priorities for Preventing and Treating Alzheimer's Disease and Related Dementias Public Workshop, Hybrid. January 16–17, 2024.

Kiyota, T., J. Machhi, Y. Lu, B. Dyavarshetty, M. Nemati, I. Yokoyama, R. L. Mosley, and H. E. Gendelman. 2018. Granulocyte-macrophage colony-stimulating factor neuroprotective activities in Alzheimer's disease mice. *Journal of Neuroimmunology* 319:80-92.

Klionsky, D. J., and S. D. Emr. 2000. Autophagy as a regulated pathway of cellular degradation. *Science* 290(5497):1717-1721.

Koivisto, J., and A. Malik. 2021. Gamification for older adults: A systematic literature review. *Gerontologist* 61(7):e360-e372.

Krzeczkowska, A., D. M. Spalding, W. J. McGeown, A. J. Gow, M. C. Carlson, and L. A. B. Nicholls. 2021. A systematic review of the impacts of intergenerational engagement on older adults' cognitive, social, and health outcomes. *Ageing Research Reviews* 71:101400.

Kulmala, J., T. Ngandu, S. Havulinna, E. Levälahti, J. Lehtisalo, A. Solomon, R. Antikainen, T. Laatikainen, P. Pippola, M. Peltonen, R. Rauramaa, H. Soininen, T. Strandberg, J. Tuomilehto, and M. Kivipelto. 2019. The effect of multidomain lifestyle intervention on daily functioning in older people. *Journal of the American Geriatric Society* 67(6):1138-1144.

Kwak, K. A., S. P. Lee, J. Y. Yang, and Y. S. Park. 2018. Current perspectives regarding stem cell-based therapy for Alzheimer's disease. *Stem Cells International* 2018:6392986.

Largent, E. A., and H. F. Lynch. 2017. Paying research participants: The outsized influence of "undue influence." *IRB* 39(4):1-9.

Laske, C., H. R. Sohrabi, S. M. Frost, K. López-de-Ipiña, P. Garrard, M. Buscema, J. Dauwels, S. R. Soekadar, S. Mueller, C. Linnemann, S. A. Bridenbaugh, Y. Kanagasingam, R. N. Martins, and S. E. O'Bryant. 2015. Innovative diagnostic tools for early detection of Alzheimer's disease. *Alzheimer's & Dementia* 11(5):561-578.

Lazar, A. A., B. F. Cole, M. Bonetti, and R. D. Gelber. 2010. Evaluation of treatment-effect heterogeneity using biomarkers measured on a continuous scale: Subpopulation treatment effect pattern plot. *Journal of Clinical Oncology* 28(29):4539-4544.

Leinenga, G., X. V. To, L.-G. Bodea, J. Yousef, G. Richter-Stretton, T. Palliyaguru, A. Chicoteau, L. Dagley, F. Nasrallah, and J. Götz. 2024. Scanning ultrasound-mediated memory and functional improvements do not require amyloid-β reduction. *Molecular Psychiatry* 29(8):2408-2423.

Lelo de Larrea-Mancera, E. S., T. Stavropoulos, A. A. Carrillo, S. Cheung, Y. J. He, D. A. Eddins, M. R. Molis, F. J. Gallun, and A. R. Seitz. 2022. Remote auditory assessment using portable automated rapid testing (PART) and participant-owned devices). *Journal of the Acoustical Society of America* 152(2):807-819.

Leng, Y., and K. Yaffe. 2024. Harnessing brain pathology for dementia prevention. *JAMA Neurology* 81(3):229-231.

Lennon, M. J., G. Rigney, V. Raymont, and P. Sachdev. 2021. Genetic therapies for Alzheimer's disease: A scoping review. *Journal of Alzheimer's Disease* 84:491-504.

Li, S., and D. J. Selkoe. 2020. A mechanistic hypothesis for the impairment of synaptic plasticity by soluble Aβ oligomers from Alzheimer's brain. *Journal of Neurochemistry* 154(6):583-597.

Li, X., M. Ji, H. Zhang, Z. Liu, Y. Chai, Q. Cheng, Y. Yang, D. Cordato, and J. Gao. 2023. Non-drug therapies for Alzheimer's disease: A review. *Neurology and Therapy* 12(1):39-72.

Lian, P., X. Cai, C. Wang, K. Liu, X. Yang, Y. Wu, Z. Zhang, Z. Ma, X. Cao, and Y. Xu. 2023. Identification of metabolism-related subtypes and feature genes in Alzheimer's disease. *Journal of Translational Medicine* 21(1):628.

Liguori, C., A. Romigi, M. Nuccetelli, S. Zannino, G. Sancesario, A. Martorana, M. Albanese, N. B. Mercuri, F. Izzi, S. Bernardini, A. Nitti, G. M. Sancesario, F. Sica, M. G. Marciani, and F. Placidi. 2014. Orexinergic system dysregulation, sleep impairment, and cognitive decline in Alzheimer's disease. *JAMA Neurology* 71(12):1498-1505.

Lim, Y. Y., J. Kong, P. Maruff, J. Jaeger, E. Huang, and E. Ratti. 2022. Longitudinal cognitive decline in patients with mild cognitive impairment or dementia due to Alzheimer's disease. *Journal of Prevention of Alzheimer's Disease* 9(1):178-183.

Lin, H., L. Zhang, D. Lin, W. Chen, Y. Zhu, C. Chen, K. C. Chan, Y. Liu, and W. Chen. 2018. Visual restoration after cataract surgery promotes functional and structural brain recovery. *EBioMedicine* 30:52-61.

Liu, Q., N. Vaci, I. Koychev, A. Kormilitzin, Z. Li, A. Cipriani, and A. Nevado-Holgado. 2022. Personalised treatment for cognitive impairment in dementia: Development and validation of an artificial intelligence model. *BMC Medicine* 20(1):45.

Liu, Z., Q. Liang, Y. Ren, C. Guo, X. Ge, L. Wang, Q. Cheng, P. Luo, Y. Zhang, and X. Han. 2023. Immunosenescence: Molecular mechanisms and diseases. *Signal Transduction and Targeted Therapy* 8(1):200.

Livingston, G., J. Huntley, A. Sommerlad, D. Ames, C. Ballard, S. Banerjee, C. Brayne, A. Burns, J. Cohen-Mansfield, C. Cooper, S. G. Costafreda, A. Dias, N. Fox, L. N. Gitlin, R. Howard, H. C. Kales, M. Kivimäki, E. B. Larson, A. Ogunniyi, V. Orgeta, K. Ritchie, K. Rockwood, E. L. Sampson, Q. Samus, L. S. Schneider, G. Selbæk, L. Teri, and N.

Mukadam. 2020. Dementia prevention, intervention, and care: 2020 report of the Lancet Commission. *Lancet* 396(10248):413-446.

Livingston, G., J. Huntley, K. Y. Liu, S. G. Costafreda, G. Selbæk, S. Alladi, D. Ames, S. Banerjee, A. Burns, C. Brayne, N. C. Fox, C. P. Ferri, L. N. Gitlin, R. Howard, H. C. Kales, M. Kivimäki, E. B. Larson, N. Nakasujja, K. Rockwood, Q. Samus, K. Shirai, A. Singh-Manoux, L. S. Schneider, S. Walsh, Y. Yao, A. Sommerlad, and N. Mukadam. 2024. Dementia prevention, intervention, and care: 2024 report of the Lancet Standing Commission. *Lancet* 404(10452):572-628.

Llano, D. A., S. S. Kwok, and V. Devanarayan. 2021. Reported hearing loss in Alzheimer's disease is associated with loss of brainstem and cerebellar volume. *Frontiers in Human Neuroscience* 15:739754.

Loera-Valencia, R., A. Piras, M. A. M. Ismail, S. Manchanda, H. Eyjolfsdottir, T. C. Saido, J. Johansson, M. Eriksdotter, B. Winblad, and P. Nilsson. 2018. Targeting Alzheimer's disease with gene and cell therapies. *Journal of Internal Medicine* 284(1):2-36.

Logue, M. W., M. Schu, B. N. Vardarajan, J. Farrell, D. A. Bennett, J. D. Buxbaum, G. S. Byrd, N. Ertekin-Taner, D. Evans, T. Foroud, A. Goate, N. R. Graff-Radford, M. I. Kamboh, W. A. Kukull, J. J. Manly, and Alzheimer Disease Genetics Collaborative. 2014. Two rare *AKAP9* variants are associated with Alzheimer's disease in African Americans. *Alzheimer's & Dementia* 10(6):609-618.e611.

Loomis, S. J., R. Miller, C. Castrillo-Viguera, K. Umans, W. Cheng, J. O'Gorman, R. Hughes, S. Budd Haeberlein, and C. D. Whelan. 2024. Genome-wide association studies of ARIA from the aducanumab phase 3 ENGAGE and EMERGE studies. *Neurology* 102(3):e207919.

López-Ortiz, S., S. Lista, P. L. Valenzuela, J. Pinto-Fraga, R. Carmona, F. Caraci, G. Caruso, N. Toschi, E. Emanuele, A. Gabelle, R. Nisticò, F. Garaci, A. Lucia, and A. Santos-Lozano. 2023. Effects of physical activity and exercise interventions on Alzheimer's disease: An umbrella review of existing meta-analyses. *Journal of Neurology* 270(2):711-725.

López-Otín, C., M. A. Blasco, L. Partridge, M. Serrano, and G. Kroemer. 2023. Hallmarks of aging: An expanding universe. *Cell* 186(2):243-278.

Lourida, I., E. Hannon, T. J. Littlejohns, K. M. Langa, E. Hypponen, E. Kuzma, and D. J. Llewellyn. 2019. Association of lifestyle and genetic risk with incidence of dementia. *JAMA* 322(5):430-437.

Luchsinger, J. A., Y. Ma, C. A. Christophi, H. Florez, S. H. Golden, H. Hazuda, J. Crandall, E. Venditti, K. Watson, S. Jeffries, J. J. Manly, F. X. Pi-Sunyer, and Diabetes Prevention Program Research Group. 2017. Metformin, lifestyle intervention, and cognition in the diabetes prevention program outcomes study. *Diabetes Care* 40(7):958-965.

MacDonald, S., A. S. Shah, and B. Tousi. 2022. Current therapies and drug development pipeline in Lewy body dementia: An update. *Drugs & Aging* 39(7):505-522.

Maharani, A., P. Dawes, J. Nazroo, G. Tampubolon, and N. Pendleton. 2018. Cataract surgery and age-related cognitive decline: A 13-year follow-up of the English Longitudinal Study of Ageing. *PLoS ONE* 13(10):e0204833.

Majumder, S., A. Richardson, R. Strong, and S. Oddo. 2011. Inducing autophagy by rapamycin before, but not after, the formation of plaques and tangles ameliorates cognitive deficits. *PLoS ONE* 6(9):e25416.

Mamo, S. K., N. S. Reed, C. Price, D. Occhipinti, A. Pletnikova, F. R. Lin, and E. S. Oh. 2018. Hearing loss treatment in older adults with cognitive impairment: A systematic review. *Journal of Speech, Language, and Hearing Research* 61(10):2589-2603.

Márquez, F., and M. A. Yassa. 2019. Neuroimaging biomarkers for Alzheimer's disease. *Molecular Neurodegeneration* 14(1):21.

McGuinness, B., D. Craig, R. Bullock, and P. Passmore. 2016. Statins for the prevention of dementia. *Cochrane Database of Systematic Reviews* 2016(1):CD003160.

McKenzie, A. T., S. Moyon, M. Wang, I. Katsyv, W. M. Song, X. Zhou, E. B. Dammer, D. M. Duong, J. Aaker, Y. Zhao, N. Beckmann, P. Wang, J. Zhu, J. J. Lah, N. T. Seyfried, A. I. Levey, P. Katsel, V. Haroutunian, E. E. Schadt, B. Popko, P. Casaccia, and B. Zhang. 2017. Multiscale network modeling of oligodendrocytes reveals molecular components of myelin dysregulation in Alzheimer's disease. *Molecular Neurodegeneration* 12(1):82.

McKenzie, A. T., M. Wang, M. E. Hauberg, J. F. Fullard, A. Kozlenkov, A. Keenan, Y. L. Hurd, S. Dracheva, P. Casaccia, P. Roussos, and B. Zhang. 2018. Brain cell type specific gene expression and co-expression network architectures. *Scientific Reports* 8(1):8868.

McMaster, M., S. Kim, L. Clare, S. J. Torres, N. Cherbuin, C. D'Este, and K. J. Anstey. 2020. Lifestyle risk factors and cognitive outcomes from the multidomain dementia risk reduction randomized controlled trial, Body Brain Life for Cognitive Decline (BBL-CD). *Journal of the American Geriatrics Society* 68(11):2629-2637.

Meng, X., S. Fang, S. Zhang, H. Li, D. Ma, Y. Ye, J. Su, and J. Sun. 2022. Multidomain lifestyle interventions for cognition and the risk of dementia: A systematic review and meta-analysis. *International Journal of Nursing Studies* 130:104236.

Meyer, P. F., J. Tremblay-Mercier, J. Leoutsakos, C. Madjar, M. E. Lafaille-Magnan, M. Savard, P. Rosa-Neto, J. Poirier, P. Etienne, and J. Breitner. 2019. INTREPAD: A randomized trial of naproxen to slow progress of presymptomatic Alzheimer disease. *Neurology* 92(18):e2070-e2080.

Miah, J., P. Dawes, S. Edwards, I. Leroi, B. Starling, and S. Parsons. 2019. Patient and public involvement in dementia research in the European Union: A scoping review. *BMC Geriatrics* 19(1):220.

Michailidis, M., D. A. Tata, D. Moraitou, D. Kavvadas, S. Karachrysafi, T. Papamitsou, P. Vareltzis, and V. Papaliagkas. 2022. Antidiabetic drugs in the treatment of Alzheimer's disease. *International Journal of Molecular Sciences* 23(9):4641.

Mielke, M. 2024. Sex and gender differences in Alzheimer's disease and Alzheimer's disease related dementias. Commissioned Paper for the Committee on Research Priorities for Preventing and Treating Alzheimer's Disease and Related Dementias.

Miller, J. B., and W. B. Barr. 2017. The technology crisis in neuropsychology. *Archives in Clinical Neuropsychology* 32(5):541-554.

Min, Y., X. Wang, O. Is, T. A. Patel, J. Gao, J. S. Reddy, Z. S. Quicksall, T. Nguyen, S. Lin, F. Q. Tutor-New, J. L. Chalk, A. O. Mitchell, J. E. Crook, P. T. Nelson, L. J. Van Eldik, T. E. Golde, M. M. Carrasquillo, D. W. Dickson, K. Zhang, M. Allen, and N. Ertekin-Taner. 2023. Cross species systems biology discovers glial *DDR2*, *STOM*, and *KANK2* as therapeutic targets in progressive supranuclear palsy. *Nature Communications* 14(1):6801.

Minen, M. T., A. Gopal, G. Sahyoun, E. Stieglitz, and J. Torous. 2021. The functionality, evidence, and privacy issues around smartphone apps for the top neuropsychiatric conditions. *Journal of Neuropsychiatry and Clinical Neuroscience* 33(1):72-79.

Mintun, M. A., A. C. Lo, C. Duggan Evans, A. M. Wessels, P. A. Ardayfio, S. W. Andersen, S. Shcherbinin, J. D. Sparks, J. R. Sims, M. Brys, L. G. Apostolova, and D. M. Skovronsky. 2021. Donanemab in early Alzheimer's disease. *New England Journal of Medicine* 384(18):1691-1704.

Mitchell, A. K., R. Ehrenkranz, S. Franzen, S. H. Han, M. Shakur, M. McGowan, and H. A. Massett. 2024. Analysis of eligibility criteria in Alzheimer's and related dementias clinical trials. *Scientific Reports* 14:15036.

Miyata, K., T. Yoshikawa, M. Morikawa, M. Mine, N. Okamoto, N. Kurumatani, and N. Ogata. 2018. Effect of cataract surgery on cognitive function in elderly: Results of Fujiwara-kyo Eye Study. *PLoS ONE* 13(2):e0192677.

Mohler, J., B. Najafi, M. Fain, and K. S. Ramos. 2015. Precision medicine: A wider definition. *Journal of the American Geriatrics Society* 63(9):1971-1972.

Mohs, R. C., and N. H. Greig. 2017. Drug discovery and development: Role of basic biological research. *Alzheimer's & Dementia (N Y)* 3(4):651-657.

Montori, V. M., M. M. Ruissen, I. G. Hargraves, J. P. Brito, and M. Kunneman. 2023. Shared decision-making as a method of care. *BMJ Evidence-Based Medicine* 28(4):213-217.

Morris, J. K., E. D. Vidoni, D. K. Johnson, A. Van Sciver, J. D. Mahnken, R. A. Honea, H. M. Wilkins, W. M. Brooks, S. A. Billinger, R. H. Swerdlow, and J. M. Burns. 2017. Aerobic exercise for Alzheimer's disease: A randomized controlled pilot trial. *PLoS ONE* 12(2):e0170547.

Morton, H., S. Kshirsagar, E. Orlov, L. E. Bunquin, N. Sawant, L. Boleng, M. George, T. Basu, B. Ramasubramanian, J. A. Pradeepkiran, S. Kumar, M. Vijayan, A. P. Reddy, and P. H. Reddy. 2021. Defective mitophagy and synaptic degeneration in Alzheimer's disease: Focus on aging, mitochondria and synapse. *Free Radical Biology and Medicine* 172:652-667.

Mostafavi, S., C. Gaiteri, S. E. Sullivan, C. C. White, S. Tasaki, J. Xu, M. Taga, H. U. Klein, E. Patrick, V. Komashko, C. McCabe, R. Smith, E. M. Bradshaw, D. E. Root, A. Regev, L. Yu, L. B. Chibnik, J. A. Schneider, T. L. Young-Pearse, D. A. Bennett, and P. L. De Jager. 2018. A molecular network of the aging human brain provides insights into the pathology and cognitive decline of Alzheimer's disease. *Nature Neuroscience* 21(6):811-819.

Moussa, C., M. Hebron, X. Huang, J. Ahn, R. A. Rissman, P. S. Aisen, and R. S. Turner. 2017. Resveratrol regulates neuro-inflammation and induces adaptive immunity in Alzheimer's disease. *Journal of Neuroinflammation* 14(1):1.

Mukherjee, S., L. Heath, C. Preuss, S. Jayadev, G. A. Garden, A. K. Greenwood, S. K. Sieberts, P. L. De Jager, N. Ertekin-Taner, G. W. Carter, L. M. Mangravite, and B. A. Logsdon. 2020. Molecular estimation of neurodegeneration pseudotime in older brains. *Nature Communications* 11(1):5781.

Mummery, C. J., A. Börjesson-Hanson, D. J. Blackburn, E. G. B. Vijverberg, P. P. De Deyn, S. Ducharme, M. Jonsson, A. Schneider, J. O. Rinne, A. C. Ludolph, R. Bodenschatz, H. Kordasiewicz, E. E. Swayze, B. Fitzsimmons, L. Mignon, K. M. Moore, C. Yun, T. Baumann, D. Li, D. A. Norris, R. Crean, D. L. Graham, E. Huang, E. Ratti, C. F. Bennett, C. Junge, and R. M. Lane. 2023. Tau-targeting antisense oligonucleotide MAPT$_{Rx}$ in mild Alzheimer's disease: A phase 1b, randomized, placebo-controlled trial. *Nature Medicine* 29(6):1437-1447.

Muñoz-Jiménez, M., A. Zaarkti, J. A. García-Arnés, and N. García-Casares. 2020. Antidiabetic drugs in Alzheimer's disease and mild cognitive impairment: A systematic review. *Dementia and Geriatric Cognitive Disorders* 49(5):423-434.

Myles, P. S., E. Williamson, J. Oakley, and A. Forbes. 2014. Ethical and scientific considerations for patient enrollment into concurrent clinical trials. *Trials* 15:470.

N'Songo, A., M. M. Carrasquillo, X. Wang, J. D. Burgess, T. Nguyen, Y. W. Asmann, D. J. Serie, S. G. Younkin, M. Allen, O. Pedraza, R. Duara, M. T. Greig Custo, N. R. Graff-Radford, and N. Ertekin-Taner. 2017. African American exome sequencing identifies potential risk variants at Alzheimer disease loci. *Neurology Genetics* 3(2):e141.

Nag, S., L. L. Barnes, L. Yu, R. S. Wilson, D. A. Bennett, and J. A. Schneider. 2020. Limbic-predominant age-related TDP-43 encephalopathy in black and white decedents. *Neurology* 95(15):e2056-e2064.

NASEM (National Academies of Sciences, Engineering, and Medicine). 2017. *Preventing cognitive decline and dementia: A way forward*. Edited by A. I. Leshner, S. Landis, C. Stroud and A. Downey. Washington, DC: The National Academies Press.

NASEM. 2020. *Social isolation and loneliness in older adults: Opportunities for the health care system*. Washington, DC: The National Academies Press.

NASEM. 2021. *Implications for behavioral and social research of preclinical markers of Alzheimer's disease and related dementias: Proceedings of a workshop—in brief.* Edited by E. H. Forstag. Washington, DC: The National Academies Press.

NASEM. 2024. *Preventing and treating Alzheimer's disease and related dementias: Promising research and opportunities to accelerate progress: Proceedings of a workshop—in brief.* Edited by O. Yost and A. Downey. Washington, DC: The National Academies Press.

Neff, R. A., M. Wang, S. Vatansever, L. Guo, C. Ming, Q. Wang, E. Wang, E. Horgusluoglu-Moloch, W. M. Song, A. Li, E. L. Castranio, J. Tcw, L. Ho, A. Goate, V. Fossati, S. Noggle, S. Gandy, M. E. Ehrlich, P. Katsel, E. Schadt, D. Cai, K. J. Brennand, V. Haroutunian, and B. Zhang. 2021. Molecular subtyping of Alzheimer's disease using RNA sequencing data reveals novel mechanisms and targets. *Science Advances* 7(2):eabb5398.

Neumann, P. J., L. P. Garrison, and R. J. Willke. 2022. The history and future of the "ISPOR value flower": Addressing limitations of conventional cost-effectiveness analysis. *Value Health* 25(4):558-565.

Ngandu, T., J. Lehtisalo, A. Solomon, E. Levälahti, S. Ahtiluoto, R. Antikainen, L. Bäckman, T. Hänninen, A. Jula, T. Laatikainen, J. Lindström, F. Mangialasche, T. Paajanen, S. Pajala, M. Peltonen, R. Rauramaa, A. Stigsdotter-Neely, T. Strandberg, J. Tuomilehto, H. Soininen, and M. Kivipelto. 2015. A 2 year multidomain intervention of diet, exercise, cognitive training, and vascular risk monitoring versus control to prevent cognitive decline in at-risk elderly people (FINGER): A randomised controlled trial. *Lancet* 385(9984):2255-2263.

Nguyen, L., K. Murphy, and G. Andrews. 2022. A game a day keeps cognitive decline away? A systematic review and meta-analysis of commercially-available brain training programs in healthy and cognitively impaired older adults. *Neuropsychology Review* 32(3):601-630.

NIA (National Institute of Aging). n.d. *Recruitment: Logistical barriers (milestone 12.C).* https://www.nia.nih.gov/research/milestones/translational-clinical-research/trial-innovation/milestone-12-c (accessed August 19, 2024).

NIA. 2022. *Gaps and opportunities for real-world data infrastructure.* https://www.nia.nih.gov/sites/default/files/2022-09/workshop_report_nia-real-world-data-workshop.pdf (accessed September 25, 2024).

NIA. 2024. *Clinically meaningful outcomes in AD/ADRD trials.* https://www.nia.nih.gov/research/dbsr/workshops/clinically-meaningful-outcomes-ad-adrd-trials#summary (accessed August 22, 2024).

NIH (National Institutes of Health). 2021. *Notice of special interest (NOSI): Improving patient adherence to treatment and prevention regimens to promote health.* https://grants.nih.gov/grants/guide/notice-files/NOT-OD-21-100.html (accessed August 20, 2024).

NIH. 2023. *Seamless early-stage clinical drug development (phase 1 to 2a) for novel therapeutic agents for the spectrum of Alzheimer's disease (AD) and AD-related dementias (ADRD) (UG3/UH3 clinical trial required).* https://grants.nih.gov/grants/guide/pa-files/PAR-23-274.html?utm_source=OLPIA+Stakeholders&utm_campaign=589f1ebb3d-EMAIL_CAMPAIGN_2023_12_11_08_31&utm_medium=email&utm_term=0_-589f1ebb3d-%5BLIST_EMAIL_ID%5D (accessed August 20, 2023).

NIH. 2024. *Safety and efficacy of amyloid-beta directed antibody therapy in mild cognitive impairment and dementia with evidence of Lewy body dementia and amyloid-beta pathology (U01—Clinical trial required).* https://grants.nih.gov/grants/guide/rfa-files/RFA-NS-25-010.html (accesed October 28, 2024).

NIH Collaboratory. n.d. *The embedded pragmatic clinical trial ecosystem.* https://rethinkingclinicaltrials.org/chapters/design/what-is-a-pragmatic-clinical-trial/the-embedded-pct-ecosystem/ (accessed August 20, 2024).

NIHR (National Institute for Health and Care Research). 2019. *PPI (patient and public involvement) resources for applicants to NIHR research programmes*. https://www.nihr.ac.uk/ppi-patient-and-public-involvement-resources-applicants-nihr-research-programmes (accessed October 22, 2024).

Nixon, R. A. 2020. The aging lysosome: An essential catalyst for late-onset neurodegenerative diseases. *Biochimica Biophysica Acta Proteins and Proteomics* 1868(9):140443.

Nixon, R. A., and D. C. Rubinsztein. 2024. Mechanisms of autophagy–lysosome dysfunction in neurodegenerative diseases. *Nature Reviews Molecular Cell Biology* 25:926-946..

Nørgaard, C. H., S. Friedrich, C. T. Hansen, T. Gerds, C. Ballard, D. V. Møller, L. B. Knudsen, K. Kvist, B. Zinman, E. Holm, C. Torp-Pedersen, and L. S. Mørch. 2022. Treatment with glucagon-like peptide-1 receptor agonists and incidence of dementia: Data from pooled double-blind randomized controlled trials and nationwide disease and prescription registers. *Alzheimer's & Dementia: Translational Research & Clinical Interventions* 8(1):e12268.

Oatman, S. R., J. S. Reddy, Z. Quicksall, M. M. Carrasquillo, X. Wang, C. C. Liu, Y. Yamazaki, T. T. Nguyen, K. Malphrus, M. Heckman, K. Biswas, K. Nho, M. Baker, Y. A. Martens, N. Zhao, J. P. Kim, S. L. Risacher, R. Rademakers, A. J. Saykin, M. DeTure, M. E. Murray, T. Kanekiyo, Alzheimer's Disease Neuroimaging Initiative, D. W. Dickson, G. Bu, M. Allen, and N. Ertekin-Taner. 2023. Genome-wide association study of brain biochemical phenotypes reveals distinct genetic architecture of Alzheimer's disease related proteins. *Molecular Neurodegeneration* 18(1):2.

Öhman, F., J. Hassenstab, D. Berron, M. Scholl, and K. V. Papp. 2021. Current advances in digital cognitive assessment for preclinical Alzheimer's disease. *Alzheimer's & Dementia (Amsterdam, Netherlands)* 13(1):e12217.

Olmastroni, E., G. Molari, N. De Beni, O. Colpani, F. Galimberti, M. Gazzotti, A. Zambon, A. L. Catapano, and M. Casula. 2022. Statin use and risk of dementia or Alzheimer's disease: A systematic review and meta-analysis of observational studies. *European Journal of Preventive Cardiology* 29(5):804-814.

Papaioannou, T., A. Voinescu, K. Petrini, and D. Stanton Fraser. 2022. Efficacy and moderators of virtual reality for cognitive training in people with dementia and mild cognitive impairment: A systematic review and meta-analysis. *Journal of Alzheimer's Disease* 88(4):1341-1370.

Park, D. C., and G. N. Bischof. 2013. The aging mind: Neuroplasticity in response to cognitive training. *Dialogues in Clinical Neuroscience* 15(1):109-119.

Park, J. J. H., O. Harari, L. Dron, R. T. Lester, K. Thorlund, and E. J. Mills. 2020. An overview of platform trials with a checklist for clinical readers. *Journal of Clinical Epidemiology* 125:1-8.

Patel, T., T. P. Carnwath, X. Wang, M. Allen, S. J. Lincoln, L. J. Lewis-Tuffin, Z. S. Quicksall, S. Lin, F. Q. Tutor-New, C. C. G. Ho, Y. Min, K. G. Malphrus, T. T. Nguyen, E. Martin, C. A. Garcia, R. M. Alkharboosh, S. Grewal, K. Chaichana, R. Wharen, H. Guerrero-Cazares, A. Quinones-Hinojosa, and N. Ertekin-Taner. 2022. Transcriptional landscape of human microglia implicates age, sex, and *APOE*-related immunometabolic pathway perturbations. *Aging Cell* 21(5):e13606.

Patrick, E., M. Taga, A. Ergun, B. Ng, W. Casazza, M. Cimpean, C. Yung, J. A. Schneider, D. A. Bennett, C. Gaiteri, P. L. De Jager, E. M. Bradshaw, and S. Mostafavi. 2020. Deconvolving the contributions of cell-type heterogeneity on cortical gene expression. *PLoS Computer Biology* 16(8):e1008120.

Paul, K. C., M. Haan, E. R. Mayeda, and B. R. Ritz. 2019. Ambient air pollution, noise, and late-life cognitive decline and dementia risk. *Annual Review of Public Health* 40:203-220.

Paulsen, R. 2024. *UsAgainstAlzheimer's*. Presentation at the Committee on Research Priorities for Preventing and Treating Alzheimer's Disease and Related Dementias Public Workshop, Hybrid. January 16–17, 2024.

Pellegrini, M., F. Bernabei, C. Schiavi, and G. Giannaccare. 2020. Impact of cataract surgery on depression and cognitive function: Systematic review and meta-analysis. *Clinical Experiments in Ophthalmology* 48(5):593-601.

Petek, B., H. Häbel, H. Xu, M. Villa-Lopez, I. Kalar, M. T. Hoang, S. Maioli, J. B. Pereira, S. Mostafaei, B. Winblad, M. Gregoric Kramberger, M. Eriksdotter, and S. Garcia-Ptacek. 2023. Statins and cognitive decline in patients with Alzheimer's and mixed dementia: A longitudinal registry-based cohort study. *Alzheimer's Research & Therapy* 15(1):220.

Peters, R., N. Beckett, F. Forette, J. Tuomilehto, R. Clarke, C. Ritchie, A. Waldman, I. Walton, R. Poulter, S. Ma, M. Comsa, L. Burch, A. Fletcher, and C. Bulpitt. 2008. Incident dementia and blood pressure lowering in the Hypertension in the Very Elderly Trial Cognitive Function Assessment (HYVET-COG): A double-blind, placebo controlled trial. *Lancet Neurology* 7(8):683-689.

Peters, R., J. Warwick, K. J. Anstey, and C. S. Anderson. 2019. Blood pressure and dementia. *Neurology* 92(21):1017-1018.

Petersen, J. 2023. A meta-analytic review of the effects of intergenerational programs for youth and older adults. *Educational Gerontology* 49(3):175-189.

Piendel, L., M. Vališ, and J. Hort. 2023. An update on mobile applications collecting data among subjects with or at risk of Alzheimer's disease. *Frontiers in Aging Neuroscience* 15:1134096.

Potter, H., J. H. Woodcock, T. D. Boyd, C. M. Coughlan, J. R. O'Shaughnessy, M. T. Borges, A. A. Thaker, B. A. Raj, K. Adamszuk, D. Scott, V. Adame, P. Anton, H. J. Chial, H. Gray, J. Daniels, M. E. Stocker, and S. H. Sillau. 2021a. Safety and efficacy of sargramostim (GM-CSF) in the treatment of Alzheimer's disease. *Alzheimer's & Dementia (N Y)* 7(1):e12158.

Potter, D. A., C. A. Herrera-Ponzanelli, D. Hinojosa, R. Castillo, I. Hernandez-Cruz, V. A. Arrieta, M. J. Franklin, and D. Yee. 2021b. Recent advances in neoadjuvant therapy for breast cancer. *Faculty Reviews* 10:2.

Prins, N. D., W. de Haan, A. Gardner, K. Blackburn, H. M. Chu, J. E. Galvin, and J. J. Alam. 2024. Phase 2a learnings incorporated into RewinD-LB, a phase 2b clinical trial of neflamapimod in dementia with Lewy bodies. *Journal of Prevention of Alzheimer's Disease* 11(3):549-557.

Pugh, M. A. M. 2023. TRAILBLAZER-ALZ 3—a deeper dive into time-to-event trials. *Alzheimer's & Dementia* 19(S21):e070865.

QLHC (Quantum Leap Healthcare Collaborative). 2024. *What is I-SPY and I-SPY Trials?*. https://www.quantumleaphealth.org/for-investigators/i-spy-trials/ (accessed August 20, 2024).

Rafii, M. S., R. A. Sperling, M. C. Donohue, J. Zhou, C. Roberts, M. C. Irizarry, S. Dhadda, G. Sethuraman, L. D. Kramer, C. J. Swanson, D. Li, S. Krause, R. A. Rissman, S. Walter, R. Raman, K. A. Johnson, and P. S. Aisen. 2023. The AHEAD 3-45 Study: Design of a prevention trial for Alzheimer's disease. *Alzheimer's & Dementia* 19(4):1227-1233.

Raman, R., Y. T. Quiroz, O. Langford, J. Choi, M. Ritchie, M. Baumgartner, D. Rentz, N. T. Aggarwal, P. Aisen, R. Sperling, and J. D. Grill. 2021. Disparities by race and ethnicity among adults recruited for a preclinical Alzheimer's disease trial. *JAMA Network Open* 4(7):e2114364.

Raman, R., P. S. Aisen, M. C. Carillo, M. Detke, J. D. Grill, O. C. Okonkwo, M. Rivera-Mindt, M. Sabbagh, B. Vellas, M. Weiner, and R. Sperling. 2022. Tackling a major deficiency of diversity in Alzheimer's disease therapeutic trials: A CTAD Task Force report. *Journal of Prevention of Alzheimer's Disease* 9(3):388-392.

Ramos, I. N., K. N. Ramos, and K. S. Ramos. 2019a. Driving the precision medicine highway: Community health workers and patient navigators. *Journal of Translational Medicine* 17(1):85.

Ramos, K. S., E. C. Bowers, M. A. Tavera-Garcia, and I. N. Ramos. 2019b. Precision prevention: A focused response to shifting paradigms in healthcare. *Experiments in Biological Medicine (Maywood)* 244(3):207-212.

Rawji, K. S., M. K. Mishra, N. J. Michaels, S. Rivest, P. K. Stys, and V. W. Yong. 2016. Immunosenescence of microglia and macrophages: Impact on the ageing central nervous system. *Brain* 139(Pt 3):653-661.

Ray, J., G. Popli, and G. Fell. 2018. Association of cognition and age-related hearing impairment in the English Longitudinal Study of Ageing. *JAMA Otolaryngology and Head and Neck Surgery* 144(10):876-882.

Reardon, S. 2023. Alzheimer's drug trials plagued by lack of racial diversity. *Nature* 620(7973):256-257.

Rebok, G. W., K. Ball, L. T. Guey, R. N. Jones, H.-Y. Kim, J. W. King, M. Marsiske, J. N. Morris, S. L. Tennstedt, F. W. Unverzagt, and S. L. Willis. 2014. Ten-year effects of the advanced cognitive training for independent and vital elderly cognitive training trial on cognition and everyday functioning in older adults. *Journal of the American Geriatrics Society* 62(1):16-24.

Rebok, G. W., A. Gellert, N. B. Coe, O. J. Clay, G. Wallace, J. M. Parisi, A. T. Aiken-Morgan, M. Crowe, K. Ball, R. J. Thorpe, M. Marsiske, L. B. Zahodne, C. Felix, and S. L. Willis. 2023. Effects of cognitive training on Alzheimer's disease and related dementias: The moderating role of social determinants of health. *Journal of Aging and Health* 35(9 Suppl):40S-50S.

Reddy, J. S., M. Allen, C. C. G. Ho, S. R. Oatman, O. Is, Z. S. Quicksall, X. Wang, J. Jin, T. A. Patel, T. P. Carnwath, T. T. Nguyen, K. G. Malphrus, S. J. Lincoln, M. M. Carrasquillo, J. E. Crook, T. Kanekiyo, M. E. Murray, G. Bu, D. W. Dickson, and N. Ertekin-Taner. 2021. Genome-wide analysis identifies a novel *LINC-PINT* splice variant associated with vascular amyloid pathology in Alzheimer's disease. *Acta Neuropathologica Communications* 9(1):93.

Reddy, J. S., J. Jin, S. J. Lincoln, C. C. G. Ho, J. E. Crook, X. Wang, K. G. Malphrus, T. Nguyen, N. Tamvaka, M. T. Greig-Custo, J. A. Lucas, N. R. Graff-Radford, N. Ertekin-Taner, and M. M. Carrasquillo. 2022. Transcript levels in plasma contribute substantial predictive value as potential Alzheimer's disease biomarkers in African Americans. *EBioMedicine*, 78:103929.

Reddy, J. S., L. Heath, A. V. Linden, M. Allen, K. P. Lopes, F. Seifar, E. Wang, Y. Ma, W. L. Poehlman, Z. S. Quicksall, A. Runnels, Y. Wang, D. M. Duong, L. Yin, K. Xu, E. S. Modeste, A. Shantaraman, E. B. Dammer, L. Ping, S. R. Oatman, J. Scanlan, C. Ho, M. M. Carrasquillo, M. Atik, G. Yepez, A. O. Mitchell, T. T. Nguyen, X. Chen, D. X. Marquez, H. Reddy, H. Xiao, S. Seshadri, R. Mayeux, S. Prokop, E. B. Lee, G. E. Serrano, T. G. Beach, A. F. Teich, V. Haroutunian, E. J. Fox, M. Gearing, A. Wingo, T. Wingo, J. J. Lah, A. I. Levey, D. W. Dickson, L. L. Barnes, P. De Jager, B. Zhang, D. Bennett, N. T. Seyfried, A. K. Greenwood, and N. Ertekin-Taner. 2024. Bridging the gap: Multi-omics profiling of brain tissue in Alzheimer's disease and older controls in multi-ethnic populations. *Alzheimer's Dementia* 20(10):7174-7192.

Reitz, C. 2016. Toward precision medicine in Alzheimer's disease. *Annals of Translational Medicine* 4(6):107.

Reitz, C., G. Jun, A. Naj, R. Rajbhandary, B. N. Vardarajan, L. S. Wang, O. Valladares, C. F. Lin, E. B. Larson, N. R. Graff-Radford, D. Evans, P. L. De Jager, P. K. Crane, J. D. Buxbaum, J. R. Murrell, T. Raj, N. Ertekin-Taner, M. Logue, C. T. Baldwin, R. C. Green, L. L. Barnes, L. B. Cantwell, M. D. Fallin, R. C. Go, P. Griffith, T. O. Obisesan, J. J. Manly, K. L.

Lunetta, M. I. Kamboh, O. L. Lopez, D. A. Bennett, H. Hendrie, K. S. Hall, A. M. Goate, G. S. Byrd, W. A. Kukull, T. M. Foroud, J. L. Haines, L. A. Farrer, M. A. Pericak-Vance, G. D. Schellenberg, R. Mayeux, and Alzheimer Disease Genetics Consortium. 2013. Variants in the ATP-binding cassette transporter (*ABCA7*), apolipoprotein E ε4, and the risk of late-onset Alzheimer disease in African Americans. *JAMA* 309(14):1483-1492.

Religa, D., S.-M. Fereshtehnejad, P. Cermakova, A.-K. Edlund, S. Garcia-Ptacek, N. Granqvist, A. Hallbäck, K. Kåwe, B. Farahmand, L. Kilander, U.-B. Mattsson, K. Nägga, P. Nordström, H. Wijk, A. Wimo, B. Winblad, and M. Eriksdotter. 2015. SveDem, the Swedish Dementia Registry—a tool for improving the quality of diagnostics, treatment and care of dementia patients in clinical practice. *PLoS ONE* 10(2):e0116538.

Rezai, A. R., P. F. D'Haese, V. Finomore, J. Carpenter, M. Ranjan, K. Wilhelmsen, R. I. Mehta, P. Wang, U. Najib, C. Vieira Ligo Teixeira, T. Arsiwala, A. Tarabishy, P. Tirumalai, D. O. Claassen, S. Hodder, and M. W. Haut. 2024. Ultrasound blood–brain barrier opening and aducanumab in Alzheimer's disease. *New England Journal of Medicine* 390(1):55-62.

Riessland, M., and M. E. Orr. 2023. Translating the biology of aging into new therapeutics for Alzheimer's disease: Senolytics. *Journal of Prevention of Alzheimer's Disease* 10(4):633-646.

Ritchie, C. W., G. M. Terrera, and T. J. Quinn. 2015. Dementia trials and dementia tribulations: Methodological and analytical challenges in dementia research. *Alzheimer's Research & Therapy* 7(1):31.

Rizzolo, P., V. Silvestri, M. Falchetti, and L. Ottini. 2011. Inherited and acquired alterations in development of breast cancer. *Applied Clinical Genetics* 4:145-158.

Rocchi, A., S. Yamamoto, T. Ting, Y. Fan, K. Sadleir, Y. Wang, W. Zhang, S. Huang, B. Levine, R. Vassar, and C. He. 2017. A *Becn1* mutation mediates hyperactive autophagic sequestration of amyloid oligomers and improved cognition in Alzheimer's disease. *PLoS Genetics* 13(8):e1006962.

Rommer, P. S., G. Bsteh, T. Zrzavy, R. Hoeftberger, and T. Berger. 2022. Immunosenescence in neurological diseases—Is there enough evidence? *Biomedicines* 10(11):2864.

Rosenberg, A., F. Mangialasche, T. Ngandu, A. Solomon, and M. Kivipelto. 2020. Multidomain interventions to prevent cognitive impairment, Alzheimer's disease, and dementia: From FINGER to world-wide FINGERS. *Journal of Prevention of Alzheimer's Disease* 7(1):29-36.

Ruangritchankul, S., P. Chantharit, S. Srisuma, and L. C. Gray. 2021. Adverse drug reactions of acetylcholinesterase inhibitors in older people living with dementia: A comprehensive literature review. *Therapeutics and Clinical Risk Management* 17:927-949.

Salinas, J., A. S. Beiser, J. K. Samra, A. O'Donnell, C. S. DeCarli, M. M. Gonzales, H. J. Aparicio, and S. Seshadri. 2022. Association of loneliness with 10-year dementia risk and early markers of vulnerability for neurocognitive decline. *Neurology* 98(13):e1337-e1348.

Salloway, S. P., J. Sevingy, K. Budur, J. T. Pederson, R. B. DeMattos, P. Von Rosenstiel, A. Paez, R. Evans, C. J. Weber, J. A. Hendrix, S. Worley, L. J. Bain, and M. C. Carrillo. 2020. Advancing combination therapy for Alzheimer's disease. *Alzheimer's & Dementia: Translational Research & Clinical Interventions* 6(1):e12073.

Salzman, T., Y. Sarquis-Adamson, S. Son, M. Montero-Odasso, and S. Fraser. 2022. Associations of multidomain interventions with improvements in cognition in mild cognitive impairment: A systematic review and meta-analysis. *JAMA Network Open* 5(5):e226744.

Sanders, M. E., E. Kant, A. L. Smit, and I. Stegeman. 2021. The effect of hearing aids on cognitive function: A systematic review. *PLoS ONE* 16(12):e0261207.

Sarkar, S., N. Das, and K. Sambamurti. 2024. Development of early biomarkers of Alzheimer's disease: A precision medicine perspective. In *Comprehensive precision medicine*, 1st ed., Vol. 2, edited by K. S. Ramos. Elsevier, pp. 511-525.

Saunders, S., G. Muniz-Terrera, S. Sheehan, C. W. Ritchie, and S. Luz. 2021. A UK-wide study employing natural language processing to determine what matters to people about brain health to improve drug development: The Electronic Person-Specific Outcome Measure (ePSOM) programme. *Journal of Prevention of Alzheimer's Disease* 8(4):448-456.

Say, R. E., and R. Thomson. 2003. The importance of patient preferences in treatment decisions—challenges for doctors. *BMJ* 327(7414):542-545.

Seckl, J. 2024. 11β-hydroxysteroid dehydrogenase and the brain: Not (yet) lost in translation. *Journal of Internal Medicine* 295(1):20-37.

Seifar, F., E. J. Fox, A. Shantaraman, Y. Liu, E. B. Dammer, E. Modeste, D. M. Duong, L. Yin, A. N. Trautwig, Q. Guo, K. Xu, L. Ping, J. S. Reddy, M. Allen, Z. Quicksall, L. Heath, J. Scanlan, E. Wang, M. Wang, A. V. Linden, W. Poehlman, X. Chen, S. Baheti, C. Ho, T. Nguyen, G. Yepez, A. O. Mitchell, S. R. Oatman, X. Wang, M. M. Carrasquillo, A. Runnels, T. Beach, G. E. Serrano, D. W. Dickson, E. B. Lee, T. E. Golde, S. Prokop, L. L. Barnes, B. Zhang, V. Haroutunian, M. Gearing, J. J. Lah, P. Jager, D. A. Bennett, A. Greenwood, N. Ertekin-Taner, A. I. Levey, A. Wingo, T. Wingo, and N. T. Seyfried. 2024. Large-scale deep proteomic analysis in Alzheimer's disease brain regions across race and ethnicity. Update in *Alzheimer's & Dementia* 20(12):8878-8897

Sevigny, J., O. Uspenskaya, L. D. Heckman, L. C. Wong, D. A. Hatch, A. Tewari, R. Vandenberghe, D. J. Irwin, D. Saracino, I. Le Ber, R. Ahmed, J. D. Rohrer, A. L. Boxer, S. Boland, P. Sheehan, A. Brandes, S. R. Burstein, B. M. Shykind, S. Kamalakaran, C. W. Daniels, E. D. Litwack, E. Mahoney, J. Velaga, I. McNamara, P. Sondergaard, S. A. Sajjad, Y. M. Kobayashi, A. Abeliovich, and F. Hefti. 2024. Progranulin AAV gene therapy for frontotemporal dementia: Translational studies and phase 1/2 trial interim results. *Nature Medicine* 30(5):1406-1415.

Shakhnovich, V. 2018. It's time to reverse our thinking: The reverse translation research paradigm. *Clinical and Translational Science* 11(2):98-99.

Shanks, H. R. C., K. Chen, E. M. Reiman, K. Blennow, J. L. Cummings, S. M. Massa, F. M. Longo, A. Börjesson-Hanson, M. Windisch, and T. W. Schmitz. 2024. p75 Neurotrophin receptor modulation in mild to moderate Alzheimer disease: A randomized, placebo-controlled phase 2a trial. *Nature Medicine* 30(6):1761-1770.

Sierra, C. 2020. Hypertension and the risk of dementia. *Frontiers in Cardiovascular Medicine* 7:5.

Silva, P. J., V. M. Schaibley, and K. S. Ramos. 2018. Academic medical centers as innovation ecosystems to address population -omics challenges in precision medicine. *Journal of Translational Medicine* 16(1):28.

Silva, A. C., D. D. Lobo, I. M. Martins, S. M. Lopes, C. Henriques, S. P. Duarte, J.-C. Dodart, R. J. Nobre, and L. Pereira de Almeida. 2020. Antisense oligonucleotide therapeutics in neurodegenerative diseases: The case of polyglutamine disorders. *Brain* 143(2):407-429.

Simmons, M., S. Hetrick, and A. Jorm. 2010. Shared decision-making: Benefits, barriers and current opportunities for application. *Australasian Psychiatry* 18(5):394-397.

Sliwinski, M. J., J. A. Mogle, J. Hyun, E. Munoz, J. M. Smyth, and R. B. Lipton. 2018. Reliability and validity of ambulatory cognitive assessments. *Assessment* 25(1):14-30.

Smith, M. 2024. *Cure Alzheimer's Fund.* Presentation at the Committee on Research Priorities for Preventing and Treating Alzheimer's Disease and Related Dementias Public Workshop, Hybrid. January 16-17, 2024.

Smith, D., J. Lovell, C. Weller, B. Kennedy, M. Winbolt, C. Young, and J. Ibrahim. 2017. A systematic review of medication non-adherence in persons with dementia or cognitive impairment. *PLoS ONE* 12(2):e0170651.

Solomon, A., H. Turunen, T. Ngandu, M. Peltonen, E. Levälahti, S. Helisalmi, R. Antikainen, L. Bäckman, T. Hänninen, A. Jula, T. Laatikainen, J. Lehtisalo, J. Lindström, T. Paajanen, S. Pajala, A. Stigsdotter-Neely, T. Strandberg, J. Tuomilehto, H. Soininen, and M. Kivipelto.

2018. Effect of the apolipoprotein E genotype on cognitive change during a multidomain lifestyle intervention: A subgroup analysis of a randomized clinical trial. *JAMA Neurology* 75(4):462-470.

Solopova, E., W. Romero-Fernandez, H. Harmsen, L. Ventura-Antunes, E. Wang, A. Shostak, J. Maldonado, M. J. Donahue, D. Schultz, T. M. Coyne, A. Charidimou, and M. Schrag. 2023. Fatal iatrogenic cerebral β-amyloid-related arteritis in a woman treated with lecanemab for Alzheimer's disease. *Nature Communications* 14(1):8220.

Song, S., Y. Stern, and Y. Gu. 2022. Modifiable lifestyle factors and cognitive reserve: A systematic review of current evidence. *Ageing Research Reviews* 74:101551.

Sperling, R. A., C. R. Jack, Jr., S. E. Black, M. P. Frosch, S. M. Greenberg, B. T. Hyman, P. Scheltens, M. C. Carrillo, W. Thies, M. M. Bednar, R. S. Black, H. R. Brashear, M. Grundman, E. R. Siemers, H. H. Feldman, and R. J. Schindler. 2011. Amyloid-related imaging abnormalities in amyloid-modifying therapeutic trials: Recommendations from the Alzheimer's Association Research Roundtable Workgroup. *Alzheimer's & Dementia* 7(4):367-385.

Sperling, R., S. Salloway, D. J. Brooks, D. Tampieri, J. Barakos, N. C. Fox, M. Raskind, M. Sabbagh, L. S. Honig, A. P. Porsteinsson, I. Lieburg, H. M. Arrighi, K. A. Morris, Y. Lu, E. Liu, K. M. Gregg, H. R. Brashear, G. G. Kinney, R. Black, M. Grundman. 2012. Amyloid-related imaging abnormalities in patients with Alzheimer's disease treated with bapineuzumab: A retrospective analysis. *Lancet Neurology* 11(3):241-249.

Sperling, R. A., D. M. Rentz, K. A. Johnson, J. Karlawish, M. Donohue, D. P. Salmon, and P. Aisen. 2014. The A4 study: Stopping AD before symptoms begin? *Science Translational Medicine* 6(228):228fs213.

Spierer, O., N. Fischer, A. Barak, and M. Belkin. 2016. Correlation between vision and cognitive function in the elderly: A cross-sectional study. *Medicine (Baltimore)* 95(3):e2423.

SPRINT MIND Investigators. 2019. Effect of intensive vs standard blood pressure control on probable dementia: A randomized clinical trial. *JAMA* 321(6):553-561.

Stallard, N., J. Whitehead, S. Todd, and A. Whitehead. 2001. Stopping rules for phase II studies. *British Journal of Clinical Pharmacology* 51(6):523-529.

Stites, S. D., A. Gurian, C. Coykendall, E. A. Largent, K. Harkins, J. Karlawish, and N. B. Coe. 2023. Gender of study partners and research participants associated with differences in study partner ratings of cognition and activity level. *Journals of Gerontology Series B: Psychological Sciences and Social Sciences* 78(8):1318-1329.

Strayhorn, J. C., C. M. Cleland, D. J. Vanness, L. Wilton, M. Gwadz, and L. M. Collins. 2024. Using decision analysis for intervention value efficiency to select optimized interventions in the multiphase optimization strategy. *Health and Psychology* 43(2):89-100.

Strickland, S. L., H. Morel, C. Prusinski, M. Allen, T. A. Patel, M. M. Carrasquillo, O. J. Conway, S. J. Lincoln, J. S. Reddy, T. Nguyen, K. G. Malphrus, A. I. Soto, R. L. Walton, J. E. Crook, M. E. Murray, B. F. Boeve, R. C. Petersen, J. A. Lucas, T. J. Ferman, R. J. Uitti, Z. K. Wszolek, O. A. Ross, N. R. Graff-Radford, D. W. Dickson, and N. Ertekin-Taner. 2020. Association of *ABI3* and *PLCG2* missense variants with disease risk and neuropathology in Lewy body disease and progressive supranuclear palsy. *Acta Neuropathologica Communications* 8(1):172.

Sun, J., and S. Roy. 2021. Gene-based therapies for neurodegenerative diseases. *Nature Neuroscience* 24(3):297-311.

Sun, L., A. Wu, G. R. Bean, I. S. Hagemann, and C.-Y. Lin. 2021. Molecular testing in breast cancer: Current status and future directions. *Journal of Molecular Diagnostics* 23(11):1422-1432.

Sun, Y.-Y., Z. Wang, H.-Y. Zhou, and H.-C. Huang. 2022. Sleep–wake disorders in Alzheimer's disease: A review. *ACS Chemical Neuroscience* 13(10):1467-1478.

Sutin, A. R., Y. Stephan, M. Luchetti, and A. Terracciano. 2020. Loneliness and risk of dementia. *Journals of Gerontology: Series B: Psychological Sciences and Social Sciences* 75(7):1414-1422.

Taylor, J. C., H. W. Heuer, A. L. Clark, A. B. Wise, M. Manoochehri, L. Forsberg, C. Mester, M. Rao, D. Brushaber, J. Kramer, A. E. Welch, J. Kornak, W. Kremers, B. Appleby, B. C. Dickerson, K. Domoto-Reilly, J. A. Fields, N. Ghoshal, N. Graff-Radford, M. Grossman, M. G. Hall, E. D. Huey, D. Irwin, M. I. Lapid, I. Litvan, I. R. Mackenzie, J. C. Masdeu, M. F. Mendez, N. Nevler, C. U. Onyike, B. Pascual, P. Pressman, K. P. Rankin, B. Ratnasiri, J. C. Rojas, M. C. Tartaglia, B. Wong, M. L. Gorno-Tempini, B. F. Boeve, H. J. Rosen, A. L. Boxer, and A. M. Staffaroni. 2023. Feasibility and acceptability of remote smartphone cognitive testing in frontotemporal dementia research. *Alzheimer's & Dementia (Amsterdam, Netherlands)* 15(2):e12423.

Taylor-Rowan, M., S. Edwards, A. H. Noel-Storr, J. McCleery, P. K. Myint, R. Soiza, C. Stewart, Y. K. Loke, and T. J. Quinn. 2021. Anticholinergic burden (prognostic factor) for prediction of dementia or cognitive decline in older adults with no known cognitive syndrome. *Cochrane Database of Systematic Reviews* 5(5):CD013540.

Tedeschi, D. V., A. F. da Cunha, M. R. Cominetti, and R. V. Pedroso. 2021. Efficacy of gene therapy to restore cognition in Alzheimer's disease: A systematic review. *Current Gene Therapy* 21(3):246-257.

Tejera, D., D. Mercan, J. M. Sanchez-Caro, M. Hanan, D. Greenberg, H. Soreq, E. Latz, D. Golenbock, and M. T. Heneka. 2019. Systemic inflammation impairs microglial Aβ clearance through NLRP3 inflammasome. *EMBO Journal* 38(17):e101064.

Temple, S. 2023. Advancing cell therapy for neurodegenerative diseases. *Cell Stem Cell* 30(5):512-529.

Tennstedt, S. L., and F. W. Unverzagt. 2013. The ACTIVE study: Study overview and major findings. *Journal of Aging Health* 25(8 Suppl):3s-20s.

Thunborg, C., A. Rosenberg, M. Barbera, N. Coley, M. Ekblom, Ö. Ekblom, N. Levak, A. Solomon, and M. Kivipelto. 2021. Physical activity and sedentary time in a multimodal lifestyle intervention in prodromal Alzheimer's disease: The MIND-ADMINI pilot trial. *Alzheimer's & Dementia* 17(S10):e054890.

Thunell, J., Y. Chen, G. Joyce, D. Barthold, P. G. Shekelle, R. D. Brinton, and J. Zissimopoulos. 2021. Drug therapies for chronic conditions and risk of Alzheimer's disease and related dementias: A scoping review. *Alzheimer's & Dementia* 17(1):41-48.

Tijms, B. M., E. M. Vromen, O. Mjaavatten, H. Holstege, L. M. Reus, S. van der Lee, K. E. J. Wesenhagen, L. Lorenzini, L. Vermunt, V. Venkatraghavan, N. Tesi, J. Tomassen, A. den Braber, J. Goossens, E. Vanmechelen, F. Barkhof, Y. A. L. Pijnenburg, W. M. van der Flier, C. E. Teunissen, F. S. Berven, and P. J. Visser. 2024. Cerebrospinal fluid proteomics in patients with Alzheimer's disease reveals five molecular subtypes with distinct genetic risk profiles. *Nature Aging* 4(1):33-47.

Tochel, C., M. Smith, H. Baldwin, A. Gustavsson, A. Ly, C. Bexelius, M. Nelson, C. Bintener, E. Fantoni, J. Garre-Olmo, O. Janssen, C. Jindra, I. F. Jorgensen, A. McKeown, B. Ozturk, A. Ponjoan, M. H. Potashman, C. Reed, E. Roncancio-Diaz, S. Vos, and C. Sudlow. 2019. What outcomes are important to patients with mild cognitive impairment or Alzheimer's disease, their caregivers, and health-care professionals? A systematic review. *Alzheimer's and Dementia: Diagnosis, Assessment and Disease Monitoring* 11:231-247.

Toledo, J. B., M. Arnold, G. Kastenmuller, R. Chang, R. A. Baillie, X. Han, M. Thambisetty, J. D. Tenenbaum, K. Suhre, J. W. Thompson, L. S. John-Williams, S. MahmoudianDehkordi, D. M. Rotroff, J. R. Jack, A. Motsinger-Reif, S. L. Risacher, C. Blach, J. E. Lucas, T. Massaro, G. Louie, H. Zhu, G. Dallmann, K. Klavins, T. Koal, S. Kim, K. Nho, L. Shen, R. Casanova, S. Varma, C. Legido-Quigley, M. A. Moseley, K. Zhu, M. Y. R.

Henrion, S. J. van der Lee, A. C. Harms, A. Demirkan, T. Hankemeier, C. M. van Duijn, J. Q. Trojanowski, L. M. Shaw, A. J. Saykin, M. W. Weiner, P. M. Doraiswamy, R. Kaddurah-Daouk, Alzheimer's Disease Neuroimaging Initiative, and the Alzheimer Disease Metabolomics Collaborative. 2017. Metabolic network failures in Alzheimer's disease: A biochemical road map. *Alzheimer's & Dementia* 13(9):965-984.

Toledo, J. B., C. Abdelnour, R. S. Weil, D. Ferreira, F. Rodriguez-Porcel, A. Pilotto, K. A. Wyman-Chick, M. J. Grothe, J. P. M. Kane, A. Taylor, A. Rongve, S. Scholz, J. B. Leverenz, B. F. Boeve, D. Aarsland, I. G. McKeith, S. Lewis, I. Leroi, J. P. Taylor; and ISTAART Lewy body dementias Trial Methods Working Group. 2023. Dementia with Lewy bodies: Impact of co-pathologies and implications for clinical trial design. *Alzheimer's & Dementia* 19(1):318-332.

Trudler, D., S. Sanz-Blasco, Y. S. Eisele, S. Ghatak, K. Bodhinathan, M. W. Akhtar, W. P. Lynch, J. C. Piña-Crespo, M. Talantova, J. W. Kelly, and S. A. Lipton. 2021. α–Synuclein oligomers induce glutamate release from astrocytes and excessive extrasynaptic NMDAR activity in neurons, thus contributing to synapse loss. *Journal of Neuroscience* 41(10):2264-2273.

Tulliani, N., M. Bissett, P. Fahey, R. Bye, and K. P. Y. Liu. 2022. Efficacy of cognitive remediation on activities of daily living in individuals with mild cognitive impairment or early-stage dementia: A systematic review and meta-analysis. *Systematic Reviews* 11(1):156.

Tullo, D., Y. Feng, A. Pahor, J. M. Cote, A. R. Seitz, and S. M. Jaeggi. 2023. Investigating the role of individual differences in adherence to cognitive training. *Journal of Cognition* 6(1):48.

Turner, R. S., R. G. Thomas, S. Craft, C. H. van Dyck, J. Mintzer, B. A. Reynolds, J. B. Brewer, R. A. Rissman, R. Raman, P. S. Aisen, Society for the Alzheimer's Disease Cooperative, J. Mintzer, B. A. Reynolds, J. Karlawish, D. Galasko, J. Heidebrink, N. Aggarwal, N. Graff-Radford, M. Sano, R. Petersen, K. Bell, R. Doody, A. Smith, C. Bernick, A. Porteinsson, P. Tariot, R. Mulnard, A. Lerner, L. Schneider, J. Burns, M. Raskind, S. Ferris, G. Jicha, M. Quiceno, T. Obisesan, P. Rosenberg, D. Weintraub, K. Kieburtz, B. Miller, R. Kryscio, and G. Alexopoulis. 2015. A randomized, double-blind, placebo-controlled trial of resveratrol for Alzheimer's disease. *Neurology* 85(16):1383-1391.

Turunen, M., L. Hokkanen, L. Bäckman, A. Stigsdotter-Neely, T. Hänninen, T. Paajanen, H. Soininen, M. Kivipelto, and T. Ngandu. 2019. Computer-based cognitive training for older adults: Determinants of adherence. *PLoS ONE* 14(7):e0219541.

Umar, N., D. Litaker, M.-L. Schaarschmidt, W. K. Peitsch, A. Schmieder, and D. D. Terris. 2012. Outcomes associated with matching patients' treatment preferences to physicians' recommendations: Study methodology. *BMC Health Services Research* 12(1):1.

U.S. Preventive Services Task Force. 2021. Screening for hearing loss in older adults: US Preventive Services Task Force recommendation statement. *JAMA* 325(12):1196-1201.

Valiukas, Z., R. Ephraim, K. Tangalakis, M. Davidson, V. Apostolopoulos, and J. Feehan. 2022. Immunotherapies for Alzheimer's disease—a review. *Vaccines (Basel)* 10(9):1527.

van Dyck, C. H., C. J. Swanson, P. Aisen, R. J. Bateman, C. Chen, M. Gee, M. Kanekiyo, D. Li, L. Reyderman, S. Cohen, L. Froelich, S. Katayama, M. Sabbagh, B. Vellas, D. Watson, S. Dhadda, M. Irizarry, L. D. Kramer, and T. Iwatsubo. 2023. Lecanemab in early Alzheimer's disease. *New England Journal of Medicine* 388(1):9-21.

van Dyck, C. H., A. P. Mecca, R. S. O'Dell, H. H. Bartlett, N. G. Diepenbrock, Y. Huang, M. E. Hamby, M. Grundman, S. M. Catalano, A. O. Caggiano, and R. E. Carson. 2024. A pilot study to evaluate the effect of CT1812 treatment on synaptic density and other biomarkers in Alzheimer's disease. *Alzheimer's Research & Therapy* 16(1):20.

Van Eldik, L. J., M. C. Carrillo, P. E. Cole, D. Feuerbach, B. D. Greenberg, J. A. Hendrix, M. Kennedy, N. Kozauer, R. A. Margolin, J. L. Molinuevo, R. Mueller, R. M. Ransohoff, D. M. Wilcock, L. Bain, and K. Bales. 2016. The roles of inflammation and immune mechanisms in Alzheimer's disease. *Alzheimer's & Dementia (N Y)* 2(2):99-109.

Vemuri, P., J. Fields, J. Peter, and S. Klöppel. 2016. Cognitive interventions in Alzheimer's and Parkinson's diseases: Emerging mechanisms and role of imaging. *Current Opinion in Neurology* 29(4):405-411.

Vijiaratnam, N., and T. Foltynie. 2023. How should we be using biomarkers in trials of disease modification in Parkinson's disease? *Brain* 146(12):4845-4869.

Vrahatis, A. G., K. Skolariki, M. G. Krokidis, K. Lazaros, T. P. Exarchos, and P. Vlamos. 2023. Revolutionizing the early detection of Alzheimer's disease through non-invasive biomarkers: The role of artificial intelligence and deep learning. *Sensors* 23(9):4184.

Wan, Y. W., R. Al-Ouran, C. G. Mangleburg, T. M. Perumal, T. V. Lee, K. Allison, V. Swarup, C. C. Funk, C. Gaiteri, M. Allen, M. Wang, S. M. Neuner, C. C. Kaczorowski, V. M. Philip, G. R. Howell, H. Martini-Stoica, H. Zheng, H. Mei, X. Zhong, J. W. Kim, V. L. Dawson, T. M. Dawson, P. C. Pao, L. H. Tsai, J. V. Haure-Mirande, M. E. Ehrlich, P. Chakrabarty, Y. Levites, X. Wang, E. B. Dammer, G. Srivastava, S. Mukherjee, S. K. Sieberts, L. Omberg, K. D. Dang, J. A. Eddy, P. Snyder, Y. Chae, S. Amberkar, W. Wei, W. Hide, C. Preuss, A. Ergun, P. J. Ebert, D. C. Airey, S. Mostafavi, L. Yu, H. U. Klein, C. Accelerating Medicines Partnership-Alzheimer's Disease, G. W. Carter, D. A. Collier, T. E. Golde, A. I. Levey, D. A. Bennett, K. Estrada, T. M. Townsend, B. Zhang, E. Schadt, P. L. De Jager, N. D. Price, N. Ertekin-Taner, Z. Liu, J. M. Shulman, L. M. Mangravite, and B. A. Logsdon. 2020. Meta-analysis of the Alzheimer's disease human brain transcriptome and functional dissection in mouse models. *Cell Reports* 32(2):107908.

Wang, H., and D. Yee. 2019. I-SPY 2: A neoadjuvant adaptive clinical trial designed to improve outcomes in high-risk breast cancer. *Current Breast Cancer Reports* 11(4):303-310.

Wang, C., and D. M. Holtzman. 2020. Bidirectional relationship between sleep and Alzheimer's disease: Role of amyloid, tau, and other factors. *Neuropsychopharmacology* 45(1):104-120.

Wang, X., M. Allen, S. Li, Z. S. Quicksall, T. A. Patel, T. P. Carnwath, J. S. Reddy, M. M. Carrasquillo, S. J. Lincoln, T. T. Nguyen, K. G. Malphrus, D. W. Dickson, J. E. Crook, Y. W. Asmann, and N. Ertekin-Taner. 2020. Deciphering cellular transcriptional alterations in Alzheimer's disease brains. *Molecular Neurodegeneration* 15(1):38.

Wang, W.-W., R. Han, H.-J. He, Z. Wang, X.-Q. Luan, J. Li, L. Feng, S.-Y. Chen, Y. Aman, and C.-L. Xie. 2021. Delineating the role of mitophagy inducers for Alzheimer's disease patients. *Aging and Disease* 12(3):852-867.

Wang, X. C., C. L. Chu, H. C. Li, K. Lu, C. J. Liu, Y. F. Cai, S. J. Quan, and S. J. Zhang. 2022a. Efficacy and safety of hypoglycemic drugs in improving cognitive function in patients with Alzheimer's disease and mild cognitive impairment: A systematic review and network meta-analysis. *Frontiers in Neurology* 13:1018027.

Wang, X., M. Allen, O. Is, J. S. Reddy, F. Q. Tutor-New, M. Castanedes Casey, M. M. Carrasquillo, S. R. Oatman, Y. Min, Y. W. Asmann, C. Funk, T. Nguyen, C. C. Ho, K. G. Malphrus, N. T. Seyfried, A. I. Levey, S. G. Younkin, M. E. Murray, D. W. Dickson, N. D. Price, T. E. Golde, and N. Ertekin-Taner. 2022b. Alzheimer's disease and progressive supranuclear palsy share similar transcriptomic changes in distinct brain regions. *Journal of Clinical Investigation* 132(2):e149904.

Wang, C., S. Zong, X. Cui, X. Wang, S. Wu, L. Wang, Y. Liu, and Z. Lu. 2023. The effects of microglia-associated neuroinflammation on Alzheimer's disease. *Frontiers in Immunology* 14:1117172.

Weinstein, G., K. L. Davis-Plourde, S. Conner, J. J. Himali, A. S. Beiser, A. Lee, A. M. Rawlings, S. Sedaghat, J. Ding, E. Moshier, C. M. van Duijn, M. S. Beeri, E. Selvin, M. A. Ikram, L. J. Launer, M. N. Haan, and S. Seshadri. 2019. Association of metformin, sulfonylurea and insulin use with brain structure and function and risk of dementia and Alzheimer's disease: Pooled analysis from 5 cohorts. *PLoS ONE* 14(2):e0212293.

WHO (World Health Organization). 2022. *Optimizing brain health across the life course: WHO position paper.* https://www.who.int/publications/i/item/9789240054561 (accessed August 13, 2024).

Wilfling, D., S. Calo, M. N. Dichter, G. Meyer, R. Möhler, and S. Köpke. 2023. Non-pharmacological interventions for sleep disturbances in people with dementia. *Cochrane Database of Systematic Reviews* 1(1):CD011881.

Withington, C. G., and R. S. Turner. 2022. Amyloid-related imaging abnormalities with anti-amyloid antibodies for the treatment of dementia due to Alzheimer's disease. *Frontiers in Neurology* 13:862369.

Wolters, F. J., L. B. Chibnik, R. Waziry, R. Anderson, C. Berr, A. Beiser, J. C. Bis, D. Blacker, D. Bos, C. Brayne, J. F. Dartigues, S. K. L. Darweesh, K. L. Davis-Plourde, F. de Wolf, S. Debette, C. Dufouil, M. Fornage, J. Goudsmit, L. Grasset, V. Gudnason, C. Hadjichrysanthou, C. Helmer, M. A. Ikram, M. K. Ikram, E. Joas, S. Kern, L. H. Kuller, L. Launer, O. L. Lopez, F. E. Matthews, K. McRae-McKee, O. Meirelles, T. H. Mosley, Jr., M. P. Pase, B. M. Psaty, C. L. Satizabal, S. Seshadri, I. Skoog, B. C. M. Stephan, H. Wetterberg, M. M. Wong, A. Zettergren, and A. Hofman. 2020. Twenty-seven-year time trends in dementia incidence in Europe and the United States: The Alzheimer Cohorts Consortium. *Neurology* 95(5):e519-e531.

Woodcock, J., and L. M. LaVange. 2017. Master protocols to study multiple therapies, multiple diseases, or both. *New England Journal of Medicine* 377(1):62-70.

Xu, H., R. Yang, X. Qi, C. Dintica, R. Song, D. A. Bennett, and W. Xu. 2019. Association of lifespan cognitive reserve indicator with dementia risk in the presence of brain pathologies. *JAMA Neurology* 76(10):1184-1191.

Yaffe, K., E. Vittinghoff, S. Dublin, C. B. Peltz, L. E. Fleckenstein, D. E. Rosenberg, D. E. Barnes, B. H. Balderson, and E. B. Larson. 2024. Effect of personalized risk-reduction strategies on cognition and dementia risk profile among older adults: The SMARRT randomized clinical trial. *JAMA Internal Medicine* 184(1):54-62.

Yancey, A. K., A. N. Ortega, and S. K. Kumanyika. 2006. Effective recruitment and retention of minority research participants. *Annual Review of Public Health* 27:1-28.

Yang, H. S., C. C. White, H. U. Klein, K. Lu, C. Gaiteri, Y. Ma, D. Felsky, S. Mostafavi, V. A. Petyuk, R. A. Sperling, N. Ertekin-Taner, J. A. Schneider, D. A. Bennett, and P. L. De Jager. 2020. Genetics of gene expression in the aging human brain reveal TDP-43 proteinopathy pathophysiology. *Neuron* 107(3):496-508.e496.

Yang, J., H. Zhao, and S. Qu. 2024. Phytochemicals targeting mitophagy: Therapeutic opportunities and prospects for treating Alzheimer's disease. *Biomedicine & Pharmacotherapy* 177:117144.

Yip, W.-K., M. Bonetti, B. F. Cole, W. Barcella, X. V. Wang, A. Lazar, and R. D. Gelber. 2016. Subpopulation treatment effect pattern plot (STEPP) analysis for continuous, binary, and count outcomes. *Clinical Trials* 13(4):382-390.

Yoshida, Y., K. Ono, S. Sekimoto, R. Umeya, and Y. Hiratsuka. 2024. Impact of cataract surgery on cognitive impairment in older people. *Acta Ophthalmology* 102(4):e602-e611.

Yu, J. C., J. P. Hlávka, E. Joe, F. J. Richmond, and D. N. Lakdawalla. 2022. Impact of non-binding FDA guidances on primary endpoint selection in Alzheimer's disease trials. *Alzheimer's & Dementia (N Y)* 8(1):e12280.

Yu, X., T. C. Cho, A. C. Westrick, C. Chen, K. M. Langa, and L. C. Kobayashi. 2023. Association of cumulative loneliness with all-cause mortality among middle-aged and older adults in the United States, 1996 to 2019. *Proceedings of the National Academy of Science USA* 120(51):e2306819120.

Yu, Y., R. Chen, K. Mao, M. Deng, and Z. Li. 2024. The role of glial cells in synaptic dysfunction: Insights into Alzheimer's disease mechanisms. *Aging Disorders* 15(2):459-479.

Zammit, G., Y. Dauvilliers, S. Pain, D. Sebök Kinter, Y. Mansour, and D. Kunz. 2020. Daridorexant, a new dual orexin receptor antagonist, in elderly subjects with insomnia disorder. *Neurology* 94(21):e2222-e2232.

Zhang, H., J. Huntley, R. Bhome, B. Holmes, J. Cahill, R. L. Gould, H. Wang, X. Yu, and R. Howard. 2019a. Effect of computerised cognitive training on cognitive outcomes in mild cognitive impairment: A systematic review and meta-analysis. *BMJ Open* 9(8):e027062.

Zhang, P., Y. Kishimoto, I. Grammatikakis, K. Gottimukkala, R. G. Cutler, S. Zhang, K. Abdelmohsen, V. A. Bohr, J. Misra Sen, M. Gorospe, and M. P. Mattson. 2019b. Senolytic therapy alleviates Aβ-associated oligodendrocyte progenitor cell senescence and cognitive deficits in an Alzheimer's disease model. *Nature Neuroscience* 22(5):719-728.

Zhang, J. H., X. Y. Zhang, Y. Q. Sun, R. H. Lv, M. Chen, and M. Li. 2022. Metformin use is associated with a reduced risk of cognitive impairment in adults with diabetes mellitus: A systematic review and meta-analysis. *Frontiers in Neuroscience* 16:984559.

Zhang, X., Q. Li, W. Cong, S. Mu, R. Zhan, S. Zhong, M. Zhao, C. Zhao, K. Kang, and Z. Zhou. 2023. Effect of physical activity on risk of Alzheimer's disease: A systematic review and meta-analysis of twenty-nine prospective cohort studies. *Ageing Research and Reviews* 92:102127.

Zhao, Y., J. K. Zhan, and Y. Liu. 2020. A perspective on roles played by immunosenescence in the pathobiology of Alzheimer's disease. *Aging and Disease* 11(6):1594-1607.

Zheng, G., R. Xia, W. Zhou, J. Tao, and L. Chen. 2016. Aerobic exercise ameliorates cognitive function in older adults with mild cognitive impairment: A systematic review and meta-analysis of randomised controlled trials. *British Journal of Sports Medicine* 50(23):1443-1450.

Zhong, D., L. Chen, Y. Feng, R. Song, L. Huang, J. Liu, and L. Zhang. 2021. Effects of virtual reality cognitive training in individuals with mild cognitive impairment: A systematic review and meta-analysis. *International Journal of Geriatric Psychiatry* 36(12):1829-1847.

Zhou, M., and S. Tang. 2022. Effect of a dual orexin receptor antagonist on Alzheimer's disease: Sleep disorders and cognition. *Frontiers in Medicine (Lausanne)* 9:984227.

Zhu, C. W., H. Grossman, J. Neugroschl, S. Parker, A. Burden, X. Luo, and M. Sano. 2018. A randomized, double-blind, placebo-controlled trial of resveratrol with glucose and malate (RGM) to slow the progression of Alzheimer's disease: A pilot study. *Alzheimer's & Dementia (N Y)* 4:609-616.

5

Advancing Research Priorities for Preventing and Treating Alzheimer's Disease and Related Dementias

Accelerating the development of effective preventive and treatment interventions for Alzheimer's disease and related dementias (AD/ADRD) that can preserve cognitive function and improve quality of life is a global public health priority. In the last decade, spurred by the National Alzheimer's Project Act, the National Institutes of Health (NIH) has invested billions of dollars to support research on detecting, understanding, and developing interventions for AD/ADRD. The committee reviewed this broad research landscape, working to identify areas of promise and priorities for future investments, and found that the investments by NIH and others have led to many scientific advances and created a foundation of knowledge from which much more can be learned. However, the pace of progress has not matched the growing urgency for interventions that can prevent, slow, or cure AD/ADRD and reduce the societal impact of these diseases.

This final chapter presents the committee's recommendations for accelerating progress on the research priorities identified in Chapters 2, 3, and 4 with the goal of advancing the science needed to develop effective preventive and therapeutic strategies. The identified research priorities represent areas of scientific inquiry with the greatest promise to catalyze significant advances and maximize return on investment. These research priorities are summarized in Recommendation 1 and detailed in Table 5-1. The committee's Recommendations 2–10 are aimed at overcoming key barriers to progress on those research priorities (see Figure 5-1). Addressing both the research priorities and the recommendations will require sustained and dedicated resources and need to be guided at all stages by those with lived

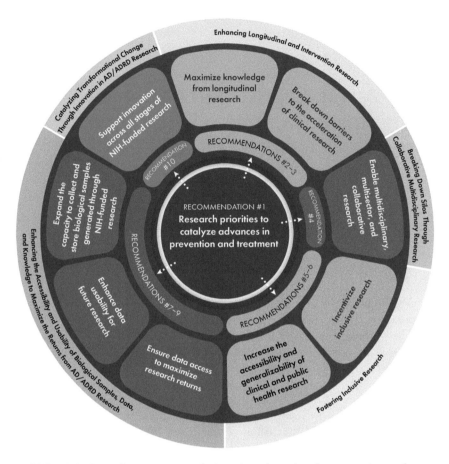

FIGURE 5-1 Committee recommendations for advancing the prevention and treatment of AD/ADRD.

experience to ensure synergy between scientific priorities and the priorities of those directly affected by dementia.

ADVANCING KEY SCIENTIFIC PRIORITIES RELATED TO PREVENTING AND TREATING AD/ADRD

The past few decades have brought significant advances in the understanding of AD/ADRD and in the development of tools and methods that can drive further progress. Notable milestones include the ability to detect specific AD-related pathologies (amyloid and tau) years before symptoms emerge, the discovery of many new genes linked to AD/ADRD that shed

light on pathogenic mechanisms, and the recognition that pathologies previously thought to distinguish different forms of dementia often co-occur
(NIH, 2023a). While encouraged, the committee also found notable gaps
in scientific knowledge and research capabilities during its review of the
AD/ADRD research landscape. The following scientific gaps represent key
bottlenecks that significantly impede progress toward preventing and treating AD/ADRD.

- There is a lack of rigorous evidence to support the identification of effective public health strategies for preventing AD/ADRD.
  Epidemiological research has yielded a large set of dementia risk
  factors (e.g., health behaviors, social isolation, socioeconomic
  disadvantage) based on statistical correlations. However, gaps
  in longitudinal data, data infrastructure, and study designs have
  resulted in limited understanding of causal relationships and the
  identification of exposures and system-level factors that, if mitigated, would have the greatest effect on the incidence of dementia.
  This impedes the development of effective public health approaches
  that could be implemented at a population scale to promote brain
  health across the life course and prevent AD/ADRD in diverse and
  especially disproportionately affected populations.
- There is an incomplete understanding of the biological basis and
  multiple etiologies underlying cognitive decline and dementia, as
  well as the mechanisms of resilience. There is still much that is not
  understood about AD/ADRD, conditions that may be characterized
  by decades of life-course health insults to brain and peripheral systems contributing to the development and detectable progression
  of neuropathology in the absence of clinical symptoms. Key knowledge gaps include how life-course exposures and other risk factors
  relate to pathobiology in diverse populations and the connections
  between molecular pathways that contribute to AD/ADRD and
  resilience (the maintenance of cognitive function despite the presence of brain pathology). This lack of understanding impedes drug
  discovery and the development of effective preventive and therapeutic intervention strategies. It also makes it difficult to predict
  the effect of risk factor reduction and drugs focused on single-
  pathology targets on dementia incidence.
- There is a lack of effective, validated, and accessible tools and methods (e.g., novel biomarker tests, digital assessment technologies) for
  detecting early changes in brain health and accurately diagnosing,
  subtyping, and monitoring AD/ADRD in diverse populations, This
  foundational capability is essential to trace how the natural history
  of AD/ADRD differs from "healthy" brain aging. Progress made

in the development of tools for AD needs to be expanded beyond amyloid and tau and extended to the multiple etiologies leading to dementia. The current capability gap impedes efforts to measure disease incidence and prevalence, to intervene early when chances of preventing and mitigating disease are greatest, to detect when treatments modify the trajectory of AD/ADRD, and to target specific interventions to the right populations (precision medicine).

Within each of these major scientific gaps of knowledge, there is also promising research that suggests opportunities to break current bottlenecks as new discoveries emerge. The discovery of imaging and fluid biomarkers for AD has catalyzed a shift in phenotyping procedures used in research and needs to be tested now in clinical practice. With the identification of risk genes/loci and the discovery of additional biomarkers, particularly for related dementias, current barriers to early detection, diagnosis, prognosis (e.g., the likelihood of progression to clinical dementia), and longitudinal monitoring may be overcome, and it will be possible to quantify and better understand multiple etiology dementia. The combination of digital tools and computational methods such as artificial intelligence/machine learning (AI/ML) that may be able to identify changes in traits (e.g., speech, gait, sleep behavior) that may precede current measures of cognitive decline similarly shows promise for enabling early detection of changes in brain health, early diagnosis, and prognosis (Amini et al., 2024). Digital tools have also opened new opportunities for passive and remote data collection and are changing the way investigators engage with study participants, particularly those from underresourced and underrepresented populations, and the public (Kaye et al., 2021).

Investments in basic science and longitudinal cohort studies have led to a significant expansion of the therapeutic pipeline with novel promising interventions that are not specific to any single dementia type by uncovering shared molecular pathways contributing to AD/ADRD (e.g., autophagic and lysosomal, immune, metabolic, mylelination), as well as resilience factors (Cummings et al., 2024). Multiomics methods[1] are creating new opportunities to evaluate disease mechanisms in diverse populations (Reddy et al., 2024) and to identify molecular disease subtypes and endophenotypes (Fang et al., 2020), thereby creating the foundation for precision medicine approaches to prevention and treatment in the future. Increased understanding of the links between AD/ADRD and chronic diseases such as hypertension and diabetes (Nagar et al., 2022), along with encouraging

---

[1] Multiomics methods involve the integrative analysis of multiple "omics" datasets, such as those generated from genomic, proteomic, transcriptomic, epigenomic, and metabolomic methods.

evidence for multicomponent interventions focused on health behaviors, has highlighted the potential for public health strategies to reduce dementia risk.

Scientific Priorities for Advancing the Prevention and Treatment of AD/ADRD

Building on the aforementioned examples of momentum and lines of promising research, the committee identified 11 research priorities and associated near- and medium-term scientific questions that it believes should be a focus of NIH-funded AD/ADRD biomedical research for the next 3 to 10 years. These research priorities, which are summarized in Recommendation 1 and detailed in Table 5-1, fall into three broad areas:

1. Quantify brain health across the life course and accurately predict risk of, screen for, diagnose, and monitor AD/ADRD.
2. Build a more comprehensive and integrated understanding of the disease biology and mechanistic pathways that contribute to AD/ADRD development and resilience over the life course.
3. Catalyze advances in interventions for the prevention and treatment of AD/ADRD spanning from precision medicine to public health strategies.

TABLE 5-1 Committee-Identified Research Priorities to Advance the Prevention and Treatment of Alzheimer's Disease and Related Dementias (AD/ADRD)

Research Priority	Key Scientific Questions	Near-Term Research Opportunities to Address Key Scientific Questions
Research priorities to quantify brain health across the life course and accurately predict risk of, screen for, diagnose, and monitor AD/ADRD		
2-1: Develop better tools, including novel biomarker tests and digital assessment technologies, to monitor brain health across the life course and screen, predict, and diagnose AD/ADRD at scale.	• How can brain health be precisely measured at scale across a diverse population (universally scalable)? • Can diagnostic biomarkers help identify potential causes for changes in personalized brain health? • Which data are essential to collect across the life course? • What alternative measures can assess changes in cognition and other related behaviors (e.g., ability to learn)? • How can existing cohorts be used to understand key transition points in brain health across the life course?	• Establish criteria to evaluate the diagnostic and clinical utility of newly developed tools (e.g., cognitive, clinical, fluid or digital biomarkers, imaging). • Discover and validate novel measures that capture early changes in brain health from a person's baseline. • Discover and validate new diagnostic, prognostic, predictive, and treatment response biomarkers (molecular and digital). • Carry out analyses within and across existing cohorts, including those cohorts developed to characterize brain health and those created for examining other health outcomes. • Perform large-scale, multiomics cohort studies of peripheral and brain signatures in diverse populations. • Perform large-scale cohort studies of digital signatures in diverse subpopulations.
2-2: Implement advances in clinical research methods and tools to generate data from real-world clinical practice settings that can inform future research.	• What are the facilitators of and barriers to the adoption of clinical research tools and methods? • How does the performance of novel tools (e.g., biomarker-based diagnostics, digital health technologies) differ across real-world settings and research settings? • What are the harms and benefits of identifying those with a specific pathology but who may never develop any symptoms?	• Rapidly implement novel tools (e.g., biomarker tests, digital technologies) in current, cross-institute studies. • Educate about the use and utility of emerging tools and technologies. • Evaluate potential harms of false positive or incorrect diagnoses and stigma related to early diagnoses before meaningful cognitive or other clinical symptoms manifest.

- How are the risks and benefits of biomarker testing and preclinical diagnosis balanced?
- How can the negative social and legal consequences of early detection or diagnosis of AD/ADRD be mitigated?

Research priorities to build a more comprehensive and integrated understanding of the disease biology and mechanistic pathways that contribute to AD/ADRD development and resilience over the life course

3-1: Identify factors driving AD/ADRD risk in diverse populations, particularly understudied and disproportionately affected groups, to better understand disease heterogeneity—including molecular subtypes and disparities in environmental exposures—and to identify prevention opportunities and advance health research equity.	• What are the determinants of AD/ADRD risk in diverse population groups (e.g., racial/ethnic, sex/gender, socioeconomic, geographic)? • Why are differences in pathology observed in diverse populations, and how does that influence risk of clinical disease? • What are the relative roles of modifiable social, economic, environmental, clinical, and behavioral mechanisms that might contribute to population differences in AD/ADRD? • How does the ability to modify risk factors vary across populations and their socioeconomic contexts? • What can be learned from the observed heterogeneity in severity (e.g., level of cognitive decline) and patterns of cognitive and other clinical symptoms among people who have similar levels of AD/ADRD-related pathology? • What genetic and other multiomics factors determine individuals' responses to interventions, modifiers, and exposures (e.g., exercise, diet, air pollution)? • What is required to increase interest in brain donation in diverse populations?	• Carry out a comprehensive survey of genetic and multiomics architecture in diverse well-characterized populations, using existing cohorts and infrastructure, to identify genomic determinants of risk. • Generate data to inform polygenic risk scores in people of non-European ancestry. • Use artificial intelligence and other computational tools to integrate multiple data types (e.g., multiomics, social, environmental) and identify commonalities across disease types and diverse populations and translate risk factors into biological mechanisms. • Across diverse populations, evaluate variations in the associations of life-course social, behavioral, and environmental exposure with longitudinal cognitive and biomarker data. • Identify opportunities to use natural experiments to evaluate exposure effects across the life course on clinical and biomarker outcomes in diverse populations.

continued

TABLE 5-1 Continued

Research Priority	Key Scientific Questions	Near-Term Research Opportunities to Address Key Scientific Questions
3-2: Characterize the exposome and gene–environment interactions across the life course to gain insights into biological mechanisms and identify opportunities to reduce AD/ADRD risk and increase resilience.	• Are there sensitive or critical periods across the life course when social, behavioral, or environmental exposures have a greater effect on different etiologic processes driving AD/ADRD risk? • What is the role of early- and midlife exposures in resilience and disease progression and do these vary for specific pathologies? • Do early- and midlife exposures result in brain circuitry changes that affect later life, and are these modifiable? • Which exposures have the largest effects on AD/ADRD risk and resilience (e.g., affect the largest proportion of the population) and should be prioritized for future investigations? • Are the gene–environment interactions that influence AD/ADRD risk and resilience different among diverse populations?	• Identify profiles (e.g., biochemical, multiomics) that reflect and capture individuals' exposures and link them to AD/ADRD outcomes to better understand exposome risk factors. • Investigate gene–exposure interactions using exposure data that are already available. • Link complex combinations of life-course social, behavioral, and environmental exposure measures to evaluate how these exposures synergistically influence longitudinal cognitive and biomarker data across diverse populations. • Evaluate how features of the social and environmental exposome or gene–environment interactions influence specific pathologies contributing to AD/ADRD using a life-course framework.
3-3: Elucidate the genetic and other biological mechanisms underlying resilience and resistance to identify novel targets and effective strategies for AD/ADRD prevention and treatment.	• What are the key factors that contribute to the resilience observed in positive or negative outliers (e.g., exceptional cases, including supercentenarians)? • What can be learned from individuals who do not develop pathologies (resistance) and those who develop pathologies but do not develop clinical symptoms within their lifetimes (resilience)? • What changes occur over time (i.e., with aging) in the way the brain deals with pathology (brain plasticity and adaptability), and is that process modifiable? • How do interactions between organ systems, including brain–body axes, contribute to resilience?	• Apply human tissue models from diverse groups of patients, including those with related dementias, and animal models to elucidate genes, multiomics factors, and molecular processes contributing to AD/ADRD resilience. • Investigate the role of brain–body axes (e.g., brain–gut and brain–renal axes) in resilience. • Establish a collection of resilient brains (organ collection) as a basis for the systematic comparative analysis of the causes of selective vulnerability and selective resilience and resistance to identify key factors and determinants of vulnerability and resilience, including a focus on disease-decisive factors.

| 3-4: Develop integrated molecular and cellular causal models to guide the identification of common mechanisms underlying AD/ADRD and their validation as novel targets for prevention and treatment. | • What are the primary interactions and sequential cascading effects that translate molecular and cellular dysregulation into disease?
• How do distinct pathologic processes combine to culminate in clinical manifestations of AD/ADRD?
• When do the different molecular factors and processes begin to disturb cellular, organ, or system function that leads, eventually, to disease onset (age dependent)? Considering multiple etiologic processes contributing to AD/ADRD individually and jointly, is there a particular point of no return?
• How do the different cell types in the brain (e.g., glial cells, endothelial cells, neurons) interact with each other on a timescale, ultimately leading to neurodegeneration?
• How do genome-wide association studies (GWAS)-based risk genes set the stage for alterations in brain cell physiology, predisposing the brain to dysfunction and disease later in life?
• What is the functional effect of defined identified risk genes or defined groups of risk genes on neuronal and glial physiology and function?
• How do exposome factors affect physiology of cell types contributing to disease?
• How do amyloid-independent interventions (e.g., lysosomal stabilizers, autophagy inducers, neuroprotective compounds) change cellular biology?
• What are the molecular and cellular mechanisms mediating interactions between organ systems, including brain–body axes, that lead to brain pathologies? | • Identify the earliest biological changes related to pathologic processes.
• Investigate the function of glial, endothelial, neuronal, and other relevant types of brain cells during aging employing aged cell types and aged cell cultures.
• Study the interactions of the different types of cells and mediators and the consequences of such interactions in appropriate cell and tissue models to identify a potential point of no return.
• Include *aging* as the central risk factor of many dementia types into all cellular and molecular studies (e.g., aged glial cells, induced neurons from older individuals) and employ multiomics technologies.
• Generate a framework based on grouping certain GWAS risk loci, identify functionally causal genes in these loci, and study their cellular and molecular effect on functions.
• Systematically study the functional consequences of AD/ADRD risk genes in cellular models (extending beyond *APOE4* studies to a wider array of risk genes derived from GWAS and other omics studies).
• Study the effect of exosomal factors (individually and in combination) on the physiology of glial and endothelial cells, neurons, and other relevant brain cell types in cellular and animal models.
• Analyze the effect of experimental approaches and compounds on molecular pathways beyond those involved in the amyloid cascade, and employ amyloid-independent cellular and in vivo models. |

continued

TABLE 5-1 Continued

Research Priority	Key Scientific Questions	Near-Term Research Opportunities to Address Key Scientific Questions
3-4: Continued	• How do molecular and cellular mechanisms that contribute to development of neuropsychiatric symptoms interact with those that underlie the development of neuropathology? • Are there important differences in pathologic, molecular, and multiomics features that are shared across AD and related dementias?	• Employ comparative studies using histology and multiomics to identify commonalities among AD and related dementias. • Evaluate mediating and modifying pathways linking genetic and genomic risk factors and biomarker measures of disease with clinical manifestations. • Investigate the role of the brain–body axes (e.g., brain–gut and brain–renal axes) in the development of AD/ADRD pathology.

Research priorities to catalyze advances in interventions for the prevention and treatment of AD/ADRD spanning from precision medicine to public health strategies

Research Priority	Key Scientific Questions	Near-Term Research Opportunities to Address Key Scientific Questions
4-1: Integrate innovative approaches and novel tools into the planning, design, and execution of studies to accelerate the identification of effective interventions.	• What outcomes and biomarkers can be used to assess the interactive effects of mixed pathologies (e.g., vascular, α-synuclein, TDP-43, and AD pathology)? • What biological markers can be used to show that the intended pathway is engaged and the therapy is having the expected effect? • How can trial design be improved to determine whether late-stage trial failures are the result of ineffective interventions versus limitations in trial designs or execution? • How can trials be designed to incorporate and test innovative methodologies in ways that do not pose risks to the primary objective of the trial and the timely execution of clinical research?	• Incorporate innovative substudies into ongoing clinical trials to pilot novel approaches (e.g., new biomarkers as secondary outcomes, digital tools for remote data collection). • Create mechanisms to share successes and failures from innovative operational trial design aspects. • Optimize proof-of-concept trials with informative biomarkers and outcomes. • Identify and evaluate causal evidence on the role of past and ongoing public health initiatives, clinical care changes, and policy changes on AD/ADRD prevention at a population level (e.g., trial emulations using real-world data). • Use existing data (e.g., electronic health data) to identify subpopulations.

	• What innovative approaches can be used to increase the value of observational studies to inform prevention, including short- and long-term effects? • Can risk profiles based on biomarker testing of asymptomatic individuals decrease required sample sizes and accelerate trials?	• Use platform randomized trials to evaluate multiple interventions in parallel. • Conduct long-term follow-up of early- and midlife prevention strategies using networked data infrastructure. • Develop and use social determinants of health metrics in clinical research.
4-2: Advance the development and evaluation of combination therapies (including pharmacologic and nonpharmacologic approaches) to better address the multifactorial nature of AD/ADRD.	• Which combinations of interventions (drug combinations and combinations of drugs and nonpharmaceutical interventions [NPIs]) will work synergistically to prevent AD/ADRD or slow its clinical progression? • What are the long-term effects of combination interventions? • How does the sequencing of interventions affect their combined effectiveness and safety? • How do different combinations of interventions interact, and how can their effects be maximized? • Can combination interventions targeting multiple mechanistic pathways improve the effectiveness of treatment for people with mixed pathologies? • For combination trials that include NPIs, how can the trial be designed with adequate blinding and appropriate control groups? What are the relevant endpoints?	• Explore and understand the independent and/or synergistic mechanisms of multidomain interventions and combination therapies.
4-3: Evaluate precision medicine approaches for the prevention and treatment of AD/ADRD to better identify interventions likely to benefit specific groups of individuals.	• Can an understanding of the exposome guide population stratification to facilitate precision approaches to AD/ADRD interventions? • What criteria and molecular or multiomics factors and biomarkers are appropriate for use in (1) identifying subtypes and endophenotypes and (2) stratifying populations at a population and an individual level?	• Integrate findings from multiomic approaches and other modalities to characterize AD/ADRD subtypes that can be used to identify commonalities and stratify across different subtypes. • Use innovative research designs (e.g., platform trials, personalized interventions) that support precision medicine approaches.

continued

TABLE 5-1 Continued

Research Priority	Key Scientific Questions	Near-Term Research Opportunities to Address Key Scientific Questions
4-3: Continued	• Does giving people more agency in how they implement interventions (e.g., personalized approaches to NPIs) affect trial outcomes?	• Conduct intervention trials that include study populations living with multiple pathologies. • Invest in longer-term studies of postintervention outcomes in diverse populations, including in populations with different comorbidities and levels of adherence. • Conduct follow-up studies of individuals treated with anti-amyloid antibodies to better understand the effects of copathologies on patient symptoms and to identify key targets to include in combination interventions. • Collaborate with safety registries to evaluate safety outcomes from real-world evidence.
4-4: Advance the adoption of standardized outcomes for assessing interventions that are sensitive, person-centered, clinically meaningful, and reflect the priorities of those at risk for or living with AD/ADRD.	• What outcomes matter most for people living with AD/ADRD and their caregivers and care partners? • How do intermediate outcomes such as biomarkers and risk scores translate to outcomes that are clinically meaningful? • What metrics are most important for assessing quality of life, well-being, and functional outcomes in diverse populations? • What are the continued clinical and biological outcomes in those who received an intervention? • How can study designs incorporate research questions around maximizing adherence to interventions?	• Develop and validate intermediate outcomes, including biomarkers and risk scores, that are robustly linked to cognitive, functional, or quality-of-life outcomes. • Use metrics that can be personalized for desired individual outcomes. • Conduct ethnographic and other similar studies to identify person-centered outcomes for use in clinical research. • Engage clinicians (e.g., primary care providers, geriatricians) and people living with AD/ADRD in the identification of clinically meaningful outcomes for use in clinical research. • Evaluate factors that influence adherence to interventions and how it affects outcomes.

4-5: Evaluate the causal effects of public health approaches on overall dementia incidence and incidence in understudied and/or disproportionately affected populations.	• What is the potential effect of a population approach (e.g., modifying exposure to an adverse environmental or social factor or behavior) on dementia incidence and inequalities relative to a precision medicine or high-risk individual-level approach (i.e., targeting risk reduction in individuals with the highest level of an adverse risk factor)? • Considering mediating mechanisms and spillover effects, what are the most effective strategies for population interventions to reduce dementia incidence? • What interventions can be most easily scaled to reduce risk of dementia at a population level in the near and medium terms?	• Estimate population-attributable fractions associated with identified risk factors for all-cause dementia risk, dementia subtypes, and on social inequalities in dementia risk. • Compare plausible population-attributable fractions for AD/ADRD cases prevented associated with high-risk/precision medicine versus population approaches. • Evaluate the evidence for causality of known risk factors with high population prevalence, with specificity regarding dose, duration, timing (age), and other possible sources of heterogeneity in exposure effects. • Evaluate whether there are important distinct determinants of dementia that are common in groups historically underrepresented in AD/ADRD research (e.g., Black, Latino, Asian, or Indigenous populations; rural populations; and individuals from low socioeconomic backgrounds) and may be targets for public health approaches. • Evaluate how specific policies or interventions that can be scaled to large populations influence dementia risk overall and inequalities in dementia risk. • Evaluate how changes in existing policies shaping social and environmental determinants of health (e.g., policies shaping food security, economic security, healthy housing access, educational experiences across the life course, safe working conditions, retirement policies, violence exposure, air pollution and other environmental toxins, and community climate resilience) influence biomarkers associated with AD/ADRD risk and clinical AD/ADRD.

continued

TABLE 5-1 Continued

Research Priority	Key Scientific Questions	Near-Term Research Opportunities to Address Key Scientific Questions
4-5: Continued		• Contrast the near- and medium-term impact of clinical care strategies (e.g., hypertension treatment, access to amyloid-targeting therapies, or management of comorbid conditions and infectious diseases) versus behavior change strategies (e.g., dietary or physical activity interventions) versus policy interventions (e.g., changes in retirement age or clean air and water standards). • Incorporate estimates of spillover effects of modifying risk factors and of prevented dementia cases on family and other social network members.

NOTE: The numbering of research priorities in this table reflects the numbering in the report chapters.

Recommendation 1: Research priorities to catalyze advances in prevention and treatment

The National Institutes of Health (NIH) should focus on the research priorities and associated near- and medium-term scientific questions detailed in Table 5-1 to advance a person-centered, multidisciplinary, and integrative research approach that will catalyze advances in the prevention and treatment of Alzheimer's disease and related dementias (AD/ADRD). These research priorities cover the following areas:

- Develop better tools, including novel biomarker tests and digital assessment technologies, to monitor brain health across the life course and screen, predict, and diagnose AD/ADRD at scale (Research Priority 2-1)
- Implement advances in clinical research methods and tools to generate data from real-world clinical practice settings that can inform future research (Research Priority 2-2)
- Identify factors driving AD/ADRD risk in diverse populations, particularly understudied and disproportionately affected groups, to better understand disease heterogeneity—including molecular subtypes and disparities in environmental exposures—and to identify prevention opportunities and advance health research equity (Research Priority 3-1)
- Characterize the exposome and gene–environment interactions across the life course to gain insights into biological mechanisms and identify opportunities to reduce AD/ADRD risk and increase resilience (Research Priority 3-2)
- Elucidate the genetic and other biological mechanisms underlying resilience and resistance to identify novel targets and effective strategies for AD/ADRD prevention and treatment (Research Priority 3-3)
- Develop integrated molecular and cellular causal models to guide the identification of common mechanisms underlying AD/ADRD and their validation as novel targets for prevention and treatment (Research Priority 3-4)
- Integrate innovative approaches and novel tools into the planning, design, and execution of studies to accelerate the identification of effective interventions (Research Priority 4-1)
- Advance the development and evaluation of combination therapies (including pharmacological and nonpharmacological approaches) to better address the multifactorial nature of AD/ADRD (Research Priority 4-2)
- Evaluate precision medicine approaches for the prevention and treatment of AD/ADRD to better identify interventions likely to benefit specific groups of individuals (Research Priority 4-3)

- Advance the adoption of standardized outcomes for assessing interventions that are sensitive, person-centered, clinically meaningful, and reflect the priorities of those at risk for or living with AD/ADRD (Research Priority 4-4)
- Evaluate the causal effects of public health approaches on overall dementia incidence and incidence in understudied and/or disproportionately affected populations. (Research Priority 4-5)

The committee acknowledges that NIH has already made investments in each of these priority research areas to varying degrees. Given the breadth of the NIH AD/ADRD research portfolio, it is unsurprising that the committee did not identify any research priorities for which there had been no prior NIH investment. In some cases, research priorities identified by the committee, such as the development of biomarkers for monitoring brain health and the identification of factors driving risk in diverse populations, are already the focus of major NIH-funded research programs and initiatives, many of which are described in this report. Other identified research priorities, such as the characterization of the exposome and gene–environment interactions, the development of integrated molecular and cellular causal models, and the development of digital tools, represent scientific areas of more recent or limited NIH investment. Relatedly, efforts to achieve associated near-term research opportunities, which are detailed in the right-hand column of Table 5-1, may indeed be underway but have not yet been fully realized. Significant investment in the totality of the priority research areas is needed to address the knowledge gaps laid out in this report. Critically, beyond financial investment, success in tackling each of these research priorities will require an emphasis on the intentional expansion of research efforts beyond AD and the inclusion of diverse and understudied and/or disproportionately affected populations.

Importantly, Table 5-1 is not intended as a prescribed research agenda. Nor is the identification of these priority areas meant to imply that lines of scientific inquiry outside of these areas are not of value or that work in all other areas should be suspended. There is a great deal of uncertainty in the process for scientific investigation regarding which discoveries from current research will lead to transformational advances in the future and no guarantees can be offered regarding the ultimate fruitfulness of any specific line of inquiry. The committee's intention, however, is that the priorities will be used as a guide in the rebalancing of NIH funding for AD/ADRD. Closing the scientific knowledge gaps raised by these priorities can occur by working to answer the committee's proposed scientific questions and acting on opportunities to overcome barriers to progress, as detailed in the recommendations that follow.

Opportunities to Enhance Longitudinal and Intervention Research to Advance Key Scientific Priorities for Preventing and Treating AD/ADRD

Studies that follow individuals longitudinally and test interventions across time are needed to address the research priorities and associated scientific questions identified in Table 5-1. This section highlights opportunities to ensure such research has the greatest possible impact by maximizing the insights that can be gleaned and accelerating the pace of discovery.

Leveraging Longitudinal Research

Longitudinal cohort studies represent an important mechanism for identifying data that provide a comprehensive view of brain health and AD/ADRD development over the life course (including risk and resilience factors). Knowledge gained from such studies can be translated into protocols and sensitive tools (e.g., digital health technologies, biomarker assays) that can be deployed in research and practice for ongoing clinical monitoring and AD/ADRD prediction, detection, prognostication, and diagnosis.

Numerous cohorts have been established specifically for the study of cognitive impairment and dementia. The constituents of such cohorts often are limited to upper age ranges, and such studies will generally collect measures (e.g., exposures, health data) determined a priori to be specific to AD/ADRD. With the growing understanding of AD/ADRD as conditions that develop over the life course, there has been recognition of opportunities to use data relevant to brain health and AD/ADRD generated through longitudinal research focused on other health conditions (e.g., the Bogalusa Heart Study, which focuses on cardiovascular disease), as discussed in Chapter 2. Integrating those data with AD/ADRD outcomes can help to fill current data gaps (e.g., data for younger age ranges and populations underrepresented in AD/ADRD research), expand the set of measures that can be linked to brain health trajectories, and yield important insights on prevention and treatment strategies while newer AD/ADRD-focused cohort studies remain ongoing.

NIH has made significant investments in recent years to expand and better use its existing support for longitudinal research related to aging, resilience, and AD/ADRD. Such investments have included

- the creation of new cohorts (e.g., the ARTFL-LEFFTDS Longitudinal Frontotemporal Lobar Degeneration [ALLFTD] study) and the augmentation of existing cohorts (e.g., the Longevity Consortium) to better understand AD/ADRD risk and resilience across diverse populations;
- the integration of AD/ADRD research into existing cohorts established for examining other health outcomes (e.g., funding the

Aging, Demographics, and Memory Study as a supplement to the Health and Retirement Study); and

- collaborative efforts to harmonize outcomes (e.g., the Harmonized Cognitive Assessment Protocol) to facilitate cross-study comparisons and multicohort analyses.

Recognizing these prior investments, the committee encourages NIH to continue and expand support for longitudinal AD/ADRD research that can fill data gaps and address the scientific questions included in Table 5-1. In addition to establishing new cohorts that can meet the need for diverse and representative populations in dementia research, this should include a concerted effort to identify other existing cohorts—including those funded by agencies other than the National Institute on Aging (NIA) and the National Institute of Neurological Disorders and Stroke (NINDS), as well as international studies—to which a focus on AD/ADRD could be added through supplemental funding and other appropriate NIH funding mechanisms. Such efforts may provide an opportunity to pilot novel tools such as biomarker tests and digital technologies. Additionally, NIH should ensure funding opportunities are designed to maximize the insights from longitudinal research through attention to data accessibility and harmonization and the collection and storage of data (e.g., digital, exposure) and biosamples (see Recommendations 7, 8, and 9). Proactive coordination and planning through the convening of investigators from different cohort studies, before study initiation whenever possible, can help to identify approaches that would enable data access, interoperability, and harmonization.

Recommendation 2: Maximize knowledge from longitudinal research
To maximize knowledge from longitudinal research and enable future discoveries, the National Institutes of Health should prioritize investments in longitudinal research to address existing knowledge gaps regarding factors that influence brain health over the life course. These efforts should include the following:

- Invest in data infrastructure (see Recommendation 7), data harmonization (see Recommendation 8), and the cultivation of specialized expertise to enable the collection of data and conduct of analyses within and across existing cohorts, including those cohorts developed to characterize brain health and those created for examining other health outcomes.
- Create new, multidimensionally diverse (e.g., multilanguage, ethnoracial, geographic, socioeconomic) cohorts.
- Strategically add data points important to assessing brain health into existing cohorts constituted for research on other health conditions.

- Routinely collect early- and midlife exposure data (e.g., residential and work history, environmental toxicants, nutrition, education) from cohort study participants.
- Ensure that the data generated from shared biological samples are stored, searchable, and sharable.

Accelerating Translational and Clinical Intervention Research

Decades of research and hundreds of clinical trials have yielded only a limited number of treatments for Alzheimer's disease (AD) that offer modest clinical benefits (Boxer and Sperling, 2023; Cummings et al., 2024; Kim et al., 2022), and no treatments have been approved by the U.S. Food and Drug Administration (FDA) for related dementias (Liu et al., 2019; MacDonald et al., 2022; Nag et al., 2020), beyond those for managing symptoms. Evidence for some nonpharmacological approaches to preventing cognitive decline and dementia (physical activity, cognitive training), while encouraging, has been inconclusive (NASEM, 2017), leaving the public with much uncertainty about steps they should take to protect their cognitive function as they age. This lack of progress toward effective strategies for preventing and treating AD/ADRD reflects the complex and multifactorial pathobiology of this group of diseases, but it also underscores the need to accelerate the translational research yielding novel targets for interventions and to expand and improve the efficiency of clinical trials.

Many entities (government, private, philanthropic, and academic) contribute to research for advancing interventions for AD/ADRD with complementary resources and expertise. NIH plays a critical role in this complex research ecosystem by funding research on interventions and certain trial designs that may be less appealing to industry owing to financial risk or the lack of financial incentives, incentivizing industry participation in collaborative efforts designed to develop and bring new and combination interventions to scale (see Recommendation 10), and supporting basic and translational research (e.g., target identification and validation) that feeds into the private-sector drug development pipeline. As discussed in Chapter 3, NIH has made significant infrastructure investments (e.g., Accelerating Medicines Partnership® Program for Alzheimer's Disease [AMP-AD], Target Enablement to Accelerate Therapy Development for Alzheimer's Disease [TREAT-AD], Model Organism Development and Evaluation for Late-onset Alzheimer's Disease [MODEL-AD]) to generate a pipeline that can translate discoveries from basic research into candidates that can be evaluated in clinical trials. With the necessary infrastructure in place, there is now an opportunity to scale and diversify these efforts to a broader set of risk factors and pathways (e.g., neuroinflammation, cellular senescence, lysosomal dysfunction, mitochondrial dysfunction).

There has been notable growth in innovation in clinical trials in the last couple of decades, particularly outside of AD/ADRD, highlighting opportunities to learn from the successes and lessons from other fields. As discussed in Chapter 4, NIH infrastructure investments, such as the Alzheimer's Clinical Trials Consortium, the Alzheimer's Prevention Initiative, and the Dominantly Inherited Alzheimer Network Trials Unit, have facilitated increased collaboration with industry, philanthropy, and other partners (e.g., by using public–private partnerships) and innovation in AD/ADRD clinical trials (e.g., decentralization of trials, piloting platform trials, virtual engagement of participants, and digital data collection). However, to accelerate the pace of discovery, these efforts need to be expanded to a much greater scale as NIH continues to support clinical research to evaluate AD/ADRD interventions in the coming years.

Drug discovery can take 15–20 years, and a long-term focus on the mechanisms involved in AD/ADRD to allow multiple targets to be tested through clinical proof-of-concept (phase 1b and 2) trials is critically important. Expanded support (e.g., via R61/R33 mechanisms) for the validation of novel targets or effective strategies for the prevention and treatment of AD/ADRD is needed to ensure that an adequate number of validated targets (roughly 50 per year) can serve as input to the pipeline with the goal of yielding promising candidates that could be transitioned to clinical trials (within academia or industry).

As drug discovery and target validation efforts are scaled, phase 1b and phase 2 clinical trials in particular need to be expanded. Increasing the quantity and quality of small phase 1b and phase 2 proof-of-concept trials with a focus on mechanisms, informative biomarkers (e.g., target engagement, biomarkers for copathologies), and outcomes (e.g., pharmacokinetics and pharmacodynamics, surrogate outcomes) is needed to smooth the transition to and better guide decision making for larger, later-stage trials. Importantly, as the incorporation of additional biomarkers and imaging for pathologies associated with related dementias (e.g., TDP-43, alpha-synuclein) becomes more feasible, including them within each early-phase study, even those clinical trials of single therapeutic agents targeting a different pathology, would be highly informative of potential links among copathologies. In the meantime, banking of biological samples can enable future measurement of these pathologies.

In anticipation of the increased demand for clinical trial investigators, attention is needed to address current gaps in the workforce (e.g., investigators with specialized expertise in pharmacology trials). Ensuring investigators new to conducting trials use existing training programs with best practices can help to improve the rigor of earlier-stage trials. The NIA and Alzheimer's Association-funded Institute on Methods and Protocols for Advancement of Clinical Trials in ADRD (IMPACT-AD), for example, provides multidisciplinary training for current and future principal investigators on the design, conduct, and analysis of clinical trials. IMPACT-AD also works to strengthen the broader clinical trial workforce through dedicated training opportunities for clinician-researchers and clinical trial support staff (Berkness et al., 2021).

The expanded use of innovative clinical trial designs, described in Chapter 4, has the potential to significantly accelerate clinical research. Master protocols—trial protocols for use with multiple substudies (FDA, 2022)—and platform, combination, and adaptive trial designs create efficiencies and enable a shift away from a clinical research paradigm focused on testing individual interventions in single populations sequentially.

Additional opportunities to improve trial efficiency can be realized by ensuring a trial-ready pool of research participants and a ready clinical trial infrastructure. Recruitment and enrollment represent major bottlenecks in the clinical trial pipeline (Langbaum et al., 2023). As has been done in the cancer field, NIH-funded Alzheimer's Disease Research Centers (ADRCs) and other AD/ADRD-focused centers should be evaluated and held accountable for enrolling participants in clinical trials.

A key strategy to improve trial efficiency at the recruitment phase is to reduce screen failure.[2] With master protocols, a single recruitment pool can be used to populate multiple substudies. Volunteers that may be ineligible for one substudy could potentially be enrolled in a different substudy under the same protocol. Highly phenotyped and increasingly diverse cohorts represent invaluable pools of prescreened participants (Gregory et al., 2022). Examples include ALLFTD (discussed in Chapter 2) and the North American Prodromal Synucleinopathy (NAPS) study, which enrolls people with rapid eye movement (REM) sleep behavior disorders who are at risk of developing LBD, Parkinson's, or other neurological disorders (NAPS Consortium, 2024). Similarly, the Trial-Ready Cohort-Down Syndrome collects longitudinal data (e.g., blood and cognitive tests, imaging) on people with Down syndrome to fast-track the enrollment process as soon as they are eligible and matched with a qualifying clinical study (TRC-DS, 2024). While biases in the cohort populations need to be considered, drawing from such pools could accelerate startup.

Finally, there needs to be consideration of opportunities to use technology to move from screen fail to screen enroll. While registries[3] are one mechanism to track volunteers who did not meet screening criteria but

---

[2] Screen failure occurs when a potential participant is screened for but is not able to enroll in the trial (Parekh et al., 2022).

[3] NIA maintains a list of registries and matching services for AD/ADRD clinical trials at https://www.nia.nih.gov/health/clinical-trials-and-studies/registries-and-matching-services-clinical-trials (accessed October 19, 2024).

may be eligible for other studies (e.g., people who exhibit signs of cognitive impairment but fail the screen for AD pathology), other technologies, such as social engagement platforms, should be explored. There is also a need for studies on best practices for community screening and referral.[4]

A ready clinical trial infrastructure can help to speed up other aspects of the startup phase. These include centralized support functions, such as centralized institutional review boards (now required by NIH for most multisite trials) and contracting; systems for decentralized screening (online or at local community centers); and systems for electronic and staged consent processes. The development of clinical trial networks that use a hub-and-spoke model to centralize some core infrastructure can reduce the pragmatic challenges and burdens for investigators at trial sites embedded in communities (e.g., federally qualified health centers). To support the development of such networks, ADRCs could play a role in creating registries of regional clinical trial sites, and NIH-funded clinical trial consortia, if adequately supported, could provide training for clinical trial sites to disseminate knowledge, standards, and best practices.

Recommendation 3: Break down barriers to the acceleration of clinical research
The National Institutes of Health (NIH) should continue to lead efforts across a multiplicity of relevant entities (e.g., pharmaceutical and biotechnology companies, academia, foundations) to accelerate the movement of promising interventions for Alzheimer's disease and related dementias (AD/ADRD) into clinical trials and to expand the use of innovative approaches to improve the efficiency of clinical trials. These efforts should include the following:

- Organize NIH investments in basic and translational research related to potential molecular targets for intervention into a portfolio to create a pipeline of validated targets that can be transitioned into drug development.
- Expand the use of innovative trial designs (e.g., master protocols, platform, combination, adaptive trials) and increase investment in both early-phase (phase 1b and 2) proof-of-concept trials and later-stage pragmatic trials.
- Identify and promulgate best practices for decreasing the barriers to, and time for, the clinical trial startup phase (e.g., decentralized participant screening, creation and use of pre-screened cohorts and screen-enroll mechanisms, use of electronic

---

[4] While beyond the scope of this report, it should be noted that an important issue that arises with regards to screening of individuals for participation in clinical research is the return of screening results to the individuals (NASEM, 2018).

consenting procedures, centralized contracting, and institutional review board processes).

- Continue investing in innovative funding models, such as public–private partnerships, shared funding for global trials, and combined-phase funding, that support the progression of candidate interventions across the early-stage clinical research pipeline.
- Maximize coordination between NIH-funded AD/ADRD clinical trial programs and NIH-funded AD/ADRD centers (e.g., Alzheimer's Disease Research Centers) and evaluate these centers for representative participant clinical trial enrollment.

STRATEGIES FOR ADDRESSING CROSSCUTTING BARRIERS THAT IMPEDE PROGRESS ON AD/ADRD SCIENTIFIC PRIORITIES

The committee was asked to identify key barriers to advancing AD/ADRD prevention and treatment and to highlight opportunities to address these barriers to catalyze advances across the field. In its examination of the AD/ADRD research landscape, several impediments to progress were consistently identified across the continuum from basic to clinical research. These crosscutting barriers include

- siloing within the AD/ADRD field and across related domains of research (e.g., aging, neurodegenerative diseases more broadly, exposure science);
- insufficient population representativeness and generalizability of research;
- inadequate infrastructure and support for management and analysis of data, samples, and knowledge generated from AD/ADRD research; and
- inadequate support for innovative methods capable of realizing transformational progress.

The sections below discuss opportunities and strategies for addressing these barriers. As detailed in each of the sections, the committee recognizes the significant NIH investment to address each of these key barriers. Examples of NIH activities highlighted in the sections below are meant to be illustrative and do not represent a comprehensive cataloging of such efforts as the committee was not charged with a review of NIH's programs. It should also be acknowledged that many barriers are not unique to dementia research, and other scientific fields are also working to overcome similar challenges. Accordingly, in considering the implementation of the recommendations below, NIH and other research funders should continuously monitor the broader research landscape for examples of how such challenges have been successfully tackled in other fields and consider opportunities to apply those strategies in AD/ADRD research.

Breaking Down Silos Through Collaborative, Multidisciplinary Research

The heterogeneity of AD/ADRD, the prevalence of mixed pathologies, and the multifactorial and intersecting nature of the diverse pathways that lead to disease all suggest that the path to effective strategies for preventing and treating this group of neurodegenerative diseases lies in collaborative, multidisciplinary research. Yet, throughout its information-gathering process the committee encountered numerous silos, commonly reinforced by funding structures, that impede efforts to elucidate the biological basis of AD/ADRD and advance prevention and treatment. Current funding strategies that target individual diseases, which have historically favored AD, fail to address the reality of overlapping and mixed pathologies that contribute to neurodegenerative disease, and they have contributed to the current dearth of effective therapies for related dementias. There have been few efforts to develop a larger integrated model of aging and neurodegenerative disease despite clear overlap in research endeavors and shared mechanisms (see Chapter 3). As discussed in Chapter 4, research on pharmacological and non-pharmacological interventions are not well integrated, and as a result there have been few efforts to date to evaluate the effect of combination approaches despite a high likelihood that risk reduction and drug therapies will both be necessary elements of a strategy to reduce the incidence and impact of dementia. Moreover, the efforts of federal agencies supporting related areas of research are not adequately coordinated, resulting in missed opportunities to leverage synergies and effectively use existing investments in studies and infrastructure. Innovative funding strategies, such as multi-institute research consortia and public–private partnerships, and other incentives, as well as the application of collaborative research mechanisms, and greater coordination and integration of research and infrastructure are needed to address the current siloing of research and accelerate the development of interventions for preventing and treating AD/ADRD. Disincentives to team approaches, such as academic promotion structures, also need to be addressed.

Funding opportunities that encourage collaboration across disease areas by bringing together multidisciplinary teams have the potential to accelerate the development of not only interventions that target common underlying mechanisms but also disease-agnostic resilience mechanisms, as discussed in Chapter 3. Supporting collaboration across disciplines also facilitates the application of approaches and technologies to address research questions and technical challenges in novel ways. Multi-institute research consortia represent one mechanism for fostering collaborative research and bridging the divide between basic and clinical research (Gladman et al., 2019). For example, the Biomarkers for Vascular Contributions to Cognitive Impairment and Dementia Consortium (MarkVCID) was established to advance the discovery and validation of biomarkers for small vessel diseases of the brain involved in cognitive impairment and dementia, as cerebrovascular small vessel disease is a commonly identified pathology in mixed dementia (Greenberg, 2017; MarkVCID, 2017). Ultimately, the consortium seeks to deliver biomarker kits that can be used in intervention trials, thereby translating basic science findings into clinical research (Gladman et al., 2019). Diverse VCID is another example of a multi-institute research program focused on understanding the role that cerebrovascular disease plays in AD/ADRD for diverse populations with the goal of improving diagnosis and treatment (Diverse VCID, 2024). Multi-institute consortia often have the benefit of effectively using existing, mature research infrastructure to scale up research efforts. Coordinating centers play a key role in such consortia to centralize resources and facilitate harmonization, coordination, and data sharing across the multiple participating research institutions. When supported by multiple funders, research consortia also provide opportunities to align and better use existing resources and future investments across funding organizations.

Multi-institute research collaborations should not be limited to U.S. institutions. Dementia is a global challenge—the burden of which is borne in large part by people living in low- and middle-income countries (LMICs)—and it will not be overcome by the siloed efforts of individual countries (Nature Medicine, 2023). From a health equity perspective, international collaborations can help to address the problems of overrepresentation of some populations in AD/ADRD research and the underrepresentation of many global populations living outside North America and Western Europe. Underrepresented populations include those within LMICs but also in some high-income countries (e.g., within Asia and the Middle East). Such global collaborations can also help to uncover rare genetic variants and answer important scientific questions regarding the relative contributions of genetic ancestry and sociocultural factors (e.g., social determinants of health) to dementia risk and resilience. It should be acknowledged, however, that current international laws and regulations, including but not limited to the General Data Protection Regulation of the European Union, pose a formidable impediment to the reciprocal exchange of data and biological samples with researchers from other countries. While not insurmountable (and not limited to AD/ADRD), these issues are complex and require careful legal analysis. Investigator-level relationships can lead to some workarounds, but ultimately these barriers need to be addressed at the level of national governmental leaders. As a major global funder of biomedical (including AD/ADRD) research and intellectual leader, NIH can spearhead efforts to overcome these barriers by engaging its counterparts in other countries and the broader research community to understand their needs and jointly develop practical mid- to long-term solutions. Such solutions will need to address mechanisms for data access (e.g., cloud-based mechanisms, federated learning platforms) and security (e.g., encryption, use of synthetic data), and the more challenging issues of biosample sharing.

Public–private partnerships create unique opportunities for cross-discipline collaboration (within the United States and globally) and are established specifically to more effectively leverage the respective talents of investigators in academia and industry toward a shared goal. A notable example in the AD/ADRD field is AMP-AD (see Box 3-4 in Chapter 3). Government and philanthropic funding for such partnerships can incentivize industry engagement in activities that might otherwise be considered too financially risky, as well as encouraging innovation (e.g., innovative trial designs) (Boxer and Sperling, 2023). While there are multiple mechanisms for establishing public–private partnerships, the Foundation for the National Institutes of Health (FNIH)—a nonprofit organization—specifically focuses on convening partners, including NIH, academic institutions, industry, philanthropy, and advocacy organizations (FNIH, 2023) and may be positioned to facilitate collaboration without creating financial conflicts of interest for academic researchers. Current gap areas that may benefit from public–private partnerships include efforts to develop combination interventions that include pharmacological and nonpharmacological components (see Chapter 4), and the development of a platform for real-world data collection (see Chapter 2).

Challenge programs are another powerful mechanism for facilitating interdisciplinary approaches while simultaneously pushing boundaries and driving further innovation in AD/ADRD research. Such programs often set ambitious goals and use prize money to incentivize investigators to tackle complex problems from novel perspectives. By encouraging rapid iteration and establishing feedback loops, challenge programs can push researchers to develop and refine ideas and strategies in relatively short periods of time. A recent example is the Pioneering Research for Early Prediction of Alzheimer's and Related Dementias Eureka (PREPARE) Challenge, a multiphase competition that was launched by NIA in fiscal year 2023 with support from the NASA Tournament Lab (Driven Data, 2024).[5] The objective of the challenge is to spur innovation in data science to advance solutions for accurate prediction of AD/ADRD in diverse and historically underrepresented populations. PREPARE is designed to bring teams together to explore how AI/ML and other computing approaches can be used to collect and analyze data

---

[5] More information on the PREPARE challenge is available at https://www.drivendata.org/competitions/253/competition-nih-alzheimers-adrd-1/ (accessed July 2, 2024).

in ways that could advance the development of tools and technologies for clinical and research use in predicting disease. By encouraging team science approaches and risk taking, challenge programs such as PREPARE stimulate creativity within the scientific community and accelerate the translation of discoveries into tangible solutions. They can also serve as a means of bringing new talent into a field. Moreover, these initiatives often cultivate a culture of innovation within the research workforce by establishing a supportive ecosystem where participants can exchange ideas, bring to bear diverse expertise, and forge partnerships that transcend institutional and geographic boundaries. While challenge programs are not the answer to every knowledge gap, NIH should continue to employ this model where applicable.

Collaborative research mechanisms that engage people living with AD/ADRD and members of the community in which the study is being conducted are critical to ensuring that research on prevention and treatment strategies is conducted in alignment with what is important to those living with, or who are at risk for, the diseases. Such mechanisms come in many forms with the level of engagement varying across a continuum, from advisory bodies (e.g., patient and community advisory boards, focus groups) to community-based participatory research and coproduction models featuring shared decision making between researchers and participants at all phases (Reyes et al., 2023; UK Research and Innovation, 2024). The mechanism employed should be informed by the nature of the study. Advocacy and other organizations that serve people with AD/ADRD and their care partners are also key partners and can facilitate opportunities for the engagement of people with lived experience in research. The benefits are myriad and include enhancing understanding of the experiences, needs, and values of those being asked to participate in research; improving equity in AD/ADRD research; facilitating recruitment and retention of hard-to-reach populations; and informing researchers as to the acceptability and feasibility of both the intervention strategies and the research methods (Kowe et al., 2022; Reyes et al., 2023).

Coordination and collaboration at the program and project level is facilitated and may be incentivized by analogous efforts at the federal level. Collaboration among NIH institutes, centers, and offices and with other federal agencies, such as the Centers for Disease Control and Prevention (CDC), the Centers for Medicare & Medicaid Services (CMS), and the Department of Veteran's Affairs, occurs through a variety of mechanisms with variable levels of formality (e.g., National Alzheimer's Project Act Federal SubGroup, NIH-Wide Microphysiological Systems working group) (NIH, n.d, 2024a).

Greater coordination is needed to reduce siloing across the existing major NIH research investments to leverage the knowledge that has been generated by these individual efforts to advance the AD/ADRD field more broadly. For example, AMP-AD functions in parallel to the AMP for Parkinson's Disease and Related Disorders (AMP-PDRD) and the AMP for Amyotrophic Lateral Sclerosis (AMP-ALS). Similarly, other major AD/ADRD-related programs for genetics research, biobanking, and data infrastructure funded by NIA, NINDS, and other NIH institutes are not well integrated. Breaking down these silos to maximize return on these research investments will require action beyond that which can be driven at the investigator level and will instead require NIH and others leading these programs to actively incentivize opportunities for coordination and integration and the breakdown of any logistical and technical barriers.

Recognizing the existing mechanisms already in place and the challenges of establishing new interagency bodies (e.g., time for agency personnel), the committee encourages NIA, NINDS, and other NIH funders of AD/ADRD research to identify further opportunities to maximally leverage the strengths, resources, and unique capacities of other agencies to advance shared focus areas. For example, existing federal-level collaboration and cofunding among NIA, NINDS, and the National Institute of Environmental Health Sciences (NIEHS) related to exposome research and precision environmental health approaches to AD/ADRD risk reduction and disease prevention (Stetler, 2023) could create new opportunities and incentives for environmental scientists at NIEHS-funded centers to work with ADRCs to advance exposome research related to AD/ADRD. Expanded collaboration across NIA, NINDS, and the National Institute of Mental Health (e.g., building on the joint investments in the Psych-AD program[6] [NIH, 2023b] and other cofunding opportunities [NIH, 2023c]) can accelerate efforts to elucidate interactions between mechanistic pathways contributing to the development of neuropsychiatric symptoms and those underlying the development of AD/ADRD neuropathology. Such efforts may uncover novel targets or strategies for intervention.

Examples of collaborations with other federal agencies might include (1) collaborating with the U.S. Census Bureau to expand access to federal statistical research data centers (FSRDCs) and facilitate the linkage of multiple data types relevant to AD/ADRD within the FSRDCs, (2) working with CMS or FDA to tie expedited review processes for industry to data sharing policies, and (3) working with the CDC to generate a more robust evidence base for public health-level interventions.

---

[6] More information about Psych-AD is available on the AD-Knowledge Portal at https://adknowledgeportal.synapse.org/Explore/Programs/DetailsPage?Program=Psych-AD (accessed October 19, 2024).

Recommendation 4: Enable multidisciplinary, multisector, and collaborative research
The National Institutes of Health (NIH) should expand mechanisms and leverage existing resources to break down silos and encourage multidisciplinary and integrative Alzheimer's disease and related dementias (AD/ADRD) research efforts, including the following:

- Expand trans-NIH initiatives and cofunded projects focused on healthy aging and neurodegenerative diseases to reduce the siloing of research efforts by individual institutes and centers, better cross-link and use existing resources, and address inconsistencies in data sharing policies across NIH institutes and centers while prioritizing data access.
- Prioritize research funding for projects with multidisciplinary research teams (e.g., basic and clinical researchers, population scientists, data scientists and artificial intelligence specialists, and those with lived experience) that address community-informed research questions.
- Expand collaborations globally, including but not limited to low- and middle-income countries and other countries less often involved in such collaborations, for both longitudinal research and clinical trials to better understand the biology of AD/ADRD and enhance the generalizability of findings to diverse populations.
- The National Institute on Aging and the National Institute of Neurological Disorders and Stroke should collaborate with the National Center for Advancing Translational Sciences and others to speed up the translation of research advances to clinical and public health practice and, in turn, expand new research inquiries through the collection of real-world evidence.

Fostering Inclusive Research

A recurring challenge noted throughout the previous chapters of this report is the inadequate diversity of participants included in AD/ADRD research. Lack of representation of specific subpopulations in clinical research is not a problem unique to dementia. Across numerous domains of biomedical research, there are large population groups that are less able to benefit from investments in clinical research and the resulting discoveries because they were not adequately represented in the studies that yielded those discoveries (NASEM, 2022). The result is limited generalizability of clinical research findings to the broader target population, impaired trust in the research enterprise, reduced understanding of the biological phenomena under study, clinical trial failures at later stages, and the compounding of existing health disparities. As noted in a recent National Academies report, "An equitable clinical research enterprise would include trials and studies that match the demographics of the disease burden under study" (NASEM, 2022, p. 1).

As discussed in Chapter 1, the impacts of dementia are not experienced uniformly across the U.S. population (Brewster et al., 2019) or globally. In the United States, racial and ethnic disparities have continued to persist despite overall decreases in clinical dementia prevalence. Black and Hispanic people are more likely to develop clinical dementia compared to non-Hispanic White people (Chen and Zissimopoulos, 2018), and the lifetime risk for women is about twice that of men (Mielke, 2024). The prevalence of AD/ADRD is also increased in rural and lower-income areas (Powell et al., 2020; Wing et al., 2020). And yet, the populations that are disproportionately affected by dementia are persistently underrepresented in AD/ADRD research, both in observational studies and clinical trials (Gilmore-Bykovskyi et al., 2019; Godbole et al., 2023; Lim et al., 2023). The cascading effects on dementia research are myriad and include

- the limited understanding of the contributing factors (e.g., rare genetic variants) and pathways that increase risk and causally contribute to AD/ADRD in diverse populations, which may result in a focus on risk-reduction strategies and intervention targets that are not likely to be effective for some groups who are at higher risk of dementia;
- effects on the establishment of biomarker cutoffs for diagnosis and normative comparisons; and
- the limited generalizability of research findings (i.e., external validity) (Gianattasio et al., 2021), including safety and efficacy data from clinical trials (Canevelli et al., 2019; Franzen et al., 2022), which raises concerns regarding the potential to implement interventions that are ineffective or even unsafe for certain population groups.

Representative studies that incorporate measures of social determinants of health along with multiomics, cardiometabolic, AD and other dementia biomarkers, and cognition are urgently needed. Intensifying investment in understanding factors that contribute to cognitive decline and impairment in underserved populations will enable the implementation of comprehensive, innovative, accessible, and affordable therapies that will mitigate multiple mechanisms driving AD/ADRD.

Increasing the participation of underrepresented populations in dementia research has been a focus of past recommendations to NIH (NASEM, 2017, 2021), and it is clear that NIA, NINDS, and other funders of dementia research are committed to and actively working on closing this gap (Hodes,

2023). Several of the research implementation milestones established by NIH to support the goals of the National Plan to Address Alzheimer's Disease (see Chapter 1) specifically address increasing the inclusion of diverse and underrepresented populations in AD/ADRD research.[7] Many other milestones include a focus on diverse and higher-risk special populations (e.g., individuals with Down Syndrome). Additionally, NIA has indicated that investigator requests to submit large grant applications (i.e., grant application with direct costs totaling $500,000 or more for a single year of support) will receive priority review if they

> (1) include proposed planned enrollment tables representative of the population affected by the disease/condition, and (2) are appropriately inclusive of racial and ethnic minority groups; participants across the lifespan; as well as other populations experiencing health disparities (Santora, 2023).

Given the multiple, interrelated factors that are associated with chronic underrepresentation of certain populations (e.g., some ethnic/racial, people with low socioeconomic or educational attainment), achieving greater inclusivity and accessibility in AD/ADRD research will require a multipronged approach. While many of the barriers are well known and NIH appropriately continues to support research to further elucidate these factors (Ashford et al., 2022, 2023; Mindt et al., 2023), such an approach will benefit from the regular analysis of recruitment, enrollment, and retainment outcomes. For example, the identification of factors that result in studies falling short of recruitment goals can help to identify strategies (e.g., oversampling, use of sampling frames) that can be used to overcome persisting impediments while avoiding the introduction of bias from the use of different recruitment practices for different subpopulations (Raman et al., 2021). Such efforts will ultimately help to build the science of recruitment. The implementation of standardized common data elements for recruitment- and enrollment-based factors could enable better ascertainment of biases at specific stages in the recruitment and screening processes (Manly et al., 2021).

Selection processes—resulting from targeted outreach, selective enrollment, and highly patterned attrition—make it difficult to understand how observations in a selected sample (i.e., study population) relate to the general

---

[7] Implementation milestones specifically focused on inclusion of diverse and underrepresented populations in AD/ADRD research include Milestone 1.C: Population Studies: Diverse cohorts; Milestone 12.A: Recruitment: Diverse community partnerships; Milestone 12.K: Health Equity: Inclusion and retention of underrepresented populations in clinical research; and Milestone 12.L: Health Equity: Inclusion of diverse communities in AD/ADRD research. The AD/ADRD research implementation milestone database is available at https://www.nia.nih.gov/research/milestones (accessed July 1, 2024).

population of older adults (Gibbons et al., 2024). Statistical methods can enable generalization from a highly selected sample to more general target populations based on shared variables measured in the selected sample and the target population. Key to these approaches is having measurements that are identical in the highly selected sample and the target population. Many key demographics (e.g., race, ethnicity, age, gender) are measured with standardized questions, but some important characteristics, such as education and measures of health or cognition, may be measured differently across data sources. There has been little attention to using the same measures as are available in a surveillance-type study of the target population (e.g., the U.S. Census or the National Health and Nutrition Examination Survey), which could help generalize estimates from the highly selected sample to a more representative group. Thus, there is a need for standardized benchmark measurements to be incorporated into new and ongoing studies to evaluate and correct for selection bias.

One novel mechanism that may enable broad reach to a diverse population and mitigate some biases introduced by current recruitment practices is the establishment of an opt-in option for newly age-eligible individuals at the time of Medicare or Medicaid enrollment to receive information on AD/ADRD studies and invitations to contribute to research. While mailings to Medicare beneficiaries are already used in clinical trial recruitment strategies (Grill and Galvin, 2014), such an initiative could better target trial information to enrollees based on areas of interest and baseline data. Enrollees who opt in could be asked for a blood sample, a baseline digital cognitive test, and to fill out a basic life history questionnaire, all of which could be included in a repository. Screening and other data could be provided back to those who opt in as an incentive. Importantly, Medicare and Medicaid already cover routine costs that accompany clinical trial participation, a step that improved equitable access to clinical trials (Takvorian et al., 2021). A collaborative effort by NIH and CMS to establish the infrastructure for such an initiative would further advance health research equity and help to scale up efforts to improve the representativeness of AD/ADRD research.

In 2018, NIA released a National Strategy for Recruitment and Participation in Alzheimer's and Related Dementias Clinical Research[8] that aims to meet the goal of engaging "broad segments of the public in the Alzheimer's and related dementias research enterprise, with a particular focus on underrepresented communities, so studies with an aim to better understand and eventually cure these disorders can successfully and more quickly enroll and retain individuals" (NIA, 2024a). This strategy and its

---

[8] The National Strategy, along with the associated planning guide and online toolbox, is available at https://www.nia.nih.gov/research/recruitment-strategy (accessed July 1, 2024).

related planning guide outline best practices and potential resources for study sites and researchers in overcoming barriers to engaging with and retaining diverse and underrepresented populations in clinical research (NIA, 2024a). Practices highlighted in the strategy align well with those that have been emphasized in the published literature (Brewster et al., 2019; Davis and Bekker, 2022; Mindt et al., 2023) and were discussed with the committee during its public workshop (NASEM, 2024). Examples include the following:

- Establish relationships with communities, employing culturally and linguistically appropriate modalities and content during outreach efforts, and build trust.
- Incorporate community voices into all phases of the study (e.g., through such mechanisms as community advisory boards, community-science partnership boards, and community-based participatory methods).
- Embed trials in communities (particularly those with populations at increased risk), for example by working with federally qualified health centers.
- Take trial activities to the participants by expanding opportunities for virtual engagement, use of in-home testing kits (e.g., for blood sample collection), and digital/remote data collection to increase accessibility.
- Give back to communities, and compensate participants for their time.

To support such efforts, NIA also created an online toolbox of resources—the Alzheimer's and Dementia Outreach, Recruitment, and Engagement Resources (ADORE)—that is based on the recommendations and practices outlined in the planning guide. Resources from this searchable repository include videos specific to diverse and underrepresented communities, outreach materials that can be adapted for use in local communities, and resources from other centers and organizations that can be used to improve recruitment and retention. Knowledge regarding the engagement of diverse populations in research can continue to be evaluated and practices optimized through the use of community-based participatory research projects and other approaches.

While these NIH efforts connect researchers to resources that can support more inclusive research, costs associated with employing these best practices may remain a barrier to adoption. The committee found limited examples of supplemental funding from NIH to expand the participation of underrepresented groups (NINDS, 2021, 2024). Ensuring adequate resources are budgeted for community engagement, recruitment, and the development of culturally appropriate research tools is critical to furthering inclusive AD/ADRD research. Additional funding, including through supplemental funding, could be provided by NIH for recruitment of diverse populations and specific clinical trial financial needs not well covered by project budgets (e.g., transportation for participants, additional medical supplies needed by participants). Strategies for using technological advances to bring these best practices to scale in a cost-effective manner also need to be considered.

Building a diverse research workforce at all levels is another critical factor that was emphasized in the national strategy and planning guide (NIA, 2018, 2019a). Effectively engaging with communities requires insights into, and sensitivity to, the different perspectives and cultures represented therein. This cannot be achieved without a diverse and multidisciplinary study team (NASEM, 2021). Recognizing that inadequate diversity of the scientific workforce is a broader issue that transcends individual studies, NIH established and recently expanded the Resource Centers for Minority Aging Research program, which aims to provide career development (e.g., training, mentorship) to early-career scientists from diverse backgrounds who conduct research related to aging, AD/ADRD, and health disparities in older adults in the areas of social, behavioral, psychological, and economic research (NIA, 2024b). Acknowledging the work NIH is already doing to foster a diverse research workforce, continued efforts are needed to understand and mitigate the barriers to entry and ongoing career advancement into leadership positions. This will include system-level research on barriers, metrics for evaluation, and the expansion of such existing support mechanisms as paid internships and mentorships, collaborative research partnerships, competitive stipends, and salary support to retain researchers in academia).

The development of a diverse research workforce requires early-career professionals to choose to enter and advance their careers in the field. Inadequate compensation for trainees and postdoctoral researchers under NIH-funded awards, however, represents a significant financial barrier to entry into the biomedical research field that may deter pursuit of academic research careers and limit diversity within the research workforce (NIH ACD Working Group, 2023; Sainburg, 2023). Ph.D. training represents a financial burden, even when participating in a fully funded program or prestigious institutional or individual NIH-funded awards (e.g., T32, F31 or F99). Financial stressors extend into postdoctoral training with the rising costs of housing, childcare, and the desire to maintain a reasonable quality of life frequently cited as major career concerns. Between 2020 and 2022, there was a nearly 10 percent decrease in the number of NIH-funded postdoctoral researchers in the health and science fields in the United States (Gewin, 2023). The current NIH structure for postdoctoral stipends results in wages that are below the cost of living in major metropolitan areas and current rules for supplementing stipends from NIH training awards to bring compensation up to a living wage requires the use of non-federal funds, which represents an additional barrier (NIH Office of Extramural Research, 2024; Sainburg, 2023). Relatedly, compensation following training years, in comparison to compensation that could be received in private industry with similar expertise, may not entice early-career researchers to initiate or continue to pursue a career in academic research (Sainburg, 2023). These early financial pressures, in combination with other factors (e.g., uncertain career prospects), disproportionately affect marginalized groups and act as impediments at all career stages to the development of a strong and diverse biomedical research workforce. These factors need to be better understood and swiftly addressed in the context of the AD/ADRD field.

Importantly, endeavors to foster a diverse research workforce need to be focused on overcoming systemic barriers, such as ethnic and racial disparities in the awarding of federal research funding (Ginther et al., 2011; Nguyen et al., 2023) and the lack of research infrastructure and protected faculty time for research at such institutions as historically Black colleges and universities and tribal colleges and universities. Such efforts not only help to address challenges related to underrepresentation in research but ensure that the scientific workforce benefits from the nation's rich diversity of people and their broad range of perspectives and experiences.

Efforts to increase inclusive AD/ADRD research have largely focused on recruitment practices, with less attention given to other factors such as eligibility (Franzen et al., 2022) and retention (Gilmore-Bykovskyi et al., 2019). Exclusion based on eligibility requirements can have the undesirable effect of disengaging people who otherwise would have been interested and willing to participate in research and potentially limiting generalizability to the broader target population, as might be the case when comorbidities such as active depression and diabetes are used as exclusion criteria (Mitchell et al., 2024; Ritchie et al., 2015). Understanding that some eligibility criteria may be instituted to protect the safety of research participants, particularly in the context of clinical trials, consideration should be given to ways to overcome or work around common factors that contribute to attrition at the screening stage (e.g., waiving caregiver/care partner requirements if adequate cognitive function can be demonstrated through ongoing evaluation), particularly for members of underrepresented groups. For example, recent FDA guidance on enhancing the diversity of clinical trial populations suggests considering whether criteria used in earlier-phase trials can be eliminated or modified in later-stage studies (FDA, 2020). There also needs to be consideration as to how gaps in knowledge regarding AD/ADRD in diverse populations may exacerbate underrepresentation caused by eligibility requirements. In developing inclusion and exclusion criteria, study investigators also need to be cognizant of sex and gender differences and how those might influence recruitment and retention.

Accountability—for NIH and NIH-funded investigators—will be a key determinant of future success in these endeavors. On the front end, funding requirements can be used as policy levers to ensure inclusivity is a priority for investigators and considered from the outset of the study. For instance, in some cases restrictions on initiating data collection could be imposed until recruitment goals are met. On the back end, there also needs to be routine tracking of sociodemographic features such as gender, race/ethnicity, socioeconomic status, and geographic region of participants enrolled in NIH-funded AD/ADRD studies.

NIA's Clinical Research Operations & Management System, a system for reporting, tracking, and management of enrollment data and study documents from NIA-funded clinical trials (NIA, 2023a), can aid in monitoring progress toward recruitment goals for the inclusion of underrepresented groups. Such data can inform the implementation and enforcement of policies to address the enrollment of diverse populations and help to identify best practices from successful studies. However, reporting requirements need to be broadened beyond clinical trials to include all study types involving human participants.

While there is some evidence to suggest that the efforts of NIH and those of the broader scientific community are starting to move the needle with regards to representation in AD/ADRD research, progress has been slow. Some measures of diversity in AD/ADRD-related studies are improving as compared to past decades (Lim et al., 2023), but this may not be consistent across all types of research (Franzen et al., 2022) or populations. It is imperative that NIH and AD/ADRD researchers continue to prioritize and incentivize inclusive research and increase accessibility for populations that are historically underrepresented despite being disproportionately affected by dementia.

Recommendation 5: Incentivize inclusive research
The National Institutes of Health should incentivize and guide the use of inclusive research practices to increase the accessibility of clinical and public health research and ensure that study populations are representative of populations at risk for and living with Alzheimer's disease and related dementias (AD/ADRD). These efforts should include the following:
- Strengthen requirements for the recruitment of diverse populations as a condition for initiating data collection (e.g., use of sampling frames as a best practice for targeted and intentional outreach).
- Support research to further understand participant and institutional barriers to involvement in clinical research at all levels.

- Develop social determinants of health metrics to be used as measures of diversity.
- Incentivize the incorporation of standardized benchmark measurements that can be used to evaluate and correct selection bias into new and ongoing research studies.
- Work with the Centers for Medicare & Medicaid Services to explore Medicare and Medicaid enrollment as opportunities for data collection and for enrollees to receive information about participation in AD/ADRD research studies using an opt-in model.
- Support initiatives to identify and overcome barriers to entry and continued professional advancement for a diverse clinical research workforce.

Recommendation 6: Increase the accessibility and generalizability of clinical and public health research
Investigators supported by the National Institutes of Health (NIH) should adopt inclusive research practices to increase the accessibility of clinical and public health research and ensure that study populations are representative of populations at risk for and living with Alzheimer's disease and related dementias (AD/ADRD). To increase research accessibility and generalizability, NIH-supported investigators should do the following:

- Reduce barriers to research participation (e.g., directing ineligible research volunteers to other studies, offering fair compensation, expanding opportunities for virtual participation and passive and/or remote data collection, using in-home testing kits).
- Eliminate unnecessarily restrictive exclusion criteria that screen out diversity in the study population.
- Invest in the development of long-term, mutually beneficial relationships between research institutions and communities, and embed trials sites in communities with underrepresented populations (decentralized trials).
- Meaningfully engage and incorporate the perspectives of research participants and their communities throughout the research design and execution process (e.g., through patient or community advisory councils, codesigning research, community-based participatory research methods, use of community members such as *promotoras* or health navigators to collect data).

Enhancing the Accessibility and Usability of Biological Samples, Data, and Knowledge to Maximize the Returns from AD/ADRD Research

The billions of dollars in funding from NIH and others that has supported scientific investigations in the dementia field and the development of a robust AD/ADRD research infrastructure represents a significant national investment. Careful stewardship of that investment requires attention to opportunities to maximize returns in the form of knowledge, scientific progress, and, ultimately, benefit to society, including those at risk for or living with AD/ADRD. This involves ensuring that the products of research—including biological samples, raw data, and findings—are accessible to, and usable by, the broader scientific community for the purpose of knowledge generation. When data and samples are siloed and sequestered within individual research groups, the kind of collaborative and integrative research called for by the committee cannot be achieved. Sharing processes are likely to differ for finite biological samples as compared to raw data collected through digital technologies (e.g., voice recordings, data from wearable devices and in-home sensors) that can be used indefinitely and simultaneously by multiple data users without losing value over time. Also critical is the compilation and synthesis of knowledge in such a manner that it can be easily accessed and used to draw insights to guide future research and inform clinical care.

Data Access and Usability

The usability of data for future research generally depends on their accessibility, ability to be linked to or compared with other data, and the availability of tools that enable analysis. Small but meaningful signals may only be detectable when data are aggregated into large datasets. Thus, the ability to aggregate data and analyze large datasets with powerful computational tools will enable the generation of new scientific insights (NIA, 2023b). Such capabilities have been significant focus areas for NIH. NIH has affirmed its commitment to open science and open-source principles (Jorgenson, 2023) and is working to apply the FAIR (findable, accessible, interoperable, and reusable) principles in its efforts to create a more integrated data ecosystem to support AD/ADRD research (NIA, 2023b; Wilkinson et al., 2016).

In 2020, NIH released an updated policy on data management and sharing, which went into effect in 2023 (NIH, 2020). The data management and sharing policy requires investigators to submit a data management and sharing plan as a component of an award application and to comply with the plan following NIH approval. The plan is required to specify how scientific data and associated metadata will be managed and shared, with consideration to potential restrictions or limitations on data sharing (NIH, 2020).

In recognition of the gap between the requirements for data sharing and real-world practices, NIH is also investing in research to better understand the factors that pose barriers to or facilitate data sharing (NIH RePORTER, 2023a). Such barriers may include concerns regarding the inability to control how data will be used, potential effects on the ability of the original investigators to publish their analyses of the data, the need to protect participant privacy and confidentiality, and the substantial resources and effort required to share data (Alzheimer Europe, n.d.; Arias et al., 2024). Such barriers point to the importance of data infrastructure and adequate financial support to cover costs, as well as culture, for aligning data sharing practices with current policy.

Cultural barriers to data sharing are a broader issue within the scientific community and beyond the scope of this report. Still, it is worth emphasizing the need for incentives to drive meaningful compliance with existing policies and ensuring consistency across data sharing policies (e.g., across different NIH institutes and centers). Academic reward systems in particular need to place greater value on data sharing. For instance, reuse of datasets could be given similar status as publication citations, but this necessitates a system to ensure original data generators are credited when their data are reused (Pierce et al., 2019).

Reflecting the substantial breadth of NIH-funded AD/ADRD research initiatives, AD/ADRD data infrastructure investments by NIH have included a number of different platforms and repositories to support data storage and accessibility (see Box 5-1). For example,

- All ADRC data (e.g., fluid biomarker, neuroimaging, neuro-pathology, and clinical data) are stored in the National Alzheimer's Coordinating Center (NACC). Such data, including those derived from NIH-supported longitudinal cohort studies, have been critical to fluid and imaging biomarker discovery efforts.
- Data generated by the Alzheimer's Disease Sequencing Project (ADSP) consortia (the AI/ML Consortium, the Phenotype Harmonization Consortium, and the Functional Genomics Consortium) and projects are deposited in NIA data repositories, including the NIA Genetics of Alzheimer's Disease Data Storage Site (NIAGADS).
- Multiomics data collected through such programs as AMP-AD and MODEL-AD are stored in the AD Knowledge Portal and are informing drug development, beginning with target identification and validation and continuing through all phases of clinical trials (Hodes and Buckholtz, 2016; NIA, 2023c).

A key challenge before NIH is to link its major data hubs (e.g., NIAGADS, NACC, Laboratory of Neuro Imaging [LONI]/ADNI, AD Knowledge Portal)

BOX 5-1
Select NIH-Supported Efforts to Strengthen Data Infrastructure and Promote Data Access and Usability for Alzheimer's Disease and Related Dementias (AD/ADRD) Research

AD Knowledge Portal: The National Institute on Aging (NIA)-supported AD Knowledge Portal is a centralized platform maintained by Sage Bionetworks that connects investigators to data, resources, and tools generated from the programs that make up NIA's Alzheimer's Disease Translational Research Program (see Chapter 3) (AD Knowledge Portal, 2024a). Some of these programs include the AMP-AD, TREAT-AD, M²OVE-AD, MODEL-AD, and Resilience-AD. The portal provides information on available data from studies associated with these programs, as well as computational tools and target-enabling resources, among other resources (AD Knowledge Portal, 2024b). The portal also supports the integration of a number of external data analysis platforms to better facilitate the usability and interoperability of data from the portal (AD Knowledge Portal, 2024c). Additionally, the portal provides information about, and navigation to, additional resources and tools that can be found on other platforms (e.g., the Alzheimer's Disease Preclinical Efficiency Database, Agora, AD Atlas, NIAGADS) (AD Knowledge Portal, 2024a).

Agora: Agora is an NIA-funded, interactive web platform managed by Sage Bionetworks that hosts high-dimensional transcriptomic, proteomic, and metabolomic data and novel drug targets for AD. The over 900 novel drug targets included on the platform were nominated by researchers working in the AD/ADRD field, including researchers involved with AMP-AD (see Box 3-4) and TREAT-AD (see Box 3-5) (Agora, 2024a). The web application provides several different interfaces that can be used by investigators to explore genes and targets, such as a gene comparison tool through which detailed expression information can be viewed and compared (Agora, 2024b).

National Institute on Aging Genetics of Alzheimer's Disease Data Storage Site (NIAGADS): NIAGADS is supported by a cooperative agreement between NIA and the University of Pennsylvania and serves as a national repository for genotypic data (e.g., data from genome-wide association studies, next-generation sequencing, targeted genome sequencing) to facilitate research on including the discovery of new therapeutic approaches (NIAGADS, 2024a). All NIA-funded studies of genetics of late-onset AD are required to deposit data at NIAGADS and/or a different site approved by NIA (2023d). As of October 2024, the continuously updated repository includes 128 datasets and over 23 types of data (NIAGADS, 2024b). In addition to storing and facilitating access to and the exploration of these data, NIAGADS connects investigators

BOX 5-1 Continued

to other datasets stored on other platforms (e.g., imaging data from the Alzheimer's Disease Neuroimaging Initiative) (NIAGADS, 2024a).

National Alzheimer's Coordinating Center (NACC): NACC is an NIA-funded resource and hub for research coordination housed at the University of Washington that serves as a centralized data repository for ADRCs (NACC, 2024a), which contribute data from enrolled participants to the NACC uniform dataset (UDS) (NACC, 2024b). The UDS contains data from all participants enrolled by the ADRCs since 2005; importantly, these data do not represent a representative sample of the U.S. population. In 2012, NACC launched a voluntary Frontotemporal Lobar Degeneration module, followed by similar modules for Lewy body disease and Down syndrome in 2017 and 2020, respectively (NACC, 2024b). The NACC data platform is undergoing significant modernization to enable greater integration of data streams and data linking across different repositories (e.g., National Centralized Repository for Alzheimer's Disease and Related Dementias, NIAGADS) with ADRC data, as well as providing tools to facilitate data searching, visualization, and access by investigators (NACC, 2024c).

into an agile, integrated data ecosystem while preserving the autonomy of the individual platforms and their respective strengths and networks (NIA, 2023b), with an emphasis on the inclusion of repositories with data on related dementias. This integrated system should enable researchers without deep data analytics expertise to locate, access, and query existing data from NIH-funded research and, when available, data submitted by other investigators. This is a formidable undertaking but critical to maximizing insights from AD/ADRD research and returns from NIH's various investments. Insights captured during recent NIH-hosted workshops on the topics of data infrastructure and interoperability (NIA, 2023b, 2024c) can guide these efforts.

Given the diversity of data types, data sources, and constraints such as privacy protection needs, there is no single solution to data management and accessibility. For example, although AI/ML models may facilitate the sharing and processing of digital data, commercially available platforms lack transparency and have associated privacy and security concerns. It will be important for NIH to work with investigators to identify solutions to data access challenges. While many datasets can and should be made publicly available, for others, such as clinical datasets with protected health information generated by private health systems, data accessibility may need to be achieved through other means (e.g., federated data analyses). One solution to data that cannot be shared is to enable code generated by external investigators (generated, for example, using a synthetic dataset) to be run using a secure system that outputs the results from the executed program without allowing the investigator to see the data being analyzed. Consideration could also be given to categorizing data into access levels. At the lowest level would be those data that can be made freely available without any permission process to access them. Higher levels would involve increasingly more stringent access permission processes based on the sensitivity of the data and privacy/confidentiality concerns. For datasets that include both sensitive and nonsensitive data, such an approach may improve access to those data that are not sensitive by reducing hurdles associated with permission processes.

Accessibility is necessary but not sufficient to ensure that data from past AD/ADRD research are usable to the fullest extent possible. A key challenge has been the lack of interoperability and comparability of data from different studies, which impedes data integration and cross-study analyses. Investments in basic and preclinical research and longitudinal cohort studies have resulted in the generation of large and diverse (e.g., genetic, exposome, functional omics) datasets that can guide the development of effective interventions for AD/ADRD. A notable challenge, however, is the harmonization and integration of data to make them available and ready for analysis so that the many potential targets can be comparatively evaluated and prioritized for intervention development, with consideration of the needs of diverse populations.

One way NIH has sought to make data more comparable is through the standardization and harmonization of data collection tools and outcome measures (e.g., common data elements [CDEs]). The NINDS Common Data Elements project, for instance, had resulted in the creation of data standards for neuroscientific clinical research, including both general and disease-specific CDEs (NINDS, n.d.). Another example of such efforts is the Harmonized Cognitive Assessment Protocol (HCAP) (see Box 2-11 in Chapter 2), the design of which was led by the investigators of the Health and Retirement Study with the goal of creating a flexible instrument for detailed cognitive assessment of older adults that would be comparable across populations in diverse contexts (e.g., cultural, educational, social, economic, political) (Gross et al., 2023). In the digital data space, NIH is seeking to develop standards for wearable/sensor data and automated scripts that can convert raw data into a standardized format to facilitate integration with other patient data types (e.g., clinical, molecular, digital) (NIA, 2019b, 2024d). The status of these efforts is unclear, however, and expansion of data standardization and harmonization remains a priority. In February 2023, NIA convened an expert meeting to explore the use of

CDEs to harmonize data from real-world-data (RWD) sources, such as health care claims and electronic health records, with the goal of accelerating AD/ADRD research (Lieberthal et al., 2023). Looking to the future, new harmonization methods will be required to meet the needs of a broad range of analytic approaches (e.g., biostatistics/epidemiology, data science/AI, and other emerging methods such as quantum computing) used for both structured and unstructured data (e.g., digital images and raw digital data streams such as voice recordings).

With the growing volume and diversity of data being generated through AD/ADRD research, data integration and analysis are requiring increasingly complex tools and analytic methods. Such capabilities will be needed to advance precision medicine approaches, for example, by enabling the extraction of patterns that could guide population stratification, matching of subgroups to interventions, and life-course timing for those interventions. AI/ML and other computational methods (e.g., network analysis) hold great promise for enabling the linkage and subsequent extraction of insights from large and complex datasets to inform intervention strategies. These methods need to be biologically informed and relevant to clinical phenotypes, which will require close collaborations between AI/data scientists and biomedical researchers (Recommendation 4).

Academia is well suited to the experimentation and small-scale, proof-of-concept development that can lead to novel analytic tools but may lack access to the computational resources available in private industry (NASEM, 2024). Thus, there is a need for national-level resources that can support the development of novel, open-source data acquisition, ingestion, cleaning, processing, and harmonization tools to deliver data in a sufficient form for different analytic methods. Some initiatives that could meet this need are already underway. The National Artificial Intelligence Research Resource (NAIRR) pilot, an NSF-led, multipartner effort—including federal agencies and private-sector, nonprofit, and philanthropic partners—to develop a proof of concept for shared national AI research resources, represents a first step in in this direction. As part of the NAIRR pilot, NIH will co-lead with the DOE an operational focus area on data privacy and security and "provide open and controlled-access to NIH computing and data platforms and biomedical datasets to support health care-focused AI research (NSF, 2024).

Additionally, in 2021, NIA awarded funds for the creation of Artificial Intelligence and Technology Collaboratories (AITCs), which serve as national resources to "promote the development and implementation of artificial intelligence approaches and technology through demonstration projects to improve care and health outcomes for older Americans, including persons living with dementia and their caregivers" (NIA, 2023e). The AITCs are developing approaches for the analysis of raw digital data; creating policies and best practices for the incorporation of AI in partnership with industry, venture capitalists, and health care systems; and piloting new tools and technologies in collaboration with these partners and the NIA Small Business Programs (NIA, 2023e). The AITCs operate through pilot awards and are intended to create an ecosystem that fosters innovation and transdisciplinary collaboration spanning academia and industry (Abadir et al., 2024; NIH RePORTER, 2023b). In the longer term, NIH will need to evaluate the success of such innovative models and their potential role in broader efforts to use AI/ML and other technologies to accelerate data integration and knowledge generation.

Recommendation 7: Ensure data access to maximize research returns
Using the National Institutes of Health (NIH) Data Management and Sharing Policy as a foundation, NIH should convene and support an NIH workgroup to work with NIH-funded investigators to identify and implement solutions to barriers that impede access to data from Alzheimer's disease and related dementias research. Specific issues that should be addressed by the NIH workgroup include but are not limited to the following:
- the need for a centralized and continuously updated NIH-managed system for locating and searching existing data sources across different (NIH and non-NIH) data platforms;
- provision of incentives and clear procedures for ensuring compliance with the Data Management and Sharing Policy;
- approaches to maximize access to data from initiatives funded by multiple NIH institutes and centers;
- incentivization of transparent reporting and the synthesis of findings from negative studies, including observational studies and clinical trials, ideally with accompanying data release;
- provision of project-specific supplemental funding, including additional administrative supplements, commensurate with the anticipated level of data and code sharing;
- formulation of guidance for subsets of data within any given dataset to be categorized into access levels based on the access controls needed to protect sensitive data (e.g., participant health information) such that the portion of data requiring no permission for use can be made publicly available;
- return of derived data and analysis code from data users, as well as the return of newly collected data from ancillary studies, to the parent study while respecting the need to protect intellectual property and innovation;
- approaches to facilitate access to data from international collaborations; and

- expansion of capacity for storing raw digital data (e.g., unstructured data such as images and high-velocity voice recordings and sensor data).

Recommendation 8: Enhance data usability for future research
To enable the usability of data generated by Alzheimer's disease and related dementias research funded by the National Institutes of Health (NIH), NIH should do the following:
- Invest in data harmonization and interoperability efforts (e.g., use of common data elements) across data platforms and through collaborations across institutions and organizations, ensuring that levels of harmonization are aligned with the needs of different analytic approaches.
- Set requirements for user-intuitive data dictionaries.
- Explore new approaches, such as natural language processing, to automate the integration of different data types (e.g., clinical phenotype, multiomics data, exposure data).
- Fund the development and dissemination of novel open-source tools and analytic methods (e.g., large language models and other artificial intelligence/machine learning methods, statistical transport methods, data fusion approaches, synthetic data) to collect, link, explore, and query existing data and support efficient analyses when data privacy rules create barriers.
- Provide dedicated grants for investigators working in settings with proprietary data that are difficult to share (e.g., major clinical datasets) focused on data curation or supporting analyses by external researchers.

Biobanking

The continued evolution of technology, tools, and analytic methods will create new opportunities to analyze previously stored biological samples in ways that may not be possible to predict at present. Such future analyses may lead to the development of novel therapeutics or biomarkers. Consideration of this future value of biological samples collected from research participants or donated by other members of the public is important when investing in infrastructure and plans for collection and storage. For example, attention needs to be given to the harmonized collection and storage of pre- and postmortem samples from across cohorts so that variation in collection and storage procedures does not introduce undesired variability that compromises the comparability of data from the later analyses of those samples. Furthermore, stored samples have little value if they are not accessible to the scientific community. Ensuring accessibility entails the development of transparent inventories of samples that are available to external investigators and clear processes for sample requests and decision making on sample sharing. As described earlier, access to biological samples from international collaborations remains a priority barrier to be addressed.

NIH has made substantial investments in infrastructure for biobanking, as described in Chapter 2. However, critical gaps remain, and initiatives and resources appear fragmented. Research institutions outside of the ADRCs may lack the pathology laboratory infrastructure to collect certain valuable samples (e.g., well-characterized brain tissue) from decedents enrolled in longitudinal studies. With adequate support, ADRCs and other large NIH-funded programs such as the Alzheimer's Clinical Trials Consortium could expand autopsy and brain collection services to participants enrolled in studies at other institutions. Such a system may help to address the current dearth of samples from diverse participants but would need to ensure that costs for autopsy and transportation to and from the donation site do not fall on the research participants or their families. Additionally, capacity to store biosamples, also a cost-intensive undertaking, is limited. As a result, precious samples may be discarded at the completion of studies. Repositories may be sent sample collections with little advance notice and through processes that are ad hoc.

Maximizing the use and value of biological samples will require a more structured and standardized system for collection, archiving, and access. Biosample sharing systems should also require the return of results from analyses of shared samples back to the parent study so that these new data are made available along with any previously generated phenotypic and other data related to the shared sample (see Recommendation 2). This will ensure future requests for biosamples are made in the context of knowing what has already been measured and will avoid duplicate measurements on precious samples.

Technologies that have enabled the digitization and computational analysis of histopathological samples are transforming the practice of neuropathology. The portability and rapid transferability of digital image files in comparison to traditional slides enhances the accessibility of these valuable data sources (Scalco et al., 2023). The capability to use AI/ML for analysis of whole slide images opens opportunities to shift to quantitative measurement of the neuroanatomic distribution of pathologies (Shakir and Dugger, 2022). This kind of scalable quantitative method has the potential to allow deeper phenotyping of AD/ADRD and the correlation of specific clinical phenotypes to patterns of neuropathology. Incorporation of digital pathology methods into cohort studies is just getting underway, and digitization of existing slide inventories at ADRCs has been slow. ADRC personnel have reported a lack of resource support for digital pathology and ML (Scalco et al., 2023). NIH can advance AD/ADRD disease phenotyping and the current understanding of the neuropathologic landscape by ensuring adequate support for the implementation and refinement of digital pathology methods. Importantly, infrastructure support needs to go beyond equipment (e.g., slide scanners, data storage/servers) and include the full range of expertise needed for implementation (e.g., pathologists, ML engineers, information technology personnel, statisticians, and database managers) (Shakir and Dugger, 2022). These efforts should be guided by the existing ADRC Digital Pathology Working Group (Scalco et al., 2023).

Recommendation 9: Expand the capacity to collect and store biological samples generated through National Institutes of Health (NIH)-funded research
The National Institute on Aging, along with the National Institute of Neurological Disorders and Stroke, should expand support for the collection and storage of valuable biological samples from NIH-funded Alzheimer's disease and related dementias research in a manner that maximizes opportunities for future use. This should include the following:
- Provide supplements to researchers that meet the actual cost of storing and sharing samples following study completion.
- Expand support for the collection and storage of highly characterized biological samples (e.g., antemortem and postmortem blood and cerebrospinal fluid, donated brains) from participants of any longitudinal research studies and clinical trials, and from the public.
- Use standardized sample collection, assessment, and storage practices with careful consideration of the implications of different storage approaches for future value.
- Facilitate access to biological samples from international collaborations.
- Support digitized neuropathology to enable quantitative analysis using artificial intelligence and other computational methods.

Catalyze Transformational Change Through Innovation in AD/ADRD Research

Accelerating progress in AD/ADRD prevention and treatment will require transformational change that can only be achieved through greater support for innovation in NIH-supported research. Such efforts may look different at different stages in the research continuum and would include the following:

- Basic research: developing and applying novel models and tools, seeking potential points of connection and commonalities with related fields (e.g., aging, other neurodegenerative diseases).
- Translational research: increasing the viability of innovative research targets and approaches.
- Clinical research: adopting innovative trial designs and participant recruitment and engagement mechanisms.
- Population research: identifying and integrating novel data sources that can be used to evaluate population-level strategies (e.g., policies or exposures that vary across larger geographic units) and effects on inequalities.

The current system for peer review at NIH favors investigators and projects for which there are strong track records and evidence for likely success based on existing preliminary data. Although the current process has many advantages, it is not ideally suited to promoting innovation and truly novel methods. Incentives and novel strategies are needed to promote more disruptive research approaches that may lead to significant steps forward.

Agencies such as the Defense Advanced Research Projects Agency and the Advanced Research Projects Agency for Health (ARPA-H) are specifically focused on high-risk, high-reward research to generate innovative solutions to complex problems. While the committee's charge is to recommend research priorities for NIH, ARPA-H, with its focus on accelerating better health outcomes, holds promise for advancing the kind of transformational research that is needed to accelerate the prevention and treatment of AD/ADRD. Indeed, the Advisory Council on Alzheimer's Research, Care, and Services recommended that ARPA-H "implement a dementia portfolio that enables the translation and demonstration of scientific breakthroughs in the diagnosis, treatment, and management of dementias and facilitates efficient translation of evidence to patient care" (Advisory Council on Alzheimer's Research, Care, and Services, 2024, p. 21).

As an example of its potential for breakthroughs in dementia treatment, in April 2024 ARPA-H forayed into the field of neurodegenerative diseases with its funding of a new project on Cell Therapies for Neuroinflammation and Neurodegeneration (CT-NEURO) (ARPA-H, 2024a). The CT-NEURO program aims to develop an immune cell-based, disease-agnostic platform that can deliver therapeutics to the brain and central nervous system to treat diverse neurological conditions, including neurodegeneration. As projects such as CT-NEURO come to completion, NIH should be prepared to transition relevant innovations into its portfolio of ongoing AD/ADRD research. For example, another potential ARPA-H project of relevance is the advancement of digital histopathology capabilities including automated analysis using AI/ML (NASEM, 2024). While envisioned as supporting the

Cancer Moonshot initiative, such a capability also has clear relevance to neurodegenerative disease research and practice (see Recommendation 9).

Of note, because ARPA-H-funded research is time delimited by design, transition of the resulting scientific and technological breakthroughs into real-world application is an integral part of the life cycle of ARPA-H projects and programs. The Project Accelerator Transition Innovation Office (PATIO) helps ARPA-H awardees identify investors and customers but also works with CMS and FDA to develop strategies for regulatory approval (e.g., for technologies that may not fit into traditional FDA pathways) and reimbursement (ARPA-H, 2024b). This approach creates the necessary demand–pull conditions to ensure innovations reach the market (Pannu et al., 2023). The absence of a similar transition model for innovative technologies (e.g., digital technologies for AD/ADRD diagnosis) arising from NIH-funded research serves as a barrier to the financial sustainability of the innovative product and future product development.

The NIH Small Business Innovation Research (SBIR) and Small Business Technology Transfer (STTR) funding mechanisms and the NIH Blueprint for Neuroscience Research program provide some support for converting research ideas into commercially viable products. For example, in addition to providing funding for drug discovery and development, the Blueprint Neurotherapeutics Network offers access to consultants with extensive industry drug development experience (NIH, 2024b). Such mechanisms, however, fall short of addressing the needs around nontraditional regulatory pathways and reimbursement, gaps that warrant NIH attention.

Funding mechanisms such as SBIR/STTR and NIH Blueprint function to derisk investment in innovation. The phased funding in SBIR, for example, enables awardees to establish the scientific merit, feasibility, and commercialization of the proposed research in phase 1 (approximately 0.5–2 years) prior to receipt of a larger and longer-term (1–3 years) funding award for phase 2 (NIH, 2024c). A fast-track path allows a single application to cover both phases. Some philanthropic funders also seek to derisk novel approaches by funding proof-of-concept research and pilot-scale projects to generate the initial data needed to secure longer-term funding, including follow-on awards from NIH (FNIH, 2023).

These kinds of phased funding approaches, which can involve a review of a priori-specified milestones prior to transition to phase 2 (NASEM, 2015), could be adapted to further promote innovative and high-risk AD/ADRD research. For example, partnerships between NIH and philanthropic groups could create a seamless transition from philanthropic proof-of-concept funding to NIH grant funding. Additionally, NIH and the FNIH could collaborate to build private–public partnerships for fast-tracked phase 1–2 high-risk research opportunities. In such a model, NIH could fund phase 1 with the goal of lowering the risk for the phase 2 component, which would be focused on scalability and could largely be funded through industry. Public–private partnerships enable the leveraging of the respective talents of industry and academia and best-in-class practices (e.g., data infrastructure and knowledge management, social engagement) from other sectors.

Other funding mechanisms to support innovation could include supplements focused on critical scientific areas or technologies and R56 awards (or similar) focused on high-risk, high-reward research. The R56 mechanism would allow discrete pieces of an R01 application that include novel ideas to be funded in cases where the full application did not meet criteria for an R01 award.

Recommendation 10: Support innovation across all stages of National Institutes of Health (NIH)-funded research
NIH should use existing funding structures and other incentive mechanisms to stimulate innovation across all stages of Alzheimer's disease and related dementias (AD/ADRD) research. This could include the following:

- Implement advances and tools generated by the Advanced Research Projects Agency for Health and others into NIH-funded AD/ADRD research, including advances that are specific to dementia and those that can be applied from other fields.
- Field a program-wide review of the opportunities and barriers to interdisciplinary and transformational research at NIH-funded AD/ADRD centers and infrastructure programs (e.g., the Alzheimer's Disease Research Centers) and their capacity to prioritize the inclusion of diverse populations and foster innovative research with high potential for population impact.
- Capitalize on the best-in-class practices and technologies of other fields that are applicable to, and may address, current AD/ADRD research needs (e.g., data infrastructure and knowledge management, social engagement for recruitment).
- Prioritize support for research inquiries that have clear potential for future scalability and uptake.
- Build partnerships with foundations and other research funders to coordinate seamless funding pathways for fast-tracked phase 1–2 high-risk research opportunities.
- Identify and provide short-term funding for specific, highly innovative components of otherwise unsuccessful new and competing award applications.
- Identify past funded projects in the NIH portfolio that have progressed to real-world clinical implementation and adapt the grant review process to include criteria that promotes real-world clinical implementation.

CONCLUDING REMARKS

The last decade of research has seen encouraging progress in the capability to detect early signals of changes in brain health, to understand the pathophysiologic mechanisms underlying AD/ADRD, and to develop and evaluate preventive and therapeutic interventions. Accelerating progress in AD/ADRD prevention and treatment will require transformation and new direction. With continued strategic research investments as outlined by the committee, there is good reason to hope that the coming years will see significant progress in the capability to prevent and treat AD/ADRD. Through the continued and collaborative efforts of NIH, academic researchers, private industry, health care professionals, funders, policy makers, advocates, and people living with cognitive and other forms of impairment from AD/ADRD, it is possible to envision a future where dementia is not inevitable for millions of people across the globe but is preventable and treatable.

REFERENCES

Abadir, P., E. Oh, R. Chellappa, N. Choudhry, G. Demiris, D. Ganesan, J. Karlawish, B. Marlin, R. M. Li, N. Dehak, A. Arbaje, M. Unberath, T. Cudjoe, C. Chute, J. H. Moore, P. Phan, Q. Samus, N. L. Schoenborn, A. Battle, and J. D. Walston. 2024. Artificial intelligence and technology collaboratories: Innovating aging research and Alzheimer's care. *Alzheimer's & Dementia* 20(4):3074-3079.

AD Knowledge Portal. 2024a. *Welcome to the AD Knowledge Portal.* https://adknowledgeportal.synapse.org/ (accessed August 22, 2024).

AD Knowledge Portal. 2024b. *Explore.* https://adknowledgeportal.synapse.org/Explore/Studies (accessed October 29, 2024).

AD Knowledge Portal. 2024c. *Analysis platforms.* https://adknowledgeportal.synapse.org/Analysis%20Platforms (accessed August 22, 2024).

Advisory Council on Alzheimer's Research, Care, and Services. 2024. *Public members of the Advisory Council on Alzheimer's Research, Care, and Services: 2024 recommendations.* https://aspe.hhs.gov/collaborations-committees-advisory-groups/napa/napa-documents/napa-recommendations (Accessed on November 11, 2024).

Agora. 2024a. *About.* https://agora.adknowledgeportal.org/about (accessed August 22, 2024).

Agora. 2024b. *Gene comparison tool.* https://agora.adknowledgeportal.org/genes/comparison (accessed August 22, 2024).

Alzheimer Europe. n.d. Data sharing in dementia research—the EU landscape. https://www.alzheimer-europe.org/policy/positions/data-sharing-dementia-research-eu-landscape?language_content_entity=en (accessed September 19, 2024).

Amini, S., B. Hao, J. Yang, C. Karjadi, V. B. Kolachalama, R. Au, and I. C. Paschalidis. 2024. Prediction of Alzheimer's disease progression within 6 years using speech: A novel approach leveraging language models. *Alzheimer's & Dementia* 20(8):5262-5270.

Arias, J. J., A. M. Tyler, L. M. Beskow, M. C. Carillo, S. Dickinson, J. Goldman, M. A. Majumder, M. M. Mello, H. M. Snyder, and J. S. Yokoyama. 2024. Data stewardship in FTLD research: Investigator and research participant views. *Alzheimer's & Dementia* 20(4):2886-2893.

ARPA-H (Advanced Research Projects Agency for Health). 2024a. *ARPA-H funds project to develop treatments for neurodegenerative diseases.* https://arpa-h.gov/news-and-events/arpa-h-funds-project-develop-treatments-neurodegenerative-diseases (accessed August 21, 2024).

ARPA-H. 2024b. *Project Accelerator Transition Innovation Office (PATIO).* https://arpa-h.gov/engage-and-transition/patio (accessed August 21, 2024).

Ashford, M. T., R. Raman, G. Miller, M. C. Donohue, O. C. Okonkwo, M. R. Mindt, R. L. Nosheny, G. A. Coker, R. C. Petersen, P. S. Aisen, M. W. Weiner, and the Alzheimer's Disease Neuroimaging Initiative. 2022. Screening and enrollment of underrepresented ethnocultural and educational populations in the Alzheimer's Disease Neuroimaging Initiative (ADNI). *Alzheimer's & Dementia* 18(12):2603-2613.

Ashford, M. T., D. Zhu, J. Bride, E. McLean, A. Aaronson, C. Conti, C. Cypress, P. Griffin, R. Ross, T. Duncan, X. Deng, A. Ulbricht, J. Fockler, M. R. Camacho, D. Flenniken, D. Truran, S. R. Mackin, C. Hill, M. W. Weiner, D. Byrd, R. W. Turner II, H. Cham, M. Rivera Mindt, and R. L. Nosheny. 2023. Understanding online registry facilitators and barriers experienced by Black brain health registry participants: The Community Engaged Digital Alzheimer's Research (CEDAR) Study. *Journal of Prevention of Alzheimer's Disease* 10(3):551-561.

Berkness, T., M. C. Carrillo, R. Sperling, R. Petersen, P. Aisen, C. Flournoy, H. Snyder, R. Raman, and J. D. Grill. 2021. The Institute on Methods and Protocols for Advancement of Clinical Trials in ADRD (IMPACT-AD): A novel clinical trials training program. *Journal of Prevention of Alzheimer's Disease* 8(3):286-291.

Boxer, A. L., and R. Sperling. 2023. Accelerating Alzheimer's therapeutic development: The past and future of clinical trials. *Cell* 186(22):4757-4772.

Brewster, P., L. Barnes, M. Haan, J. K. Johnson, J. J. Manly, A. M. Napoles, R. A. Whitmer, L. Carvajal-Carmona, D. Early, S. Farias, E. R. Mayeda, R. Melrose, O. L. Meyer, A. Zeki Al Hazzouri, L. Hinton, and D. Mungas. 2019. Progress and future challenges in aging and diversity research in the United States. *Alzheimer's & Dementia* 15(7):995-1003.

Canevelli, M., G. Bruno, G. Grande, F. Quarata, R. Raganato, F. Remiddi, M. Valletta, V. Zaccaria, N. Vanacore, and M. Cesari. 2019. Race reporting and disparities in clinical trials on Alzheimer's disease: A systematic review. *Neuroscience & Biobehavioral Reviews* 101:122-128.

Chen, C., and J. M. Zissimopoulos. 2018. Racial and ethnic differences in trends in dementia prevalence and risk factors in the United States. *Alzheimer's & Dementia (N Y)* 4:510-520.

Cummings, J., Y. Zhou, G. Lee, K. Zhong, J. Fonseca, and F. Cheng. 2024. Alzheimer's disease drug development pipeline: 2024. *Alzheimer's & Dementia: Translational Research & Clinical Interventions* 10(2):e12465.

Davis, R., and P. Bekker. 2022. Recruitment of older adults with dementia for research: An integrative review. *Research into Gerontological Nursing* 15(5):255-264.

Diverse VCID. 2024. *Who we are.* https://diversevcid.ucdavis.edu/our-goal (accessed August 22, 2024).

Driven Data. 2024. *PREPARE: Pioneering Research for Early Prediction of Alzheimer's and Related Dementias EUREKA Challenge.* https://www.drivendata.org/competitions/253/competition-nih-alzheimers-adrd-1/ (accessed November 9, 2024).

Fang, J., A. A. Pieper, R. Nussinov, G. Lee, L. Bekris, J. B. Leverenz, J. Cummings, and F. Cheng. 2020. Harnessing endophenotypes and network medicine for Alzheimer's drug repurposing. *Medical Research Review* 40(6):2386-2426.

FDA (Food and Drug Administration). 2020. *Enhancing the diversity of clinical trial populations—eligibility criteria, enrollment practices, and trial designs guidance for industry.* https://www.fda.gov/regulatory-information/search-fda-guidance-documents/enhancing-diversity-clinical-trial-populations-eligibility-criteria-enrollment-practices-and-trial?utm_medium=email&utm_source=govdelivery (accessed August 21, 2024).

FDA. 2022. *Master protocols: Efficient clinical trial design strategies to expedite development of oncology drugs and biologics guidance for industry.* https://www.fda.gov/regulatory-information/search-fda-guidance-documents/master-protocols-efficient-clinical-trial-design-strategies-expedite-development-oncology-drugs-and (accessed August 21, 2024).

FNIH (Foundation for the National Institutes of Health). 2023. *Our mission.* https://fnih.org/who-we-are/ (accessed August 21, 2024).

Franzen, S., J. E. Smith, E. van den Berg, M. Rivera Mindt, R. L. van Bruchem-Visser, E. L. Abner, L. S. Schneider, N. D. Prins, G. M. Babulal, and J. M. Papma. 2022. Diversity in Alzheimer's disease drug trials: The importance of eligibility criteria. *Alzheimer's & Dementia* 18(4):810-823.

Gewin, V. 2023. Postdoctoral researchers warn NIH that cost-of-living pressures are gutting the workforce. *Nature,* June 29.

Gianattasio, K. Z., E. E. Bennett, J. Wei, M. L. Mehrotra, T. Mosley, R. F. Gottesman, D. F. Wong, E. A. Stuart, M. E. Griswold, D. Couper, M. M. Glymour, M. C. Power, and the Alzheimer's Disease Neuroimaging Initiative. 2021. Generalizability of findings from a clinical sample to a community-based sample: A comparison of ADNI and ARIC. *Alzheimer's & Dementia* 17(8):1265-1276.

Gibbons, L., T. Mobley, E. Mayeda, C. Lee, N. Gatto, A. LaCroix, L. McEvoy, P. Crane, and E. Hayes-Larson. 2024. How generalizable are findings from a community-based prospective cohort study? Extending estimates from the Adult Changes in Thought Study to its source population. *Journal of Alzheimer's Disease* 100(1):163-174.

Gilmore-Bykovskyi, A. L., Y. Jin, C. Gleason, S. Flowers-Benton, L. M. Block, P. Dilworth-Anderson, L. L. Barnes, M. N. Shah, and M. Zuelsdorff. 2019. Recruitment and retention of underrepresented populations in Alzheimer's disease research: A systematic review. *Alzheimer's & Dementia (N Y)* 5:751-770.

Ginther, D., S. W., J. Schnell, B. Masimore, F. Liu, L. Haak, and R. Kington. 2011. Race, ethnicity, and NIH reserach awards. *Science* 333(6045):1015-1019.

Gladman, J. T., R. A. Corriveau, S. Debette, M. Dichgans, S. M. Greenberg, P. S. Sachdev, J. M. Wardlaw, and G. J. Biessels. 2019. Vascular contributions to cognitive impairment and dementia: Research consortia that focus on etiology and treatable targets to lessen the burden of dementia worldwide. *Alzheimer's & Dementia (N Y)* 5:789-796.

Godbole, N., S. C. Kwon, J. M. Beasley, T. Roberts, J. Kranick, J. Smilowitz, A. Park, S. E. Sherman, C. Trinh-Shevrin, and J. Chodosh. 2023. Assessing equitable inclusion of underrepresented older adults in Alzheimer's disease, related cognitive disorders, and aging-related research: A scoping review. *Gerontologist* 63(6):1067-1077.

Greenberg, S. M. 2017. William M. Feinberg award for excellence in clinical stroke: Big pictures and small vessels. *Stroke* 48(9):2628-2631.

Gregory, S., S. Saunders, and C. W. Ritchie. 2022. Science disconnected: The translational gap between basic science, clinical trials, and patient care in Alzheimer's disease. *Lancet Healthy Longevity* 3(11):e797-e803.

Grill, J. D., and J. E. Galvin. 2014. Facilitating Alzheimer disease research recruitment. *Alzheimer's Disease & Associated Disorders* 28(1):1-8.

Gross, A. L., C. Li, E. M. Briceno, M. Arce Renteria, R. N. Jones, K. M. Langa, J. J. Manly, E. Nichols, D. Weir, R. Wong, L. Berkman, J. Lee, and L. C. Kobayashi. 2023. Harmonisation of later-life cognitive function across national contexts: Results from the harmonized cognitive assessment protocols. *Lancet Healthy Longevity* 4(10):e573-e583.

Hodes, R. J. 2023. *NIA's commitment to inclusion.* https://www.nia.nih.gov/research/blog/2023/11/nias-commitment-inclusion (accessed August 21, 2024, 2024).

Hodes, R. J., and N. Buckholtz. 2016. Accelerating Medicines Partnership: Alzheimer's Disease (AMP-AD) knowledge portal aids Alzheimer's drug discovery through open data sharing. *Expert Opinions on Therapeutic Targets* 20(4):389-391.

Jorgenson, L. 2023. *Advancing the promise of open science: We want to hear from you!* https://osp.od.nih.gov/advancing-the-promise-of-open-science/ (accessed August 22, 2024).

Kaye, J., P. Aisen, R. Amariglio, R. Au, C. Ballard, M. Carrillo, H. Fillit, T. Iwatsubo, G. Jimenez-Maggiora, S. Lovestone, F. Natanegara, K. Papp, M. E. Soto, M. Weiner, B. Vellas, and the EU/US CTAD Task Force. 2021. Using digital tools to advance Alzheimer's drug trials during a pandemic: The EU/U.S. CTAD Task Force. *Journal of Prevention of Alzheimer's Disease* 8(4):513-519.

Kim, C. K., Y. R. Lee, L. Ong, M. Gold, A. Kalali, and J. Sarkar. 2022. Alzheimer's disease: Key insights from two decades of clinical trial failures. *Journal of Alzheimer's Disease* 87(1):83-100.

Kowe, A., H. Panjaitan, O. A. Klein, M. Boccardi, M. Roes, S. Teupen, and S. Teipel. 2022. The impact of participatory dementia research on researchers: A systematic review. *Dementia (London)* 21(3):1012-1031.

Langbaum, J. B., J. Zissimopoulos, R. Au, N. Bose, C. J. Edgar, E. Ehrenberg, H. Fillit, C. V. Hill, L. Hughes, M. Irizarry, S. Kremen, D. Lakdawalla, N. Lynn, K. Malzbender, T. Maruyama, H. A. Massett, D. Patel, D. Peneva, E. M. Reiman, K. Romero, C. Routledge, M. W. Weiner, S. Weninger, and P. S. Aisen. 2023. Recommendations to address key recruitment challenges of Alzheimer's disease clinical trials. *Alzheimer's & Dementia* 19(2):696-707.

Lieberthal, R., N. Vakil, and M. Wilson. 2023. *Deriving common data elements from real-word data for Alzheimer's disease related dementias.* McLean, VA: MITRE Corp.

Lim, A. C., L. L. Barnes, G. H. Weissberger, M. Lamar, A. Nguyen, L. Fenton, J. Herrera, and D. S. Han. 2023. Quantification of race/ethnicity representation in Alzheimer's disease neuroimaging research in the USA: A systematic review. *Communications Medicine* 3:101.

Liu, M. N., C. I. Lau, and C. P. Lin. 2019. Precision medicine for frontotemporal dementia. *Frontiers in Psychiatry* 10:75.

MacDonald, S., A. S. Shah, and B. Tousi. 2022. Current therapies and drug development pipeline in Lewy body dementia: An update. *Drugs & Aging* 39(7):505-522.

Manly, J. J., A. Gilmore-Bykovskyi, and K. D. Deters. 2021. Inclusion of underrepresented groups in preclinical Alzheimer's disease trials—opportunities abound. *JAMA Network Open* 4(7):e2114606.

MarkVCID. 2017. *MarkVCID consortium overview.* https://markvcid.partners.org/about/m2-consortium-overview (accessed August 21, 2024).

Mielke, M. 2024. Sex and gender differences in Alzheimer's disease and Alzheimer's disease related dementias. Commissioned Paper for the Committee on Research Priorities for Preventing and Treating Alzheimer's Disease and Related Dementias.

Mindt, M. R., O. Okonkwo, M. W. Weiner, D. P. Veitch, P. Aisen, M. Ashford, G. Coker, M. C. Donohue, K. M. Langa, G. Miller, R. Petersen, R. Raman, and R. Nosheny. 2023. Improving generalizability and study design of Alzheimer's disease cohort studies in the United States by including under-represented populations. *Alzheimer's & Dementia* 19(4):1549-1557.

Mitchell, A. K., R. Ehrenkranz, S. Franzen, S. H. Han, M. Shakur, M. McGowan, and H. A. Massett. 2024. Analysis of eligibility criteria in Alzheimer's and related dementias clinical trials. *Scientific Reports* 14(1):15036.

NACC (National Alzheimer's Coordinating Center). 2024a. *National Alzheimer's Coordinating Center.* https://naccdata.org/ (accessed October 25, 2024).

NACC. 2024b. *About NACC Data.* https://naccdata.org/requesting-data/nacc-data (accessed October 25, 2024).

NACC. 2024c. *NACC's Data Platform.* https://naccdata.org/adrc-resources/nacc-data-platform (accessed October 25, 2024).

Nag, S., L. L. Barnes, L. Yu, R. S. Wilson, D. A. Bennett, and J. A. Schneider. 2020. Limbic-predominant age-related TDP-43 encephalopathy in black and white decedents. *Neurology* 95(15):e2056-e2064.

Nagar, S. D., P. Pemu, J. Qian, E. Boerwinkle, M. Cicek, C. R. Clark, E. Cohn, K. Gebo, R. Loperena, K. Mayo, S. Mockrin, L. Ohno-Machado, A. H. Ramirez, S. Schully, A. Able, A. Green, S. Zuchner, S. Consortium, I. K. Jordan, and R. Meller. 2022. Investigation of hypertension and type 2 diabetes as risk factors for dementia in the All of Us cohort. *Scientific Reports* 12(1):19797.

NAPS Consortium. 2024. *About NAPS.* https://www.naps-rbd.org/about-the-consortium (accessed October 29, 2024).

NASEM (National Academies of Sciences, Engineering, and Medicine). 2015. *SBIR/STTR at the National Institutes of Health.* Washington, DC: The National Academies Press.

NASEM. 2017. *Preventing cognitive decline and dementia: A way forward.* Edited by A. I. Leshner, S. Landis, C. Stroud and A. Downey. Washington, DC: The National Academies Press.

NASEM. 2018. *Returning individual research results to participants: Guidance for a new research paradigm.* Washington, DC: The National Academies Press.

NASEM. 2021. *Reducing the impact of dementia in America: A decadal survey of the behavioral and social sciences.* Washington, DC: The National Academies Press.

NASEM. 2022. *Improving representation in clinical trials and research: Building research equity for women and underrepresented groups,* edited by K. Bibbins-Domingo and A. Helman. Washington, DC: The National Academies Press.

NASEM. 2024. *Preventing and treating Alzheimer's disease and related dementias: Promising research and opportunities to accelerate progress: Proceedings of a workshop—in brief,* edited by O. Yost and A. Downey. Washington, DC: The National Academies Press.

Nature Medicine. 2023. Dementia research needs a global approach. *Nature Medicine* 29:279. https://doi.org/10.1038/s41591-023-02249-z.

Nguyen, M., S. I. Chaudhry, M. M. Desai, K. Dzirasa, J. E. Cavazos, and D. Boatright. 2023. Gender, racial, and ethnic and inequities in receipt of multiple National Institutes of Health research project grants. *JAMA Network Open* 6(2):e230855.

NIA (National Institute on Aging). 2018. *Together we make a difference: National strategy for recruitment and participation in Alzheimer's and related dementias clinical research.* NIA. www.nia.nih.gov/sites/default/files/2018-10/alzheimers-disease-recruitment-strategy-final. pdf (accessed on October 25, 2024).

NIA. 2019a. *Alzheimer's disease and related dementias: Clinical studies recruitment planning guide.* NIA.

NIA. 2019b. *National Institute on Aging workshop on applying digital technology for early diagnosis and monitoring of Alzheimer's disease and related dementias.* https://www.nia. nih.gov/research/dn/workshops/workshop-applying-digital-technology-early-diagnosis-and-monitoring (accessed September 19, 2024).

NIA. 2023a. *NIA's clinical research operations & management system (CROMS).* https:// www.nia.nih.gov/research/grants-funding/nias-clinical-research-operations-management-system-croms (accessed August 21, 2024).

NIA. 2023b. *NIH AD/ADRD platforms workshop: FAIRness within and across infrastructures. Workshop summary. June 20-21, 2023.*

NIA. 2023c. *Research enterprise.* https://www.nia.nih.gov/report-2019-2020-scientific-advances-prevention-treatment-and-care-dementia/research-enterprise (accessed August 22, 2024).

NIA. 2023d. *Alzheimer's disease genomics sharing plan.* https://www.nia.nih.gov/research/dn/ alzheimers-disease-genomics-sharing-plan (accessed October 25, 2024).

NIA. 2023e. *Artificial intelligence and technology collaboratories for aging research*. https://
www.nia.nih.gov/research/dbsr/artificial-intelligence-and-technology-collaboratories-
aging-research (accessed August 21, 2024).

NIA, 2024a. *National strategy for recruitment and participation in Alzheimer's and related
dementias clinical research*. https://www.nia.nih.gov/research/recruitment-strategy (accessed October 29, 2024).

NIA. 2024b. *Resource centers for minority aging research (2023-2028)*. https://www.nia.nih.
gov/research/dbsr/resource-centers-minority-aging-research-rcmar (accessed August 21,
2024, 2024).

NIA. 2024c. *The NIH aging and AD/ADRD omics data resources: A path to interoperability*.
https://www.nia.nih.gov/research/dn/workshops/nih-aging-and-ad-adrd-omics-data-
resources-path-interoperability (accessed August 22, 2024).

NIA. 2024d. *Enabling tech: Wearable technologies (milestone 11.C)*. https://www.nia.nih.
gov/research/milestones/diagnosis-assessment-and-disease-monitoring/enabling-tech-
wearable-technologies (accessed August 21, 2024, 2024).

NIAGADS (National Institute on Aging Genetics of Alzheimer's Disease Data Storage Site).
2024a. *About*. https://www.niagads.org/about/ (accessed November 11, 2024).

NIAGADS. 2024b. *Qualified access data*. https://www.niagads.org/qualified-access-data/ (accessed November 11, 2024).

NIH (National Institutes of Health). n.d. *Collaboration details*. https://crs.od.nih.gov/CRSPublic/
View.aspx?Id=8704 (accessed August 21, 2024).

NIH. 2020. *Final NIH policy for data management and sharing*. https://grants.nih.gov/grants/
guide/notice-files/NOT-OD-21-013.html (accessed August 22, 2024).

NIH. 2023a. *NIH professional judgment budget for Alzheimer's disease and related dementias
for fiscal year 2023*. https://www.nia.nih.gov/sites/default/files/2021-08/nih_ad-adrd_bypass_
budget_fy23.pdf (accessed September 19, 2024).

NIH. 2023b. *Advancements build momentum: 10 years of Alzheimer's disease and related
dementias research*. NIH Scientific Progress Report.

NIH. 2023c. *Novel mechanism research on neuropsychiatric symptoms (NPS) in Alzheimer's
dementia (R01 clinical trial optional)*. https://grants.nih.gov/grants/guide/pa-files/PAR-23-
207.html (accessed October 29, 2024).

NIH. 2024a. *Tissue chip program collaborations and partnerships*. https://ncats.nih.gov/
research/research-activities/tissue-chip/collaborations (accessed August 21, 2024).

NIH. 2024b. *Blueprint neurotherapeutics network (BPN) for small molecules*. https://
neuroscienceblueprint.nih.gov/neurotherapeutics/bpn-small-molecules (accessed August 21,
2024).

NIH. 2024c. *Understanding SBIR and STTR*. https://seed.nih.gov/small-business-funding/
small-business-program-basics/understanding-sbir-sttr (accessed October 29, 2024).

NIH ACD Working Group (NIH Advisory Committee to the Director Working Group on Re-
Envisioning NIH-Supported Postdoctoral Training). 2023. *Report to the NIH Advisory
Committee to the Director*.

NIH Office of Extramural Research, 2024. *NIH grants policy statement*. https://grants.
nih.gov/grants/policy/nihgps/html5/section_11/11.3.10_stipend_supplementation__
compensation__and_other_income.htm (accessed on October 25, 2024).

NIH RePORTER. 2023a. *Identifying barriers to optimizing data sharing and accelerate discovery in Alzheimer's disease and related dementia research*. https://reporter.nih.gov/search/
Yx1EJNc3W0-s33aUvMdY3A/project-details/10568214 (accessed August 22, 2024).

NIH RePORTER. 2023b. *Utilizing technology and AI approaches to facilitate independence
and resilience in older adults*. https://reporter.nih.gov/search/9mSA_KiHAk-InwQPU18rSg/
project-details/10274370 (accessed August 21, 2024, 2024).

NINDS (National Institute of Neurological Disorders and Stroke). n.d. *Project overview.* https://www.commondataelements.ninds.nih.gov/ProjReview (accessed October 29, 2024).

NINDS. 2021. *Notice of special interest (NOSI): Administrative supplements to promote diversity for NINDS Alzheimer's disease and Alzheimer's disease-related dementias (AD/ADRD) awardees.* https://grants.nih.gov/grants/guide/notice-files/NOT-NS-21-047.html (accessed August 21, 2024).

NINDS. 2024. *Notice of special interest (NOSI): Administrative supplements to promote diversity for NINDS ADRD awardees.* https://grants.nih.gov/grants/guide/notice-files/NOT-NS-24-071.html (accessed August 21, 2024).

NSF (National Science Foundation). 2024. *National artificial intelligence research resource pilot.* https://new.nsf.gov/focus-areas/artificial-intelligence/nairr#nairr-pilot-partners-and-contributors-890 (accessed October 29, 2024).

Pannu, J., J. Schmitt, and J. Swett. 2023. *ARPA-H should zero in on pandemic prevention.* https://issues.org/arpa-h-pandemic-prevention-pannu-schmitt-swett/ (accessed August 21, 2024, 2024).

Parekh, D., V. M. Patil, K. Nawale, V. Noronha, N. Menon, S. More, S. Goud, S. Jain, V. Mathrudev, Z. Peelay, S. Dhumal, S. Jogdhankar, and K. Prabhash. 2022. Audit of screen failure in 15 randomised studies from a low and middle-income country. *Ecancermedicalscience* 16:1476.

Pierce, H., A. Dev, E. Statham, and B. E. Bierer. 2019. Credit data generators for data reuse. *Nature* 570(7759):30-32.

Powell, W. R., W. R. Buckingham, J. L. Larson, L. Vilen, M. Yu, M. S. Salamat, B. B. Bendlin, R. A. Rissman, and A. J. H. Kind. 2020. Association of neighborhood-level disadvantage with Alzheimer disease neuropathology. *JAMA Network Open* 3(6):e207559.

Raman, R., Y. T. Quiroz, O. Langford, J. Choi, M. Ritchie, M. Baumgartner, D. Rentz, N. T. Aggarwal, P. Aisen, R. Sperling, and J. D. Grill. 2021. Disparities by race and ethnicity among adults recruited for a preclinical Alzheimer disease trial. *JAMA Network Open* 4(7):e2114364.

Reddy, J. S., L. Heath, A. V. Linden, M. Allen, K. P. Lopes, F. Seifar, E. Wang, Y. Ma, W. L. Poehlman, Z. S. Quicksall, A. Runnels, Y. Wang, D. M. Duong, L. Yin, K. Xu, E. S. Modeste, A. Shantaraman, E. B. Dammer, L. Ping, S. R. Oatman, J. Scanlan, C. Ho, M. M. Carrasquillo, M. Atik, G. Yepez, A. O. Mitchell, T. T. Nguyen, X. Chen, D. X. Marquez, H. Reddy, H. Xiao, S. Seshadri, R. Mayeux, S. Prokop, E. B. Lee, G. E. Serrano, T. G. Beach, A. F. Teich, V. Haroutunian, E. J. Fox, M. Gearing, A. Wingo, T. Wingo, J. J. Lah, A. I. Levey, D. W. Dickson, L. L. Barnes, P. De Jager, B. Zhang, D. Bennett, N. T. Seyfried, A. K. Greenwood, and N. Ertekin-Taner. 2024. Bridging the gap: Multi-omics profiling of brain tissue in Alzheimer's disease and older controls in multi-ethnic populations. *Alzheimer's & Dementia* 20(10):7174-7192.

Reyes, L., C. J. Scher, and E. A. Greenfield. 2023. Participatory research approaches in Alzheimer's disease and related dementias literature: A scoping review. *Innovation in Aging* 7(7):igad091.

Ritchie, C. W., G. M. Terrera, and T. J. Quinn. 2015. Dementia trials and dementia tribulations: Methodological and analytical challenges in dementia research. *Alzheimer's Research & Therapy* 7(1):31.

Sainburg, T. 2023. American postdoctoral salaries do not account for growing disparities in cost of living. *Research Policy* 52(3):104714.

Santora, K. 2023. *NIA new deadlines: Awaiting receipt of application (ARA) for large budget grant applications.* https://www.nia.nih.gov/research/blog/2023/11/nia-new-deadlines-awaiting-receipt-application-ara-large-budget-grant (accessed August 21, 2024).

Scalco, R., Y. Hamsafar, C. L. White, J. A. Schneider, R. R. Reichard, S. Prokop, R. J. Perrin, P. T. Nelson, S. Mooney, A. P. Lieberman, W. A. Kukull, J. Kofler, C. D. Keene, A. Kapasi, D. J. Irwin, D. A. Gutman, M. E. Flanagan, J. F. Crary, K. C. Chan, M. E. Murray, and B. N. Dugger. 2023. The status of digital pathology and associated infrastructure within Alzheimer's disease centers. *Journal of Neuropathology & Experimental Neurology* 82(3):202-211.

Shakir, M. N., and B. N. Dugger. 2022. Advances in deep neuropathological phenotyping of Alzheimer disease: Past, present, and future. *Journal of Neuropathology & Experimental Neurology* 81(1):2-15.

Stetler, C. 2023. *NIH to fund exposome research coordinating center.* https://factor.niehs.nih. gov/2023/10/science-highlights/nih-funding-to-support-exposome-research-coordinating-center (accessed August 21, 2024, 2024).

Takvorian, S., C. Guerra, and W. Schpero. 2021. A hidden opportunity — Medicaid's role in supporting equitable access to clinical trials. *New England Journal of Medicine* 384(21):1975-1978.

TRC-DS. 2024. *About TRC-DS.* https://www.trcds.org/about/ (accessed October 29, 2024).

UK Research and Innovation. 2024. *Co-production in research.* https://www.ukri.org/manage-your-award/good-research-resource-hub/research-co-production/ (accessed August 21, 2024, 2024).

Wilkinson, M. D., M. Dumontier, I. J. Aalbersberg, G. Appleton, M. Axton, A. Baak, N. Blomberg, J. W. Boiten, L. B. da Silva Santos, P. E. Bourne, J. Bouwman, A. J. Brookes, T. Clark, M. Crosas, I. Dillo, O. Dumon, S. Edmunds, C. T. Evelo, R. Finkers, A. Gonzalez-Beltran, A. J. Gray, P. Groth, C. Goble, J. S. Grethe, J. Heringa, P. A. C. 't Hoen, R. Hooft, T. Kuhn, R. Kok, J. Kok, S. J. Lusher, M. E. Martone, A. Mons, A. L. Packer, B. Persson, P. Rocca-Serra, M. Roos, R. van Schaik, S. A. Sansone, E. Schultes, T. Sengstag, T. Slater, G. Strawn, M. A. Swertz, M. Thompson, J. van der Lei, E. van Mulligen, J. Velterop, A. Waagmeester, P. Wittenburg, K. Wolstencroft, J. Zhao, and B. Mons. 2016. The FAIR guiding principles for scientific data management and stewardship. *Scientific Data* 3:160018.

Wing, J., D. A. Levine, A. Ramamurthy, and C. Reider. 2020. Alzheimer's disease and related disorders prevalence differs by Appalachian residence in Ohio. *Journal of Alzheimer's Disease* 76(4):1309-1316.

Appendix A

Scoping Review Methods

The committee was asked to examine and assess the current state of biomedical research related to Alzheimer's disease and related dementias (AD/ADRD), including evidence on interventions aimed at preventing, delaying, and treating AD/ADRD. This appendix presents the rationale and methods for a scoping review of published systematic reviews that aided the committee in addressing this element of its Statement of Task. A systematic review of the recent primary literature was not feasible given the available time and budget. The use of previously published systematic reviews was useful for developing an overarching view of the landscape of AD/ADRD intervention research; however, the committee acknowledges the potential for biases and the inherent limitations of this approach. These include the potential for a compounding of biases from individual systematic reviews (e.g., accumulation of publication and selection biases), variation in the quality of the included reviews, variation in the quality of primary literature included in those systematic reviews, overlap in the primary studies included, and inclusion of outdated information (Ballard and Montgomery, 2017). Additionally, because a limited number of systematic reviews were selected for the scoping review and given the potential lag between publication of primary studies and the conduct of systematic reviews synthesizing the body of evidence, the failure to identify a systematic review for a given intervention or population may not indicate a lack of primary evidence. This represents an important limitation when using a scoping review of existing systematic reviews for a gap analysis.

To the extent possible, the review protocol sought to directly address some of these limitations. However, for these reasons, the committee determined that the scoping review would not be appropriate for drawing conclusions on the effectiveness of a given intervention. Importantly, this exercise does not represent the entirety of the research efforts included in the report, which is the product of extensive literature searches, input from experts in public sessions, feedback from the public, and committee expertise. The findings from the scoping review were used to inform the committee's description of the research landscape and provide some evidence on emerging and established pharmacological and nonpharmacological interventions described in Chapter 4. Details about the articles included and excluded from the scoping review and more details about the methods used to carry out the scoping review can be found below.

RATIONALE AND OBJECTIVES

Recent approvals of three therapeutics to treat Alzheimer's disease (AD) have increased optimism that the tremendous investment in research for AD/ADRD over the last decade may be yielding tangible returns. Despite this optimism, these therapies come with high costs and significant risks and may provide modest benefits to only a small proportion of the millions of people living with AD in the United States. There remains a clear need for the development of a broader array of effective interventions to prevent, delay, and treat AD/ADRD across the entirety of the population. This scoping review included recently published systematic reviews to identify current gaps in research related to interventions for preventing, delaying, and treating AD/ADRD. Tools for screening and diagnosis of AD/ADRD were not included in this review of interventions. The understanding of the AD/ADRD research landscape afforded by the scoping review supported the development of the committee's conclusions and recommendations for priority research areas and the creation of scientific research questions that could be addressed by the National Institutes of Health in the next 3–10 years.

The primary objective of this review was to evaluate the recent research landscape for gaps and develop an understanding of the state of the evidence for interventions for the prevention, delay, or treatment of AD/ADRD and the limitations of that evidence. The review considered interventions across three categories: pharmacological, nonpharmacological, and combinations of both. Research of interest for this review included studies in humans that are focused on interventions to prevent, delay, or treat AD/ADRD. Owing to the complex nature of AD/ADRD and the breadth of conditions involved, the population of interest included all individuals who are currently living with AD or a related dementia and individuals who are at risk of AD/ADRD (all individuals who expect to reach older age). Interventions of interest included those aimed at preventing AD/ADRD from developing and treatments aimed at delaying the onset or slowing or halting the progression of AD/ADRD. Articles not of interest to this review included research conducted using animal or in vitro models, research on neurodegenerative diseases outside of the scope of the committee's work, and research on the care of people living with dementia and interventions for caregivers and care partners. More detailed information on inclusion and exclusion criteria, as well as the operational process for carrying out the steps of the review, is described in the methods section below.

METHODS

All systematic reviews included in the scoping review were published between January 1, 2017, and February 20, 2024, written in English, and peer reviewed. The included systematic reviews focused on the assessment of an intervention (including individual- and population-level strategies) in human participants to prevent, delay, or slow AD/ADRD and included interventions that are pharmacological or nonpharmacological, as well as combinations of both.

Articles were excluded if they did not meet the criteria listed above. This included articles that do not assess the effectiveness of an intervention in humans and articles classified as perspectives or opinions or as conference papers. Articles were excluded if they exclusively focused on conditions and outcomes unrelated to the defined dementia types within the scope of the committee's work. Excluded neurodegenerative conditions and their associated outcomes included dementia related to human immunodeficiency virus/acquired immunodeficiency syndrome, dementia as a result of traumatic brain injury, dementia as a result of incident stroke (although vascular contributions to dementia are included), Huntington's disease, amyotrophic lateral sclerosis, multiple system atrophy, and Parkinson's disease. Importantly, all articles solely focused on care partners and caregivers as the population of interest or on outcomes associated with caregivers (e.g., depression or anxiety in caregivers) were excluded as these outcomes are outside the committee's charge. In accordance with the Statement of Task, articles focused on care interventions (e.g., care coordination, pain management) were also excluded.

The following definitions were used:
- *AD/ADRD*, for the purposes of the committee's report, includes all causes of neurodegeneration that are included in the study scope, including AD, Lewy body dementia (LBD), frontotemporal dementia (FTD), limbic-predominant age-related TDP-43 encephalopathy, vascular dementia, and multiple etiology dementia.

- *Dementia* is an umbrella term used to describe the grouping of neurodegenerative disorders included within the study scope.
- *Clinical dementia* is impairment that meets the clinical criteria for a diagnosis of dementia.
- *Mild cognitive impairment* is a status that denotes a level of deterioration from normal cognitive function that is identifiable (e.g., by the individuals themselves, close contacts, or clinicians) but that does not significantly impair functions related to activities of daily living.
- *Intervention* refers to any program or treatment applied to an individual or at a population level (whether pharmacological or not) that is designed to prevent or modify the condition under investigation. These can include interventions aimed at the prevention or delay of onset and are not limited to pharmacological treatments. Interventions may also include nonpharmacological neuroprotective strategies implemented at any stage in the life course to prevent pathophysiologic processes. Given the current incomplete neurobiological understanding of AD/ADRD, the distinction between interventions that prevent, delay, and treat cognitive decline and interventions to prevent and treat neuropsychiatric symptoms may not be as clear as may be assumed.
- *Cognitive outcomes* include changes that can be measured in the brain and are associated with impaired cognition that can be perceived by the person living with the condition and their loved ones. Cognitive outcomes can include changes in language processing and use, attention, executive function, and visual perception that can be identified with cognitive tests, as well as intermediate outcome measures, such as biomarkers (e.g., amyloid, tau).
- *Functional outcomes* include changes in an individual's physical or social function in their daily living. These outcomes can be conceptualized as the ability to perform self-care, self-maintenance, and daily physical activities. Common measures include activities of daily living, which include basic, daily tasks, and instrumental activities of daily living. Examples of some measurable functional outcomes include mobility (e.g., gait, risk of falls), personal hygiene (e.g., ability to bathe and use the toilet), dressing, preparing meals and feeding, using transportation, managing finances, using communication devices, and managing medications.
- *Neuropsychiatric, behavioral, and quality-of-life outcomes* include those noncognitive core features of AD/ADRD that are included within the diagnostic criteria for these conditions. The severity of these symptoms is often used as outcome measures and may include aggression, challenging or unpredictable behavior, agitation,

personality changes/mood, sleep changes and disruptions, apathy, anxiety, insecurity, hallucinations, delusions/other psychotic behavior, disinhibition, and depression, among others.

- *Systematic review* is a review of a clearly formulated question that uses systematic and explicit methods to identify, select, and critically appraise relevant research, and to collect and analyze data from the studies that are included in the review. Statistical methods (meta-analysis) may or may not be used to analyze and summarize the results of the included studies.

Information Sources, Search, and Screening

To identify articles meeting the inclusion criteria of the scoping review, PubMed and Embase were searched for articles published between January 2017 and January 2024. This search was carried out on February 20, 2024. Search strategies were drafted by National Academies program staff based on committee-developed search terms and criteria and were reviewed by a trained research librarian. Search results from both databases were imported into PICO Portal and duplicates were removed.

Two National Academies staff members performed the initial title/abstract screening, beginning in February 2024, with one staff member serving as the adjudicator for any records for which inclusion or exclusion was unclear. The first 50 abstracts went through dual review to test and calibrate the screening process, and the remainder of the abstracts were divided among the two reviewers for a single reviewer title/abstract screening. The 824 records included after title/abstract screening were then passed to the PICO Portal team, a consulting group contracted by the committee, for full-text review and quality assessment.

Quality Assessment and Systematic Review Selection Process

The review selection process was developed in consultation with the PICO Portal team, which included consultants from evidence-based practice centers. The selection process sought to bring to the attention of the committee the most current and high-quality reviews by identifying the presence or absence of key methodological characteristics as determined through a series of questions. This simplified quality assessment process confirmed whether the article represents a true systematic review and that a minimum set of quality criteria were met (see Box A-1). The PICO Portal consultant team then provided those articles that met these quality criteria to the National Academies team for further assessment and selection. Articles meeting the criteria were organized by dementia type (e.g., LBD, FTD, AD), outcomes assessed, and intervention type to facilitate the selection

---

BOX A-1
Overview of Quality Assessment Process

1. Was >1 source searched?
   a. No, only one source was searched
   b. Yes, two or more sources were searched
   c. No information provided
2. Was a named RoB tool used? (Did the study assess RoB of each individual study with a named tool?) (If answered "No" for Q1, please skip this question and subsequent ones)
   a. No. A named RoB tool was not used to assess each study.
   b. Yes. A named RoB tool was used to assess each study.
   c. No information provided
3. Was protocol registered? (Was the protocol used for this systematic review prepublished or registered? Please enter a registration # in the Notes field if provided.) (If answered "No" for Q1 or Q2, please skip this question.)
   a. No
   b. Yes
4. Latest search date
   This information will be entered as text: [Year-Month-Day]

NOTE: RoB = risk of bias

---

of the recent, high-quality reviews representing the current research landscape for inclusion in the scoping review. Additionally, primary research articles included in the systematic reviews were compared to limit overlap where possible. Sixty-five articles were ultimately selected for data extraction, which represented a spectrum of different interventions and types of dementia. The PICO Portal then completed the data extraction from these selected articles.

SCOPING REVIEW ANALYSIS

Descriptive summaries of the 65 articles included in the scoping review are presented in Tables A-1 and A-2 for pharmacological and nonpharmacological interventions, respectively (systematic reviews that included both nonpharmacological and pharmacological interventions are indicated in the tables). The systematic reviews were used in the development of a gap analysis related to the current state of the evidence on interventions for preventing and treating AD/ADRD, which is presented in Chapter 4. Where relevant, they also informed the description of the evidence for interventions identified as promising by the committee, also presented in Chapter 4.

TABLE A-1 Description of Selected Systematic Reviews of
Pharmacological Interventions Included in the Scoping Review

Author, Year	Publication Dates of Studies Reviewed[a]	Population[b]	Total Studies Included[c]	Included Study Designs
Adesuyan et al., 2022	2001–2018	Adults age 40 years or older with hypertension and normal cognition	9	Cohort studies; case–control studies
Battle et al., 2021	2002–2010	Persons living with vascular dementia or other vascular cognitive impairment	8	RCTs
Blackman et al., 2021*	1993–2020	Persons living with MCI or mild to moderate AD dementia	16	RCTs; crossover trials; prospective cohort studies
Cardinali et al., 2021	1994–2019	Postmenopausal women living with or at risk for AD	25	Controlled clinical trials; observational studies
Corasaniti et al., 2024*	2011–2023	Persons living with dementia of any etiology	10	Clinical trials; retrospective studies

Primary Outcome Categories Assessed[d]	Relevant Interventions Assessed[e]
Prevention of AD	Individual or combined antihypertensive agents: • angiotensin-converting enzyme inhibitor • angiotensin II receptor blocker • beta blockers • calcium channel blockers • diuretics
Cognitive function; functional outcomes	Cholinesterase inhibitors: • donepezil • rivastigmine • galantamine
Neuropsychiatric and behavioral symptoms (sleep)	Interventions to improve the duration or quality of sleep: • cognitive behavioral therapy for insomnia • a multicomponent group-based therapy • a structured limbs exercise program • aromatherapy • phase-locked loop acoustic stimulation • transcranial stimulation • suvorexant • melatonin • donepezil • galantamine • rivastigmine • tetrahydroaminoacridine • continuous positive airway pressure
Cognitive function; neuropsychiatric and behavioral symptoms; prevention of AD	Hormone therapy
Cognitive function; neuropsychiatric and behavioral symptoms	Autophagy inducers: • metformin • TBI-287 • masitinib • resveratrol • spermidine

continued

TABLE A-1 Continued

Author, Year	Publication Dates of Studies Reviewed[a]	Population[b]	Total Studies Included[c]	Included Study Designs
Cunningham et al., 2021	1991–2019	Adults with hypertension without prior cerebrovascular disease	12	RCTs
Chu et al., 2021	1999–2019	Persons living with DLB	29	RCTs; uncontrolled single-arm trials
Dallaire-Theroux et al., 2021	2010–2019	Adults age 40 years or older with hypertension and without prior dementia diagnosis	7 (5 completed and included in authors' analysis)	RCTs
d'Angremont et al., 2023	2000–2016	Persons living with AD and DLB	19 (14 in AD and DLB populations)	RCTs
Ebell et al., 2024	2009–2023	Persons living with cognitive impairment or AD, or at high risk for AD	19	RCTs
Gomez-Soria et al., 2023b	2003–2021	Adults over 65 years of age who are cognitively healthy or living with MCI or dementia	30	RCTs; non-randomized controlled clinical trials; observational studies; pre-post studies

Primary Outcome Categories Assessed[d]	Relevant Interventions Assessed[e]
Prevention of cognitive impairment or dementia	Antihypertensive agents: • angiotensin-converting enzyme inhibitors • angiotensin receptor blockers • beta-adrenergic blockers • combined alpha and beta blockers • calcium channel blockers • diuretics • alpha-adrenergic blockers • central sympatholytics • direct vasodilators • peripheral adrenergic antagonists • sympathomimetics
Cognitive function; neuropsychiatric and behavioral symptoms	Aripiprazole; armodafinil; citalopram; donepezil; galantamine; levodopa; memantine; olanzapine; quetiapine; risperidone; rivastigmine; yokukansan; zonisamide
Prevention of cognitive decline, MCI, and dementia	Standard versus intensive blood pressure control
Neuropsychiatric and behavioral symptoms	Cholinesterase inhibitors: • donepezil • rivastigmine • galantamine
Cognitive function; functional outcomes	Monoclonal antibodies targeting amyloid
Neuropsychiatric and behavioral symptoms; functional outcomes; quality of life	Cognitive stimulation, alone or in combination with acetylcholinesterase inhibitors

continued

TABLE A-1 Continued

Author, Year	Publication Dates of Studies Reviewed[a]	Population[b]	Total Studies Included[c]	Included Study Designs
Gómez-Soria et al., 2023a	2003–2021	Adults age 65 years or older who are cognitively healthy or living with MCI or dementia	33	RCTs; non-randomized controlled clinical trials; observational studies; pre-post studies
Huang et al., 2023b	1998–2018	Persons living with dementia	59	RCTs
Huang et al., 2023a	2003–2020	Persons living with FTD	7	RCTs
Kitt et al., 2023	2007–2023	Adults without prior dementia diagnosis	11	RCTs

Primary Outcome Categories Assessed[d]	Relevant Interventions Assessed[e]
Cognitive function	Cognitive stimulation, alone or in combination with acetylcholinesterase inhibitors
Neuropsychiatric and behavioral symptoms	Cognitive enhancers: • donepezil • memantine • galantamine • rivastigmine Antipsychotics: • risperidone • haloperidol • olanzapine • aripiprazole • quetiapine • pimavanserin; Antidepressants: • citalopram • escitalopram • trazodone; Mood stabilizers: • divalproex • topiramate
Neuropsychiatric and behavioral symptoms; cognitive function; functional outcomes	Oxytocin, trazodone, paroxetine, piracetam, memantine, tolcapone
Prevention of dementia or cognitive impairment	Antiplatelet therapy

continued

TABLE A-1 Continued

Author, Year	Publication Dates of Studies Reviewed[a]	Population[b]	Total Studies Included[c]	Included Study Designs
Kuate Defo et al., 2024	2011–2022	Adults diagnosed with diabetes and without prior dementia diagnosis	127 (27 primary studies included in authors' quantitative analysis and 100 review articles included in authors' qualitative review)	Cohort studies; case–control studies
Kwan et al., 2022	2014–2018	Adults with cerebral small vessel disease and without prior dementia diagnosis	3	RCTs
Lyu et al., 2023	2003–2023	Persons living with AD	41 (35 with relevant outcomes)	RCTs
McShane et al., 2019	1991–2016	Persons living with AD, vascular, mixed, or other types of dementia	44	RCTs

Primary Outcome Categories Assessed[d]	Relevant Interventions Assessed[e]
Prevention of dementia	Antidiabetic medications: • metformin • thiazolidinediones (including pioglitazone) • dipeptidyl peptidase-4 inhibitors • α-glucosidase inhibitors • meglitinides • insulin • sulphonylureas • glucagon-like peptide-1 receptor agonists • sodium-glucose cotransporter-2 inhibitors
Cognitive function; functional outcomes	Antithrombotic therapy
Cognitive function	Anti-amyloid-β drugs including Active immunotherapy drugs: • ACC-001 • AD02 • AN1792 • CAD106 Passive immunotherapy drugs: • aducanumab • bapineuzumab • crenezumab • donanemab • gantenerumab • lecanemab • ponezumab • solanezumab Small-molecule drugs: • tramiprosate • clioquinol • ELND005 • PBT2
Cognitive function; functional outcomes; neuropsychiatric and behavioral symptoms	Memantine

continued

TABLE A-1 Continued

Author, Year	Publication Dates of Studies Reviewed[a]	Population[b]	Total Studies Included[c]	Included Study Designs
Muhlbauer et al., 2021	1995–2020	Persons living with AD, vascular dementia, or mixed dementia (AD and vascular)	24	RCTs
Nimmons et al., 2024*	1982–2023	Persons living with dementia	31	RCTs
Olmastroni et al., 2022	2000–2020	Adults at risk for dementia	46	Cohort studies; case-control studies

Primary Outcome Categories Assessed[d]	Relevant Interventions Assessed[e]
Neuropsychiatric and behavioral symptoms	Typical antipsychotics: • haloperidol • thiothixene Atypical antipsychotics: • brexpiprazol • risperidone • olanzapine • aripiprazole • quetiapine • pimavanserin • tiapride
Neuropsychiatric and behavioral symptoms	Nonpharmacological interventions: • music therapy, • cognitive approaches (e.g., cognitive behavioral therapy, cognitive training) • muscular approaches (e.g., hand motor therapy, massage) • sensory stimulation (e.g., Snoezelen, stimulating robotic animals) • stimulating cognitive and physical activities; • Gingko biloba • probiotics Pharmacological interventions: • antidepressants • antipsychotics
Prevention of AD and dementia	Statins

continued

TABLE A-1 Continued

Author, Year	Publication Dates of Studies Reviewed[a]	Population[b]	Total Studies Included[c]	Included Study Designs
Profyri et al., 2022*	1999–2021	Persons living with severe dementia	30 (23 not related to care or caregiver interventions)	RCTs
Sun et al., 2023	2001–2022	Adults without prior dementia diagnosis	6	Cohort studies
Tao et al., 2024	1995–2023	Adults at risk for dementia and AD	22	Cohort studies; cross-sectional studies; RCTs
Tedeschi et al., 2021	2018–2020	Persons living with AD	34 (2 using relevant [clinical] study design)	Clinical trials
Terao and Kodama, 2024	2013–2023	Persons living with MCI and AD	7	RCTs
van Middelaar et al., 2018*	1996–2017	Adults without prior dementia diagnosis	9	RCTs

Primary Outcome Categories Assessed[d]	Relevant Interventions Assessed[e]
Cognitive function; neuropsychiatric and behavioral symptoms; functional outcomes; mortality	Nonpharmacological interventions: • multisensory stimulation • essential oils • bright light treatment • combination of physical activity, multisensory stimulation, and reminiscence • activity schedules to balance arousal levels • animal-assisted activities, • music therapy Pharmacological interventions: • donepezil • galantamine • GRF6019 • memantine • olanzapine • risperidone • analgesics for depression • sertraline
Prevention of dementia	Influenza vaccination
Prevention of AD and dementia	Aspirin
Cognitive function	Gene therapy: Adeno-associated virus-nerve growth factor
Cognitive function	Passive anti-amyloid beta immunotherapies: • donanemab • lecanemab • aducanumab Lithium
Prevention of all-cause dementia, AD, and vascular dementia	Blood-pressure-lowering interventions: • antihypertensive medications, • lifestyle changes Combination interventions

continued

TABLE A-1 Continued

Author, Year	Publication Dates of Studies Reviewed[a]	Population[b]	Total Studies Included[c]	Included Study Designs
Wang et al., 2022a	2006–2021	Persons living with AD or MCI	16	RCTs
Watts et al., 2023*		Persons living with DLB	135**	RCTs; nonrandomized trials; open-label trials; longitudinal studies; case series; case reports
Zhan et al., 2021*	2003–2020	Persons living with vascular cognitive impairment	23	RCTs
Zhang et al., 2022	2012–2021	Persons living with dementia	22	RCTs
Zheng et al., 2022	2003–2021	Persons living with mild to moderate cognitive impairment	34	RCTs

*Indicates systematic review that assessed both nonpharmacological and pharmacological interventions.

[a] Publication date range for primary articles included in listed systematic reviews is only inclusive of primary articles relevant to the focus of this scoping review (population, intervention types, outcomes of interest).

[b] Populations listed are only those relevant to the focus of this scoping review (e.g., if primary studies included in a systematic review were focused on Parkinson's dementia, that population was not described in the table).

[c] When a systematic review included primary studies that were not a focus of this scoping review (e.g., wrong population, care- or caregiver-focused interventions), the number of relevant included studies for that systematic review is provided in parentheses.

Primary Outcome Categories Assessed[d]	Relevant Interventions Assessed[e]
Cognitive function, functional outcomes	Hypoglycemic drugs: • intranasal insulin • metformin • glucagon-like peptide-1 • dipeptidyl peptidase-4 inhibitor (sitagliptin) • pioglitazone • rosiglitazone
Cognitive function; neuropsychiatric and behavioral symptoms; mortality	Donepezil; rivastigmine; galantamine; memantine; modafinil/armodafinil; clozapine; quetiapine; risperidone; olanzapine; aripiprazole; dopamine antagonists; herbal medications (yokukasan, Feru-guard); ramelteon; clonazepam; antidepressants (citalopram, paroxetine)
Cognitive function; functional outcomes	Gingko biloba extract alone or in combination with pharmacologic treatments (donepezil, nimodipine, huperzine, oxiracetam, piracetam, butylphthalide, ergoloid mesylate)
Cognitive function; neuropsychiatric symptoms; functional outcomes	Magnesium valproate when used in conjunction with other dementia treatments (donepezil, galantamine, quetiapine, olanzapine, aripiprazole)
Cognitive function	Anti-tau drugs

[d] Reported outcomes are only those noted by the systematic review authors as primary outcomes and relevant to the focus of this scoping review (e.g., motor outcomes for a Parkinson's dementia population were not reported in this table). If primary outcomes were not identified by the authors, all noted outcomes relevant to the focus of this scoping review were listed. Prevention was listed as an outcome if the systematic review included an assessment of intervention impact on relative risk or disease incidence.

[e] Described interventions are only those relevant to this scoping review. Interventions for an excluded population and care- or caregiver-focused interventions are not listed.

NOTES: AD = Alzheimer's disease; DLB = dementia with Lewy bodies; FTD = frontotemporal dementia; MCI = mild cognitive impairment; RCTs = randomized controlled trials.

TABLE A-2 Description of Selected Systematic Reviews of Nonpharmacological Interventions Included in the Scoping Review

Author, Year	Publication Dates of Studies Reviewed[a]	Population[b]	Total Studies Included[c]	Included Study Designs
Ahn and Kim, 2023	2011–2020	Persons age 60 years or older living with MCI	22	RCTs
Buele et al., 2023	1999–2022	Healthy adults and persons living with MCI or dementia	19	RCTs; non-RCT clinical trials; pilot pretest-posttest; case study
Blackman et al., 2021*	1993–2020	Persons living with MCI or mild to moderate AD dementia	16	RCTs; crossover trials; prospective cohort studies
Cai et al., 2023	2010–2021	Persons age 45 years or older living with MCI	27	RCTs
Corasaniti et al., 2024*	2011 - 2023	Persons living with dementia of any etiology	10	Clinical trials; retrospective studies
Castro et al., 2023**	2010–2020	Adults age 49 years or older at increased risk of dementia	15	RCTs
Chan et al., 2024	1994–2023	Persons living with MCI or dementia	35	RCTs

Primary Outcome Categories Assessed[d]	Relevant Interventions Assessed[e]
Cognition function	Physical activity: • aerobic • resistance • multicomponent • neuromotor
Cognitive function	VR applications based on instrumental activities of daily living for cognitive training, rehabilitation, or stimulation
Neuropsychiatric and behavioral symptoms (sleep)	Interventions to improve the duration or quality of sleep: • cognitive behavioral therapy for insomnia • a multicomponent group-based therapy • a structured limbs exercise program • aromatherapy • phase-locked loop acoustic stimulation • transcranial stimulation • suvorexant • melatonin • donepezil • galantamine • rivastigmine • tetrahydroaminoacridine • continuous positive airway pressure
Cognitive function	Mind–body exercise
Cognitive function; neuropsychiatric and behavioral symptoms	Autophagy inducers: • metformin • TBI-287 • masitinib • resveratrol • spermidine
Cognitive function; reduced dementia risk factors	Multimodal lifestyle interventions that included diet and physical activity with or without cognitive training
Cognitive function	Computerized cognitive training

continued

TABLE A-2 Continued

Author, Year	Publication Dates of Studies Reviewed[a]	Population[b]	Total Studies Included[c]	Included Study Designs
Chen et al., 2022	2008–2021	Persons living with MCI or mild to moderate AD	16	RCTs
Cho et al., 2023	2015–2021	Persons living with dementia	16 (14 not related to caregiving interventions)	RCTs
Connors et al., 2018	2002–2016	Persons living with DLB	21 (13 in DLB population not involving caregiving interventions)	RCTs; case studies; case series
Fu et al., 2022	2006–2021	Cognitively normal adults	36	RCTs; prospective cohort studies
Gomez-Soria et al., 2023b	2003–2021	Adults over 65 years of age who are cognitively healthy or living with MCI or dementia	30	RCTs; non-randomized controlled clinical trials; observational studies; pre-post studies
Gómez-Soria et al., 2023a	2003–2021	Adults age 65 years or older who are cognitively healthy or living with MCI or dementia	33	RCTs; non-randomized controlled clinical trials; observational studies; pre-post studies
Guo et al., 2024	2005–2023	Adults diagnosed with atrial fibrillation	14	RCTs; cohort studies; case-control studies

Primary Outcome Categories Assessed[d]	Relevant Interventions Assessed[e]
Cognitive function	Transcranial direct current stimulation, alone or in combination with cognitive/memory training
Neuropsychiatric and behavioral symptoms	Nonpharmacological interventions using information and communication technologies: • music therapy • reminiscence therapy • physical training • social interaction interventions using robotic pets or humanoid robots
Cognitive function; neuropsychiatric and behavioral symptoms; functional outcomes	Psychological interventions for visual hallucinations; physical exercise; gait cueing; music therapy; environmental modification for mirrored self-misidentification delusion; simulated presence; occupational therapy; electroconvulsive therapy; transcranial magnetic stimulation; transcranial direct current stimulation
Prevention of MCI, AD, and dementia; cognitive function	Mediterranean diet
Neuropsychiatric and behavioral symptoms; functional outcomes; quality of life	Cognitive stimulation, alone or in combination with acetylcholinesterase inhibitors
Cognitive function	Cognitive stimulation, alone or in combination with acetylcholinesterase inhibitors
Prevention of dementia; cognitive function	Rate-control and rhythm-control strategies, including atrial fibrillation ablation

continued

TABLE A-2 Continued

Author, Year	Publication Dates of Studies Reviewed[a]	Population[b]	Total Studies Included[c]	Included Study Designs
Hafdi et al., 2021**	2010–2020	Adults over 50 years of age without prior dementia diagnosis, including populations with known dementia risk factors and subjective cognitive symptoms or impairment	9	RCTs
Karamacoska et al., 2023	2012–2023	Adults living with subjective cognitive decline, MCI, or vascular cognitive impairment	12	RCTs
Leow et al., 2023	2013–2021	Adults age 60 years or older living with MCI	10	RCTs
Lin et al., 2022	1999–2021	Persons living with AD	67	RCTs
López-Ortiz et al., 2023	2009–2021	Adults at risk for or living with AD	21	RCTs; prospective studies; case–control studies
Miller et al., 2023	2012–2022	Persons living with MCI or dementia related to AD	16 (8 in relevant population)	RCTs

Primary Outcome Categories Assessed[d]	Relevant Interventions Assessed[e]
Prevention of dementia and MCI; cognitive function	Multimodal interventions targeting some combination of any of the following domains: • diet • physical activity • weight loss • blood pressure control • diabetes management • blood lipids • smoking • alcohol intake • cognitive training • social activities
Cognitive function	Physical activity: • aerobic exercise • resistance training • mind-body exercise
Cognitive function; neuropsychiatric and behavioral symptoms	Mindfulness-based interventions (e.g., guided meditation, psychoeducation related to mindfulness)
Cognitive function	Acupuncture treatments: • needle-acupuncture • electro-acupuncture • scalp-acupuncture • body acupressure • auricular acupressure • moxibustion • transcutaneous electrical acupoint stimulation
Prevention of AD; cognitive function; functional outcomes; quality of life; neuropsychiatric and behavioral symptoms	Physical activity and exercise
Cognitive function	Repetitive transcranial magnetic stimulation targeting the dorsolateral prefrontal cortex

continued

TABLE A-2 Continued

Author, Year	Publication Dates of Studies Reviewed[a]	Population[b]	Total Studies Included[c]	Included Study Designs
Morrin et al., 2018	2003–2016	Persons living with LBD	15 (8 in relevant population)	Uncontrolled trials; case reports
Nimmons et al., 2024*	1982–2023	Persons living with dementia	31	RCTs
Papaioannou et al., 2022	1999–2021	Persons living with MCI or dementia	20	RCTs
Profyri et al., 2022*	1999–2021	Persons living with severe dementia	30 (23 not related to care or caregiver interventions)	RCTs
Ren et al., 2024	2012–2022	Persons over 60 years of age living with MCI or dementia	21	RCTs

Primary Outcome Categories Assessed[d]	Relevant Interventions Assessed[e]
Cognitive function; neuropsychiatric and behavioral symptoms; functional outcomes	Electroconvulsive therapy; repetitive transcranial magnetic stimulation; transcranial direct current stimulation; physical exercise; environmental intervention for "mirror sign"
Neuropsychiatric and behavioral symptoms	Nonpharmacological interventions: • music therapy, • cognitive approaches (e.g., cognitive behavioral therapy, cognitive training) • muscular approaches (e.g., hand motor therapy, massage) • sensory stimulation (e.g., Snoezelen, stimulating robotic animals) • stimulating cognitive and physical activities; • Gingko biloba • probiotics Pharmacological interventions: • antidepressants • antipsychotics
Cognitive function	Virtual reality applications used for cognitive training
Cognitive function; neuropsychiatric and behavioral symptoms; functional outcomes; mortality	Nonpharmacological interventions: • multisensory stimulation • essential oils • bright light treatment • combination of physical activity, multisensory stimulation, and reminiscence • activity schedules to balance arousal levels • animal-assisted activities, • music therapy Pharmacological interventions: • donepezil • galantamine • GRF6019 • memantine • olanzapine • risperidone • analgesics for depression • sertraline
Cognitive function	Virtual reality-based cognitive rehabilitation training

continued

TABLE A-2 Continued

Author, Year	Publication Dates of Studies Reviewed[a]	Population[b]	Total Studies Included[c]	Included Study Designs
Rostamzadeh et al., 2022	2007–2021	Persons living with subjective cognitive decline and MCI who are at risk of AD dementia	32	RCTs; non-randomized trials; case reports
Salzman et al., 2022**	2011–2021	Persons age 65 years or older living with MCI	28	RCTs
Shoesmith et al., 2023	2001–2021	Persons living with dementia	51	RCTs; non-randomized trials; cohort studies; pre-post studies; case studies; qualitative studies; mixed method study
Talar et al., 2022**	2022–2021	Adults age 60 years or older who are cognitively healthy or living with MCI or dementia	74	RCTs
Tosatti et al., 2022	2006–2018	Adults living with AD	4	RCTs
Townsend et al., 2023	2006–2022	Adults age 18 years or older	93	RCTs; prospective studies

Primary Outcome Categories Assessed[d]	Relevant Interventions Assessed[e]
Cognitive function; neuropsychiatric and behavioral symptoms; quality of life	Psychotherapeutic and psychoeducational interventions, alone or in combination with other nonpharmacologic interventions (e.g., physical activity, cognitive training)
Cognitive function	Multimodal interventions targeting some combination of any of the following domains: • physical activities • cognitive activities • social activities • mind-body activities • acupressure and acupuncture • nutritional supplements • education • transcranial direct current stimulation • music with movement
Neuropsychiatric and behavioral symptoms; quality of life	Animal-assisted interventions and robotic animal interventions
Cognitive function	Aerobic exercise and transcranial direct current stimulation, alone or in combination
Cognitive function; functional outcomes	Resveratrol supplementation
Cognitive function; prevention of MCI, AD, and dementia	Whole dietary patterns

continued

TABLE A-2 Continued

Author, Year	Publication Dates of Studies Reviewed[a]	Population[b]	Total Studies Included[c]	Included Study Designs
Tulliani et al., 2022	2013–2022	Persons age 60 years or older living with MCI or early-stage dementia	13	RCTs
van Middelaar et al., 2018*	1996–2017	Adults without prior dementia diagnosis	9	RCTs
Wang et al., 2023	2015–2023	Persons living with MCI or AD	17	RCTs
Wang et al., 2022b	1998–2019	Adults who are cognitively healthy or living with MCI, AD, vascular dementia, or dementia with other causes	95	RCTs; cohort studies; cross-sectional studies
Watts et al., 2023*		Persons living with DLB	135***	RCTs; nonrandomized trials; open-label trials; longitudinal studies; case series; case reports
Wei et al., 2023	1997–2021	Participants with and without dementia	48	Cohort studies; prospective nested case-control studies
Wilfling et al., 2023	1999–2019	Persons living with dementia	19 (17 not related to care or caregiver interventions)	RCTs

Primary Outcome Categories Assessed[d]	Relevant Interventions Assessed[e]
Functional outcomes	Cognitive remediation including the following alone or in combination: • cognitive training • cognitive rehabilitation • cognitive stimulation
Prevention of all-cause dementia, AD, and vascular dementia	Blood-pressure-lowering interventions: • antihypertensive medications, • lifestyle changes • combination interventions
Cognitive function	Repetitive transcranial magnetic stimulation or transcranial direct current stimulation
Cognitive function; prevention of dementia	B vitamin supplementation
Cognitive function; neuropsychiatric and behavioral symptoms; mortality	Donepezil; rivastigmine; galantamine; memantine; modafinil/armodafinil; clozapine; quetiapine; risperidone; olanzapine; aripiprazole; dopamine antagonists; herbal medications (yokukasan, Feru-guard); ramelteon; clonazepam; antidepressants (citalopram, paroxetine)
Cognitive function; prevention of dementia, AD, or cognitive decline	Omega-3 fatty acids
Neuropsychiatric and behavioral symptoms (sleep)	Nonpharmacologic interventions to improve sleep: • light therapy • physical activities • social activities • practices to improve sleep routines and decrease sleep disruptions • massage • transcranial electrostimulation

continued

TABLE A-2 Continued

Author, Year	Publication Dates of Studies Reviewed[a]	Population[b]	Total Studies Included[c]	Included Study Designs
Xue et al., 2023**	2013–2022	Persons living with MCI or dementia	29	RCTs
Zeng et al., 2023	2011–2021	Persons living with AD or a related dementia	18	RCTs
Zhan et al., 2021*	2003–2020	Persons living with vascular cognitive impairment	23	RCTs
Zhang et al., 2023	1995–2023	Cognitively normal adults	29	Cohort studies

*Indicates the inclusion of a systematic review that assessed both nonpharmacological and pharmacological interventions.

**Includes assessment of multimodal or multicomponent approaches.

*** Indicates that the number of primary studies that were relevant to the focus of this scoping review could not be determined.

[a] Publication date range for primary articles included in listed systematic reviews is only inclusive of primary articles relevant to the focus of this scoping review (population, intervention types, outcomes of interest).

[b] Populations listed are only those relevant to the focus of this scoping review (e.g., if primary studies included in a systematic review were focused on Parkinson's dementia, that population was not described in the table).

[c] When a systematic review included primary studies that were not a focus of this scoping review (e.g., wrong population, care- or caregiver-focused interventions), the number of relevant included studies for that systematic review is provided in parentheses.

Primary Outcome Categories Assessed[d]	Relevant Interventions Assessed[e]
Cognitive function; neuropsychiatric and behavioral symptoms; functional outcomes	Combined exercise (e.g., aerobic, strength) and cognitive interventions (e.g., cognitive training, cognitive stimulation)
Cognitive function	Physical activity interventions: • aerobic exercise • resistance training • combined exercise
Cognitive function; functional outcomes	Gingko biloba extract alone or in combination with pharmacologic treatments (donepezil, nimodipine, huperzine, oxiracetam, piracetam, butylphthalide, ergoloid mesylate)
Prevention of AD	Physical activity

[d] Reported outcomes are only those noted by the systematic review authors as primary outcomes and relevant to the focus of this scoping review (e.g., motor outcomes for a Parkinson's dementia population were not reported in this table). If primary outcomes were not identified by the authors, all noted outcomes relevant to the focus of this scoping review were listed. Prevention was listed as an outcome if the systematic review included an assessment of intervention impact on relative risk or disease incidence.

[e] Described interventions are only those relevant to this scoping review. Interventions for an excluded population and care- or caregiver-focused interventions are not listed.

NOTES: AD = Alzheimer's disease; DLB = dementia with Lewy bodies; FTD = frontotemporal dementia; LBD = Lewy body dementia; MCI = mild cognitive impairment; RCTs = randomized controlled trials.

REFERENCES

Adesuyan, M., Y. H. Jani, D. Alsugeir, E. C. L. Cheung, C. S. L. Chui, R. Howard, I. C. K. Wong, and R. Brauer. 2022. Antihypertensive agents and incident Alzheimer's disease: A systematic review and meta-analysis of observational studies. *Journal of Prevention of Alzheimer's Disease* 9(4):715-724.

Ahn, J., and M. Kim. 2023. Effects of exercise therapy on global cognitive function and depression in older adults with mild cognitive impairment: A systematic review and meta-analysis. *Archives of Gerontology and Geriatrics* 106:104855.

Ballard, M., and P. Montgomery. 2017. Risk of bias in overviews of reviews: A scoping review of methodological guidance and four-item checklist. *Research Synthesis Methods* 8(1):92-108.

Battle, C. E., A. H. Abdul-Rahim, S. D. Shenkin, J. Hewitt, and T. J. Quinn. 2021. Cholinesterase inhibitors for vascular dementia and other vascular cognitive impairments: A network meta-analysis. *Cochrane Database Systematic Reviews* 2(2):CD013306.

Blackman, J., M. Swirski, J. Clynes, S. Harding, Y. Leng, and E. Coulthard. 2021. Pharmacological and non-pharmacological interventions to enhance sleep in mild cognitive impairment and mild Alzheimer's disease: A systematic review. *Journal of Sleep Research* 30(4):e13229.

Buele, J., J. L. Varela-Aldas, and G. Palacios-Navarro. 2023. Virtual reality applications based on instrumental activities of daily living (IADLS) for cognitive intervention in older adults: A systematic review. *Journal of NeuroEngineering and Rehabilitation* 20(1):168.

Cai, H., K. Zhang, M. Wang, X. Li, F. Ran, and Y. Han. 2023. Effects of mind-body exercise on cognitive performance in middle-aged and older adults with mild cognitive impairment: A meta-analysis study. *Medicine (Baltimore)* 102(34):e34905.

Cardinali, C. A. E. F., Y. A. Martins, and A. S. Torrão. 2021. Use of hormone therapy in postmenopausal women with Alzheimer's disease: A systematic review. *Drugs & Aging* 38(9):769-791.

Castro, C. B., L. M. Costa, C. B. Dias, J. Chen, H. Hillebrandt, S. L. Gardener, B. M. Brown, R. L. Loo, M. L. Garg, S. R. Rainey-Smith, R. N. Martins, and H. R. Sohrabi. 2023. Multi-domain interventions for dementia prevention—a systematic review. *Journal of Nutrition, Health and Aging* 27(12):1271-1280.

Chan, A. T. C., R. T. F. Ip, J. Y. S. Tran, J. Y. C. Chan, and K. K. F. Tsoi. 2024. Computerized cognitive training for memory functions in mild cognitive impairment or dementia: A systematic review and meta-analysis. *NPJ Digital Medicine* 7(1):1.

Chen, J., Z. Wang, Q. Chen, Y. Fu, and K. Zheng. 2022. Transcranial direct current stimulation enhances cognitive function in patients with mild cognitive impairment and early/mid Alzheimer's disease: A systematic review and meta-analysis. *Brain Science* 12(5):562.

Cho, E., J. Shin, J. W. Seok, H. Lee, K. H. Lee, J. Jang, S. J. Heo, and B. Kang. 2023. The effectiveness of non-pharmacological interventions using information and communication technologies for behavioral and psychological symptoms of dementia: A systematic review and meta-analysis. *International Journal of Nursing Studies* 138:104392.

Chu, C. S., F. C. Yang, P. T. Tseng, B. Stubbs, A. Dag, A. F. Carvalho, T. Thompson, Y. K. Tu, T. C. Yeh, D. J. Li, C. K. Tsai, T. Y. Chen, M. Ikeda, C. S. Liang, and K. P. Su. 2021. Treatment efficacy and acceptabilityof pharmacotherapies for dementia with lewy bodies: A systematic review and network meta-analysis. *Archives of Gerontology and Geriatrics* 96:104474.

Connors, M. H., L. Quinto, I. McKeith, H. Brodaty, L. Allan, C. Bamford, A. Thomas, J. P. Taylor, and J. T. O'Brien. 2018. Non-pharmacological interventions for Lewy body dementia: A systematic review. *Psychological Medicine* 48(11):1749-1758.

Corasaniti, M. T., G. Bagetta, P. Nicotera, S. Maione, P. Tonin, F. Guida, and D. Scuteri. 2024. Exploitation of autophagy inducers in the management of dementia: A systematic review. *International Journal of Molecular Sciences* 25(2):1264.

Cunningham, E. L., S. A. Todd, P. Passmore, R. Bullock, and B. McGuinness. 2021. Pharmacological treatment of hypertension in people without prior cerebrovascular disease for the prevention of cognitive impairment and dementia. *Cochrane Database of Systematic Reviews* 5(5):CD004034.

d'Angremont, E., M. J. H. Begemann, T. van Laar, and I. E. C. Sommer. 2023. Cholinesterase inhibitors for treatment of psychotic symptoms in Alzheimer disease and Parkinson disease: A meta-analysis. *JAMA Neurology* 80(8):813-823.

Dallaire-Theroux, C., M. H. Quesnel-Olivo, K. Brochu, F. Bergeron, S. O'Connor, A. F. Turgeon, R. J. Laforce, S. Verreault, M. C. Camden, and S. Duchesne. 2021. Evaluation of intensive vs standard blood pressure reduction and association with cognitive decline and dementia: A systematic review and meta-analysis. *JAMA Network Open* 4(11):e2134553.

Ebell, M. H., H. C. Barry, K. Baduni, and G. Grasso. 2024. Clinically important benefits and harms of monoclonal antibodies targeting amyloid for the treatment of Alzheimer disease: A systematic review and meta-analysis. *Annals of Family Medicine* 22(1):50-62.

Fu, J., L. J. Tan, J. E. Lee, and S. Shin. 2022. Association between the Mediterranean diet and cognitive health among healthy adults: A systematic review and meta-analysis. *Frontiers in Nutrition* 9:946361.

Gómez-Soria, I., I. Iguacel, A. Aguilar-Latorre, P. Peralta-Marrupe, E. Latorre, J. N. C. Zaldívar, and E. Calatayud. 2023a. Cognitive stimulation and cognitive results in older adults: A systematic review and meta-analysis. *Archives of Gerontology and Geriatrics* 104:104807.

Gomez-Soria, I., I. Iguacel, J. N. Cuenca-Zaldivar, A. Aguilar-Latorre, P. Peralta-Marrupe, E. Latorre, and E. Calatayud. 2023b. Cognitive stimulation and psychosocial results in older adults: A systematic review and meta-analysis. *Archives of Gerontology and Geriatrics* 115:105114.

Guo, J., Y. Liu, J. Jia, J. Lu, D. Wang, J. Zhang, J. Ding, and X. Zhao. 2024. Effects of rhythm-control and rate-control strategies on cognitive function and dementia in atrial fibrillation: A systematic review and meta-analysis. *Age and Ageing* 53(2):afae009.

Hafdi, M., M. P. Hoevenaar-Blom, and E. Richard. 2021. Multi-domain interventions for the prevention of dementia and cognitive decline. *Cochrane Database Systematic Reviews* 11(11):CD013572.

Huang, M. H., B. S. Zeng, P. T. Tseng, C. W. Hsu, Y. C. Wu, Y. K. Tu, B. Stubbs, A. F. Carvalho, C. S. Liang, T. Y. Chen, Y. W. Chen, and K. P. Su. 2023a. Treatment efficacy of pharmacotherapies for frontotemporal dementia: A network meta-analysis of randomized controlled trials. *American Journal of Geriatric Psychiatry* 31(12):1062-1073.

Huang, Y. Y., T. Teng, C. D. Giovane, R. Z. Wang, J. Suckling, X. N. Shen, S. D. Chen, S. Y. Huang, K. Kuo, W. J. Cai, K. L. Chen, L. Feng, C. Zhang, C. Y. Liu, C. B. Li, Q. H. Zhao, Q. Dong, X. Y. Zhou, and J. T. Yu. 2023b. Pharmacological treatment of neuropsychiatric symptoms of dementia: A network meta-analysis. *Age and Ageing* 52(6):afad091.

Karamacoska, D., A. Butt, I. H. K. Leung, R. L. Childs, N. J. Metri, V. Uruthiran, T. Tan, A. Sabag, and G. Z. Steiner-Lim. 2023. Brain function effects of exercise interventions for cognitive decline: A systematic review and meta-analysis. *Frontiers in Neuroscience* 17:1127065.

Kitt, K., R. Murphy, A. Clarke, C. Reddin, J. Ferguson, J. Bosch, W. Whiteley, M. Canavan, C. Judge, and M. O'Donnell. 2023. Antiplatelet therapy and incident cognitive impairment or dementia—A systematic review and meta-analysis of randomised clinical trials. *Age and Ageing* 52(10).

Kuate Defo, A., V. Bakula, A. Pisaturo, C. Labos, S. S. Wing, and S. S. Daskalopoulou. 2024. Diabetes, antidiabetic medications and risk of dementia: A systematic umbrella review and meta-analysis. *Diabetes, Obesity & Metabolism* 26(2):441-462.

Kwan, J., M. Hafdi, L. L. W. Chiang, P. K. Myint, L. S. Wong, and T. J. Quinn. 2022. Antithrombotic therapy to prevent cognitive decline in people with small vessel disease on neuroimaging but without dementia. *Cochrane Database Systematic Reviews* 7(7):CD012269.

Leow, Y., N. Rashid, P. Klainin-Yobas, Z. Zhang, and X. V. Wu. 2023. Effectiveness of mindfulness-based interventions on mental, cognitive outcomes and neuroplastic changes in older adults with mild cognitive impairment: A systematic review and meta-analysis. *Journal of Advanced Nursing* 79(12):4489-4505.

Lin, C. J., M. L. Yeh, S. F. Wu, Y. C. Chung, and J. C. Lee. 2022. Acupuncture-related treatments improve cognitive and physical functions in Alzheimer's disease: A systematic review and meta-analysis of randomized controlled trials. *Clinical Rehabilitation* 36(5):609-635.

López-Ortiz, S., S. Lista, P. L. Valenzuela, J. Pinto-Fraga, R. Carmona, F. Caraci, G. Caruso, N. Toschi, E. Emanuele, A. Gabelle, R. Nisticò, F. Garaci, A. Lucia, and A. Santos-Lozano. 2023. Effects of physical activity and exercise interventions on Alzheimer's disease: An umbrella review of existing meta-analyses. *Journal of Neurology* 270(2):711-725.

Lyu, D., X. Lyu, L. Huang, and B. Fang. 2023. Effects of three kinds of anti-amyloid-beta drugs on clinical, biomarker, neuroimaging outcomes and safety indexes: A systematic review and meta-analysis of phase II/III clinical trials in Alzheimer's disease. *Ageing Research Reviews* 88:101959.

McShane, R., M. J. Westby, E. Roberts, N. Minakaran, L. Schneider, L. E. Farrimond, N. Maayan, J. Ware, and J. Debarros. 2019. Memantine for dementia. *Cochrane Database Systematic Reviews* 3(3):CD003154.

Miller, A., R. J. Allen, A. A. Juma, R. Chowdhury, and M. R. Burke. 2023. Does repetitive transcranial magnetic stimulation improve cognitive function in age-related neurodegenerative diseases? A systematic review and meta-analysis. *International Journal of Geriatric Psychiatry* 38(8):e5974.

Morrin, H., T. Fang, D. Servant, D. Aarsland, and A. P. Rajkumar. 2018. Systematic review of the efficacy of non-pharmacological interventions in people with Lewy body dementia. *International Psychogeriatrics* 30(3):395-407.

Muhlbauer, V., R. Mohler, M. N. Dichter, S. U. Zuidema, S. Kopke, and H. J. Luijendijk. 2021. Antipsychotics for agitation and psychosis in people with Alzheimer's disease and vascular dementia. *Cochrane Database Systematic Reviews* 12(12):CD013304.

Nimmons, D., N. Aker, A. Burnand, K. P. Jordan, C. Cooper, N. Davies, J. Manthorpe, C. A. Chew-Graham, T. Kingstone, I. Petersen, and K. Walters. 2024. Clinical effectiveness of pharmacological and non-pharmacological treatments for the management of anxiety in community dwelling people living with dementia: A systematic review and meta-analysis. *Neuroscience & Biobehavioral Reviews* 157:105507.

Olmastroni, E., G. Molari, N. De Beni, O. Colpani, F. Galimberti, M. Gazzotti, A. Zambon, A. L. Catapano, and M. Casula. 2022. Statin use and risk of dementia or Alzheimer's disease: A systematic review and meta-analysis of observational studies. *European Journal of Preventive Cardiology* 29(5):804-814.

Papaioannou, T., A. Voinescu, K. Petrini, and D. Stanton Fraser. 2022. Efficacy and moderators of virtual reality for cognitive training in people with dementia and mild cognitive impairment: A systematic review and meta-analysis. *Journal of Alzheimer's Disease* 88:1341-1370.

Profyri, E., P. Leung, J. Huntley, and V. Orgeta. 2022. Effectiveness of treatments for people living with severe dementia: A systematic review and meta-analysis of randomised controlled clinical trials. *Ageing Research Reviews* 82.

Ren, Y., Q. Wang, H. Liu, G. Wang, and A. Lu. 2024. Effects of immersive and non-immersive virtual reality-based rehabilitation training on cognition, motor function, and daily functioning in patients with mild cognitive impairment or dementia: A systematic review and meta-analysis. *Clinical Rehabilitation* 38(3):305-321.

Rostamzadeh, A., A. Kahlert, F. Kalthegener, and F. Jessen. 2022. Psychotherapeutic interventions in individuals at risk for Alzheimer's dementia: A systematic review. *Alzheimer's Research and Therapy* 14(1):18.

Salzman, T., Y. Sarquis-Adamson, S. Son, M. Montero-Odasso, and S. Fraser. 2022. Associations of multidomain interventions with improvements in cognition in mild cognitive impairment: A systematic review and meta-analysis. *JAMA Network Open* 5(5):e226744.

Shoesmith, E., C. Surr, and E. Ratschen. 2023. Animal-assisted and robotic animal-assisted interventions within dementia care: A systematic review. *Dementia (London)* 22(3):664-693.

Sun, H., M. Liu, and J. Liu. 2023. Association of influenza vaccination and dementia risk: A meta-analysis of cohort studies. *Journal of Alzheimer's Disease* 92(2):667-678.

Talar, K., T. Vetrovsky, M. van Haren, J. Negyesi, U. Granacher, M. Vaczi, E. Martin-Arevalo, M. F. Del Olmo, E. Kalamacka, and T. Hortobagyi. 2022. The effects of aerobic exercise and transcranial direct current stimulation on cognitive function in older adults with and without cognitive impairment: A systematic review and meta-analysis. *Ageing Research Reviews* 81:101738.

Tao, T., G. Feng, and Y. Fang. 2024. Association between aspirin use and risk of dementia: A systematic review and meta-analysis. *European Geriatric Medicine* 15(1):3-18.

Tedeschi, D. V., A. F. da Cunha, M. R. Cominetti, and R. V. Pedroso. 2021. Efficacy of gene therapy to restore cognition in Alzheimer's disease: A systematic review. *Current Gene Therapy* 21(3):246-257.

Terao, I., and W. Kodama. 2024. Comparative efficacy, tolerability and acceptability of donanemab, lecanemab, aducanumab and lithium on cognitive function in mild cognitive impairment and Alzheimer's disease: A systematic review and network meta-analysis. *Ageing Reserch Reviews* 94:102203.

Tosatti, J. A. G., A. Fontes, P. Caramelli, and K. B. Gomes. 2022. Effects of resveratrol supplementation on the cognitive function of patients with Alzheimer's disease: A systematic review of randomized controlled trials. *Drugs & Aging* 39(4):285-295.

Townsend, R. F., D. Logan, R. F. O'Neill, F. Prinelli, J. V. Woodside, and C. T. McEvoy. 2023. Whole dietary patterns, cognitive decline and cognitive disorders: A systematic review of prospective and intervention studies. *Nutrients* 15(2):333.

Tulliani, N., M. Bissett, P. Fahey, R. Bye, and K. P. Y. Liu. 2022. Efficacy of cognitive remediation on activities of daily living in individuals with mild cognitive impairment or early-stage dementia: A systematic review and meta-analysis. *Systematic Reviews* 11(1):156.

van Middelaar, T., L. A. van Vught, W. A. van Gool, E. M. F. Simons, B. H. van den Born, E. P. Moll van Charante, and E. Richard. 2018. Blood pressure-lowering interventions to prevent dementia: A systematic review and meta-analysis. *Journal of Hypertension* 36(9):1780-1787.

Wang, X. C., C. L. Chu, H. C. Li, K. Lu, C. J. Liu, Y. F. Cai, S. J. Quan, and S. J. Zhang. 2022a. Efficacy and safety of hypoglycemic drugs in improving cognitive function in patients with Alzheimer's disease and mild cognitive impairment: A systematic review and network meta-analysis. *Frontiers in Neurology* 13:1018027.

Wang, Z., W. Zhu, Y. Xing, J. Jia, and Y. Tang. 2022b. B vitamins and prevention of cognitive decline and incident dementia: A systematic review and meta-analysis. *Nutrition Reviews* 80(4):931-949.

Wang, T., S. Yan, and J. Lu. 2023. The effects of noninvasive brain stimulation on cognitive function in patients with mild cognitive impairment and Alzheimer's disease using resting-state functional magnetic resonance imaging: A systematic review and meta-analysis. *CNS Neuroscience & Therapeutics* 29(11):3160-3172.

Watts, K. E., N. J. Storr, P. G. Barr, and A. P. Rajkumar. 2023. Systematic review of pharmacological interventions for people with Lewy body dementia. *Aging and Mental Health* 27(2):203-216.

Wei, B. Z., L. Li, C. W. Dong, C. C. Tan, I. Alzheimer's Disease Neuroimaging, and W. Xu. 2023. The relationship of omega-3 fatty acids with dementia and cognitive decline: Evidence from prospective cohort studies of supplementation, dietary intake, and blood markers. *American Journal of Clinical Nutrition* 117(6):1096-1109.

Wilfling, D., S. Calo, M. N. Dichter, G. Meyer, R. Mohler, and S. Kopke. 2023. Non-pharmacological interventions for sleep disturbances in people with dementia. *Cochrane Database Systematic Reviews* 1(1):CD011881.

Xue, D., P. W. C. Li, D. S. F. Yu, and R. S. Y. Lin. 2023. Combined exercise and cognitive interventions for adults with mild cognitive impairment and dementia: A systematic review and network meta-analysis. *International Journal of Nursing Studies* 147:104592.

Zeng, Y., J. Wang, X. Cai, X. Zhang, J. Zhang, M. Peng, D. Xiao, H. Ouyang, and F. Yan. 2023. Effects of physical activity interventions on executive function in older adults with dementia: A meta-analysis of randomized controlled trials. *Geriatric Nursing* 51:369-377.

Zhan, M., L. Sun, J. Liu, Z. Zeng, W. Shen, H. Li, Y. Wang, F. Han, J. Shi, X. Zeng, X. Lu, Y. Zhang, and X. Liao. 2021. *EGb* in the treatment for patients with VCI: A systematic review and meta-analysis. *Oxidative Medicine and Cellular Longevity* 2021:8787684.

Zhang, C., L. Sun, and H. Sun. 2022. Effects of magnesium valproate adjuvant therapy on patients with dementia: A systematic review and meta-analysis. *Medicine (Baltimore)* 101(31):E29642.

Zhang, X., Q. Li, W. Cong, S. Mu, R. Zhan, S. Zhong, M. Zhao, C. Zhao, K. Kang, and Z. Zhou. 2023. Effect of physical activity on risk of Alzheimer's disease: A systematic review and meta-analysis of twenty-nine prospective cohort studies. *Ageing Research Reviews* 92:102127.

Zheng, X., Y. Tang, Q. Yang, S. Wang, R. Chen, C. Tao, P. Zhang, B. Fan, J. Zhan, C. Tang, and L. Lu. 2022. Effectiveness and safety of anti-tau drugs for Alzheimer's disease: Systematic review and meta-analysis. *Journal of the American Geriatrics Society* 70(11):3281-3292.

Appendix B

Biographical Sketches of Committee Members and Staff

COMMITTEE MEMBERS

Tia Powell, M.D. (Chair), is professor of epidemiology, Division of Bioethics, and psychiatry at Albert Einstein College of Medicine and Montefiore Medical Center, and former director of the Montefiore Einstein Center for Bioethics. Dr. Powell focuses on bioethics issues related to public policy, aging, dementia, end-of-life care, and public health disasters. She served 4 years as executive director of the New York State Task Force on Life and the Law, New York State's bioethics commission. Dr. Powell has worked with the National Academies of Sciences, Engineering, and Medicine on many projects, and in 2021 chaired the report from the Committee for Reducing the Impact of Dementia in America: a Decadal Survey of Behavioral and Social Sciences. She has worked with the Centers for Disease Control, New York State and City, and various professional organizations on issues related to public health ethics and disasters. She served as a special advisor to the Agency for Healthcare Research and Quality on ethics, dementia and multiple chronic conditions. She is on the American Psychiatric Association ethics committee and is a Fellow of the New York Academy of Medicine and the Hastings Center. She wrote Dementia Reimagined: Building a Life of Joy and Dignity from Beginning to End, published by Penguin (Random House). Dr. Powell received a B.A. from Harvard College and M.D. from Yale Medical School.

Rhoda Au, Ph.D., M.B.A., is professor of anatomy and neurobiology, neurology, medicine and epidemiology at Boston University Chobanian &

Avedisian School of Medicine. She serves as one of the principal investigators of the Framingham Heart Study Brain Aging Program and is director of neuropsychology. She also serves as the director of Global Cohort Development for the Davos Alzheimer's Collaborative. Her research and work include the application of technologies to promote equal opportunity in science and to develop and validate multisensor digital biomarkers. Her long-term research objective is to enable global solutions that move the primary focus of health technologies from precision medicine to a broader emphasis on precision brain health. She graduated with her Ph.D. in cognitive psychology from the University of California, Riverside in 1985 and her M.B.A. from Boston University in 1995. In addition to these research activities, she currently advises several pharmaceutical and biotechnology companies on the development of digital biomarkers for use in clinical research in the development of novel Alzheimer's disease and related dementias (AD/ADRD) therapeutics. These include Signant Health, Biogen, and Novo Nordisk. She has previously attended advisory board meetings of companies involved in AD/ADRD research, including Kaiser Permanente, Eisai, TauRx, Merck, Novartis, and Roche, and has served as a reviewer of grants for the Alzheimer's Drug Discovery Foundation and the Alzheimer's Association. She currently serves as an advisor to several National Institutes of Health-funded studies, including the Alzheimer's Disease Neuroimaging Initiative and the Adult Changes in Thought study, and as a standing member of the Neurological, Mental and Behavioral Health study section of the National Institute on Aging. Dr. Au currently sits on the editorial review board of the *Journal of Alzheimer's Disease*. She was recently selected to receive the 2023 Melvin R. Goodes Prize for Excellence in Alzheimer's Drug Discovery from the Alzheimer's Disease Drug Discovery Foundation.

Rita Balice-Gordon, Ph.D., is chief executive officer of Muna Therapeutics, a preclinical biotech company focused on disease modifying therapies for neurodegenerative diseases. She is also a director on the Board of Collegium Pharmaceutical, a publicly traded company; a director on the Board of Capsida BioTherapeutics, a biotech company innovating new genomic medicines; and a consultant for Praesidia Therapeutics, a pharmaceutical company developing drugs for cancers and central nervous system disorders. Prior to taking on these roles, Dr. Balice-Gordon was the global head of the Rare and Neurologic Diseases Therapeutic Area at Sanofi, Inc. where she led work on research and early development stage projects for patients with neurodegenerative diseases including multiple sclerosis, Parkinson's, amyotrophic lateral sclerosis, and rare genetic disorders, including lysosomal storage diseases, inborn errors of metabolism, and renal and musculoskeletal diseases. Prior to Sanofi, she held senior leadership roles in the Neuroscience and Pain Research Unit at Pfizer. Prior to her career in biopharma, Dr. Balice-Gordon was professor of neuroscience and chair of the Neuroscience Graduate Group in the Perelman School of Medicine at the University of Pennsylvania, where she holds an appointment as adjunct professor. She was continuously funded by the National Institutes of Health (NIH) for more than 30 years, authored more than 100 scientific papers, received several awards and honors, has given hundreds of invited talks around the world, and has chaired or served on many NIH, national, and international committees, study sections, editorial boards, and research organization advisory boards. She is currently a member of the Neuroscience Forum of the National Academies of Sciences, Engineering, and Medicine. Dr. Balice-Gordon is an elected Fellow of the American Association for the Advancement of Science.

Daniel S. Barron, M.D., Ph.D., directs the Pain Intervention and Digital Research Program at Mass General Brigham, where he is funded by the National Institute on Aging (K01) to define digital markers of functional status in older patients with chronic pain conditions. His lab is also funded by the Brain and Behavior Research Foundation (originally the National Alliance for Research on Schizophrenia & Depression). He is an interventional pain physician and psychiatrist who specializes in the treatment of chronic musculoskeletal pain—specifically neck and back pain—and offers the latest evidence-based treatments that include pharmacologic, interventional, and rehabilitative therapy.

Christian Behl, Ph.D., is director of the Institute of Pathobiochemistry at the University Medical Center of the Johannes Gutenberg University Mainz, Germany, where he is full professor and chair since 2002. Dr. Behl holds a diploma in biology from the University of Würzburg, Germany, where he also received his Ph.D. in neurobiology in 1991. Following his postdoctoral research on Alzheimer's disease from 1992 to 1994 at the Salk Institute for Biological Studies, La Jolla, California, he headed an independent research group on aging and neurodegeneration at the Max-Planck-Institute for Psychiatry in Munich from 1994–2002. In Mainz, Dr. Behl has translated his long-standing interest in neurodegenerative diseases into a research focus on autophagy, proteostasis, and oxidative stress in the context of age-related neurodegeneration. One of his key research goals is to uncover molecular mechanisms that allow neurons to resist challenges occurring during neurodegenerative diseases. For the past decade, Dr. Behl has been closely following research on widening the view on Alzheimer's disease in order to improve the understanding of this complex, age-related brain disorder. He currently serves on the Scientific Advisory Board of Samsara Therapeutics. He has received several awards, including the AGNP Award for Psychopharmacology Research, and the Binder Innovation Prize of the German Society for Cell Biology. He is a member of the Board of the German Alzheimer Foundation.

Jeffrey L. Dage, Ph.D., is a senior research professor of neurology at Indiana University School of Medicine and a primary member of the Stark Neurosciences Research Institute. He received his Ph.D. from the University of Cincinnati in Ohio where he worked in the area of protein characterization using mass spectrometry. He previously worked in the pharmaceutical industry for 28 years and has contributed to many therapeutic discovery programs through the analytical measurement of biologically relevant molecules in cell culture, preclinical models, and human clinical samples. At Eli Lilly, he led the discovery and development of the first biofluid tests to measure P-tau181 and P-tau217, which could reliably predict the presence of Alzheimer's neuropathologic change and shifted the global landscape of Alzheimer's disease clinical research. He is continuing his research at Indiana University, focusing on the implementation of blood tests in clinical research as well as the discovery and development of novel biomarkers for Alzheimer's disease and related dementias. Dr. Dage provides advisory services to ALZPath, Inc. and Genotix Biotechnologies, Inc. and is a cofounder of and consultant for Monument Biosciences, all of which are involved in the development of novel treatments for Alzheimer's disease and related dementias. He has previously consulted for AbbVie and Eisai. Dr. Dage is a co-inventor of two patents relating to a fluid biomarker for diagnosing Alzheimer's disease and frontotemporal dementia and the prevention of neuronal axonal damage in Alzheimer's disease. Dr. Dage also serves as vice chair of the Biofluid Based Biomarkers Professional Interest Area for the Alzheimer's Association International Society to Advance Alzheimer's Research and Treatment and on the Scientific Program Committee of the Alzheimer's Association.

Nilüfer Ertekin-Taner, M.D., Ph.D., is chair of the Department of Neuroscience and a professor of neurology and neuroscience at the Mayo Clinic. She is a physician-scientist with seminal contributions to the field of Alzheimer's disease and related neurodegenerative conditions. Her innovative, groundbreaking work combining complex genomics and deep endophenotypes is essential for the discovery of molecular disease mechanisms, new treatments and biomarkers for these devastating and currently incurable conditions. She has pioneered the endophenotype approach in genetic studies of Alzheimer's disease and related disorders. Her laboratory applies leading-edge analytic approaches to integrate biological traits with multiomics data to discover precision medicinal therapies and biomarkers in Alzheimer's disease and related dementias. Ertekin-Taner is a principal investigator (PI) of AMP-AD and Resilience-AD and was a PI of M²OVE-AD consortia and Florida Consortium for African American Alzheimer's Disease Studies. She is the contact PI of the CLEAR-AD U19 Program comprising 13 sites and nearly 100 investigators focused on precision medicinal biomarker and therapeutic discoveries in Alzheimer's disease and related dementias. Dr. Ertekin-Taner has been continually funded by the National Institutes of Health and foundations, having served or serving as a PI on 37 grants with a total extramural grant support of about $80 million since 2008. Her lab is the leader in many national large-scale initiatives aiming to discover precision medicinal therapies in Alzheimer's and related disorders. Owing to her prolific, impactful work, Dr. Ertekin-Taner serves on numerous executive committees, advisory boards and is a frequently invited speaker. Ertekin-Taner is the recipient of numerous awards including the 2022 Alzheimer's Association Zenith Fellows Award. A board-certified neurologist, she continues to care for dementia patients. Dr. Ertekin-Taner is also a leader in education, serving as director and PI for the Mayo Clinic Center for Clinical and Translational Science KL2 Mentored Career Development Program, founding chair of the Mayo Clinic Research Pipeline K2R Program and as a mentor to more than 80 trainees to date from various career stages.

Maria Glymour, Sc.D., is a professor and chair of the Department of Epidemiology at Boston University's School of Public Health and serves on the leadership group of the Methods in Longitudinal Research on Dementia initiative. Her research focuses on how social factors experienced across the life course, from infancy to adulthood, influence cognitive function, dementia, stroke, and other health outcomes in old age. She is especially interested in education and other exposures amenable to policy interventions. She has also worked on the influence of "place" on health, for example, in understanding the excess stroke burden for individuals who grew up in the U.S. stroke belt and evaluating effects of immigration. She works with a network of colleagues on the international initiative MELODEM (Methods for Longitudinal Studies in Dementia) to foster the adoption of rigorous causal inference methods and evidence triangulation approaches to understand how to eliminate social inequalities in dementia risk and improve dementia-related outcomes. She currently serves on a National Institute on Aging advisory board for longitudinal dementia research. Dr. Glymour received her Sc.D. in social epidemiology from Harvard School of Public Health and her A.B. in biology from the University of Chicago.

Hector M. González, Ph.D., is a professor of neurosciences at the University of California, San Diego School of Medicine. He is a population neuroscientist who previously held faculty posts in departments of epidemiology and public health in Michigan. His primary professional expertise is in cognitive assessment of aging and diverse Hispanics/Latinos. Dr. González' primary research expertise is in examining modifiable health and sociocultural factors related to healthy cognitive aging, unhealthy cognitive aging, impairment, and disorders among diverse Hispanics/Latinos at the population level. Dr. González is principal investigator of the National Institutes of Health (NIH)/National Institute on Aging (NIA)–funded Study of Latinos— Investigation of Neurocognitive Aging (SOL-INCA) and leads a research program based on the life-course research framework for cognitive aging and Alzheimer's disease among diverse U.S. Latinos in order to leverage this deeply phenotyped and genotyped representative cohort. He has served as a panelist and chair of three Alzheimer's Disease and Related Dementia Summits (2016, 2019, 2022) and serves on the advisory boards of several NIA-funded Alzheimer's Disease Research Centers and studies. Dr. González's education and training are in clinical neuropsychology and epidemiology. Beginning over 20 years ago as a fellow, Dr. González assessed Mexican American patients in clinics and oversaw the cognitive assessments of 1,789 older Mexican American participants of the Sacramento Area Latino Study of Aging (SALSA). Dr. González served the National Research Council as a panelist for the 2021 Behavioral and Social Research and Clinical Practice Implications of Biomarker and other Preclinical Diagnostics of Alzheimer's Disease (AD) and AD-Related Dementias (AD/ADRD). In addition, he was a workshop panelist on the 2023 Addressing Structural Constraints Preventing Transformative Change and Highlighting Community-Driven Collaborations.

Susanne M. Jaeggi, Ph.D., is professor at Northeastern University, where she's affiliated with the Center for Cognitive and Brain Health, the Departments of Psychology, Applied Psychology, and Music. She codirects the Brain Game Center for Mental Fitness and Well Being and the SoundMind Collaboratory. Previously, she was professor in education and cognitive science at the University of California, Irvine, where she directed the Working Memory and Plasticity Lab for over a decade. She received Ph.D.s in cognitive psychology and neuroscience, as well as a "Habilitation" from the University of Bern in Switzerland, and she conducted postdoctoral work in cognitive neuroscience at the University of Michigan. Her research program focuses on understanding individual differences in executive functions and related cognitive domains, as well as their malleability across the lifespan using experimental and neuroscientific approaches. Because of the relevance of these cognitive domains for everyday foundation, her major work has focused on the development of assessments and interventions, and whether and how executive functions can be improved with both experience and targeted training. Furthermore, she aims to get a better understanding of the underlying mechanisms of learning and cognitive training and determining for what individuals and populations cognitive training is most effective and why. Her work has been funded by the National Institutes of Health (National Institute on Aging, National Institute of Mental Health), National Science Foundation, Office of Naval Research, or the Advanced Education Research and Development Fund (EF+Math Program).

Kenneth Langa, M.D., Ph.D., is the Cyrus Sturgis Professor in the Department of Internal Medicine and Institute for Social Research at the University of Michigan. He is also co-principal investigator of the Health and Retirement Study (HRS), and principal investigator of the Harmonized Cognitive Assessment Protocol Project, both funded by the National Institute on Aging. Dr. Langa's research focuses on the epidemiology and costs of chronic disease in older adults, with an emphasis on Alzheimer's disease and related dementias, and he has published more than 350 peer-reviewed articles on these topics. Dr. Langa received an M.D. and Ph.D. in public policy at the University of Chicago as a fellow in the Pew Program for Medicine, Arts, and the Social Sciences. He is a general internist and an elected member of the National Academy of Medicine (NAM). Dr. Langa was a member of the 2017 NAM Committee on Preventing Dementia and Cognitive Impairment and is a current member of the National Academy of Sciences Committee on Population.

Pamela J. Lein, Ph.D., M.S., is currently professor of neurotoxicology and chair of the Department of Molecular Biosciences at the University of California, Davis School of Veterinary Medicine with a faculty appointment in the UC Davis MIND Institute. She previously was on the faculty at Oregon Health and Science University and the Johns Hopkins University Bloomberg School of Public Health. Her research focuses on the cellular and molecular mechanisms by which environmental stressors, including toxic chemicals, contribute to neurodevelopmental and neurodegenerative disorders. Dr. Lein earned a B.S. degree in biology with honors from Cornell University, M.S. in environmental health from East Tennessee State University, and Ph.D. in pharmacology and toxicology from the University of Buffalo. Dr. Lein was selected as an American Association for the Advancement of Science (AAAS) fellow in 2023, and received the 2023 American Association of Veterinary Medical Colleges Excellence in Research Award, 2022 Distinguished Neurotoxicologist Award from the Society of Toxicology (SOT), and the 2022 Mentoring Award from the SOT Women in Toxicology Special Interest Group. Dr. Lein has held numerous leadership positions in SOT and is a member of the AAAS. She did postdoctoral training in Molecular Immunology at Roswell Park Cancer Institute. She has served on several National Academies of Sciences, Engineering, and Medicine (National Academies) committees focused on toxicological concerns, including most recently on the National Academies Committee on

Toxicology, and is currently the chair of the Board of Scientific Counselors for the National Institute of Environmental Health Sciences Division of Translational Toxicology.

Rita Doreen Monks, M.S.N., B.S.N., R.N., is a retired neuroscience nurse practitioner. She retired after a 41-year nursing career. Prior to her retirement, she was the program director of the Stroke Program at Saint Barnabas Medical Center, Livingston, New Jersey. This was a program that she personally developed. She now volunteers as an advocate and community educator for the Greater New Jersey Chapter of the Alzheimer's Association as well as a community educator and dementia advocate for several other venues. Ms. Monks is living with early-stage Alzheimer's disease and shares her experiences with the disease with interested stakeholders; this has previously included a pharmaceutical company for which she received a small honorarium. Ms. Monks advances scientific understanding of Alzheimer's disease as a participant in a randomized clinical trial for an investigational treatment for Alzheimer's disease. She recently received the Governor's Award for Volunteerism from Governor Murphy of New Jersey. She holds her R.N. diploma from Clara Maass School of Nursing; her B.S.N. from the Regents External Degree Program; and a master's degree from Seton Hall University.

Krissan Lutz Moss, R.N., B.S.N., is a retired clinical education manager and thought leader liaison. She previously worked for Genentech, California, and now volunteers with the National Council of Dementia Minds, the Lewy Body Dementia Association, and the Dementia Action Alliance, which create opportunities for dialogue and education for persons living with dementia, licensed health care professionals, researchers, families, care partners, policy makers, and communities at large about strategies for how to live well with neurocognitive disorders.

Kenneth S. Ramos, M.D., Ph.D., is professor of translational medical sciences, Alkek Chair of Medical Genetics, director of the Center for Genomic and Precision Medicine, associate vice president for health sciences, and assistant vice chancellor for health services for the Texas A&M University System. He is an accomplished physician-scientist with designations in the National Academy of Medicine (elected member) and the National Academy of Sciences (lifetime associate). He is a transformational leader recognized throughout the world for his scientific contributions in the areas of genomics, precision medicine, and toxicology. He leads several initiatives to elucidate genetic and molecular mechanisms of disease, improve health care, and reduce disease burden and health-associated costs. He is also involved in studies to evaluate functional genetic networks of human retrotransposons and their clinical utility as prognostic and diagnostic biomarkers of disease, point-of-care precision medicine approaches with a focus on pharmacogenomics in primary and specialty care practice, magnetic resonance-based and integrative interventions to promote brain health.

Reisa A. Sperling, M.D., M.M.Sc., is a neurologist focused on the detection and treatment of Alzheimer's disease at the earliest possible stage. Dr. Sperling is a professor in neurology at Harvard Medical School, director of the Center for Alzheimer Research and Treatment at Brigham and Women's Hospital, and director of Neuroimaging for the Massachusetts Aging & Disability Resource Consortia at Massachusetts General Hospital. In addition to these roles, she serves on the leadership team for the National Institutes of Health (NIH)-funded Alzheimer's Clinical Trials Consortium (ACTC) (NIH competitive award U24AG057437) and as principal investigator of several global, multicenter randomized trials of regimens to prevent cognitive decline in individuals at high risk for developing Alzheimer's disease and in those with pre-clinical disease. Two of these ACTC studies for which she is principal investigator involve public–private partnership clinical trials with Eisai and Eli Lilly. Separate from her work with the ACTC, she also applies her expertise in consultation with pharmaceutical and biotechnology companies on their clinical trial design and testing of candidates in their pipelines, including AbbVie, AC Immune, Alector, Acumen, Bristol Myers Squibb, Genentech, Janssen, Neuraly, Oligomerix, Prothena, Renew, and Vaxxinity. She has previously provided consulting services to several other companies involved in Alzheimer's disease research, including Alynylam, Cytox, JMDD, Nervgen, Neurocentria, Shionogi, Virgil Neuroscience, Ionis, and Biogen. She has served on multiple NIH, national, and international committees related to advancing the study of Alzheimer's disease and related dementias treatment and prevention. Dr. Sperling chaired the 2011 NIA-Alzheimer's Association workgroup to develop guidelines for the study of "Preclinical Alzheimer's disease." She co-led the Anti-Amyloid Treatment in Asymptomatic Alzheimer's disease (A4) and LEARN studies, and currently co-leads the AHEAD 3-45 studies. Dr. Sperling received the 2015 Potamkin Prize from the American Academy of Neurology, a Lifetime Achievement Award from Clinical Trials in Alzheimer's Disease in 2022, and was elected to the National Academy of Medicine in 2021.

Chi Udeh-Momoh, Ph.D., M.Sc., B.Sc., is a translational neuroscientist with expertise in dementia epidemiology based at Aga Khan University, Kenya, and Wake Forest University, North Carolina; and as a senior scientist with the Karolinska Institute. In her dual roles as director of the Imarisha Centre for Brain Health and Aging and lead of the Genomics and Biomarker Core at the Brain and Mind Institute Kenya, she is developing the capacity for dementia and brain-aging research, education, and care while collaborating with Mental Health and Neuroscience subject experts, clinicians, and educators from Aga Khan University, to ultimately build up neuroscience capacity and strength across global south regional partner institutions, including Pakistan. At Wake Forest University, she leads the Udeh-Momoh Lab for Global Brain Health Equity (U-M = BRAIN), focusing on translational research to advance equitable and culturally informed strategies for promoting successful aging. She is also an Atlantic Fellow for Equity in Brain Health. In 2018, she initiated the AFRICA-FINGERS project (as chief investigator) that aims to promote healthy aging and mitigate brain health and biomarker-access inequalities through culturally appropriate, sustainable multimodal intervention strategies in African populations. She is also cofounder of the Female Brain and Endocrine Research (FEMBER) consortium. Having completed a competitive CASE Ph.D. studentship in Neuroscience and Neuroendocrinology at the MRC. Centre for Synaptic Plasticity at the University of Bristol (2010–2014), her research elucidates dementia prevention biomechanistic pathways and strategies across diverse populations, adopting a translational approach to integrate human clinical studies with experimental animal models. She previously worked at Imperial College London, where components of her research received funding from industry. She currently receives competitively awarded funding for her research efforts from Wellcome Leap, the Alzheimer's Association, the Davos Alzheimer's Collaborative, and the Global Brain Health Institute. Dr. Udeh-Momoh leads multinational initiatives to address gender and racial disparities in medical research and academia and sits on the Board of Trustees of the British Society for Neuroendocrinology as the equity, diversity and inclusion lead.

Li-San Wang, Ph.D., is the Peter C. Nowell Professor and vice chair for Research at the Department of Pathology and Laboratory Medicine and founding codirector of the Penn Neurodegeneration Genomics Center at the University of Pennsylvania Perelman School of Medicine. Dr. Wang's lab focuses on the genetics and genomics of Alzheimer's disease and other neurodegenerative disorders, and informatics and algorithm development for genome-scale experiments. He is principal investigator (PI) of the National Institute on Aging Genetics of Alzheimer's Disease Data Storage Site and MPI of the Genome Center for Alzheimer's Disease (GCAD), both strategic initiatives to coordinate Alzheimer's genetics research, including Alzheimer's Disease Sequencing Project that will analyze genomic sequences of Alzheimer's patients and cognitively normal age-matched individuals to find novel genetic variants linked to the disease. He is founding PI of the Asian cohort for Alzheimer's disease, the first major international study on genetics of dementia in Asian Americans and Asian Canadians. He is a member of the external advisory board for the Framingham Heart Study

Brain Aging Program and the Adult Changes in Thought study, which are funded by the National Institute on Aging. Dr. Wang is a senior member of the International Society of Computational Biology. He received a B.S. and an M.S. in electrical engineering from National Taiwan University, and a Ph.D. in computer sciences from the University of Texas at Austin. He then received his postdoctoral training at the University of Pennsylvania for 3 years before his faculty appointment.

Julie Zissimopoulos, Ph.D., is a professor at the Sol Price School of Public Policy at the University of Southern California (USC). She is senior fellow at USC's Schaeffer Center for Health Policy and Economics where she leads a research program on aging and cognition. Additionally, she serves as the principal investigator (mPI organization) and Director of two National Institute on Aging (NIA)-funded centers: the Center for Advancing Sociodemographic and Economic Study of Alzheimer's Disease and Related Dementias and the USC's Alzheimer's Disease and Related Dementias Resource Center for Minority Aging Research. Dr. Zissimopoulos' research focuses on caregiving and health care costs associated with dementia, health disparities in dementia risk, diagnosis and detection, and medical care for individuals living with dementia. Her work also encompasses medication adherence and insurance design. Dr. Zissimopoulos actively contributes to the research community by serving as the health policy editor for *Alzheimer's & Dementia*, journal of the Alzheimer's Association. She is an advisory board member for the NIA-funded Center for Aging and Policy Studies at Syracuse University and the Center on Aging and Population Sciences at University of Texas, Austin. She also serves as an independent study monitoring officer for the University of Minnesota project, Refining a Driving Cessation Management Intervention for Person with Dementia and their Family Caregivers: CarFreeMe. Dr. Zissimopoulos served as co-chair of the NIA 2023 National Research Summit on Care, Services, and Supports for Persons Living with Dementia and Their Care Partners/Caregivers. She also served on the Committee on the Decadal Survey of Behavioral and Social Science Research on Alzheimer's Disease and Alzheimer's Disease Related Dementias for the National Academy of Sciences. She received her Ph.D. in economics from the University of California, Los Angeles.

NATIONAL ACADEMIES STAFF

Autumn S. Downey, Ph.D., is a senior program officer on the Board on Health Sciences Policy. She joined the National Academies of Sciences, Engineering, and Medicine (the National Academies) in 2012 and is currently directing a standing committee on personal protective equipment. She was formerly the director of the Standing Committee on Medical and

Epidemiological Aspects of Air Pollution on U.S. Government Employees and Their Families. National Academies consensus studies she has worked on include Nonhuman Primate Models in Biomedical Research; Frameworks for Protecting Workers and the Public from Inhalation Hazards; Meeting the Challenge of Caring for Persons Living with Dementia and Their Care Partners and Caregivers; Evidence-Based Practice for Public Health Emergency Preparedness and Response; Return of Individual-Specific Research Results Generated in Research Laboratories; Preventing Cognitive Decline and Dementia; A National Trauma Care System; Healthy, Resilient, and Sustainable Communities After Disasters; and Advancing Workforce Health at the Department of Homeland Security. Dr. Downey received her Ph.D. in molecular microbiology and immunology from the Johns Hopkins Bloomberg School of Public Health, where she also completed a postdoctoral fellowship at the school's National Center for the Study of Preparedness and Catastrophic Event Response. Prior to joining the National Academies, she was a National Research Council Postdoctoral Fellow at the National Institute of Standards and Technology, where she worked on environmental sampling for biothreat agents and the indoor microbiome.

Olivia C. Yost, M.Sc., is a program officer with the Board on Health Sciences Policy. She joined the National Academies of Sciences, Engineering, and Medicine (the National Academies) in 2015 and has worked on multiple consensus studies including: Nonhuman Primate Models in Biomedical Research; Frameworks for Protecting Workers and the Public from Inhalation Hazards; A Framework for Assessing Mortality and Morbidity After Large-Scale Disasters; Reusable Elastomeric Respirators in Health Care: Considerations for Routine and Surge Use; and Temporomandibular Disorders: Priorities for Research and Care. Prior to joining the National Academies in 2015, Ms. Yost worked as a research officer for ARCHIVE Global, where she managed evaluation activities for disease control programs in the Caribbean, West Africa, and South Asia. Ms. Yost received her M.Sc. in the Control of Infectious Diseases from the London School of Hygiene & Tropical Medicine and B.A. in history and communications from Franklin University Switzerland.

Molly Checksfield Dorries, M.P.A., P.M.P., is a senior program officer at the National Academies of Sciences, Engineering, and Medicine. She has directed several high-impact projects on diverse topics, including Alzheimer's disease and related dementias, the rising incidence of myopia, alcohol misuse and sexual assault and harassment aboard U.S. commercial vessels, behavioral economics in public policy, and veteran suicide prevention. With nearly a decade of prior experience in federal policy and advocacy, Dorries focuses on health equity and financial security issues. She holds a Master of Public Administration and is a certified Project Management Professional.

Lydia Teferra, B.A., is a research associate on the Board on Health Sciences at the National Academies. Ms. Teferra is a staff member on the Roundtable on Genomics and Precision Health and the Forum on Regenerative Medicine at the Academies. She graduated from Northwestern University in 2020 with a B.A. in psychology and global health and has been working at the National Academies for a little over one year. Prior to her time at the Academies, Ms. Teferra has also interned and volunteered for local nonprofit organizations addressing a number of public health issues. She hopes to pursue a Master's degree in Public Health in the near future.

Ashley Bologna, M.S., is a research assistant in the Health Medicine Division at the National Academies of Sciences, Engineering, and Medicine. In addition to this study, she works on projects initiated by the Committee on Personal Protective Equipment for Workplace Safety and Health. This is a standing committee at the National Academies of Sciences, Engineering, and Medicine sponsored by the National Personal Protective Technology Laboratory of the National Institute for Occupational Safety and Health. The committee provides a forum for the discussion of scientific and technical issues relevant to the development, certification, deployment, and use of personal protective equipment, standards, and related systems to ensure workplace safety and health. She earned her Master of Science in global health at Georgetown University. She also has a B.A. in international relations and political science from Virginia Wesleyan University.

Appendix C

Disclosure of Unavoidable Conflicts of Interest

The conflict-of-interest policy of the National Academies of Sciences, Engineering, and Medicine (https://www.nationalacademies.org/about/institutional-policies-and-procedures/conflict-of-interest-policies-and-procedures) prohibits the appointment of an individual to a committee like the one that authored this Consensus Study Report if the individual has a conflict of interest that is relevant to the task to be performed. An exception to this prohibition is permitted only if the National Academies determine that the conflict is unavoidable and the conflict is promptly and publicly disclosed.

When the committee that authored this report was established, a determination of whether there was a conflict of interest was made for each committee member given the individual's circumstances and the task being undertaken by the committee. A determination that an individual has a conflict of interest is not an assessment of that individual's actual behavior or character or ability to act objectively despite the conflicting interest.

Rhoda Au was determined to have a conflict of interest because of her compensated membership on the scientific advisory boards of Biogen and Novo Nordisk, which are involved in the development of interventions for the prevention and treatment of AD/ADRD, and Signant Health, which is involved in the design and conduct of digitally enabled clinical trials.

Rita Balice-Gordon was determined to have a conflict of interest because she is CEO of Muna Therapeutics, which focuses on disease modifying therapies for neurodegenerative diseases, including Alzheimer's disease.

Jeffrey Dage was determined to have a conflict of interest because he provides advisory services to companies developing novel treatments for AD/ADRD, including ALZPath, Genotix Biotechnologies, and Prevail Therapeutics. Additionally, he is a consultant for and holds stock in Monument Biosciences and holds stock in Eli Lilly and Company.

Reisa Sperling was determined to have a conflict of interest because she is a paid consultant to the following companies involved in drug development for the prevention and treatment of AD/ADRD: AC Immune, Alector, Acumen, Bristol-Myers Squib, Genentech, Janssen, Neuraly, Oligomerix, Prothena, Renew, Vaxxinity, Merck, and Biohaven.

The National Academies determined that the experience and expertise of these individuals were needed for the committee to accomplish the task for which it was established. The National Academies could not find other available individuals with the equivalent experience and expertise who did not have a conflict of interest. Therefore, the National Academies concluded that the conflict was unavoidable and publicly disclosed it on its website (www.nationalacademies.org).

Appendix D

Public Meeting Agendas

COMMITTEE ON RESEARCH PRIORITIES FOR PREVENTING AND TREATING ALZHEIMER'S DISEASE AND RELATED DEMENTIAS
OCTOBER 2, 2023
Virtual

Purpose
- Conduct committee and staff introductions.
- Hold an open session to hear from NIH on its perspective of the Statement of Task.
- Receive public comments.

All times listed in Eastern Time

PUBLIC SESSION
Session I: Presentation of the Committee's Charge

9:00 a.m.   **Welcome and Introductions for the Session**
             Tia Powell, Committee Chair

9:10 a.m.   **Remarks from NIH Leadership**
             Richard Hodes, Director, NIA
             Walter Koroshetz, Director, NINDS

9:20 a.m.   **Presentation of the Charge to the Committee**
             Melinda Kelley, Associate Director for Scientific Strategy,
             Innovation, and Management, NIA

9:35 a.m.   **Clarifying Questions on the Statement of Task**

10:00 a.m.   Break (15 min)

PUBLIC SESSION
Session II: Discussion of Study Context

10:15 a.m.   **Overview of NIH AD/ADRD Strategic Planning Activities**
             Eliezer Masliah, Director of the Division of
             Neuroscience, NIA
             Suzana Petanceska, Director, Office for Strategic
             Development and Partnerships in the Division of
             Neuroscience, NIA
             Sara Dodson, Senior Science Policy Analyst, NINDS
             Lis Nielsen, Director, Division of Behavioral and Social
             Research, NIA

11:00 a.m.   **Committee Discussion**

11:45 a.m.   **Opportunity for Public Comment and Questions** (Slido)

12:00 p.m.   **Adjourn Open Session**

COMMITTEE ON RESEARCH PRIORITIES FOR PREVENTING AND TREATING ALZHEIMER'S DISEASE AND RELATED DEMENTIAS
November 8, 2023
Virtual

Purpose
- Discuss strategies for identifying promising areas of research that have the potential to catalyze scientific breakthroughs or accelerate translation.
- Explore how the development of collaborative and interdisciplinary research efforts and other approaches can be employed to open new areas of knowledge.

All times listed in Eastern Time

PUBLIC SESSION

9:00 a.m.   **Welcome and Review of Session Objectives**
                Tia Powell, Committee Chair

9:05 a.m.   Remarks from Speakers
                Katja Brose, Science Program Officer, Chan Zuckerberg
                Initiative
                Tyler Best, Senior Advisor, Advanced Research Projects
                Agency for Health

9:35 a.m.   **Committee Discussion**

10:00 a.m.   **Adjourn Public Session**

COMMITTEE ON RESEARCH PRIORITIES FOR PREVENTING AND TREATING ALZHEIMER'S DISEASE AND RELATED DEMENTIAS

The Keck Center, 500 Fifth Street, NW
Washington, DC 20001

JANUARY 16, 2024
Keck 100 and Virtual

Meeting Objectives
- Engage a diverse group of stakeholders in exploring promising areas of AD/ADRD research that may have the potential to catalyze further scientific breakthroughs or accelerate translation of discoveries to effective preventive and therapeutic interventions.
- Explore barriers to the advancement of AD/ADRD research and opportunities and tools to address these impediments to progress.
- Investigate successes and failures experienced in other biomedical research fields, and discuss how lessons learned from these experiences could be translated to the AD/ADRD research context.

8:30 a.m.   **Welcome and Review of Meeting Objectives**
                Tia Powell, Committee Chair

OPEN SESSION
Session I: Envisioning the Future of AD/ADRD Research

Session Objectives
- Hear from funders of research aimed at preventing and treating AD/ADRD about their perspectives on future research priorities and infrastructural and technological barriers that limit progress in those priority research areas.
- Discuss opportunities to accelerate translation from basic to clinical research and catalyze advances in AD/ADRD prevention and treatment.

8:40 a.m.   **Overview of Session Objectives**
             Tia Powell, *Committee Chair, Moderator*

8:45 a.m.   **Panelist Remarks**
             Maria Carrillo, *Alzheimer's Association*
             Russ Paulsen, *UsAgainstAlzheimer's*
             Meg Smith, *Cure Alzheimer's Fund*
             Ian Kremer, *LEAD Coalition*

9:25 a.m.   **Committee Discussion**

OPEN SESSION
Session II: Lessons Learned from Successes and Failures in Other Fields

Session Objectives
- Explore the experiences in other research fields with learning from failure and opportunities to translate those lessons into successes.
- Examine the process by which research priorities evolved in other biomedical research fields over time, specific strategies used to accelerate and support translation, and efforts that were made to enhance diversity and inclusion in all aspects of research.
- Discuss the development of precision medicine approaches and the diversification of the therapeutic portfolio in the context of other diseases.

10:10 a.m.   **Overview of Session Objectives**
             Ken Ramos, *Committee Member, Moderator*

10:15 a.m.   **Panelist Remarks**
             Emelia Benjamin, *Boston University*
             Laura Esserman, *University of California, San Francisco*

10:35 a.m.   **Committee Discussion**

11:10 a.m.   **Break** (10 min)

OPEN SESSION
Session III: The Exposome and Risk and Protective Factors for AD/ADRD

Session Objectives
- Discuss modifiable risk and protective factors across diverse populations and implications for priority research on strategies for preventing and treating AD/ADRD.
- Elucidate priorities for research at the intersection of social determinants of health and AD/ADRD and how those may help to address existing disparities in AD/ADRD.
- Explore barriers and opportunities for the timely translation of knowledge on risk and protective factors to effective, accessible interventions.

11:20 a.m.   **Overview of Session Objectives**
Maria Glymour, *Committee Member, Moderator*
Pamela Lein, *Committee Member, Moderator*

11:25 a.m.   **Presentations**
Lisa Barnes, *Rush University*
Gary Miller, *Columbia University*
Maria Corrada, *University of California, Irvine*
Margaret Pericak-Vance, *University of Miami*

11:45 p.m.   Discussant Perspectives and Committee Discussion
Expert Discussants
Kirk Erickson, *University of Pittsburgh*
Amy Kind, *University of Wisconsin*
Gill Livingston, *University College London*
Jennifer Weuve, *Boston University*

12:45 p.m.   **Lunch** (45 min)

OPEN SESSION
Session IV: Molecular and Cellular Mechanisms
of Neurodegenerative Disease

Session Objectives

- Explore research priorities related to mechanistic hypotheses for AD/ADRD, including those that are shared across multiple forms of dementia and have great potential to illuminate the mechanistic underpinnings of brain health and disease and broaden approaches to AD/ADRD prevention and treatment.
- Discuss promising advances and remaining gaps in tools, technologies, and analytic methods needed to advance the identification of effective intervention strategies for AD/ADRD.

1:30 p.m.	**Overview of Session Objectives** Christian Behl, *Committee Member, Moderator*
1:35 p.m.	**Opening Remarks** Zaven Khachaturian, *Alzheimer's & Dementia*
1:45 p.m.	**Panelist Remarks** Virginia Lee, *University of Pennsylvania* Bart de Strooper, *UK Dementia Research Institute* Jürgen Götz, *University of Queensland* Bruce Lamb, *Indiana University* Ameer Taha, *University of California, Davis* Ralph Nixon, *New York University*
2:20 p.m.	**Committee Discussion**
3:00 p.m.	**Break** (15 min)

OPEN SESSION
Session V: Advancing Knowledge Across the Life Course

Session Objectives

- Identify gaps in existing cohorts (e.g., diversity of participants, lack of data on factors from earlier phases of life, cost), and discuss the importance of obtaining representative population samples from across the life course.

- Discuss opportunities for using unconventional markers and methods (e.g., digital phenotyping, plasma biomarkers, multiomics approaches) to expand understanding of the complexity of brain health and AD/ADRD disease over the life course and how these can be incorporated into longitudinal data collection efforts.
- Explore technological approaches to overcome existing infrastructure and resource barriers.

3:15 p.m.   **Overview of Session Objectives**
Nilüfer Ertekin-Taner, *Committee Member, Moderator*
Hector González, *Committee Member, Moderator*

3:20 p.m.   **Panel Discussion with Committee**
Laura Baker, *Wake Forest University*
Dawn Mechanic-Hamilton, *University of Pennsylvania*
Rachel Buckley, *Harvard Medical School*
Sid O'Bryant, *University of North Texas*
Goldie S. Byrd, *Wake Forest University*
Mark Mapstone, *University of California, Irvine*

4:10 p.m.   **Adjourn Public Session**

COMMITTEE ON RESEARCH PRIORITIES FOR PREVENTING AND TREATING ALZHEIMER'S DISEASE AND RELATED DEMENTIAS
JANUARY 17, 2024
Keck 100 and Virtual

OPEN SESSION
Day 2 Opening Remarks

8:30 a.m.   **Welcome**
Tia Powell, Committee Chair

8:35 a.m.   **The Fundamental Importance of Early and Accurate Diagnosis**
Daniel Gibbs, author and neurologist living with dementia

8:45 a.m.   **Committee Q&A**

OPEN SESSION
Session VI: Unlocking Innovation to Aid
Detection, Diagnosis, and Monitoring

Panel 1: Development and Use of Digital Technologies to Assess Human Health
Objectives:

- Explore opportunities and research priorities for the development and use of sensitive digital tools and unconventional biomarkers to catalyze advances in the monitoring of human brain health and the detection and diagnosis of AD/ADRD.
- Examine challenges and lessons learned from other fields/contexts related to the development and use of technology to assess and monitor human health.
- Discuss challenges related to the use of deep learning systems in biomedical research (e.g., black box effect).

8:50 a.m.   **Overview of Panel Objectives**
              Rhoda Au, *Committee Member, Moderator*

8:55 a.m.   **Panelist Remarks**
              Yannis Paschalidis, *Boston University*
              Jeffrey Kaye, *Oregon Health and Sciences University*
              Diane Cook, *Washington State University*

9:15 a.m.   **Committee Discussion**

Panel 2: Considerations for the Implementation of Tools to Detect, Diagnose, and Monitor AD/ADRD
Objectives:

- Consider the real-world implementation needs for tools to monitor brain health and detect and diagnose AD/ADRD, considering how these needs might inform the design and function of tools and markers in the early stages of research and development.
- Explore lessons learned from successes and failures related to the global implementation of distinct tools and markers to predict and describe human brain health.

9:55 a.m.   **Overview of Panel Objectives**
              Chi Udeh-Momoh, *Committee Member, Moderator*

10:00 a.m.   **Panelist Remarks**
             Niranjan Bose, *Gates Ventures*
             Agustín Ibáñez, *Global Brain Health Institute*
             Debby Tsuang, *University of Washington*
             Tim MacLeod, *Davos Alzheimer's Collaborative, Health System Preparedness*
             David Cutler, *Harvard University*

10:25 a.m.   **Committee Discussion**

10:55 a.m.   **Break** (10 min)

OPEN SESSION
Session VII: Addressing Barriers to Research Translation in AD/ADRD

Session Objectives
- Examine the current landscape of targets and interventions in AD/ADRD prevention and treatment research.
- Explore methods to accelerate AD/ADRD research and to successfully translate research from discovery to application by learning from past successes and failures.
- Describe approaches that could aid the development of tools to support nonclinical and clinical research and to build capacity and buy-in for open science practices.
- Discuss strategies to enhance diversity, inclusion, and engagement in AD/ADRD prevention and treatment research.

11:05 a.m.   **Overview of Session Objectives**
             Rita Balice-Gordon, *Committee Member, Moderator*

11:10 a.m.   **Opening Remarks**
             Jeffrey Cummings, *University of Nevada, Las Vegas*

11:20 a.m.   **Panelist Remarks**
             Rema Raman, *University of Southern California*
             Charlotte Teunissen, *Amsterdam University Medical Centers*
             David Bennett, *Rush University*
             Michael Irizarry, *Eisai*
             Kristine Yaffe, *University of California, San Francisco*

11:45 a.m.   **Committee Discussion**

12:15 p.m.   **Adjourn Public Session**

COMMITTEE ON RESEARCH PRIORITIES FOR PREVENTING AND TREATING ALZHEIMER'S DISEASE AND RELATED DEMENTIAS

The Keck Center, 500 Fifth Street, NW
Washington, DC 20001

APRIL 24, 2024
Virtual

Session Objectives
- Discuss research gaps and priority areas related to sex and gender differences for Alzheimer's disease and related dementias with the commissioned paper author.
- Provide input on edits to the draft commissioned paper materials.

12:30 p.m. **Welcome and Review of Session Objectives**
Tia Powell, Committee Chair

12:35 p.m. **Comments by the Commissioned Paper Author**
Michelle Mielke, Wake Forest University

1:50 p.m. **Committee Discussion**

2:15 p.m. **Adjourn Public Session**

COMMITTEE ON RESEARCH PRIORITIES FOR PREVENTING AND TREATING ALZHEIMER'S DISEASE AND RELATED DEMENTIAS

MAY 24, 2024
Virtual

Session Objectives
- Highlight recent discoveries and advances that have affected the state of the science for Lewy body dementia (LBD), frontotemporal dementia (FTD), vascular dementia, limbic-predominant age-related TDP-43 encephalopathy (LATE), and mixed etiology dementias.
- Identify priority research areas specific to these related dementias that, if addressed, could lead to significant advances in prevention and treatment.

12:00 p.m. **Welcome and Review of Session Objectives**
Tia Powell, Committee Chair

12:10 p.m.   **Committee Discussion with Subject-Matter Experts**
               Julie Schneider, Rush University
               Penny Dacks, FTD Association
               James Galvin, University of Miami

1:30 p.m.   **Adjourn Public Session**